Hartman's Nursing Assistant Care

Long-Term Care

Susan Alvare Hedman
Jetta Fuzy, RN, MS
and Suzanne Rymer, MSTE, RN-BC, LSW

THIRD EDITION

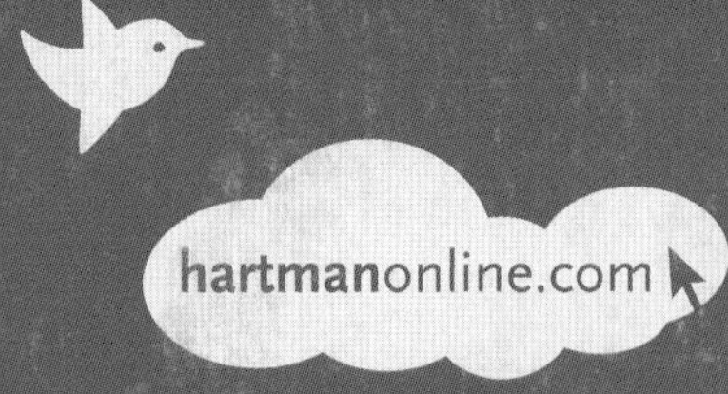

Credits

Managing Editor
Susan Alvare Hedman

Designer
Kirsten Browne

Cover Illustrator
Jo Tronc

Production
Thad Castillo

Photography
Matt Pence
Pat Berrett
Art Clifton
Dick Ruddy

Proofreaders
Kristin Calderon
Melanie Futrell

Sales/Marketing
Deborah Rinker
Kendra Robertson
Erika Walker
Belinda Midyette

Customer Service
Fran Desmond
Thomas Noble
Angela Storey
Eliza Martin
Chris Whitlock

Warehouse Coordinator
Chris Midyette

Copyright Information

8529 Indian School Road, NE
Albuquerque, New Mexico 87112
(505) 291-1274
web: hartmanonline.com
e-mail: orders@hartmanonline.com
Twitter: @HartmanPub

ISBN 978-1-60425-041-1
ISBN 978-1-60425-044-2 (Hardcover)

PRINTED IN CANADA

Notice to Readers

Though the guidelines and procedures contained in this text are based on consultations with healthcare professionals, they should not be considered absolute recommendations. The instructor and readers should follow employer, local, state, and federal guidelines concerning healthcare practices. These guidelines change, and it is the reader's responsibility to be aware of these changes and of the policies and procedures of her or his healthcare facility.

The publisher, authors, editors, and reviewers cannot accept any responsibility for errors or omissions or for any consequences from application of the information in this book and make no warranty, express or implied, with respect to the contents of the book. The publisher does not warrant or guarantee any of the products described herein or perform any analysis in connection with any of the product information contained herein.

Gender Usage

This textbook utilizes the pronouns *he*, *his*, *she*, and *her* interchangeably to denote healthcare team members and residents.

Special Thanks

We are very appreciative of the many sources who shared their informative photos with us:

Dr. Jeffrey T. Behr

The Briggs Corporation

Detecto

Dreamstime

The Eden Alternative

Exergen Corporation

Dr. Tamara D. Fishman and The Wound Care Institute

Harrisburg Area Community College

Dr. James Heilman

Hollister Incorporated

Invacare Corporation

Laerdal Medical

Dr. Jere Mammino

The Medcom Group, Ltd.

Motion Control, Inc.

North Coast Medical, Inc.

Nova Medical Products

Pavel Ševela

Phonak

RG Medical Diagnostics

Teleflex

Vancare, Inc.

Contents

Learning Objective | *Page*

24 Caring for Your Career and Yourself

Learning Objective | *Page*

Procedures

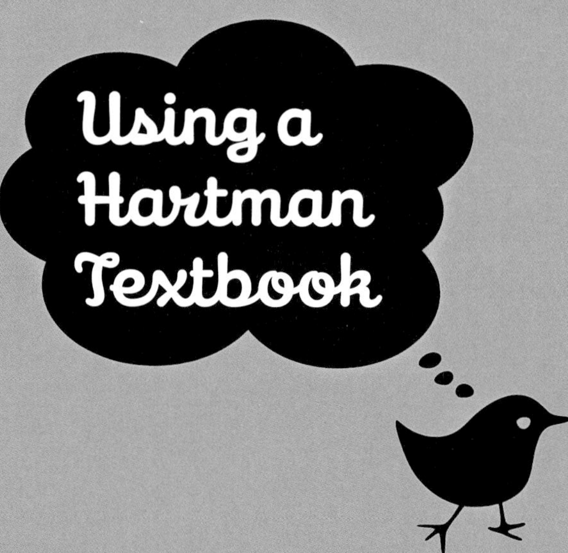

Understanding how this book is organized and what its special features are will help you make the most of this resource!

We have assigned each chapter its own colored tab. Each colored tab contains the chapter number and title, and it is on the side of every page.

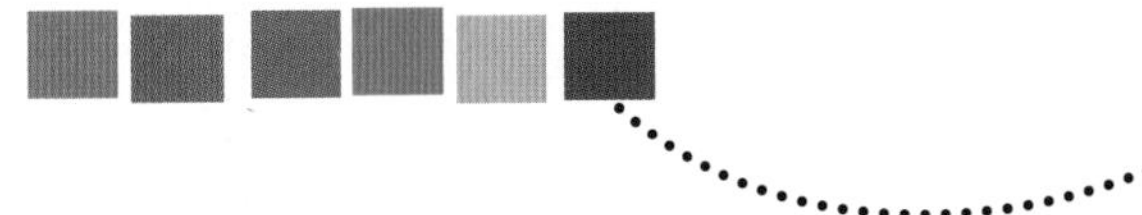

1. List examples of legal and ethical behavior

Everything in this book, the student workbook, and the instructor's teaching material is organized around learning objectives. A learning objective is a very specific piece of knowledge or a very specific skill. After reading the text, if you can do what the learning objective says, you know you have mastered the material.

---

bloodborne pathogens

Bold key terms are located throughout the text, followed by their definition. They are also listed in the glossary at the back of this book.

Making an occupied bed

All care procedures are highlighted by the same black bar for easy recognition.

Guidelines: Handwashing

Guidelines and Observing and Reporting lists are colored green for easy reference.

Residents' Rights

Call

These boxes teach important information on how to support and promote Resident's Rights, as well as how to recognize and prevent abuse and neglect.

Chapter Review

Chapter-ending questions test knowledge of the information found in the chapter. If you have trouble answering a question, you can return to the text and reread the material.

Beginning and ending steps in care procedures

For most care procedures, these steps should be performed. Understanding why they are important will help you remember to perform each step every time care is provided.

Beginning Steps	
Identify yourself by name. Identify the resident by name.	A resident's room is his home. Residents have a right to privacy. Before any procedure, knock and wait for permission to enter the resident's room. Upon entering his room, identify yourself and state your title. Residents have the right to know who is providing their care. Identify and greet the resident. This shows courtesy and respect. It also establishes correct identification. This prevents care from being performed on the wrong person.
Wash your hands.	Handwashing provides for infection prevention. Nothing fights infection in facilities like performing consistent, proper hand hygiene. Handwashing may need to be done more than once during a procedure. Practice Standard Precautions with every resident.
Explain procedure to resident. Speak clearly, slowly, and directly. Maintain face-to-face contact whenever possible.	Residents have a right to know exactly what care you will provide. It promotes understanding, cooperation, and independence. Residents are able to do more for themselves if they know what needs to happen.
Provide for the resident's privacy with a curtain, screen, or door.	Doing this maintains residents' right to privacy and dignity. Providing for privacy in a facility is not simply a courtesy; it is a legal right.
Adjust the bed to a safe level, usually waist high. Lock the bed wheels.	Locking the bed wheels is an important safety measure. It ensures that the bed will not move as you are performing care. Raising the bed helps you to remember to use good body mechanics. This prevents injury to you and to residents.

Ending Steps	
Make resident comfortable.	Make sure sheets are wrinkle-free and lie flat under the resident's body. This helps prevent pressure ulcers. Replace bedding and pillows. Check that the resident's body is in proper alignment. This promotes comfort and health after you leave the room.
Return bed to lowest position. Remove privacy measures.	Lowering the bed provides for residents' safety. Remove extra privacy measures added during the procedure. This includes anything you may have draped over and around residents, as well as privacy screens.
Place call light within resident's reach.	A call light allows residents to communicate with staff as necessary. It must always be left within the resident's reach. You must respond to call lights promptly.
Wash your hands.	Handwashing is the most important thing you can do to prevent the spread of infection.
Report any changes in the resident to the nurse. Document procedure using facility guidelines.	You will often be the person who spends the most time with a resident, so you are in the best position to note any changes in a resident's condition. Every time you provide care, observe the resident's physical and mental capabilities, as well as the condition of his or her body. For example, a change in a resident's ability to dress himself may signal a greater problem. After you have finished giving care, document the care using facility guidelines. Do not record care before it is given. If you do not document the care you gave, legally it did not happen.

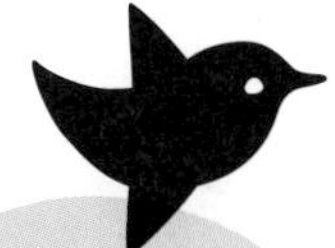

In addition to the beginning and ending steps listed above, remember to follow infection prevention guidelines. Even if a procedure in this book does not tell you to wear gloves or other PPE, there may be times when it is appropriate.

A few procedures in this book mention positioning side rails on beds, but most references to side rails have been omitted. This is due to the decline in their use because of risk of injury. Follow your facility's policies regarding side rails.

1 Understanding Healthcare Settings

1. Discuss the structure of the healthcare system and describe ways it is changing

Welcome to the world of health care. Health care is a growing field. The healthcare system refers to all the different kinds of providers, facilities, and payers involved in delivering medical care. **Providers** are people or organizations that provide health care, including doctors, nurses, clinics, and agencies. **Facilities** are places where care is delivered or administered, including hospitals, long-term care facilities, and treatment centers (such as for cancer). **Payers** are people or organizations paying for healthcare services. These include insurance companies, government programs like Medicare and Medicaid, and the individual person needing care. Together, all these people, places, and organizations make up the healthcare system.

This textbook will focus on long-term care. **Long-term care (LTC)** is given in long-term care facilities (LTCF) for people who need 24-hour skilled care. **Skilled care** is medically-necessary care given by a skilled nurse or therapist; it is available 24 hours a day. It is ordered by a doctor and involves a treatment plan. This type of care is given to people who need a high level of care for ongoing conditions. The term *nursing homes* was once widely used to refer to these facilities. Now they are often called *long-term care facilities, skilled nursing facilities, rehabilitation centers,* or *extended care facilities.*

People who live in long-term care facilities may be disabled and/or elderly. They may arrive from hospitals or other healthcare settings. Their **length of stay** (the number of days a person stays in a healthcare facility) may be short, such as a few days or months, or longer than six months. Some of these people will have a **terminal illness**, which means that the illness will eventually cause death. Other people may recover and return to their homes or to other living facilities or situations.

Most people who live in long-term care facilities have chronic conditions. This means the conditions last a long period of time, even a lifetime. Chronic conditions include physical disabilities, heart disease, and dementia. (Chapter 18 has information about these disorders and diseases.) People who live in these facilities are usually referred to as *residents* because the facility is where they reside or live. These places are their homes for the duration of their stay (Fig. 1-1).

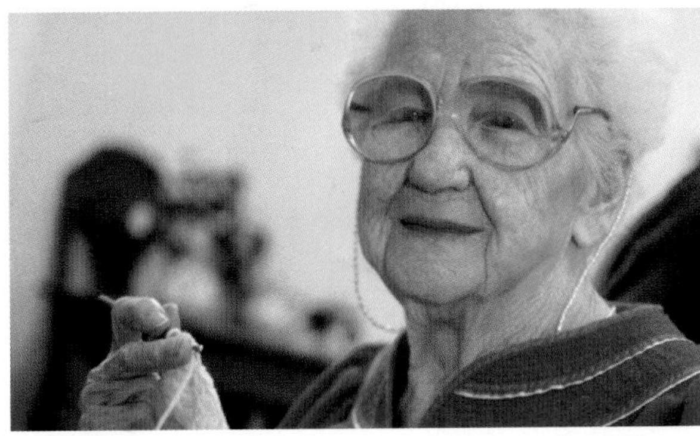

Fig. 1-1. *Long-term care is given to people who need skilled care for ongoing conditions. People who live in long-term care facilities are called* residents.

Home health care is provided in a person's home (Fig. 1-2). This type of care is also generally given to people who are older and are chronically ill but who are able to and wish to remain at home. Home care may also be needed when a person is weak after a recent hospital stay. Skilled assistance or monitoring may be required. People who receive home care are usually referred to as *clients*.

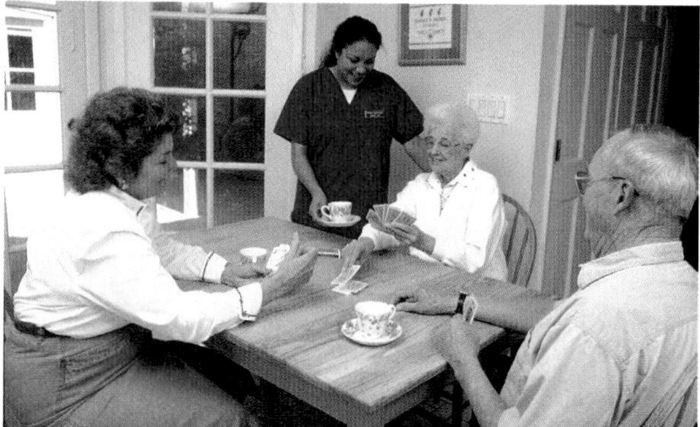

***Fig. 1-2.** Home care is performed in a person's home. People receiving home care are generally referred to as* clients.

In some ways, working as a home health aide is similar to working as a nursing assistant. Almost all care described in this textbook applies to both nursing assistants and home health aides. Most of the basic medical procedures and many of the personal care procedures are the same. Home health aides may also clean, shop for groceries, do laundry, and cook.

Home health aides may have more contact with the client's family than nursing assistants do. They also will work more independently, although a supervisor monitors their work. The advantage of home care is that clients do not have to leave home. They may have lived there for many years, and staying at home can be comforting.

People who need long-term care will have different **diagnoses**, or medical conditions determined by a doctor. The stages of illnesses or diseases affect how sick people are and how much care they will need. The jobs of nursing assistants will also vary. This is due to each person's different symptoms, abilities, and needs.

Other healthcare settings include the following:

- **Assisted living** facilities are residences for people who need some help with daily care, such as showers, meals, and dressing. Help with medications may also be given. People who live in these facilities do not need 24-hour skilled care. Assisted living facilities allow more independent living in a home-like environment. A resident can live in a single room or an apartment; however, some residents have roommates. An assisted living facility may be attached to a long-term care facility, or it may stand alone. Some assisted living facilities have *memory care* units for people who have mild dementia. **Dementia** is defined as the serious loss of mental abilities, such as thinking, remembering, reasoning, and communicating. There is more information about dementia in Chapter 19.
- **Adult day services** are for people who need some assistance and supervision during certain hours, but who do not live in the facility where care is provided. Generally, adult day services are for people who need some help but are not seriously ill or disabled. Adult day services can also provide a break for spouses, family members, and friends.
- **Acute care** is 24-hour skilled care given in hospitals and ambulatory surgical centers for people who require short-term, immediate care for illnesses or injuries (Fig. 1-3). People are also admitted for short stays for surgery.

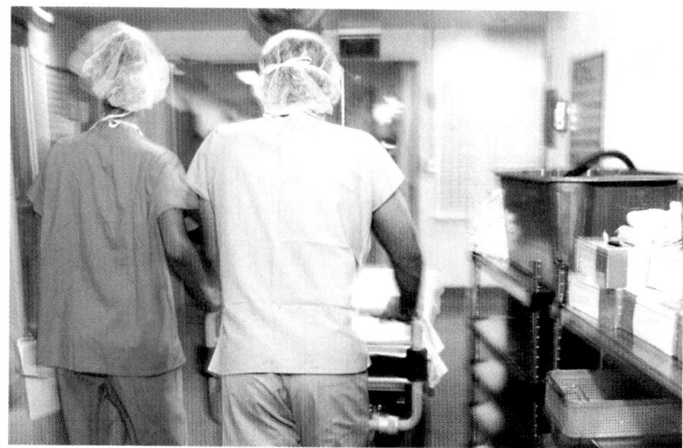

***Fig. 1-3.** Acute care is performed in hospitals for illnesses or injuries that require immediate care.*

- **Subacute care** is care given in a hospital or in a long-term care facility. It is used for people who need less care than for an acute (sudden onset, short-term) illness, but more care than for a chronic (long-term) illness. Treatment usually ends when the condition has stabilized and/or after the predetermined time period for treatment has been completed. The cost is usually less than a hospital but more than long-term care. Subacute care is covered in Chapter 22.
- **Outpatient care** is usually given for less than 24 hours. It is for people who have had treatments or surgery and need short-term skilled care.
- **Rehabilitation** is care given by specialists. Physical, occupational, and speech therapists restore or improve function after an illness or injury. Information about rehabilitation and related care is located in Chapter 21.
- **Hospice care** is given in facilities or homes for people who have approximately six months or less to live. Hospice workers give physical and emotional care and comfort while also supporting families. There is more information about hospice care in Chapter 23.

Often payers control the amount and types of healthcare services people receive. The kind of care a person receives and where he receives it may depend, in part, on who is paying for it. Traditional insurance companies offer plans that pay for the health care of plan members. Most people covered by traditional insurance are part of a plan at their place of work. The costs are paid for by the employer, the employee, or shared by both. Starting in 2014 the federal government's Patient Protection and Affordable Care Act (PPACA) will establish Affordable Insurance Exchanges. These exchanges are marketplaces for healthcare coverage and are intended to bring quality care within the reach of those who do not have access to an employer-based insurance program or who may not be able to afford their employers' programs. It is also intended to provide improved access to healthcare coverage for small businesses.

As a reaction to the increased costs of traditional insurance plans, many employers and employees belong to **health maintenance organizations (HMOs)**. HMOs require that participants use a particular doctor or group of doctors except in case of emergency. The doctors working for HMOs are paid to provide care while keeping costs down. Thus they may see more patients, order fewer tests, or cut costs in other ways.

Preferred provider organizations (PPOs) are another cost-reducing healthcare option. A PPO is a network of providers that contract to provide health services to a group of people. Employees are given incentives to use network providers. Employers are given reduced, fee-for-service rates for getting employees to participate in the network. A person in a PPO may still get health care outside the network of providers, but must pay a higher portion of the cost.

If a person becomes seriously ill, he may be admitted to a hospital. The costs of hospital care have risen greatly in recent years. To make up for these higher costs, healthcare payers are controlling who can be admitted to a hospital and for how long. After release from the hospital, many people need continuing care. This is particularly true as people are released after shorter hospital stays. Continuing care may be provided in a long-term care facility, a rehabilitation hospital, or by a home health agency. The type of care depends on the medical condition and needs of the patient or client.

Our healthcare system is constantly changing. As we develop new and better ways of caring for people, care becomes more expensive. Better health care helps people live longer, which leads to a larger elderly population that may need additional health care. New discoveries and expensive equipment have also increased healthcare costs (Fig. 1-4).

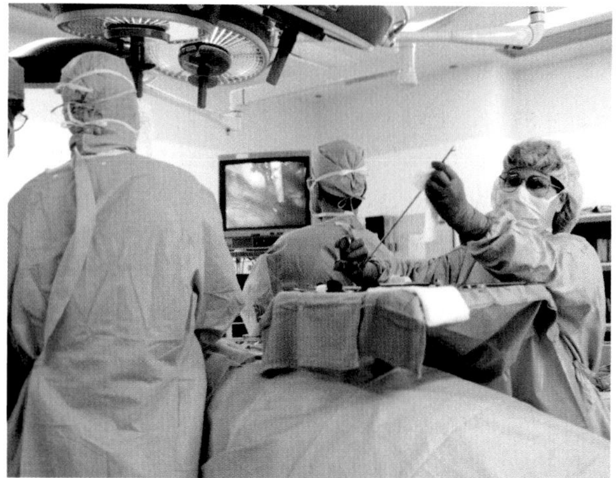

Fig. 1-4. Technology makes it possible to offer better health care, but equipment can be expensive.

HMOs and PPOs continue to replace traditional insurance plans. This affects the amount and quality of health care provided. These cost control strategies are often called **managed care**. In the past, the goal of health care was to make sick people well. Today it is to get sick people well in the most efficient (least expensive) way possible. Developments such as the PPACA's Affordable Insurance Exchanges, which are slated to begin in 2014, are sure to bring further changes to health care and healthcare coverage. The goal of these changes is to make coverage more accessible, affordable, and effective.

2. Describe a typical long-term care facility

Long-term care facilities (LTCFs) are businesses that provide skilled nursing care 24 hours a day. These facilities may offer assisted living housing, dementia care, or subacute care. Some facilities offer specialized care, while others care for all types of residents. The typical long-term care facility offers personal care for all residents and focused care for residents with special needs. Personal care includes bathing, skin, nail and hair care, and assistance with walking, eating, dressing, transferring, and toileting. All of these daily personal care tasks are called **activities of daily living**, or **ADLs**.

Other common services offered at long-term care facilities include the following:

- Physical, occupational, and speech therapy
- Wound care
- Care of different types of tubes, including **catheters** (thin tubes inserted into the body to drain fluids or inject fluids)
- Nutrition therapy
- Management of chronic diseases, such as acquired immune deficiency syndrome (AIDS), diabetes, chronic obstructive pulmonary disease (COPD), cancer, and congestive heart failure (CHF)

When specialized care is offered at long-term care facilities, the employees must have special training. Residents with similar needs may be placed in units together. Non-profit companies or for-profit companies can own long-term care facilities.

3. Describe residents who live in long-term care facilities

There are some general statements that can be made about residents in long-term care facilities. However, more important than understanding the entire population is that nursing assistants understand each individual for whom they will care. Residents' care should be based on their specific needs, illnesses, and preferences.

According to a survey conducted in 2004 by the National Center for Health Statistics, 88 percent of long-term care residents in the U.S. are over age 65. Seventy percent of residents are female. More than 90 percent are white and non-Hispanic (Fig. 1-5). This is a much larger percentage than the U.S. population as a whole. About one-third of residents come from a private residence; over 50 percent come from a hospital or other facility.

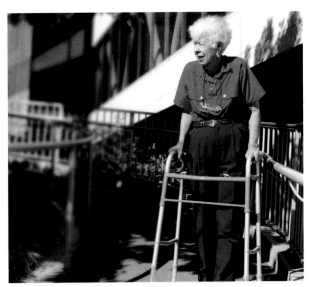

Fig. 1-5. White, non-Hispanic women make up a high percentage of residents in long-term care facilities.

The length of stay of over two-thirds of residents in long-term care is six months or longer. These residents need enough help with their activities of daily living to require 24-hour care. Often, they do not have caregivers available to give sufficient care for them to live in the community. The groups with the longest average stay are the developmentally disabled. They are often younger than 65. More information about these groups is found in Chapter 8.

The other third of residents stay for less than six months. This group generally falls into two categories. The first category is made up of residents admitted for terminal care. They will probably die in the facility. The second category is made up of residents admitted for rehabilitation or temporary illness. They will usually recover and return to the community. Care of these residents may be very different than care provided for permanent residents.

Dementia and other mental disorders are major causes of admissions to care facilities. Various studies place the number of residents with dementia between 50 and 90 percent. Many residents are admitted with other disorders as well. However, the disorders themselves are often not the main reason for admission. It is most often the lack of ability to care for oneself and the lack of a support system that leads someone to enter a facility.

A support system is vital in allowing the elderly to live outside a facility. For every elderly person living in a long-term care facility, at least two with similar disorders and disabilities live in the community.

Some residents have very little outside support from family or friends. This is one reason it is essential to care for the whole person instead of only the illness or disease. Residents have many needs besides bathing, eating, drinking, and toileting. These needs will go unmet if staff do not work to meet them.

4. Explain policies and procedures

All facilities have manuals outlining their policies and procedures. A **policy** is a course of action that should be taken every time a certain situation occurs. For example, a very basic policy is that healthcare information must remain confidential. A **procedure** is a method, or way, of doing something. For example, a facility will have a procedure for reporting information about residents. The procedure explains what form to complete, when and how often to fill it out, and to whom it is given. New employees will be told where to find a list of policies and procedures that all staff are expected to follow.

Common policies at long-term care facilities include the following:

- All resident information must remain confidential. This is not only a facility rule, it is also the law. Chapter 3 has information on confidentiality, including the Health Insurance Portability and Accountability Act (HIPAA).
- The plan of care must always be followed. Nursing assistants should perform tasks assigned by the care plan. Tasks that are not listed in the care plan or approved by the nurse should not be performed.

- Nursing assistants should not do tasks that are not listed in the job description.
- Nursing assistants must report important events or changes in residents to a nurse.
- Personal problems must not be discussed with the resident or the resident's family.
- Nursing assistants should not take money or gifts from residents or their families (Fig. 1-6).
- Nursing assistants must be on time for work. They must be dependable.

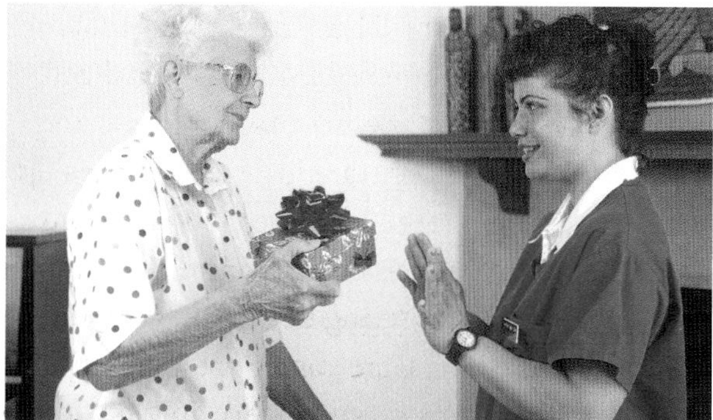

Fig. 1-6. *Nursing assistants should not accept money or gifts because it is unprofessional and may lead to conflict.*

Employers will have policies and procedures for every resident care situation. These have been developed to give quality care and protect resident safety. Written procedures may seem long and complicated, but each step is important. It is essential that nursing assistants become familiar with and always follow policies and procedures.

5. Describe the long-term care survey process

Inspections help ensure that long-term care facilities (and home health agencies) follow state and federal regulations. Inspections are performed periodically by the state agency that licenses facilities. These inspections are called surveys. They may be done more often if a facility has been cited for problems. To **cite** means to find a problem through a survey. Inspections may be done less often if the facility has a good record. Inspection teams include a variety of trained healthcare professionals.

Surveyors study how well staff care for residents. They focus on how residents' nutritional, physical, social, emotional, and spiritual needs are being met. They interview residents and their families and observe the staff's interactions with residents and the care given. They review resident charts and observe meals. Surveys are one reason the documentation done by nursing assistants is so important.

Surveyors use tags that identify specific federal regulations (F-Tags) to note any problems. When surveyors are in a facility, staff should try not to be nervous. They should give the same quality care they give every day and answer any questions to the best of their abilities. If an employee does not know the answer to a surveyor's question, she should be honest and never guess. She should tell the surveyor that she does not know the answer but will find out as quickly as possible. Then she should follow up with the surveyor after she has the answer.

The **Joint Commission** is an independent, not-for-profit organization that evaluates and accredits healthcare organizations. Its goal is to improve the safety and quality of care given to patients, clients, and residents. For an organization to receive accreditation from the Joint Commission, it must undergo a comprehensive survey process at least every three years. The survey process includes carefully checking performance in specific areas, such as patient rights, treatment, and infection prevention.

The Joint Commission's surveys are not affiliated with state inspections. Healthcare organizations are not required to participate in the Joint Commission's survey process; this is done on a voluntary basis. Organizations that are accredited by the Joint Commission include hospitals, long-term care facilities, rehabilitation centers, hospice services, home health care agencies, laboratories, and other organizations.

6. Explain Medicare and Medicaid

The **Centers for Medicare & Medicaid Services (CMS)** is a federal agency within the U.S. Department of Health and Human Services (Fig. 1-7). CMS runs two national healthcare programs—Medicare and Medicaid. They both help pay for health care and health insurance for millions of Americans. CMS has many other responsibilities as well.

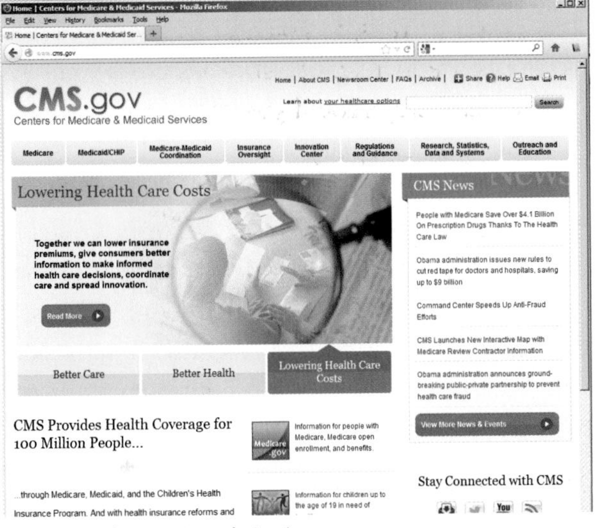
Home | Centers for Medicare & Medicaid Services - Mozilla Firefox
File Edit View History Bookmarks Tools Help
Home | Centers for Medicare & Medicaid Ser...
cms.gov
Home | About CMS | Newsroom Center | FAQs | Archive | Share Help Email Print
CMS.gov
Centers for Medicare & Medicaid Services
Learn about your healthcare options
Search
Medicare
Medicaid/CHIP
Medicare-Medicaid Coordination
Insurance Oversight
Innovation Center
Regulations and Guidance
Research, Statistics, Data and Systems
Outreach and Education
Lowering Health Care Costs
Together we can lower insurance premiums, give consumers better information to make informed health care decisions, coordinate care and spread innovation.
Read More
Better Care
Better Health
Lowering Health Care Costs
CMS News
People with Medicare Save Over $4.1 Billion On Prescription Drugs Thanks To The Health Care Law
Obama administration issues new rules to cut red tape for doctors and hospitals, saving up to $9 billion
Command Center Speeds Up Anti-Fraud Efforts
CMS Launches New Interactive Map with Medicare Review Contractor Information
Obama administration announces ground-breaking public-private partnership to prevent health care fraud
View More News & Events
CMS Provides Health Coverage for 100 Million People...
Information for people with Medicare, Medicare open enrollment, and benefits.
...through Medicare, Medicaid, and the Children's Health Insurance Program. And with health insurance reforms and
Information for children up to the age of 19 in need of
Stay Connected with CMS

Fig. 1-7. The CMS website is cms.gov.

Medicare is a health insurance program that was established in 1965 for people aged 65 or older. It also covers people of any age with permanent kidney failure or certain disabilities. Medicare has four parts. Part A helps pay for care in a hospital or skilled nursing facility or for care from a home health agency or hospice. Part B helps pay for doctor services and other medical services and equipment. Part C allows private health insurance companies to provide Medicare benefits. Part D helps pay for medications prescribed for treatment. Medicare will only pay for care it determines to be medically necessary.

Medicaid is a medical assistance program for low-income people. It is funded by both the federal government and each state. Eligibility is determined by income and special circumstances. People must qualify for this program.

Medicare and Medicaid pay long-term care facilities a fixed amount for services. This is based on the resident's needs upon admission and throughout his stay at the facility.

7. Discuss the terms *culture change* and *person-directed care* and describe Pioneer Network and The Eden Alternative

Some long-term care facilities are adopting newer models of care. These models promote meaningful environments with individualized approaches to care. **Culture change** is a term given to the process of transforming services for elders so that they are based on the values and practices of the person receiving care. Culture change involves respecting both elders and those working with them. Core values are promoting choice, dignity, respect, self-determination, and purposeful living. To honor culture change, healthcare settings may need to change their organization practices, physical environments, and relationships.

Pioneer Network was formed in 1997 by a group of people working in long-term care. Their aim was to ensure person-directed care. **Person-directed care** emphasizes the individuality of the person who needs care, and seeks to build community by recognizing and developing each person's capabilities. This group calls for a change in how elders are treated wherever they live—whether in care facilities or at home. Pioneer Network encourages a movement away from institutions and promotes caring environments. Their website, pioneernetwork.net, provides more information about this organization.

The Eden Alternative is a not-for-profit organization founded in 1991 by Dr. William Thomas. Its ongoing focus is to improve the lives of elders and their caregivers by creating environments that support growth and development, while trying to eliminate problems of loneliness, helplessness, and boredom that many elderly people suffer.

The Eden Alternative offers education, resources, and consulting services to help create meaningful environments for the elderly. Places that have adopted the Eden Alternative's philosophy are typically filled with plants and animals. Children regularly visit. The Eden Alternative strives to improve the quality of life and quality of care for the elderly (Fig. 1-8). Their website, edenalt.org, has more information.

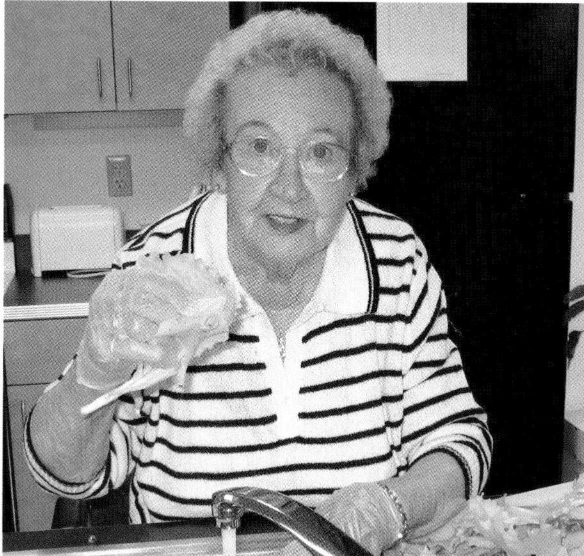

Fig. 1-8. *The Eden Alternative focuses on eliminating boredom, loneliness, and helplessness by promoting meaningful elder care.* (PHOTO COURTESY OF THE EDEN ALTERNATIVE)

Chapter Review

1. What is long-term care?
2. List one fact about each of the following healthcare settings: home health care, assisted living facilities, adult day services, acute care, subacute care, outpatient care, rehabilitation, and hospice care.
3. List five services commonly offered at long-term care facilities.
4. Who makes up the majority of residents in long-term care—men or women?
5. What are two general categories of residents who stay in a care facility for less than six months?
6. List five common policies at long-term care facilities.
7. List two ways that surveyors study how well staff care for residents in a facility.
8. Briefly describe what the Medicare and Medicaid programs do.
9. Define *culture change.*

2 The Nursing Assistant and The Care Team

1. Identify the members of the care team and describe how the care team works together to provide care

Residents will have different needs and problems. Healthcare professionals with different kinds of education and experience will help care for them. This group is known as the *care team*. Members of the care team include the following:

Nursing Assistant (NA) or Certified Nursing Assistant (CNA): The nursing assistant (NA) performs assigned tasks, such as taking vital signs, and provides or assists with routine personal care, such as bathing residents and helping with toileting. Nursing assistants must have at least 75 hours of training and in many states training exceeds 100 hours. Nursing assistants spend more time with residents than other members of the care team. That is why they act as the "eyes and ears" of the team. Observing and reporting changes in the resident's condition or abilities is a very important role of the NA (Fig. 2-1).

Registered Nurse (RN): In long-term care, a registered nurse coordinates, manages, and provides skilled nursing care. This includes administering special treatments and giving medication as prescribed by a physician. A registered nurse also assigns tasks and supervises daily care of residents by nursing assistants. A registered nurse is a licensed professional who has graduated from a two- to four-year nursing program. RNs have diplomas or college degrees and have passed a licensing examination. Registered nurses may have additional academic degrees or education in specialty areas.

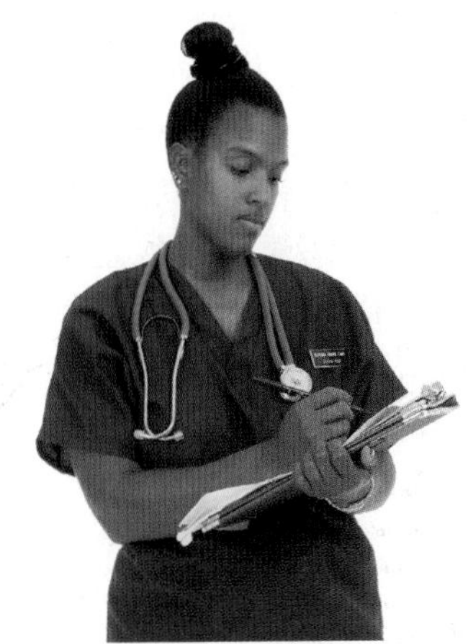

Fig. 2-1. *Observing carefully and reporting accurately are some of the most important duties performed by NAs.*

Licensed Practical Nurse (LPN) or Licensed Vocational Nurse (LVN): A licensed practical nurse or licensed vocational nurse administers medications and gives treatments. LPNs may also supervise nursing assistants' daily care of residents. A licensed practical nurse or vocational nurse is a licensed professional who has completed one to two years of education and has passed a licensing examination.

Physician or Doctor (MD [medical doctor] or DO [doctor of osteopathy]): A doctor's job is to diagnose disease or disability and prescribe treatment. Doctors have graduated from four-year medical schools, which they attended after receiving bachelor's degrees. Many doctors also attend specialized training programs after medical school (Fig. 2-2).

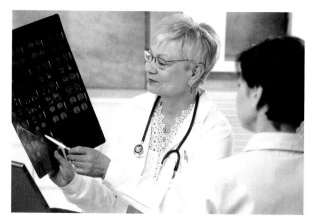

Fig. 2-2. Doctors diagnose disease and prescribe treatment.

Physical Therapist (PT): A physical therapist evaluates a person and develops a treatment plan to increase movement, improve circulation, promote healing, reduce pain, prevent disability, and help the resident regain or maintain mobility (Fig. 2-3). A PT administers therapy in the form of heat, cold, massage, ultrasound, electrical stimulation, and exercise to muscles, bones, and joints. Physical therapist education programs are mostly offered at the doctoral degree level (Doctor of Physical Therapy, or DPT). Entrance into these programs usually requires an undergraduate degree. Doctoral degree programs generally last three years. PTs have to pass national and state licensure exams before they can practice.

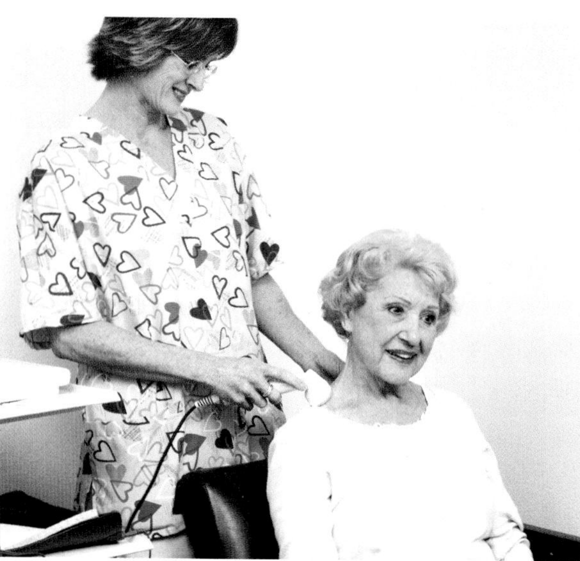

Fig. 2-3. A physical therapist will help restore specific abilities.

Occupational Therapist (OT): An occupational therapist helps residents learn to adapt to disabilities. An OT may assist in training residents to perform **activities of daily living (ADLs)**. ADLs are personal daily care tasks. They include bathing, dressing, caring for teeth, skin, nails, and hair, walking, transferring, toileting, and eating and drinking. This often involves the use of equipment called **assistive** or **adaptive devices** (Fig. 2-4). (Chapter 21 has more information.) The OT evaluates the resident's needs and plans a treatment program. Occupational therapists are required to have a minimum of a master's degree. OTs have to pass a national certification examination and most must be licensed within their state.

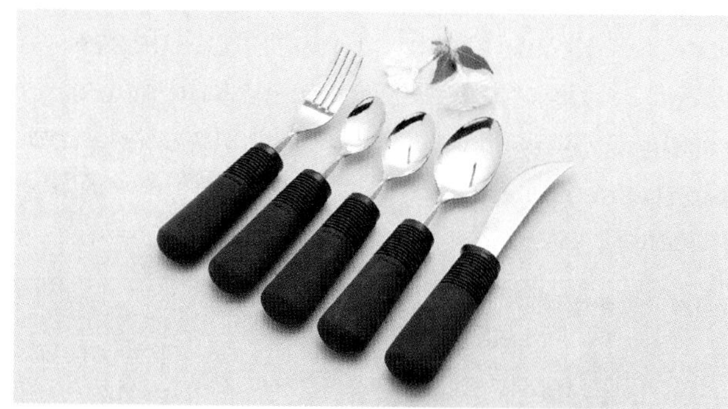

Fig. 2-4. An occupational therapist will help residents learn to use adaptive devices, such as these for eating. (PHOTO COURTESY OF NORTH COAST MEDICAL, INC., WWW.NCMEDICAL.COM, 800-821-9319)

Speech-Language Pathologist (SLP): A speech-language pathologist, or speech therapist, identifies communication disorders, addresses factors involved in recovery, and develops a plan of care to meet recovery goals. An SLP teaches exercises to help the resident improve or overcome speech problems. An SLP also evaluates a person's ability to swallow food and drink. Speech-language pathologists are required to have a master's degree in speech-language pathology. Most states require that SLPs be licensed or certified to work.

Registered Dietitian (RDT): A registered dietitian creates diets for residents with special needs. Special diets can improve health and help manage illness. RDTs may supervise the preparation and service of food and educate others about healthy nutritional habits. Registered dietitians have completed a bachelor's degree and may also have completed a postgraduate degree. Most states require that RDTs be licensed or certified.

Medical Social Worker (MSW): A medical social worker determines residents' needs and helps get them support services, such as counseling or financial assistance. He or she may help residents obtain clothing and personal items if the family is not involved or does not visit often. A medical social worker may book appointments and transportation. Generally, MSWs hold a master's degree in social work.

Activities Director: The activities director plans activities for residents to help them socialize and stay physically and mentally active. These activities are meant to improve and maintain residents' well-being and to prevent further complications from illness or disability. An activities director may have a bachelor's degree, associate's degree, or qualifying work experience. An activities director may be called a *recreational therapist* depending upon education and experience.

Resident and Resident's Family: The resident is an important member of the care team. The resident has the right to make decisions about his or her own care. The resident helps plan care and makes choices. The resident's family may also be involved in these decisions. The care team revolves around the resident and his or her condition, treatment, and progress. Without the resident, there is no care team.

2. Explain the nursing assistant's role

Nursing assistants can have many different titles. *Nurse aide, certified nurse aide, unlicensed assistive personnel, patient care technician* and *certified nursing assistant* are some examples. This textbook will use the term *nursing assistant.*

Nursing assistants (NAs) perform assigned nursing tasks, such as taking a resident's temperature. Nursing assistants also provide personal care, such as bathing residents, helping them eat and drink, and helping with hair care (Fig. 2-5). Promoting independence and self-care are other very important tasks that nursing assistants do. Other nursing assistant duties include the following:

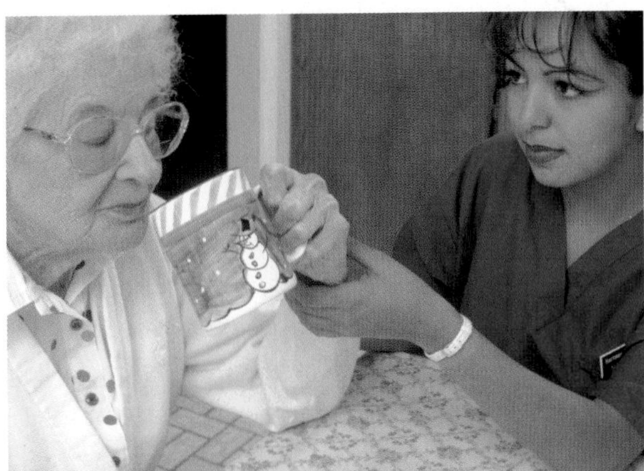

Fig. 2-5. *Encouraging residents to drink often is an important part of a nursing assistant's job.*

- Helping residents with toileting needs
- Assisting residents to move around safely
- Keeping residents' living areas neat and clean
- Encouraging residents to eat and drink
- Caring for supplies and equipment
- Helping residents dress
- Making beds
- Giving backrubs
- Helping residents with mouth care

Nursing assistants are not allowed to insert or remove tubes, change sterile dressings, or give tube feedings. Nursing assistants are usually not allowed to give medications; nurses are responsible for giving medications. However, some states allow nursing assistants to work with medications after receiving special training.

Nursing assistants spend more time with residents than other care team members. Observing changes in a resident's condition and reporting them is a very important duty of the NA. Residents' care can be revised or updated as conditions change. Another duty of the nursing assistant is writing down important information about the resident; this is called **charting**, or documenting.

Nursing assistants are part of a team of health professionals. The team includes doctors, nurses, social workers, therapists, dietitians, and specialists. The resident and resident's family are part of the team. Everyone, including the resident, works closely together to meet goals. Goals include helping residents recover from illnesses and to do as much as possible for themselves.

Residents' Rights

Responsibility for Residents

All residents are the responsibility of each nursing assistant. An NA will receive assignments to do tasks, care, and other duties for specific residents. If he sees a resident who needs help, even if the resident is not on his assignment sheet, the NA should provide the needed care.

3. Explain professionalism and list examples of professional behavior

Professional means having to do with work or a job. The opposite of professional is **personal**, which refers to life outside a job, such as family, friends, and home life. **Professionalism** is behaving properly when on the job. It includes dressing appropriately and speaking well. It also includes being on time, completing tasks, and reporting to the nurse. For a nursing assistant, professionalism also means following the care plan, making careful observations, and reporting accurately. Following policies and procedures is an important part of professionalism. Residents, coworkers, and supervisors respect employees who behave in a professional way. Professionalism helps people keep their jobs and may help them earn promotions and raises.

A professional relationship with residents includes the following:

- Keeping a positive attitude
- Doing only the assigned tasks that are in the care plan and that the NA is trained to do
- Keeping all residents' information confidential
- Being polite and cheerful at all times (Fig. 2-6)

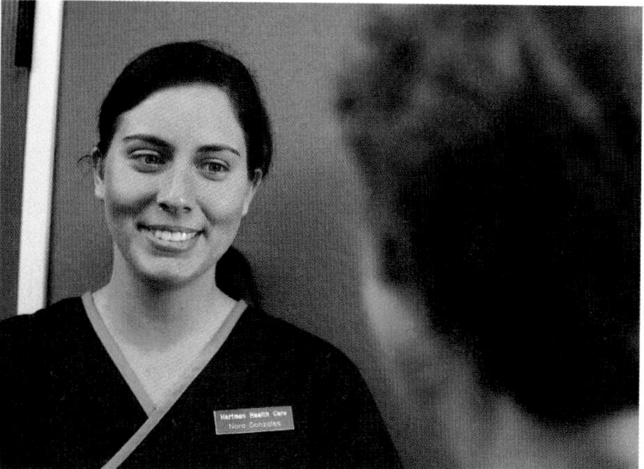

Fig. 2-6. *Nursing assistants are expected to be polite and cheerful in all circumstances.*

- Not discussing personal problems
- Not using profanity, even if a resident does
- Listening to the resident
- Calling a resident *Mr., Mrs., Ms.,* or *Miss,* and his or her last name, or by the name he or she prefers (terms such as *sweetie, honey, dearie,* etc. are disrespectful and should not be used)
- Never giving or accepting gifts
- Always explaining care before providing it
- Following practices, such as handwashing, to protect care providers and residents

A professional relationship with an employer includes the following:

- Completing tasks efficiently
- Always following all policies and procedures
- Always documenting and reporting carefully and correctly

- Reporting problems with residents or tasks
- Reporting anything that keeps a nursing assistant from completing duties
- Asking questions when the nursing assistant does not know or understand something
- Taking directions or criticism without becoming upset
- Being clean and neatly dressed and groomed
- Always being on time
- Communicating with the employer if the nursing assistant cannot report for work
- Following the chain of command
- Participating in education programs
- Being a positive role model for the facility

Nursing assistants must be

Compassionate: Being **compassionate** means being caring, concerned, considerate, empathetic, and understanding. Demonstrating **empathy** means identifying with the feelings of others. People who are compassionate understand others' problems. They care about them. Compassionate people are also sympathetic. Showing **sympathy** means sharing in the feelings and difficulties of others.

Honest: An honest person tells the truth and can be trusted. Residents need to feel that they can trust those who care for them. The care team depends on honesty in planning care. Employers count on truthful records of care and observations.

Tactful: Being **tactful** means showing sensitivity and having a sense of what is appropriate when dealing with others.

Conscientious: People who are **conscientious** try to do their best. They are guided by a sense of right and wrong. They are alert, observant, accurate, and responsible. Giving conscientious care means making accurate observations and reports, following the care plan, and taking responsibility for one's actions (Fig. 2-7). For example, taking accurate measurements of vital signs, such as temperature or pulse, is important. Other members of the care team will make treatment decisions based on the documented measurements. Without conscientious care, a resident's health and well-being are in danger.

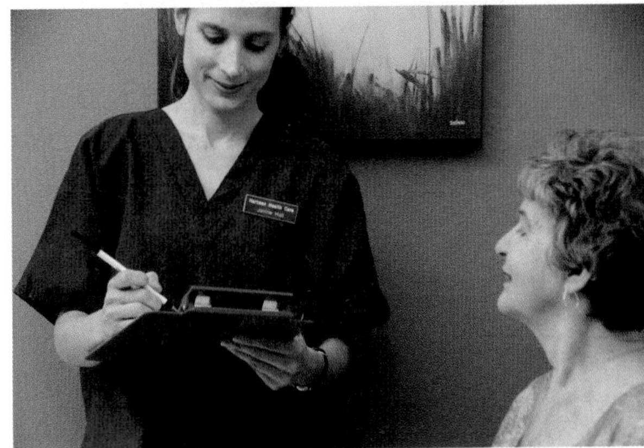

Fig. 2-7. Nursing assistants must be conscientious about documenting observations and procedures.

Dependable: Nursing assistants must be able to make and keep commitments. They must report to work on time. They must skillfully do assigned tasks, avoid too many absences, and help their peers when needed.

Respectful: Being respectful means valuing other people's individuality. This includes age, religion, culture, feelings, practices, and beliefs. People who are respectful treat others politely and kindly. They care about others' self-esteem and try not to do or say anything that will harm it. Being respectful means not gossiping and respecting the various cultures and practices of residents and others.

Unprejudiced: Nursing assistants work with many different people from different backgrounds. They must give each resident the same quality care regardless of age, gender, sexual orientation, religion, race, ethnicity, or condition.

Tolerant: Being tolerant means respecting others' beliefs and practices and not judging them. Even though nursing assistants may not like or agree with things that residents or residents' families do or have done, their job is to care for each resident as assigned, not to judge him or her. NAs should put aside their opinions and see each resident as an individual who needs their care.

4. Describe proper personal grooming habits

Regular grooming makes a person feel good about himself, and it makes a positive impression on others (Fig. 2-8). Grooming affects how confident residents feel about the care a person gives. Professional nursing assistants have the following personal grooming habits:

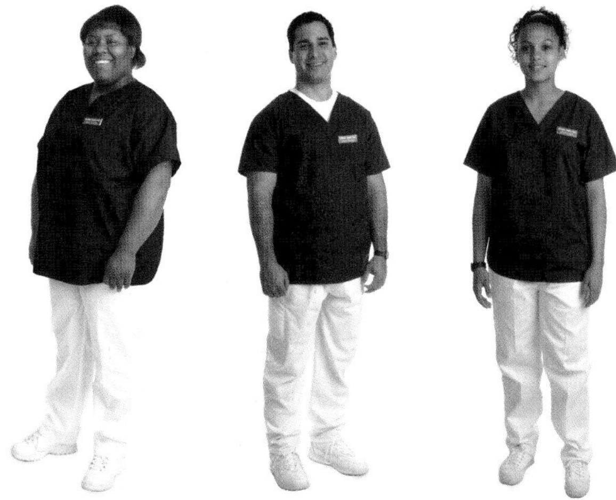

Fig. 2-8. Proper grooming includes being clean and neatly dressed. Long hair should be tied back, and shoes should be comfortable and clean.

- Bathing or showering daily and using deodorant or antiperspirant (perfume and cologne should not be used because some residents may be intolerant of some odors)
- Brushing teeth frequently and using mouthwash when necessary
- Keeping hair clean and neatly brushed or combed and tying long hair back in a bun or ponytail
- Keeping facial hair short, clean, and neat
- Dressing neatly in a uniform that has been washed and ironed
- Not wearing clothes that are too tight or too baggy, torn or stained, or too revealing (short skirts, low-cut blouses, see-through fabrics)
- Not wearing large jewelry (the main exception to this rule is wearing a simple, waterproof watch that may be used to measure vital signs and record events)
- Not having visible tattoos and body piercings (except for pierced ears)
- Wearing comfortable, clean, high-quality, closed-toe shoes.
- Keeping fingernails short, smooth, and clean
- Not wearing artificial nails, extenders, overlays, etc., because they harbor bacteria
- Wearing little or no makeup

Nursing assistants should follow any specific rules a facility has regarding their appearance.

5. Explain the chain of command and scope of practice

A nursing assistant carries out instructions given to her by a nurse. The nurse is acting on the instructions of a physician or other member of the care team. This is called the **chain of command**. It describes the line of authority and helps to make sure that residents get proper health care. The chain of command also protects employees and employers from liability. **Liability** is a legal term that means someone can be held responsible for harming someone else. For example, imagine that something a nursing assistant does for a resident harms that resident. However, what the NA did was in the care plan and was done according to policy and procedure. In this case she may not be liable, or responsible, for hurting the resident. However, if an NA does something that is not in the care plan and harms a resident, she could be held responsible. That is why it is important for team members to follow instructions in the care plan and for the facility to have a chain of command (Fig. 2-9).

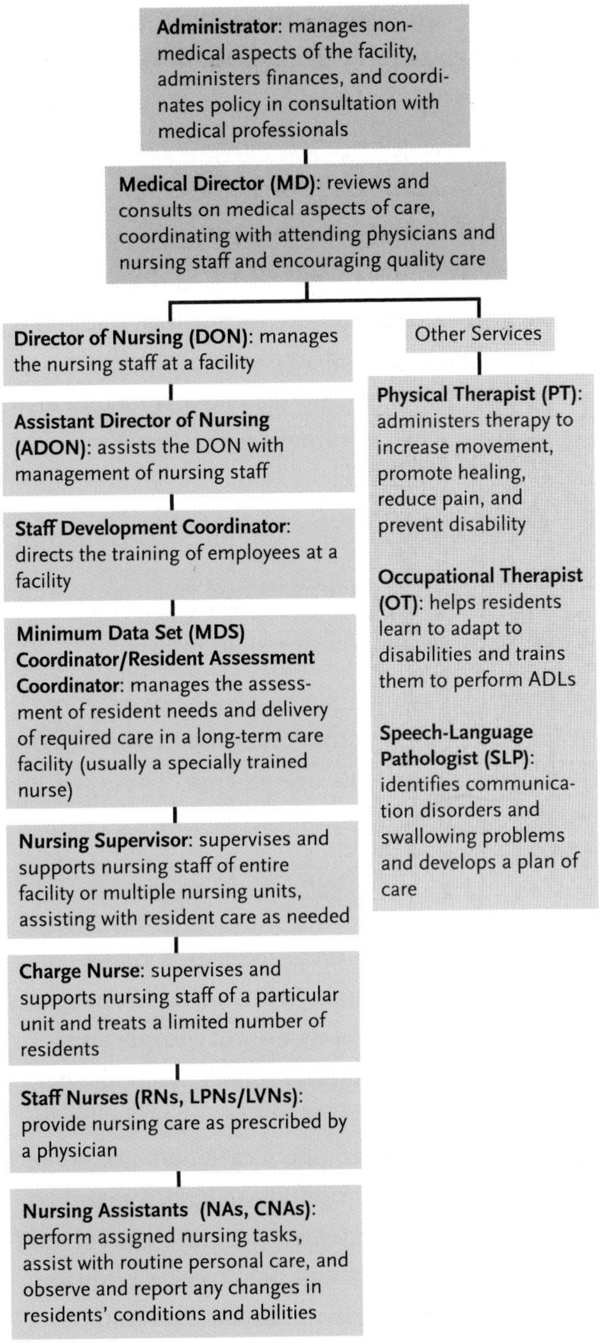

Administrator: manages non-medical aspects of the facility, administers finances, and coordinates policy in consultation with medical professionals

Medical Director (MD): reviews and consults on medical aspects of care, coordinating with attending physicians and nursing staff and encouraging quality care

Director of Nursing (DON): manages the nursing staff at a facility

Assistant Director of Nursing (ADON): assists the DON with management of nursing staff

Staff Development Coordinator: directs the training of employees at a facility

Minimum Data Set (MDS) Coordinator/Resident Assessment Coordinator: manages the assessment of resident needs and delivery of required care in a long-term care facility (usually a specially trained nurse)

Nursing Supervisor: supervises and supports nursing staff of entire facility or multiple nursing units, assisting with resident care as needed

Charge Nurse: supervises and supports nursing staff of a particular unit and treats a limited number of residents

Staff Nurses (RNs, LPNs/LVNs): provide nursing care as prescribed by a physician

Nursing Assistants (NAs, CNAs): perform assigned nursing tasks, assist with routine personal care, and observe and report any changes in residents' conditions and abilities

Other Services

Physical Therapist (PT): administers therapy to increase movement, promote healing, reduce pain, and prevent disability

Occupational Therapist (OT): helps residents learn to adapt to disabilities and trains them to perform ADLs

Speech-Language Pathologist (SLP): identifies communication disorders and swallowing problems and develops a plan of care

Fig. 2-9. *The chain of command describes the line of authority and helps ensure that the resident receives proper care.*

Nursing assistants must understand what they can and cannot do. This is important so that they do not harm residents or involve themselves or their employers in a lawsuit. Some states certify that nursing assistants are qualified to work. However, nursing assistants are not licensed healthcare providers. Everything they do in their job is assigned by a licensed healthcare professional. They work under the authority of another person's license. That is why these professionals will show great interest in what nursing assistants do and how they do it.

Every state grants the right to practice various jobs in health care through licensure. Examples include a license to practice nursing, medicine, or physical therapy. Each member of the care team works within his or her scope of practice. A **scope of practice** defines the tasks that healthcare providers are legally allowed to do and how to do them correctly.

Laws and regulations about what nursing assistants can and cannot do vary from state to state. However, some procedures are not performed by nursing assistants under any circumstances. Tasks that are outside the scope of practice of a nursing assistant include the following:

- NAs do not administer medications.
- NAs do not honor a request to do something outside the scope of practice, not listed in the care plan, or not on the assignment sheet. In this situation, an NA should explain that he cannot do the task requested. The request should then be reported to a nurse. This is true even if a nurse or doctor asks the NA to perform the task. The NA should refuse to perform the task and explain why. Refusing to do something that the NA cannot legally do is the NA's right and responsibility.
- NAs do not perform procedures that require sterile technique. For example, changing a sterile dressing on a deep, open wound requires sterile technique.
- NAs do not diagnose illnesses or prescribe treatments or medications.
- NAs do not tell the resident or the family the diagnosis or the medical treatment plan. This is the responsibility of the doctor or nurse.

An instructor or an employer may provide a list of other tasks outside the nursing assistant's scope of practice. In some cases, an NA may have received training to do a particular task but her employer does not want her to perform it. It is important that NAs know which tasks these are and not perform them. Many of these specialized tasks require more training. NAs must learn how to refuse a task for which they have not been trained or which is outside their scope of practice.

6. Discuss the resident care plan and explain its purpose

The resident care plan is individualized for each resident. It is developed to help achieve the goals of care. The nurse or doctor creates the care plan. The resident is also involved in the planning. The care plan lists the tasks that team members, including nursing assistants, must perform (Fig. 2-10). It states how often these tasks should be performed and how they should be carried out.

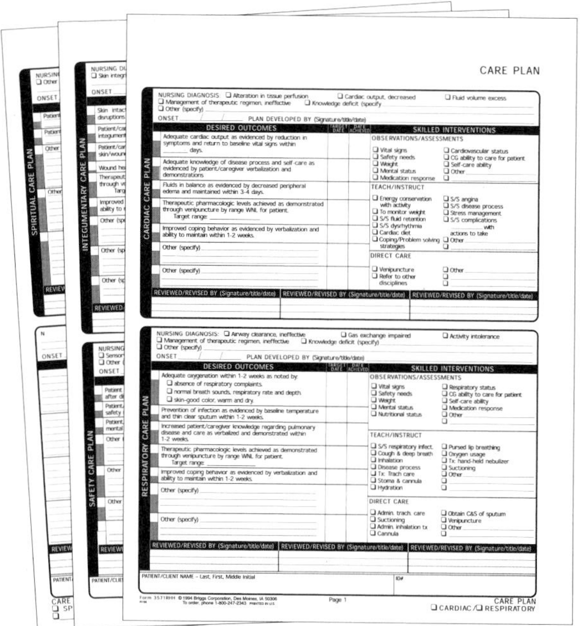

CARE PLAN

CARDIAC CARE PLAN

NURSING DIAGNOSIS: ❑ Alteration in tissue perfusion ❑ Cardiac output, decreased ❑ Fluid volume excess
❑ Management of therapeutic regimen, ineffective ❑ Knowledge deficit (specify)
❑ Other (specify)
ONSET / / PLAN DEVELOPED BY (Signature/title/date)

DESIRED OUTCOMES	TARGET DATE	DATE ACHIEVED	SKILLED INTERVENTIONS
Adequate cardiac output as evidenced by reduction in symptoms and return to baseline vital signs within ____ days.			OBSERVATIONS/ASSESSMENTS: ❑ Vital signs ❑ Safety needs ❑ Weight ❑ Mental status ❑ Medication response ❑ Cardiovascular status ❑ CG ability to care for patient ❑ Self-care ability ❑ Other ❑
Adequate knowledge of disease process and self-care as evidenced by patient/caregiver verbalization and demonstrations			
Fluids in balance as evidenced by decreased peripheral edema and maintained within 3-4 days.			TEACH/INSTRUCT: ❑ Energy conservation with activity ❑ To monitor weight ❑ S/S fluid retention ❑ S/S dysrhythmia ❑ Cardiac diet ❑ Coping/Problem solving strategies ❑ S/S angina ❑ S/S disease process ❑ Stress management ❑ S/S complications ____ with actions to take ❑ Other ❑
Therapeutic pharmacologic levels achieved as demonstrated through venipuncture by range WNL for patient. Target range: ____			
Improved coping behavior as evidenced by verbalization and ability to maintain within 1-2 weeks.			
Other (specify)			DIRECT CARE: ❑ Venipuncture ❑ Refer to other disciplines ❑ Other ❑ ❑
Other (specify)			

REVIEWED/REVISED BY (Signature/title/date) | REVIEWED/REVISED BY (Signature/title/date) | REVIEWED/REVISED BY (Signature/title/date)

RESPIRATORY CARE PLAN

NURSING DIAGNOSIS: ❑ Airway clearance, ineffective ❑ Gas exchange impaired ❑ Activity intolerance
❑ Management of therapeutic regimen, ineffective ❑ Knowledge deficit (specify)
❑ Other (specify)
ONSET / / PLAN DEVELOPED BY (Signature/title/date)

DESIRED OUTCOMES	TARGET DATE	DATE ACHIEVED	SKILLED INTERVENTIONS
Adequate oxygenation within 1-2 weeks as noted by: ❑ absence of respiratory complaints. ❑ normal breath sounds, respiratory rate and depth. ❑ skin-good color, warm and dry.			OBSERVATIONS/ASSESSMENTS: ❑ Vital signs ❑ Safety needs ❑ Weight ❑ Mental status ❑ Nutritional status ❑ Respiratory status ❑ CG ability to care for patient ❑ Self-care ability ❑ Medication response ❑ Other ❑
Prevention of infection as evidenced by baseline temperature and thin clear sputum within 1-2 weeks.			
Increased patient/caregiver knowledge regarding pulmonary disease and care as verbalized and demonstrated within 1-2 weeks.			TEACH/INSTRUCT: ❑ S/S respiratory infect. ❑ Cough & deep breath ❑ Inhalation ❑ Disease process ❑ Tx: Trach care ❑ Stoma & cannula ❑ Hydration ❑ Pursed lip breathing ❑ Oxygen usage ❑ Tx: hand-held nebulizer ❑ Suctioning ❑ Other ❑ ❑
Therapeutic pharmacologic levels achieved as demonstrated through venipuncture by range WNL for patient. Target range: ____			
Improved coping behavior as evidenced by verbalization and ability to maintain within 1-2 weeks.			
Other (specify)			DIRECT CARE: ❑ Admin. trach. care ❑ Suctioning ❑ Admin. inhalation tx ❑ Cannula ❑ Obtain C&S of sputum ❑ Venipuncture ❑ Other ❑
Other (specify)			

REVIEWED/REVISED BY (Signature/title/date) | REVIEWED/REVISED BY (Signature/title/date) | REVIEWED/REVISED BY (Signature/title/date)

PATIENT/CLIENT NAME – Last, First, Middle Initial | ID#

Form 3571RHH © 1994 Briggs Corporation, Des Moines, IA 50306 To order, phone 1-800-247-2343 PRINTED IN U.S. Page 1 CARE PLAN ❑ CARDIAC /❑ RESPIRATORY

***Fig. 2-10.** Sample resident care plans.* (REPRINTED WITH PERMISSION OF BRIGGS CORPORATION, DES MOINES, IOWA, 800-247-2343, BRIGGSCORP.COM)

The care plan is a guide to help the resident reach and maintain the best level of health possible. It must be followed very carefully. **Activities not listed on the care plan should not be performed.**

Care planning should involve input from the resident and/or the family, as well as healthcare professionals. Professionals will assess the resident's physical, financial, social, and psychological needs. After the doctor prescribes treatment, the supervisor, nurses, and other care team members create the care plan. Many factors are considered when formulating a care plan. These include the following:

- The resident's health and physical condition
- The resident's diagnosis and treatment
- The resident's goals or expectations

Multiple care plans may be necessary for some residents. In these situations, the nurse will coordinate the resident's overall care. There will be one care plan for the nursing assistant to follow. There will be separate care plans for other providers, such as the physical therapist.

It is essential that nursing assistants make observations and report them to the nurse. Sometimes even simple observations are very important. The information that NAs collect, such as vital signs, and the changes that they observe are important in determining how care plans may need to change. Because nursing assistants spend so much time with residents, they have a lot of valuable information that will help in care planning. Nursing assistants may be asked to attend care planning meetings. If they attend these meetings, it is important that they share their observations of residents. Nursing assistants who are not sure what is important to share can speak to a nurse before the meeting to find out.

7. Describe the nursing process

To communicate with other healthcare team members and to help plan and evaluate the resident's care needs, nurses use the nursing process (Fig. 2-11). The process has five steps:

- **Assessment**: getting information about the resident from many sources, including medical history, physical assessment, and environment, and reviewing this information
- **Diagnosis**: identifying the health problems after looking at all the resident's needs
- **Planning**: setting goals and creating a care plan to meet the resident's needs
- **Implementation**: putting the care plan into action; giving care
- **Evaluation**: a careful examination to see if the goals are being met

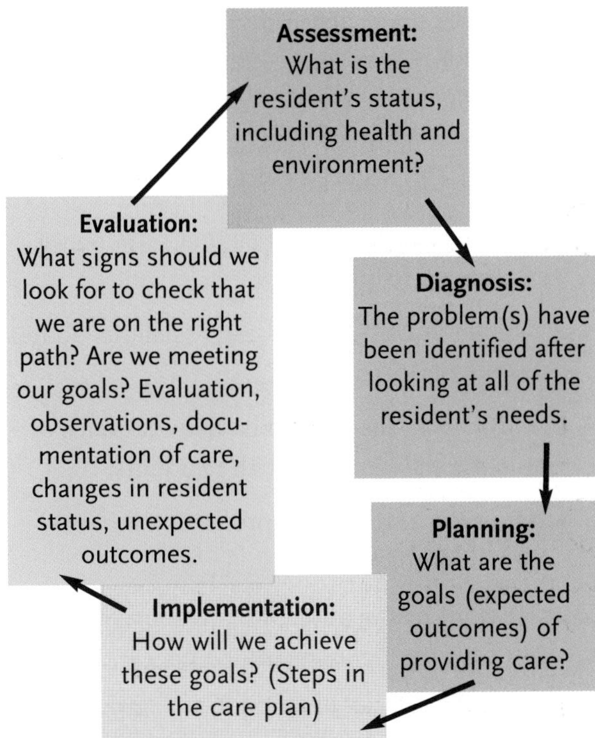

Fig. 2-11. The nursing and care planning process.

The nursing process constantly changes as new information is collected and reported. Clear communication between all team members and the resident is vital to ensure success of the process. The nursing assistant's accurate observations and reports are an important part of planning and evaluating care.

8. Describe *The Five Rights of Delegation*

When planning care, nurses decide which tasks to delegate to other team members, including nursing assistants. **Delegation** means transferring responsibility to a person for a specific task. Licensed nurses are accountable for care, including all delegated tasks. The National Council of State Boards of Nursing has identified *The Five Rights of Delegation*. This can be used as a mental checklist to help nurses in the decision-making process.

The Five Rights of Delegation are the *Right Task, Right Circumstance, Right Person, Right Direction/Communication*, and *Right Supervision/Evaluation*. Before delegating tasks, nurses consider these questions:

- Is there a match between the resident's needs and the nursing assistant's skills, abilities, and experience?
- What is the level of resident stability?
- Is the nursing assistant the right person to do the job?
- Can the nurse give appropriate direction and communication?
- Is the nurse available to give the supervision, support, and help that the nursing assistant needs?

There are questions nursing assistants may want to consider before accepting a task:

- Do I have all the information I need to do this job? Are there questions I should ask?
- Do I believe that I can do this task? Do I have the necessary skills?
- Do I have the needed supplies, equipment, and other support?
- Do I know who my supervisor is and how to reach him/her?
- Do we both understand who is doing what?

A nursing assistant should not be afraid to ask for help. She should always ask if she needs any more information or is unsure about something. If an NA feels that she does not have the skills for a task or that the task is not within her scope of practice, she should talk to the nurse.

9. Demonstrate how to manage time and assignments

Nursing assistants must manage their time well when taking care of residents. There is a variety of tasks that must be done during their shifts. Managing time properly helps NAs complete these tasks. Many of the following ideas for managing time on the job can be used to manage personal time as well:

Plan ahead. Planning is the single best way to manage time better. Sometimes it is hard even to find time to plan, but it is important to sit down and list everything that has to be done. NAs must take time to check to see if they have all the supplies needed for a procedure. Often just making the list and taking the time to re-check will help a caregiver feel better and help him focus.

The nurse creates the nursing assistant's work assignments based on the needs of residents and availability of staff. The assignments allow staff to work as team. The NA's responsibilities in completing assignments include

- Helping others when needed
- Never ignoring a resident who needs help
- Answering all call lights even when not assigned to a particular resident
- Notifying the nurse if she cannot complete an assignment

Prioritize. An NA should identify the most important things to get done and do these first.

Make a schedule. Many people find it useful to write out the hours of the day and fill in what needs to be done and when. This allows for a realistic schedule.

Combine activities. Nursing assistants can visit with residents while providing care, which combines two important tasks. It is important to work more efficiently whenever possible.

Get help. It is a simple reality that it is not possible for a nursing assistant to do everything. Sometimes NAs will need help to ensure a resident's safety, and they should not be afraid to ask for help.

Chapter Review

1. Describe what each of these care team members does: nursing assistant; registered nurse; physician; physical therapist; occupational therapist; speech-language pathologist; registered dietitian; medical social worker; activities director; and resident.
2. List six examples of duties that nursing assistants perform.
3. List two duties that nursing assistants do not usually perform.
4. Define *professionalism.* List five examples of professional behavior with residents.
5. List seven examples of professional behavior with an employer.
6. List eight personal qualities that are important for nursing assistants to have.
7. Why is it important for nursing assistants who have long hair to keep their hair tied back?
8. Why would wearing comfortable shoes be important to nursing assistants?
9. Give one reason why the chain of command is important.
10. List three tasks that are said to be outside the scope of practice of a nursing assistant.
11. Why are observing and reporting even simple observations about a resident important?

12. What are three factors considered when forming a care plan?
— the residents health & physical condition
— the residents diagnosis & treatment
— the residents goals or expectations

13. List five steps in the nursing process. assessment – info about resident from all sources
Diagnosis – what's wrong. Planning how to help.
Implementing – Doing the care
Evaluation – How did it work?

14. List *The Five Rights of Delegation.*
Right task, right circumstance, Right person,
Right direction & communication
Right supervision & evaluation

15. What should a nursing assistant do if he feels he does not have the skills necessary to perform a task? Decline to perform task & say why to the higher authority who asked.

16. List five steps in managing time and assignments.
1) PLAN AHEAD
2) PRIORITIZE
3) MAKE A SCHEDULE
4) COMBINE ACTIVITIES
5) GET HELP (Don't think you can do it all yourself.

---

1) nursing assistant: act as "ears" & "eyes" of the team. Reporting changes in resident
registered nurse: coordinates, manages & provides skilled nursing care
physician: diagnosis disease or disability & prescribe treatment
physical therapist: evaluates & developes treatment plan to increase movement, promote healing
occupational therapist: assist residents to learn ADL's. prevent disability, reduce pain, etc.
Speech-language therapist: help residents overcome speech problems
Dietitian – creates diets for residents with special needs.
medical social worker; gives counselling & aids with infor. on financial servicesetc.
Activities director: plans activities to help residents socialize, stay alert physically & mentally
Resident: Helps plan care & makes important choices. Has the right to make decisions

2) Bathing, feeding, dressing, hair care, mouth care, toileting, moving safely.
Keeping living area clean, caring for supplies, etc.

3) Giving medications, putting in tubes or taking them out, change sterile dressings etc.
tube feedings.

4) professionalism = having to do with work or a job as opposed to personal

5)
- Keep positive attitude
- being on time
- Doing only assigned tasks
- Polite & cheerful
Not discussing personal problems
No swearing
Listening to resident
Not accepting gifts
Adressing them by their real name
Explaining care before giving it.
Handwashing
- Following policies & procedures
- completing tasks efficiently
- Documenting & reporting carefully.
- Reporting problems
- Clean & neatly dressed.
- Following chain of command.

6) Compassionate
Able to sympathize
tactful
conscientious
Dependable
Honest
Respectful
Unprejudiced
Tolerant of others beliefs etc.

7) So their hair does not get in the way or fall out in food or brush someones eyes etc.
It has to do with cleanliness & the environment.

8) Because NA's are on their feet all day & support is important as well as comfort. They will feel better.

9) The chain of command helps keep order to the residents care and safety as well. It also protects employees from liability.
It helps each member of the care team to stay within their scope of practice.

10) NAS don't give meds. They don't go outside their scope of practice.
They don't do procedures with sterile technique. They cannot diagnose illnesses or prescribe treatments or medicines. They do not tell the resident or family the medical treatment plan. Only nurses & Dr's do.

11) Observing & reporting help the nurse & care team make changes to help resident. It helps them with the nursing process – Assess, Diagnosis, plan implement & evaluate care for resident.

3 Legal and Ethical Issues

1. Define the terms *law* and *ethics* and list examples of legal and ethical behavior

Ethics and laws guide behavior. **Ethics** are the knowledge of right and wrong. An ethical person has a sense of duty and responsibility toward others. He tries to do what is right. If ethics tell people what they should do, laws tell them what they must do. **Laws** are usually based on ethics. Governments establish laws to help people live peacefully together and to ensure order and safety. When someone breaks the law, he may be punished by having to pay a fine or spend time in prison.

Ethics and laws are extremely important in health care (Fig. 3-1). They protect people receiving care and guide people giving care. Nursing assistants and other healthcare providers should be guided by a code of ethics. They must know the laws that apply to their jobs. Here are guidelines that nursing assistants should follow:

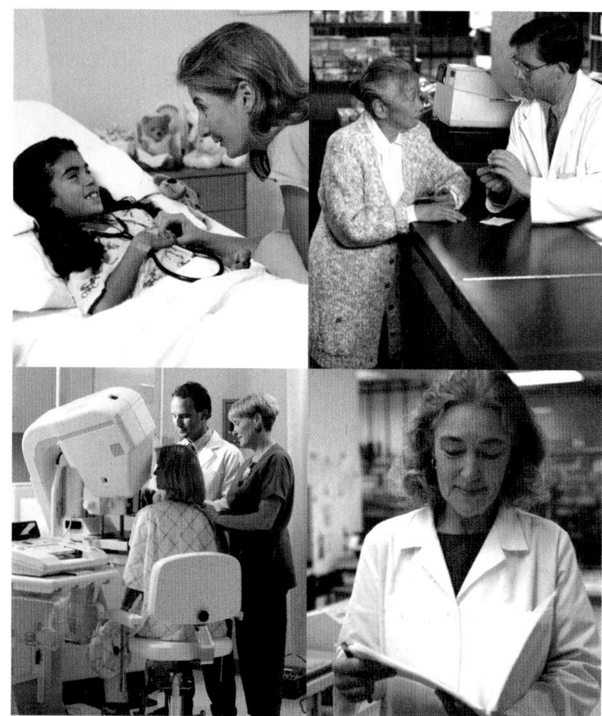

Fig. 3-1. *Behaving ethically and following the law applies to all healthcare providers.*

Guidelines: Legal and Ethical Behavior

- Be honest at all times. Stealing from a resident and lying about care provided are examples of dishonesty. Communicate honestly with all team members.
- Protect residents' privacy. Do not discuss their cases except with other members of the care team. Keeping resident information confidential is one of the Residents' Rights, which are covered later in this chapter. All team members must keep resident information confidential.
- Keep staff information confidential. Do not share information about coworkers at home or anywhere else.

- Report abuse or suspected abuse of residents, and assist residents in reporting abuse if they wish to make a complaint of abuse. This information is covered later in this chapter.
- Follow the care plan and assignments. If you make a mistake, report it promptly. This helps prevent any further problems. Reporting mistakes promotes the safety and well-being of all residents.
- Do not perform any task outside your scope of practice.
- Report all resident observations and incidents to the nurse.
- Document accurately and promptly.
- Follow rules on safety and infection prevention. Chapters 5 and 6 have information about these rules.
- Do not accept gifts or tips.
- Do not get personally or sexually involved with residents or their family members or friends.

Many organizations and companies have created a code of ethics for their members or employees to follow. These vary, but generally they focus on promoting proper conduct and high standards of practice. If a facility has its own code of ethics, all staff members will be given a copy and expected to follow it.

Crimes in Healthcare Settings

Most of the crimes that occur in the community can also occur in healthcare settings. Theft is frequently reported. Physical abuse, including hitting, punching, shoving, rough handling, and many other types of abuse can occur. Violations of Residents' Rights are reported and can be prosecuted as crimes. It is important for nursing assistants to know what to observe and how to report any illegal activity. Being vigilant can help prevent crimes and promote legal and ethical behavior in the workplace.

2. Explain the Omnibus Budget Reconciliation Act (OBRA)

Due to reports of poor care and abuse in long-term care facilities, the U.S. government passed the **Omnibus Budget Reconciliation Act (OBRA)** in 1987. It has been updated several times since. OBRA requires that the Nurse Aide Training and Competency Evaluation Program (NATCEP) set minimum standards for nursing assistant training. Nursing assistants must complete at least 75 hours of training that covers topics like communication, preventing infections, safety and emergency procedures, and how to promote residents' independence and legal rights. Training must also include specific nursing skills, such as how to take vital signs, personal care skills, and observing and reporting changes in residents' conditions. In addition, nursing assistants must know how to respond to mental health and social services needs, rehabilitative needs, and how to care for residents who are cognitively impaired.

OBRA requires that nursing assistants pass a competency evaluation (testing program) before they can be employed. They must attend regular in-service education (a minimum of 12 hours per year) to keep their skills updated.

OBRA also requires that states keep a current list of nursing assistants in a state registry. In addition, OBRA identifies standards that instructors must meet in order to train nursing assistants. OBRA sets guidelines for minimum staff requirements. It specifies the minimum services that long-term care facilities must provide.

The resident assessment requirements are another important part of OBRA. OBRA requires that complete assessments be done on every resident. The assessment forms are the same for every facility. A resident assessment system was developed in 1990 and is revised periodically. It is called the **Minimum Data Set (MDS)** (Fig. 3-2). The MDS is a detailed form with guidelines

Resident ____________ Identifier ____________ Date ____________

MINIMUM DATA SET (MDS) - Version 3.0
RESIDENT ASSESSMENT AND CARE SCREENING
Nursing Home Comprehensive (NC) Item Set

CAA's = ■ QM's = ● PPS = $

Code "-" if information unavailable or unknown

Section A Identification Information

A0050. Type of Record

Enter Code [ ]
1. **Add new record** → Continue to A0100, Facility Provider Numbers
2. **Modify existing record** → Continue to A0100, Facility Provider Numbers
3. **Inactivate existing record** → **Skip to X0150**, Type of Provider

A0100. Facility Provider Numbers

A. **National Provider Identifier (NPI):**

B. **CMS Certification Number (CCN):**

C. **State Provider Number:**

A0200. Type of Provider

Enter Code [ ]
Type of provider
1. **Nursing home (SNF/NF)**
2. **Swing Bed**

A0310. Type of Assessment CAA

Enter Code [ ][ ]
A. **Federal OBRA Reason for Assessment**
- $ 01. **Admission** assessment (required by **day 14**) 11
- $ 02. **Quarterly** review assessment
- $ 03. **Annual** assessment 1,8
- $ 04. **Significant change in status** assessment 1,8
- $ 05. **Significant correction** to **prior comprehensive** assessment 1,8
- $ 06. **Significant correction** to **prior quarterly** assessment
- $ 99. **None of the above**

Enter Code [ ][ ]
B. **PPS Assessment**

<u>**PPS Scheduled Assessments for a Medicare Part A Stay**</u>
- $ 01. **5-day** scheduled assessment
- $ 02. **14-day** scheduled assessment
- $ 03. **30-day** scheduled assessment
- $ 04. **60-day** scheduled assessment
- $ 05. **90-day** scheduled assessment
- $ 06. **Readmission/return** assessment

<u>**PPS Unscheduled Assessments for a Medicare Part A Stay**</u>
- $ 07. **Unscheduled assessment used for PPS** (OMRA, significant or clinical change, or significant correction assessment)

<u>**Not PPS Assessment**</u>
- $ 99. **None of the above**

A0310 continued on next page

QUALITY MEASURES (QM)

SHORT STAY QUALITY MEASURES:
- 76 (#0676) Residents who self report moderate to severe pain
- 78 (#0678) Residents with pressure ulcers that are new or worsened
- 80 (#0680) Residents who were assessed and appropriately given the seasonal Influenza Vaccine
- 80A (#0680A) Residents who received the seasonal Influenza Vaccine
- 80B (#0680B) Residents who were offered and declined the seasonal Influenza Vaccine
- 80C (#0680C) Residents who did not receive, due to medical contraindication, the seasonal Influenza Vaccine
- 82 (#0682) Residents accessed and appropriately given the Pneumococcal Vaccine
- 82A (#0682A) Residents who received the Pneumococcal Vaccine
- 82B (#0682B) Residents who were offered and declined the Pneumococcal Vaccine
- 82C (#0682C) Residents who did not receive, due to medical contraindication, the Pneumococcal Vaccine

LONG STAY QUALITY MEASURES
- 74 (#0674) Residents experiencing one or more falls with major injury
- 77 (#0677) Residents who self-report moderate to severe pain
- 79 (#0679) High-risk residents with pressure ulcers
- 81 (#0681) Residents assessed and appropriately given the seasonal Influenza Vaccine
- 81A (#0681A) Residents who received the seasonal Influenza Vaccine
- 81B (#0681B) Residents who were offered and declined the seasonal Influenza Vaccine
- 81C (0681C) Residents who did not receive, due to medical contraindication, the seasonal Influenza Vaccine
- 83 (#0683) Residents assessed and appropriately given the Pneumococcal Vaccine
- 83A (#0683A) Residents who received the Pneumococcal Vaccine
- 83B (#0683B) Residents who were offered and declined the Pneumococcal Vaccine
- 83C (#0683C) Residents who did not receive, due to medical contraindication, the Pneumococcal Vaccine
- 84 (#0684) Residents with a Urinary Tract Infection
- 85 (#0685) Low Risk residents who lose control of their bowel or bladder
- 86 (#0686) Residents who have/had a catheter inserted and left in their bladder
- 87 (#0687) Residents who were physically restrained
- 88 (#0688) Residents whose need for help with activities of daily living has increased
- 89 (#0689) Residents who lose too much weight
- 90 (#0690) Residents who have depressive symptoms
- 300 (#300) Prevalence of Falls
- 400 (#400) Prevalence of psychoactive medication use, in the absence of psychotic or related conditions
- 500 (#500) Prevalence of anxiety/hypnotic use
- 600 (#600) Prevalence of behavior symptoms affecting others

● Indicates responses that may impact QM items identified by a number in a solid blue oval ○ Indicates responses that may impact covariate for the QM identified by a number in an outline blue oval

CARE AREA ASSESSMENT LEGEND

1 Delirium	5 ADL Function/Rehabilitation Potential	7 Psychosocial Well-Being	11 Falls	15 Dental Care	18 Physical Restraints
2 Cognitive Loss/Dementia	6 Urinary Incontinence & Indwelling Catheter	8 Mood State	12 Nutritional Status	16 Pressure Ulcer	19 Pain
3 Visual Function		9 Behavioral Symptoms	13 Feeding Tubes	17 Psychotropic Drug Use	20 Return to Community Referral
4 Communication		10 Activities	14 Dehydration/Fluid Maintenance		

Fig. 3-2. *A sample MDS form.* (REPRINTED WITH PERMISSION OF THE BRIGGS CORPORATION, 800-247-2343, WWW.BRIGGSCORP.COM)

for assessing residents. It also lists what to do if resident problems are identified. Facilities must complete the MDS for each resident within 14 days of admission and again each year. In addition, the MDS for each resident must be reviewed every three months. A new MDS must be done when there is any significant change in the resident's condition.

OBRA made major changes in the survey process (Chapter 1). The results from surveys are available to the public and posted in the facility.

OBRA identifies important rights for residents in long-term care facilities. The next learning objective has information about these rights.

3. Explain Residents' Rights and discuss why they are important

Residents' Rights relate to how residents must be treated while living in a facility. They provide an ethical code of conduct for healthcare workers. Facilities give residents a list of these rights and review each right with them. Be familiar with these legal rights. Residents' Rights are very detailed and include the following:

Quality of life: Residents have the right to the best care available. Dignity, choice, and independence are important parts of quality of life.

Services and activities to maintain a high level of wellness: Residents must receive the correct care. Facilities must develop a care plan for residents, and their care should keep them as healthy as possible. Residents' health should not decline as a direct result of the facility's care.

The right to be fully informed about rights and services: Residents must be told what services are available and what the fee is for each service. Residents must be given a written copy of their legal rights, along with the facility's rules and regulations. Legal rights must be explained in a language they can understand. Residents must be given contact information for state agencies relating to quality of care, such as ombudsmen. When requested, survey results must be shared with residents. Residents have the right to be notified in advance of any change of room or roommate. They have the right to communicate with someone who speaks their language. They have the right to assistance for any sensory impairment, such as blindness.

The right to participate in their own care: Residents have the right to participate in planning their treatment, care, and discharge. Residents have the right to refuse medication, treatment, care, and restraints. They have the right to be told of changes in their condition. They have the right to review their medical record. Informed consent is a concept that is part of participating in one's own care. A person has the legal and ethical right to direct what happens to his or her body. Doctors also have an ethical duty to involve the person in his or her health care. **Informed consent** is the process by which a person, with the help of a doctor, makes informed decisions about his or her health care.

The right to make independent choices: Residents can make choices about their doctors, care, and treatments. They can make personal decisions, such as what to wear and how to spend their time. They can join in community activities, both inside and outside the care facility. They have a right to participate in a Resident's Council.

A Residents' Council is a group of residents who meet regularly to discuss issues related to the long-term care facility. This council gives residents a voice in facility operations. Topics of discussion may include facility policies, decisions regarding activities, concerns, and problems. The Residents' Council offers residents a chance to provide suggestions on improving the quality of care. Council executives are elected by residents. Family members are invited to attend meetings with or on behalf of residents. Staff may participate in this process when invited by council members.

The right to privacy and confidentiality: Residents have the right to privacy when care is given. Their medical and personal information cannot be shared with anyone but the care team. Residents have the right to private, unrestricted communication with anyone they choose (Fig. 3-3).

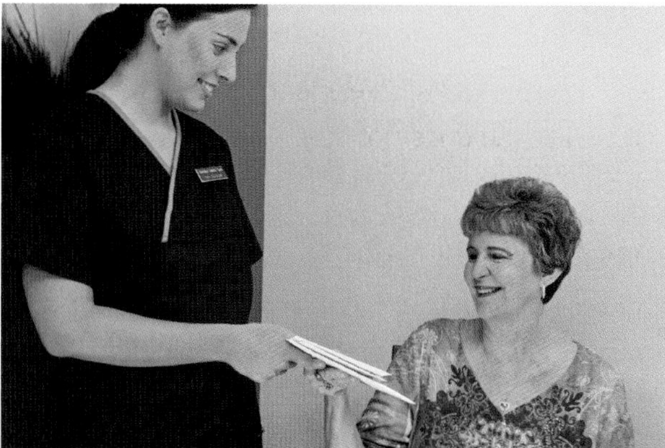

Fig. 3-3. *Residents have the right to private communication with anyone; they have the right to send and receive mail that is unopened.*

The right to dignity, respect, and freedom: Residents must be respected and treated with dignity by caregivers. They cannot be abused, mistreated, or neglected in any way.

The right to security of possessions: Residents' personal possessions must be safe at all times. They cannot be taken or used by anyone without a resident's permission. Residents have the right to manage their own finances or choose someone else to do it for them. Residents can request that the facility handle their money. If the care facility handles residents' financial affairs, residents must have access to their accounts and financial records, and they must receive quarterly statements, among other things.

Rights during transfers and discharges: Location changes must be made safely and with the resident's knowledge and consent. Residents have the right to stay in a facility unless a transfer or discharge is needed. Residents can be moved from the facility due to safety reasons (theirs or others'), if their health has improved, or if payment for care has not been received.

The right to complain: Residents have the right to make complaints and voice grievances without fear of punishment. Facilities must work quickly to try to resolve complaints.

The right to visits: Residents have the right to visits from doctors, family members, friends, clergy members, legal representatives, or any other person.

Rights with social services: The facility must provide residents with access to social services, including counseling, assistance in solving problems with others, and help contacting legal and financial professionals.

The Americans with Disabilities Act (ADA)

The Americans with Disabilities Act (ADA) became a federal law in 1990. It was passed to help people with disabilities gain skills, do jobs they want to do, and take part in desired activities. The ADA prohibits discrimination because of a disability. The law requires that employers, schools, and businesses offer equal opportunities to individuals with disabilities to use the services in society and improve their quality of life.

People with disabilities must be able to get into and around in buildings and use the bathrooms, drinking fountains, and other areas. The law requires new buildings to be accessible and older buildings to be updated when they are renovated.

Americans with disabilities have the right to education, employment, and all the services offered to the public. Schools, colleges, and many employers are not allowed to discriminate and must make reasonable accommodations, or changes, to make their services available. Examples of accommodations are providing a large screen for a computer or allowing a service dog. Providers of health care, social services, transportation, restaurants, hotels, and recreation are also not allowed to discriminate against people with disabilities. They must provide equal opportunities, which may include making some changes to their services.

4. Discuss abuse and neglect and explain how to report abuse and neglect

The healthcare community has become aware of the growing problem of elder abuse and neglect.

Abuse is purposeful mistreatment that causes physical, mental, or emotional pain or injury to someone. **Neglect** is the failure to provide needed care that results in physical, mental, or emotional harm to a person.

In their publication, *15 Questions and Answers About Elder Abuse*, published in 2005, The National Center on Elder Abuse estimated that at least one to two million elders suffer abuse or neglect in a single year. This publication also states that for every reported incident of elder abuse or neglect, as many as 14 go unreported. The National Institute of Justice's *National Elder Mistreatment Study*, released in 2009, estimates that 11 percent of older people living in community settings had experienced some form of abuse or neglect during one year. As the elderly population grows, this problem may become worse.

Elderly people may be abused intentionally or unintentionally, through ignorance, inexperience, or inability to care for them. People who abuse elders may mistreat them physically, psychologically, sexually, verbally, financially, and/or materially. They may deprive them of their rights, or they may neglect them by failing to provide food, clothing, shelter, or medical care. Some older adults may also become self-abusive or neglect their own needs. There are many forms of abuse, including the following:

Physical abuse is any treatment, intentional or unintentional, that causes harm to a person's body. This includes slapping, bruising, cutting, burning, physically restraining, pushing, shoving, or even rough handling.

Psychological abuse is emotional harm caused by threatening, scaring, humiliating, intimidating, isolating, or insulting a person, or treating him or her as a child. It also includes verbal abuse. **Verbal abuse** is the use of spoken or written words, pictures, or gestures that threaten, embarrass, or insult a person.

Sexual abuse is the forcing of a person to perform or participate in sexual acts against his or her will. This includes unwanted touching and exposing oneself to a person. It also includes the sharing of pornographic material.

Financial abuse is the improper or illegal use of a person's money, possessions, property, or other assets.

Assault is a threat to harm a person, resulting in the person feeling fearful that he or she will be harmed. Telling a resident that she will be slapped if she does not stop yelling is an example of assault.

Battery is the intentional touching of a person without his or her consent. An example is an NA hitting or pushing a resident, which is also considered physical abuse. Forcing a resident to eat a meal is another example of battery.

Domestic violence is abuse by spouses, intimate partners, or family members. It can be physical, sexual, or emotional. The victim can be a man or woman of any age or a child.

Workplace violence is abuse of staff by other staff members, residents, or visitors. It can be verbal, physical, or sexual. This includes improper touching and discussion about sexual subjects.

False imprisonment is unlawful restraint that affects a person's freedom of movement. Both the threat of being physically restrained and actually being physically restrained are types of false imprisonment. Not allowing a resident to leave the facility is also considered false imprisonment.

Involuntary seclusion is the separation of a person from others against the person's will. An example is an NA confining a resident to his room.

Sexual harassment is any unwelcome sexual advance or behavior that creates an intimidating, hostile, or offensive working environment. Requests for sexual favors, unwanted touching, and other acts of a sexual nature are examples of sexual harassment.

Substance abuse is the use of legal or illegal drugs, cigarettes, or alcohol in a way that harms oneself or others. Chapter 20 has more information on substance abuse.

Neglect can be divided into two categories: active neglect and passive neglect. **Active neglect** is the purposeful failure to provide needed care, resulting in harm to a person. Examples of active neglect are leaving a bedridden resident alone for a long time or denying the resident food, dentures, or eyeglasses. **Passive neglect** is the unintentional failure to provide needed care, resulting in physical, mental, or emotional harm to a person. The caregiver may not know how to properly care for the resident or may not understand the resident's needs.

Negligence means actions, or the failure to act or provide the proper care for a resident, resulting in unintended injury. An example of negligence is an NA forgetting to lock a resident's wheelchair before transferring her. The resident falls and is injured. **Malpractice** occurs when a person is injured due to professional misconduct through negligence, carelessness, or lack of skill.

Nursing assistants must never abuse residents in any way. They must also try to protect residents from others who abuse them. If a nursing assistant ever sees or suspects that another caregiver, family member, or resident is abusing a resident, she must report this immediately to the nurse in charge. **Reporting abuse is not an option—it is the law.**

If action is not taken, the NA should keep reporting up the chain of command until action is taken. If no appropriate action is taken at the facility level, she can call the state abuse hotline, which is an anonymous call. Nursing assistants must follow the chain of command when reporting abuse. They do not report directly to the authorities. If a life-or-death situation is witnessed, the NA should remove the resident to a safe place if possible. The NA should get help immediately or have someone go for help. The resident should not be left alone.

Observing and Reporting: Abuse and Neglect

The following injuries are considered suspicious and should be reported:

- O/R Poisoning or traumatic injury
- O/R Teeth marks
- O/R Belt buckle or strap marks
- O/R Bruises, contusions, and welts
- O/R Scars
- O/R Fractures, dislocation
- O/R Burns of unusual shape and in unusual locations, cigarette burns
- O/R Scalding burns
- O/R Scratches or puncture wounds
- O/R Scalp tenderness or patches of missing hair
- O/R Swelling in the face, broken teeth, nasal discharge
- O/R Bruises, bleeding, or discharge from the vaginal area

The following signs could indicate abuse:

- O/R Yelling obscenities
- O/R Fear, apprehension, fear of being alone
- O/R Poor self-control
- O/R Constant pain
- O/R Threatening to hurt others
- O/R Withdrawal or apathy (Fig. 3-4)

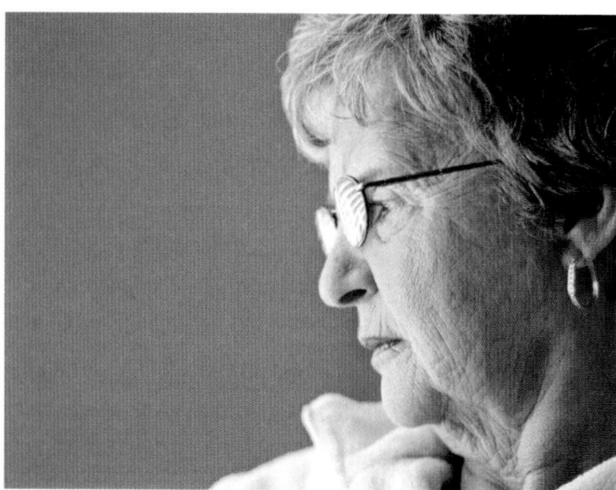

Fig. 3-4. *Withdrawing from others is an important change to report.*

- Alcohol or drug abuse
- Agitation or anxiety, signs of stress
- Low self-esteem
- Mood changes, confusion, disorientation
- Private conversations are not allowed, or the family member/caregiver is present during all conversations
- Reports of questionable care by resident or family

The following signs could indicate neglect:

- Pressure ulcers
- Body not clean
- Body lice
- Unanswered call lights
- Soiled bedding or incontinence briefs not being changed
- Poorly-fitting clothing
- Unmet needs relating to hearing aids, eyeglasses, etc.
- Weight loss, poor appetite
- Uneaten food
- Dehydration
- Fresh water or beverages not being offered regularly

Nursing assistants are in an excellent position to observe and report abuse or neglect. NAs have an ethical and legal responsibility to observe for signs of abuse and to report suspected cases to the charge nurse. Nursing assistants are considered mandated reporters and can be convicted of a crime for not reporting knowledge of abuse or neglect of residents. **Mandated reporters** are people who are legally required to report suspected or observed abuse or neglect because they have regular contact with vulnerable populations, such as the elderly in care facilities.

If abuse is suspected or observed, the NA should give the nurse as much information as possible. If residents want to make a complaint of abuse, NAs must assist them in every way. This includes telling them of the process and their rights. Nursing assistants must never retaliate against (punish) residents complaining of abuse. If an NA sees someone being cruel or abusive to a resident who made a complaint, she must report it. All care team members are responsible for residents' safety and should take this responsibility seriously.

Residents' Rights

Vulnerable Adults

Some states have Vulnerable Adults Acts or Adult Protective Services (APS) laws. These laws are written by each state and are not the same throughout the country. There are states that do not have any such laws. In general, these Vulnerable Adults Acts or Adult Protective Service laws protect individuals who because of a physical or mental impairment need help from other people for their care. The residents of long-term care facilities, assisted living, and other care facilities fit into this category.

It is important that NAs know the laws in their state. However, even if a state does not have a specific law like the ones above, residents of long-term care facilities are covered by the federal laws relating to Residents' Rights, which also forbid abuse and neglect and require reporting if these acts do occur.

Residents' Rights

Elder Justice Act

The Elder Justice Act was passed as part of the Affordable Care Act in March of 2010. It is the first federal law designed specifically to combat elder abuse. Under the Elder Justice Act, the federal Department of Health and Human Services has established an Elder Justice Coordinating Council and an Advisory Board on Elder Abuse, Neglect, and Exploitation. These groups are intended to coordinate educational resources, support, and grant funding to aid efforts to stop elder abuse.

5. List examples of behavior supporting and promoting Residents' Rights

Nursing assistants can help protect Residents' Rights by following these guidelines:

Guidelines: Protecting Residents' Rights

- Never abuse a resident physically, emotionally, verbally, or sexually.
- Watch for and immediately report any signs of abuse or neglect.
- Call the resident by the name he or she prefers.
- Involve residents in planning. Allow residents to make as many choices as possible about when, where, and how care is performed.
- Always explain a procedure to a resident before performing it.
- Do not unnecessarily expose a resident while giving care.
- Respect a resident's refusal of care. Residents have a legal right to refuse treatment and care. However, report the refusal to the nurse immediately.
- Tell the nurse if a resident has questions, concerns, or complaints about treatment or the goals of care.
- Be truthful when documenting care.
- Do not talk or gossip about residents. Keep all resident information confidential.
- Knock and ask for permission before entering a resident's room. (Fig. 3-5).

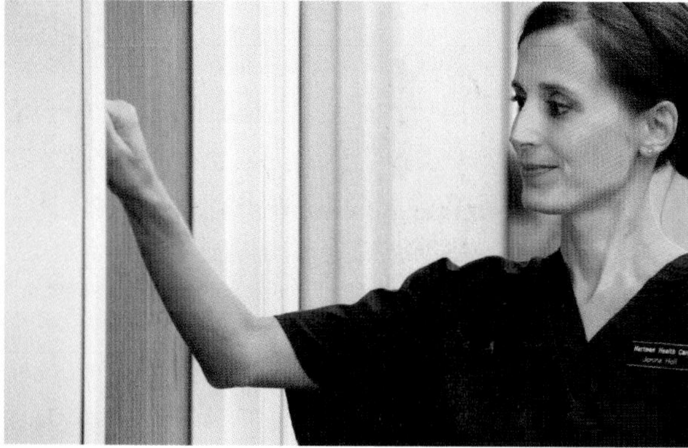

***Fig. 3-5.** Always respect residents' privacy. Knock before entering their rooms, even if the door is open.*

- Do not accept gifts or money from residents.
- Do not open a resident's mail or look through his belongings.
- Respect residents' personal possessions. Handle them gently and carefully. Keep personal items labeled and stored according to facility policy.
- Report observations about a resident's condition or care.
- Help resolve disputes by reporting them to the nurse.

Residents' Rights

Voting

People retain their legal right to vote when they are living in a care facility. They may request and receive absentee ballots. Sometimes they will be driven to the polling places to cast their vote by family, friends, or a facility employee. If an NA is asked to assist a resident with voting, he should ask the resident how she wants the NA to help. For example, a resident may want the NA to read the ballot aloud and/or mark the ballot for her. The NA should understand how to complete the ballot if asked to assist. He can ask the nurse for help if needed. The NA should not discuss his opinions with the resident, even if asked. He should not try to influence the resident in any way or discuss how the resident voted with anyone.

Maintaining Boundaries

In professional relationships, boundaries must be set. Boundaries are the limits to or within relationships. Nursing assistants, like other professionals, are guided by ethics and laws which set limits for their relationships with residents. These boundaries help support a healthy resident-staff relationship. Working closely with residents on a regular basis may make it more difficult to honor the boundaries of professional relationships. Residents may feel that nursing assistants are their friends. If a staff member and resident become personally involved with each other, it becomes more difficult to enforce rules. For instance, an NA may want to give a resident extra help or let her skip the exercise she dislikes. The resident may expect the NA to break the rules because she thinks they are friends. Emotional attachments to residents are unprofessional and may weaken an NA's judgment. NAs should be friendly, warm, and caring with residents, but should remain professional and stay within the limits of set boundaries. Facility rules and the care plan's instructions should be followed. They are in place for everyone's protection. An NA can ask her supervisor for help if a resident asks her to do things she is not allowed to do.

6. Describe what happens when a complaint of abuse is made against a nursing assistant

The Nurse Aide Training Competency Evaluation Program (NATCEP) makes the rules about training and testing nursing assistants. The state programs make sure that federal rules are followed in nursing facilities that receive payment from Medicare or Medicaid. Setting up and running the nursing assistant registry is also a part of this program. This registry keeps track of each nursing assistant working in that state.

If a nursing assistant is accused of abusing a resident, the facility will investigate according to its policies and procedures. If they determine abuse has occurred, a report must be made to the Nurse Aide Training Competency Evaluation Program.

The nursing assistant will be notified of any complaint made about him or her to NATCEP. The nursing assistant can request a hearing. NATCEP will investigate and decide whether or not to mark in the nursing assistant's record that he or she was abusive. Some states have an abuse registry and will place the nursing assistant's name on this list. Other states do not have a separate list but will add the information on the required registry of nursing assistants.

If NATCEP places the nursing assistant on the abuse registry, the nursing assistant will no longer be eligible to work in a certified nursing facility. All nursing facilities must check the registry before hiring a nursing assistant. They will be told of the abuse when they inquire.

7. Explain how disputes may be resolved and identify the ombudsman's role

An **ombudsman** is assigned by law as the legal advocate for residents. The Older Americans Act (OAA) is a federal law that requires all states to have an ombudsman program. An ombudsman visits facilities and listens to residents. He or she decides what action to take if there are problems. Ombudsmen can help resolve conflicts and settle disputes concerning residents' health, safety, welfare, and rights. The ombudsman will gather information and try to resolve the problem on the resident's behalf and may suggest ways to solve the problem. Ombudsmen provide an ongoing presence in long-term care facilities. They monitor care and conditions. Ombudsmen typically do the following tasks:

- Advocate for Residents' Rights and quality care
- Educate consumers and care providers
- Investigate and resolve complaints
- Appear in court and/or legal hearings
- Work with investigators from the police, adult protective services, and health departments to resolve complaints (Fig. 3-6)
- Give information to the public

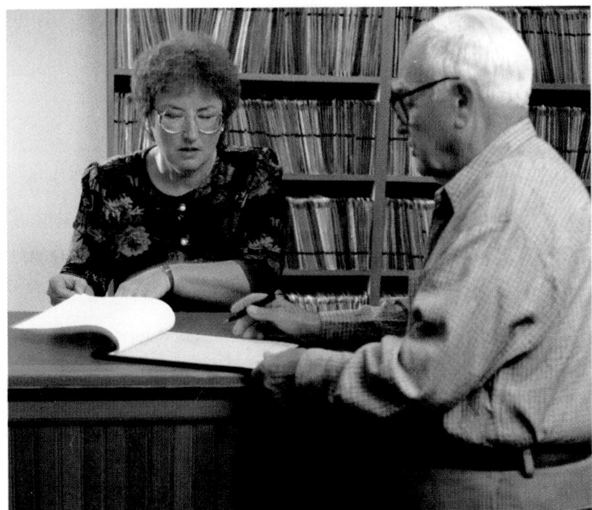

Fig. 3-6. *An ombudsman is a legal advocate for residents. He or she may work with other agencies to resolve complaints.*

Each state has a department that performs surveys and is responsible for enforcing long-term care facility laws and rules. Generally, this is the responsibility of the state's department of health. Complaints may be made directly to the state agency. Each agency has policies and procedures that are used to follow up on complaints.

8. Explain HIPAA and list ways to protect residents' privacy

To respect **confidentiality** means to keep private things private. Nursing assistants will learn confidential (private) information about residents. They may learn about a resident's state of health, finances, and personal relationships. Ethically and legally, they must protect this information. This means that nursing assistants should not share information about residents with anyone other than the care team.

Congress passed the Health Insurance Portability and Accountability Act (HIPAA) in 1996. It has been further defined and revised since then. One reason this law was passed is to help keep health information private and secure. All healthcare organizations must take special steps to protect health information. They and their employees can be fined and/or imprisoned if they do not follow rules to protect patient privacy.

Under HIPAA, a person's health information must be kept private. It is called **protected health information (PHI)**. Examples of PHI include name, address, telephone number, social security number, e-mail address, and medical record. Only people who must have information to provide care or process records should know a person's private health information (Fig. 3-7). They must make sure they protect the information so that it does not become known or used by anyone else. It must be kept confidential.

The Health Information Technology for Economic and Clinical Health (HITECH) Act became law at the end of 2009. It was enacted as a part of the American Recovery and Reinvestment Act of 2009. HITECH was created to expand the protection and security of consumers' electronic health records (EHR). HITECH increases civil and criminal penalties for sharing or accessing PHI and expands the ability to enforce these penalties. HITECH also offers incentives to providers to adopt the use of EHR.

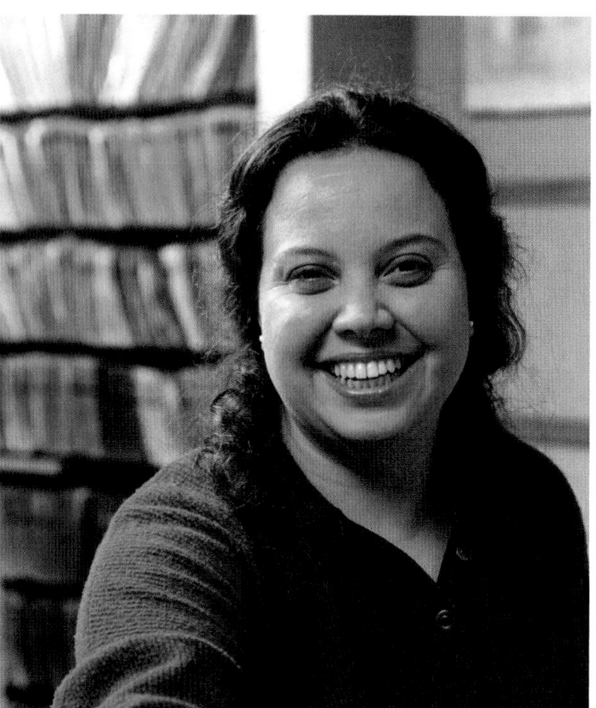

Fig. 3-7. *Special care must be taken to keep medical records confidential. Only people who provide care or process records should have access to this information.*

HIPAA applies to all healthcare providers, including doctors, nurses, nursing assistants, and any other members of the care team. NAs cannot give out any information about a resident to anyone who is not directly involved in the resident's care unless the resident gives official consent or unless the law requires it. For example, if a neighbor asks an NA how a resident is doing, she should reply, "I'm sorry, but I cannot share that information. It's confidential." That is the correct response to anyone who does not have a legal reason to know about the resident. Other ways for nursing assistants to protect privacy include these guidelines:

Guidelines: Protecting Privacy

- G Make sure you are in a private area when you are listening to or reading your messages.
- G Know with whom you are speaking on the phone. If you are not sure, get a name and number to call back after you find out it is all right to do so.

- Do not talk about residents in public places (Fig. 3-8). Public areas include elevators, grocery stores, lounges, waiting rooms, parking garages, schools, restaurants, etc.

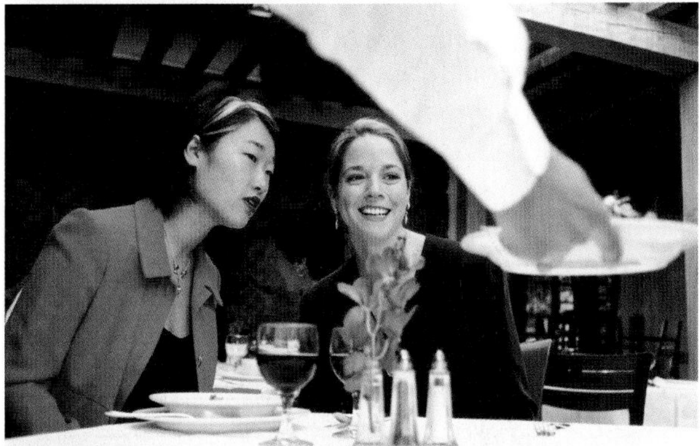

Fig. 3-8. *Do not discuss any information about residents in public places.*

- Use confidential rooms when reporting to other care team members.
- If you see a resident's family member or a former resident in public, be careful with your greeting. He or she may not want others to know about the family member or that he or she has been a resident.
- Do not bring family or friends to the facility to meet residents.
- Make sure nobody can see health or personal information on your computer screen while you are working. Log out and/or exit the web browser when you are finished with computer work.
- Do not give confidential information in e-mails; you do not know who has access to your messages.
- Do not share resident information or photos on social networking sites, such as Facebook or Twitter.
- Make sure fax numbers are correct before faxing healthcare information. Use a cover sheet with a confidentiality statement.
- Do not leave papers or documents where others may see them.
- Store, file, or shred documents according to your facility's policy. If you find documents with a resident's information, give them to the nurse.

All healthcare workers must follow HIPAA regulations no matter where they are or what they are doing. There are serious penalties for violating these regulations. Penalties differ depending upon the violation and include the following:

- Fines ranging from $100 to $250,000
- Prison sentences of up to ten years

Maintaining confidentiality is a legal and ethical obligation. It is part of respecting residents and their rights. Discussing a resident's care or personal affairs with anyone other than members of the care team violates the law.

9. Explain the Patient Self-Determination Act (PSDA) and discuss advance directives

The Patient Self-Determination Act (PSDA) is a federal law that was passed in 1990 as an amendment to OBRA. The PSDA requires all healthcare agencies that receive Medicare and Medicaid funds to provide information to adults about their rights related to advance directives during admission or enrollment. **Advance directives** are legal documents that allow people to choose what medical care they wish to have if they are unable to make those decisions themselves. Advance directives can also name someone to make medical decisions for a person if that person becomes ill or disabled. Living wills and durable powers of attorney for health care are examples of advance directives.

A **living will** outlines the medical care a person wants, or does not want, in case he or she becomes unable to make those decisions. It is called a *living will* because it takes effect while the person is still living. It may also be called a *directive to physicians, health care declaration,* or *medical directive*. A living will is not the same thing as a will. A will is a legal declaration of how a person wishes his or her possessions to be disposed of after death.

A **durable power of attorney for health care** (sometimes called a *health care proxy*) is a signed, dated, and witnessed legal document that appoints someone to make medical decisions for a person in the event he or she becomes unable to do so. This can include instructions about medical treatment that the person does not want.

A **do-not-resuscitate (DNR)** order is another tool that helps medical providers honor wishes about care. A DNR order instructs medical professionals not to perform cardiopulmonary resuscitation (CPR). CPR refers to medical procedures to restart a person's heart and breathing. A DNR order means that medical personnel will not attempt emergency CPR if breathing or the heartbeat stops.

These different types of advance directives can be used together, or a person may only use one type or none at all. Advance directives can be changed or canceled at any time, either in writing or verbally, or both.

According to the Patient Self-Determination Act, rights relating to advance directives that must be given upon admission include the following:

- The right to participate in and direct healthcare decisions
- The right to accept or refuse treatment
- The right to prepare an advance directive
- Information on the facility's policies that govern these rights

The act prohibits discriminating against a patient who does not have an advance directive. The PSDA requires documentation of patient information and ongoing community education on advance directives.

Advance Directives

Laws related to advance directives vary from state to state. Here are a few resources for locating the proper forms for a particular state:

- The National Hospice and Palliative Care Organization (NHPCO) is a nonprofit organization that represents hospice and palliative care programs in the United States. NHPCO is involved with improving care for people who are dying and their loved ones. For more information, a person can visit caringinfo.org or call 800-658-8898.
- The U.S. Living Will Registry is a privately held organization that electronically stores advance directives, organ donor information, and emergency contact information and makes them available to healthcare providers across the country 24 hours a day. For more information, a person can visit uslivingwillregistry.com or call 800-LIV-WILL (800-548-9455).

Chapter Review

1. What is the difference between ethics and laws?
2. List eight examples of legal and ethical behavior for a nursing assistant.
3. What is the minimum number of hours of training that nursing assistants must complete as required by OBRA?
4. How soon must a Minimum Data Set (MDS) be completed on new residents after admission?
5. What is the purpose of Residents' Rights?
6. If a nursing assistant sees abuse or suspects that a resident is being abused, what is her responsibility?
7. List five possible signs of abuse that should be reported by the nursing assistant. List five possible signs of neglect that should be reported by the nursing assistant.
8. If a resident wants to make a complaint of abuse, what is the nursing assistant's responsibility?

9. Pick three of the examples of behavior promoting Residents' Rights in Learning Objective 5. Describe how each example supports or promotes specific Residents' Rights.

Report abuse quickly, Explain a procedure before doing it so resident is not frightened, Call them by the name they prefer showing respect to them, Do not expose the resident (modesty) Don't gossip or talk about residents

10. What happens if a nursing assistant is accused of abusing a resident? The facility will investigate according to it's rules & policies. → If she is placed on a registry of abuse, she will no longer be able to work as a CNA

11. What is the role of an ombudsman? He works as a legal advocate for residents,

12. What is one important reason that HIPAA was passed? It was passed to keep health information private & secure,

13. List five examples of a person's protected health information (PHI). Make sure you are in a private area when you read or listen to someones Health history. Make sure you know who is asking information on the phone. Don't talk about patients in public places, Use confidential rooms when reporting to other health care team members, Do not leave paper documents where others can see them, Store, file or shred documents according to your company's policies.

14. To whom is a nursing assistant allowed to give information about a resident? Only those who are directly involved in their care (team)

15. To what members of the healthcare team is HIPAA applicable? All the entire care team — nurses, CNA's, doc, therapists etc.

16. Define *advance directives* and briefly describe two examples. are legal documents that allow people to choose what medical care they wish to have if they are not able to make that choice at the time.

Examples:
DNR = Do not resuscitate. Don't do CPR on them if needed

Health care Proxy is a signed, dated & legal document that appoints someone to make medical decision for a person when she can't make them.

17. List three rights relating to advance directives that the PSDA requires be given to a resident at the time of admission.

Patient Self-Determination Act
1) The right to participate in and direct health care decisions
2) The right to accept or refuse treatment
3) The right to prepare an advance directive
4) Policy the facility has in place about the 1st 3 rights.

7) Abuse: Teeth Marks, Bruises or welts, Dislocation or fractures, scrapes or puncture wounds, missing hair and scalp tenderness, swelling and or broken teeth etc.
Neglect: Fear of being alone. A threat to hurt others, withdrawl or apathy, Anxiety or signs of stress, pressure ulcers, Weight loss & poor appetite, missing from the person (eyeglasses, hearing aids etc.) Uncombed hair & poorly fitting clothes, Lying in poop long, unclean body odors etc.

4 Communication and Cultural Diversity

1. Define the term *communication*

Communication is the process of exchanging information with others. It is a process of sending and receiving messages. People communicate by using signs and symbols, such as words, drawings, and pictures. They also communicate through their behavior.

The simplest form of communication is a three-step process that takes place between two people (Fig. 4-1). In the first step, the sender (the person who communicates first) sends a message. In the second step, the receiver receives the message. Receiver and sender constantly switch roles as they communicate. The third step involves providing feedback. The receiver repeats the message or responds to it in some way. This lets the sender know that the message was received and understood. Feedback is especially important when working with the elderly. Nursing assistants must take time to make sure residents understand messages.

All three steps must occur before the communication process is complete. During a conversation, this process is repeated over and over.

Effective communication is a critical part of a nursing assistant's job. Nursing assistants must communicate with supervisors, the care team, residents, and family members. A resident's health depends on how well NAs communicate observations and concerns to the nurse. They must also be able to communicate clearly and respectfully in stressful or confusing situations.

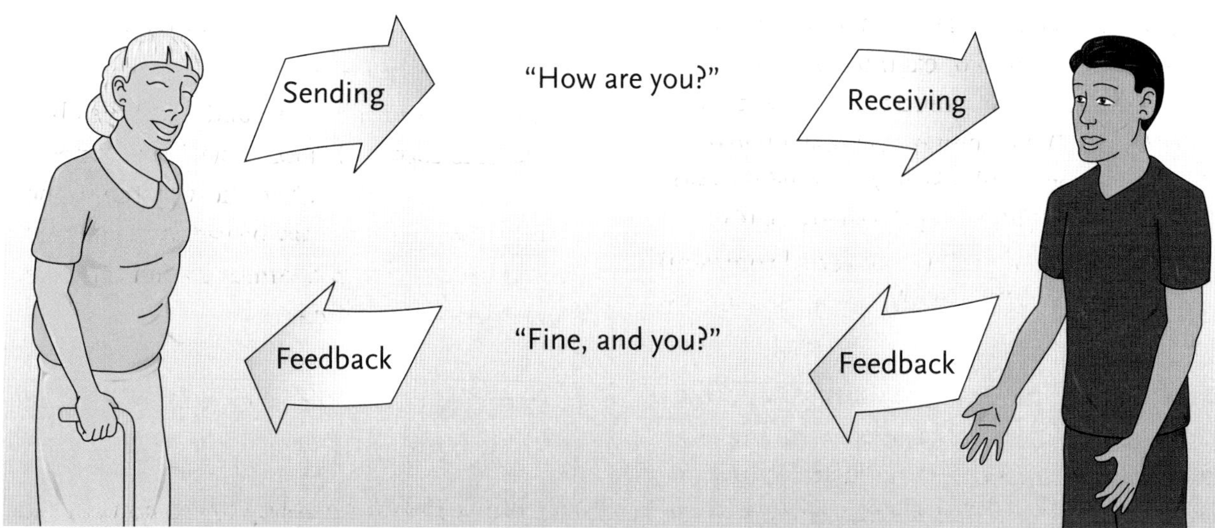

Fig. 4-1. The communication process consists of sending a message, receiving a message, and providing feedback.

2. Explain verbal and nonverbal communication

Communication is either verbal or nonverbal. **Verbal communication** involves the use of words, spoken or written. Oral reports are an example of verbal communication. When communicating verbally, it is important to use words that have the same meaning to both the sender and the receiver. Misunderstandings may occur if each person interprets the same words differently. For example, if a nursing assistant asks a resident to "turn on the light" when she needs help, the resident may not understand that the NA meant for her to push the call button.

Nonverbal communication is communicating without using words. An example of nonverbal communication is a person shrugging his shoulders. Nonverbal communication also includes how a person says something. For example, an NA says cheerfully, "I'll be right there, Mrs. Gonzales." This communicates that the NA is ready and willing to help. But saying the same phrase in a different tone or emphasizing different words can communicate frustration and annoyance: *"I'll be right there,* Mrs. Gonzales!"

Body language is another form of nonverbal communication. Body movements, facial expressions, and posture can express different attitudes or emotions. Just as with speaking, body language sends messages. Other people receive and interpret them. For example, slouching in a chair and sitting erect send two different messages (Fig. 4-2). Slouching says that a person is bored, tired, or hostile. Sitting up straight says that the person is interested and respectful. Other examples of positive nonverbal communication include smiling, nodding one's head, and looking at the person who is speaking.

Sometimes people send one message verbally and a very different message nonverbally. Nonverbal communication often illustrates how someone is feeling. This message may be quite different from what he or she is saying. For example, a resident who tells an NA, "I'm feeling fine today," but does not want to get out of bed and winces in pain, is sending two very different messages. In this case, the NA should communicate to the nurse her observation that the resident is staying in bed and appears to be wincing in pain, despite what the resident says. Paying attention to nonverbal communication helps nursing assistants give better care.

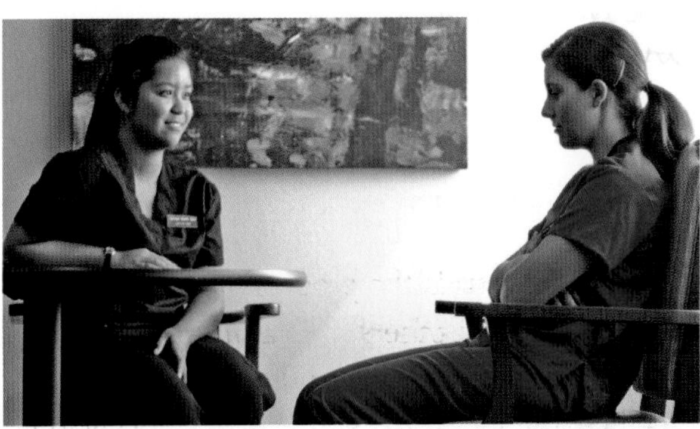

Fig. 4-2. *Body language sends messages just as words do. Which of these people seems more interested in their conversation—the person on the right who is looking down with her arms crossed or the person on the left who is sitting up straight and smiling?*

Nursing assistants must also be aware of their own verbal and nonverbal messages. If an NA says, "It's nice to see you today, Mr. Lee," but does not smile or look him in the eye, Mr. Lee may feel that the NA is not happy to see him.

When communication is confusing, the NA should try to clarify it by asking for an explanation. The NA can say, "Mrs. Jones, you've just told me something that I don't understand. Would you explain it to me?" Or the NA can state what she has observed and ask if the observation is correct. For example, "Mrs. Jones, I see that you're smiling, but I hear by the sound of your voice that you may be sad. Are you sad?" Taking time to clarify communication can help avoid misunderstandings.

3. Describe ways different cultures communicate

The term **cultural diversity** has to do with the different groups of people with varied backgrounds and experiences living together in the world. Positive responses to cultural diversity include acceptance and knowledge, not **bias**, or prejudice. A **culture** is a system of learned behaviors, practiced by a group of people, that is considered to be the tradition of that group and is passed on from one generation to the next. Each culture may have different knowledge, behaviors, beliefs, values, attitudes, religions, and customs.

Nonverbal communication may depend on personality or cultural background. Some people are more animated when they speak. They use a lot of gestures and facial expressions. Other people speak quietly or calmly, regardless of their moods. Depending on their cultural background, people may make motions with their hands when they talk. They may stand close to the person with whom they are speaking or touch the other person. People from other cultural groups stand further apart when talking. When one person moves closer, the other person may view it as a threat.

The use of touch and eye contact also varies with cultural background and personality (Fig. 4-3). For some people, touching is welcome. It expresses caring and warmth. For others, it seems threatening or harassing. In the United States, it is common to talk about "looking someone straight in the eye" or speaking "eye to eye." Eye contact is often viewed as a sign of honesty. However, in some cultures, looking someone in the eye may seem overly bold or disrespectful.

It is important for nursing assistants to be sensitive to residents' needs. Learning each resident's behavior and preferences can be a challenge. However, it is an important part of communication. It is especially vital in a multicultural society (a society made up of many cultures), such as the United States. NAs should be aware of all the messages they send and receive. Listening and observing carefully help nursing assistants better understand residents' needs and feelings.

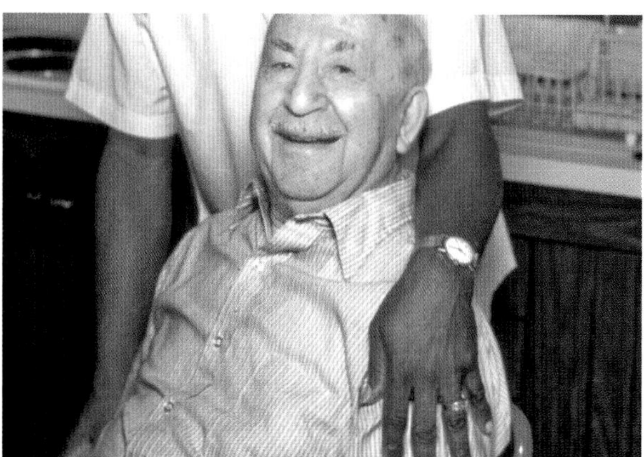

Fig. 4-3. *How a person perceives touch may depend on his cultural background.*

Residents' Rights

Culturally-Sensitive Care

Nursing assistants should focus on compassionate, respectful, and culturally-sensitive care. They should treat residents as residents wish to be treated, not as the NAs would want to be treated. Culture, age, family, background, and customs shape each person's way of thinking. What a nursing assistant wants or needs from others is probably different from what a resident wants or needs. It is important for NAs to ask questions to find out what is appropriate and to always respect residents' choices, beliefs, and behaviors.

4. Identify barriers to communication

Communication can be blocked or disrupted in many ways (Fig. 4-4). Following are some communication barriers and ways for nursing assistants to avoid them:

Resident does not hear NA, does not hear correctly, or does not understand. The NA should stand directly facing the resident. He should speak slowly and clearly. He should not shout, whisper, or mumble. The NA should speak in a low voice, using a pleasant, professional tone. If the resident wears a hearing aid, he should check to ensure that it is on and is working properly.

Resident is difficult to understand. The NA should be patient and take time to listen. He can ask the resident to repeat or explain the message, and then state the message in his own words to make sure he has understood.

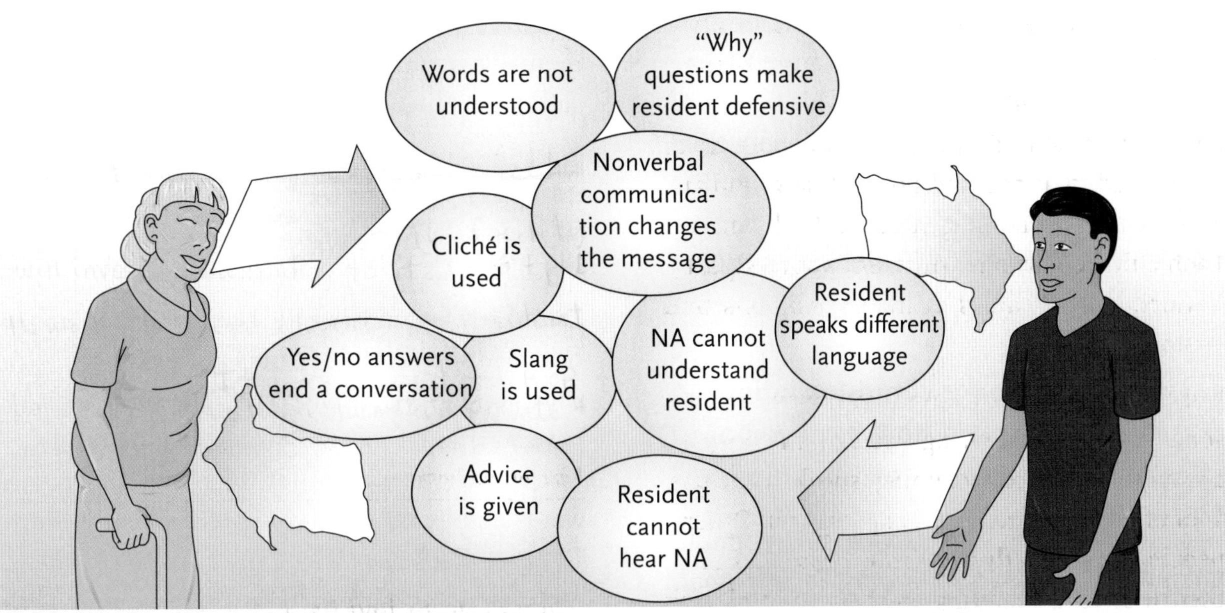

Fig. 4-4. *Barriers to communication.*

NA, resident, or others use words that are not understood. An NA should not use medical terminology with residents or their families. He should speak in simple, everyday words and ask what a word means if he is not sure.

NA uses slang or profanity. The NA should avoid using slang words and expressions. They are unprofessional and may not be understood. He should not use profanity, even if the resident does.

NA uses clichés. Clichés are phrases that are used over and over again and do not really mean anything. For example, "Everything will be fine" is a cliché. Instead of using a cliché, the NA should listen to what a resident is really saying and respond with a meaningful message. For example, if a resident is afraid of having a bath, the NA can say, "I understand that it seems scary to you. What can I do to make you feel more at ease?" instead of saying, "Oh, it'll be over before you know it."

NA responds with "Why?" The NA should avoid asking "Why?" when a resident makes a statement. "Why" questions make people feel defensive. For example, a resident may say she does not want to go for a walk today. If the NA asks, "Why not?" he may receive an angry response. Instead, he can ask, "Are you too tired to take a walk? Is there something else you want to do?" The resident may then be willing to discuss the issue.

NA gives advice. The NA should not offer his opinion or give advice. Giving medical advice is not within an NA's scope of practice. It could be dangerous.

NA asks questions that only require yes/no answers. The NA should ask open-ended questions that need more than a "yes" or "no" answer. Yes and no answers end conversation. For example, if an NA wants to know what a resident likes to eat, he should not ask, "Do you like vegetables?" Instead, he should ask, "Which vegetables do you like best?"

Resident speaks a different language. If a resident speaks a different language than the NA does, the NA should speak slowly and clearly. He should keep his messages short and simple. He should be alert for words the resident understands and also be alert for signs that the resident is only pretending to understand. He may need to use pictures or gestures to communicate. The NA can ask the resident's family, friends, or other staff members who speak the resident's language for help. He should be patient and calm.

NA or resident uses nonverbal communication. Nonverbal communication can change a message. The NA should be aware of his body language and gestures. He can look for nonverbal messages from residents and clarify them. For example, "Mr. Feldman, you say you're feeling fine but you seem to be in pain. Is that true? What can I do to help?"

5. List ways to make communication accurate and explain how to develop effective interpersonal relationships

In addition to avoiding the barriers to communication listed above, nursing assistants should use the following techniques to help send and receive clear, complete messages:

Be a good listener. The NA should allow the resident to express her ideas completely. He should concentrate on what she is saying and not interrupt. The NA should not finish the resident's sentences even if he knows what she is going to say. When she is finished, the NA should restate the message in his own words to make sure he has understood.

Provide feedback. Active listening means focusing on the person sending the message and giving feedback. Feedback might be an acknowledgment, a question, or repeating the sender's message. The NA should offer general but leading responses, such as, "Oh?" or, "Go on," or, "Hmm." By doing this, he is actively listening, providing feedback, and encouraging the sender to expand the message.

Bring up topics of concern. If the NA knows of a topic that might concern a resident, he can raise the issue in a general, non-threatening way. This lets the resident decide whether or not to discuss it. For example, if the NA observes that a resident is unusually quiet, he could say, "Mrs. Jones, you seem so quiet today." Or he may notice a certain emotion. He might say, "Mrs. Jones, you seemed upset earlier. Would you like to talk about it?"

Let some pauses happen. Using silence for a few moments at a time encourages the resident to gather her thoughts and compose messages.

Tune in to other cultures. The NA should learn the words and expressions of a resident's culture. This shows that he respects the culture and is interested in what the resident has to say. It will help the NA to understand the resident more fully. He should be careful about using new words and terms, though, because some may have a different meaning than what he thinks. The important thing is for the NA to understand words and expressions when others use them. The NA should not be judgmental; he should accept people who are different from him.

Accept a resident's religion or lack of religion. Religious differences also affect communication. Religion can be very important in people's lives, particularly when they are ill or dying. The NA should respect residents' religious beliefs, practices, or lack of beliefs, especially if they are different from his own. He should not question residents' beliefs or discuss his beliefs with residents.

Understand the importance of touch. Softly patting residents' hands or shoulders or holding their hands may communicate caring. Some people's backgrounds may make them less comfortable being touched. The NA should ask permission before touching residents. He should be sensitive to their feelings. NAs must touch residents in order to do their jobs. However, they should recognize that some residents feel more comfortable when there is little physical contact. The NA should learn about his residents and adjust care to their needs.

Ask for more. When residents report symptoms, events, or feelings, the NA should have them repeat what they have said. He should ask them for more information.

Make sure communication aids are clean and in good working order (Fig. 4-5). These include hearing aids, eyeglasses, dentures, and wrist or hand braces. The NA should tell the nurse if these items do not work properly or are dirty or damaged.

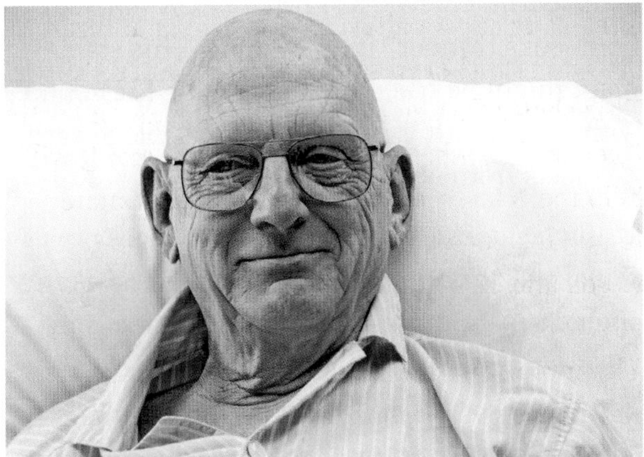

Fig. 4-5. Eyeglasses must fit well, be clean, and be in good condition. A nurse should be informed if communication aids are not clean or not working properly.

Proper Communication

When communicating with residents, the NA should remember to do the following:

- Always greet the resident by his or her preferred name.
- Identify herself.
- Focus on the topic to be discussed.
- Face the resident while speaking and avoid talking into space.
- Talk with the resident while giving care. The NA should not have personal conversations with other staff members while providing care.
- Listen and respond when the resident speaks.
- Praise the resident and smile often.
- Encourage the resident to interact with her and others.
- Be courteous.
- Tell the resident when she is leaving the room.

Residents' Rights

Names

Nursing assistants should call residents by the name the resident prefers. NAs should not refer to residents by their first names unless a resident has asked them to do so. Terms such as *sweetie, honey, dearie,* or *Gramps* are disrespectful and should not be used.

It important for nursing assistants to develop good relationships with residents, their family members, and the care team. They should not try to become friends with residents. However, they should try to develop warm professional relationships with them based on trust. In addition to the strategies already discussed, nursing assistants should use these suggestions to help develop good relationships:

Avoid changing the subject when a resident is discussing something. This is true even if the subject makes the NA feel uncomfortable or helpless. For example, a resident might say, "I'm having so much pain today." The NA should not try to avoid the topic by asking the resident if he wants to watch television. This makes the resident feel that the NA is not interested in him or what he is talking about.

Do not ignore a resident's request. Ignoring a request is considered negligent behavior. The NA should honor the request if he can. Otherwise, he can explain why the request cannot be fulfilled. These requests should always be reported to the nurse.

Do not talk down to an elderly or disabled person. An NA should talk to residents and their families as he would talk to any person. He can make adjustments if someone is visually or hearing impaired. Guidelines for visually- and hearing-impaired residents are found later in the chapter.

Sit or stand near the resident who has started the conversation. Sitting or standing near a person shows that the NA finds what he or she is saying important and worth listening to (Fig. 4-6).

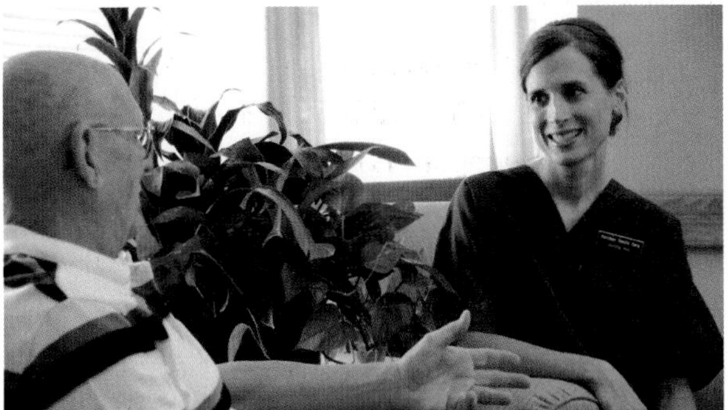

Fig. 4-6. Nursing assistants should sit near residents and look at them while they talk to show that they are interested in the conversation.

Lean forward in the chair when a resident is speaking. Leaning forward communicates interest. The NA should pay attention to his nonverbal communication. If he folds his arms in front of his body, he sends the negative message that he wishes to distance himself from the speaker.

Talk directly to the resident. The NA should not talk to other staff members while helping residents. He should not gossip about other staff members or residents.

Approach the person. Even if the NA is in another area of the room, he should approach the person who is speaking. This tells the person he is interested in what he or she has to say.

Be empathetic. The NA should try to understand and identify with what the resident is going through. This is called empathy. He can ask himself how he would feel if he were confined to bed or needed help to go to the bathroom. The NA should not tell residents he knows how they feel, because he does not know exactly how they feel. He can say things like, "I can imagine this must be difficult for you."

Have time for residents' families and friends, too. The NA should communicate with them. He should not discuss a resident's care with friends or family members, but he can listen if they want to talk. The NA should be respectful and pleasant and give privacy for visits. He should not interfere with private family business. Families are great sources of information for residents' personal preferences, history, diet, habits, and routines. The NA should ask them questions. If he sees any abusive behavior toward a resident during a visit, he should report it immediately to the nurse.

6. Explain the difference between facts and opinions

A fact is something that is definitely true. "Mr. Ford has lost four pounds this month," for example, is a fact. This fact has evidence to back it up: weighing Mr. Ford and comparing his current weight to his weight last month. An opinion is something someone believes to be true, but is not definitely true or cannot be proven. "Mr. Ford looks thinner" is an opinion. This statement might be true, but it cannot be backed up with evidence. It is important to be able to separate facts from opinions.

Using facts instead of opinions is a more professional way to communicate. Nursing assistants should separate facts and opinions when communicating with members of the care team. For example, "Mr. Morgan is acting like he had a stroke" is an opinion and could very well be wrong. Instead, the facts should be reported: "Mr. Morgan has lost strength on his right side, and his speech is slurred." When reporting opinions, nursing assistants should introduce them with, "I think...." Then it is clear that they are offering their opinion and not a fact they observed.

7. Explain objective and subjective information and describe how to observe and report accurately

When making any report, the right information must be collected before documenting it. Facts, not opinions, are most useful to the nurse and the care team. Two kinds of factual information are needed in reporting. **Objective information** is based on what a person sees, hears, touches, or smells. Objective information is collected by using the senses. It is also called *signs*. **Subjective information** is something a person cannot or did not observe, but is based on something the resident reported that may or may not be true. It is also called *symptoms*.

An example of objective information is, "Mr. McClain is holding his head and rubbing his temples." A subjective report of the same situation might be, "Mr. McClain says he has a headache." The nurse needs factual information in order to make decisions about care and treatment. Both objective and subjective reports are valuable.

In any report, what is observed (signs) and what the resident reports (symptoms) need to be clearly noted. For example, "Ms. Scott reports pain in left shoulder." Nursing assistants are not expected to make diagnoses based on signs and symptoms they observe. Their observations, however, can alert staff to possible problems. In order to report accurately, NAs must observe residents accurately. To observe accurately, they need to use as many senses as possible to gather information (Fig. 4-7). Some examples follow:

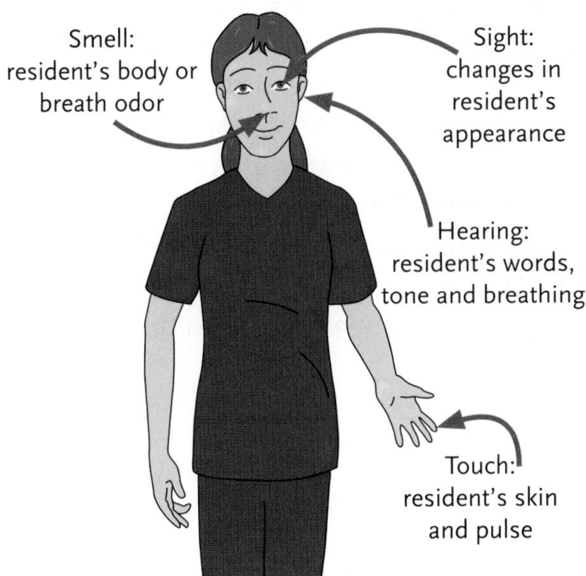

Fig. 4-7. Reporting observations means using more than one sense.

Sight. The NA should look for changes in the resident's appearance. These include rashes, redness, paleness, swelling, discharge, weakness, sunken eyes, and posture or gait (walking) changes.

Hearing. The NA should listen to what the resident says about his condition, family, or needs. Is the resident speaking clearly and making sense? Does he show emotions, such as anger, frustration, or sadness? Is his breathing normal? Does he wheeze, gasp, or cough? Is the area calm and quiet enough for him to rest as needed?

Touch. Does the resident's skin feel hot or cool, moist or dry? Is the pulse rate normal?

Smell. Are there any odors coming from the resident's body? Odors could suggest poor bathing, infections, or incontinence. **Incontinence** is the inability to control the bladder or bowels. Breath odor could suggest use of alcohol or tobacco, indigestion, or poor oral care.

Using the senses helps to make a more complete report of a resident's situation.

8. Explain how to communicate with other team members

Nursing assistants will communicate regularly with care team members, residents, and residents' families and friends. NAs should communicate freely with the charge nurse regarding residents. They should keep the nurse informed of all important issues during their shift and share information with other staff members as needed. A nursing assistant may need to share a resident's personal information with another nursing assistant to help her give care to a resident. However, the activities staff may have no need to know that same information. NAs should refer any doctor's questions to the nurse.

It is important to always respect residents' privacy. When giving information to other members of the care team, NAs should be sure that other residents or staff cannot overhear. They should be cautious when communicating with residents and their families and friends. NAs should not share new information about residents' conditions or new diagnoses. That is the nurse's or doctor's responsibility. When in doubt, NAs can ask the nurse what they can say. A resident may not want information shared with family members and that is his legal right.

The chain of command should be used to voice any complaints that NAs may have. The charge nurse should be approached first. If a complaint is not resolved, NAs can continue reporting up the chain of command. If an NA feels that her charge nurse has abused a resident, she must communicate this to the nurse's supervisor.

9. Describe basic medical terminology and abbreviations

Nursing assistants will learn medical terms for specific conditions throughout their training. For example, the medical term for a runny nose is nasal discharge; skin that is blue or gray is called **cyanotic**. Medical terms are often made up of roots, prefixes, and suffixes. A root is a part of a word that contains its basic meaning or definition. The prefix is the word part that precedes the root to help form a new word. The suffix is the word part added to the end of a root that helps form a new word. Prefixes and suffixes are called *affixes* because they are attached, or affixed, to a root. Here are some examples:

- The root *derm* or *derma* means skin. The suffix *itis* means inflammation. Dermatitis is an inflammation of the skin.
- The prefix *brady* means slow. The root *cardia* means heart. Bradycardia is slow heartbeat or pulse.
- The suffix *pathy* means disease. The root *neuro* means of the nerve or nervous system. Neuropathy is a nerve disease or disease of the nervous system.

When speaking with residents and their families, nursing assistants should use simple, non-medical terms. Medical terms may not be understood. But when speaking with the care team, using medical terminology will help nursing assistants give more complete information.

Abbreviations are another way to make communication more efficient between care team members. For example, the abbreviation *prn* means *as necessary*. *BP* means *blood pressure*. Nursing assistants should learn the standard medical abbreviations their facility uses. They can use them to report information briefly and accurately. NAs may need to know these abbreviations to read assignments or care plans. A brief list of abbreviations follows, and more are located at the end of this textbook. There may be other terms in use at a facility, so it is important for NAs to follow facility policy.

Common Abbreviations	
$\bar{a}$	before
abd	abdomen
ac, AC	before meals
ad lib	as desired
ADLs	activities of daily living
amb	ambulate, ambulatory
AP	apical pulse
b.i.d., bid	two times a day
BM	bowel movement
BP, B/P	blood pressure
$\bar{c}$	with
C	Celsius degree
c/o	complains of
CHF	congestive heart failure
CPR	cardiopulmonary resuscitation
DNR	do not resuscitate
dx, DX	diagnosis
F	Fahrenheit degree
FBS	fasting blood sugar
ft	foot
FWB	full weight-bearing
GI	gastrointestinal
H_2O	water
h, hr, hr.	hour
hs, HS	hours of sleep
inc	incontinent
I&O	intake and output
NKDA	no known drug allergies
NPO	nothing by mouth

NWB	non-weight-bearing (absolutely no weight on leg)
O_2	oxygen
OOB	out of bed
$\bar{p}$	after
pc, p.c.	after meals
PO	by mouth
prn, PRN	as necessary
PWB	partial-weight-bearing
$\bar{q}$	every
ROM	range of motion
$\bar{s}$	without
SOB	shortness of breath
stat, STAT	at once, immediately
t.i.d., tid	three times a day
TPR	temperature, pulse, respiration
v.s., VS	vital signs
w/c, W/C	wheelchair

10. Explain how to give and receive an accurate report of a resident's status

Nursing assistants must make brief and accurate oral and written reports to residents and staff. Careful observations are used to make these reports and are very important to the health and well-being of all residents. Signs and symptoms that should be reported will be discussed throughout this textbook. Some observations will need to be reported immediately to the nurse. Deciding what to report immediately involves critical thinking. Anything that endangers residents should be reported immediately, including the following:

- Falls
- Chest pain
- Severe headache
- Trouble breathing
- Abnormal pulse, respiration, or blood pressure
- Change in mental status
- Sudden weakness or loss of mobility
- High fever
- Loss of consciousness
- Change in level of consciousness
- Bleeding
- Change in resident's condition
- Bruises, abrasions, or other signs of possible abuse (Chapter 3)

Nursing assistants use oral reports to discuss their experiences with residents and observations of residents' conditions. Facts, not opinions, should be used for oral reports. It is a good idea for NAs to write notes so that important details are not forgotten. Following an oral report, NAs must document when, why, about what, and to whom an oral report was given.

Sometimes the nurse or another member of the care team will give an NA a brief oral report on one of her residents. The NA should listen carefully and take notes (Fig. 4-8). She should ask about anything she does not understand. At the end of the report, the NA can restate what she has been told to make sure she understands.

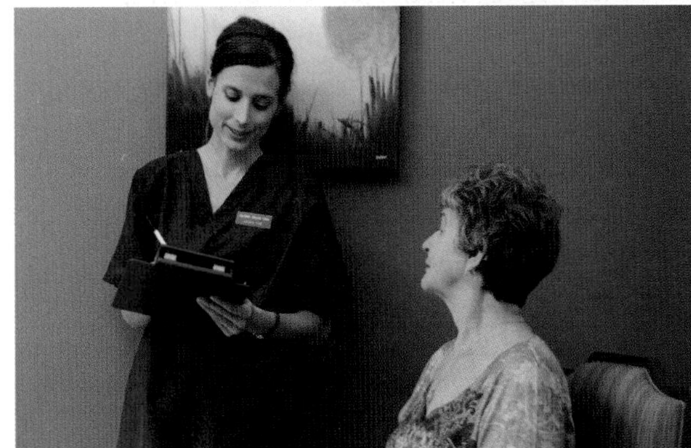

***Fig. 4-8.** Taking notes helps nursing assistants remember facts and report accurately.*

When making reports about residents, NAs must remember that all resident information is confidential. Information should only be shared with members of the care team.

11. Explain documentation and describe related terms and forms

Nursing assistants spend more time with residents than other members of the care team. They may observe things about residents that nurses or doctors have not noticed. NAs do not make diagnoses or decide on treatment. However, they have valuable information about residents that will help in care planning. Documenting accurately is the key to care planning. A thorough written record shows an NA's observations to others. It helps the NA to remember details about each resident.

Because nursing assistants see many residents during the day, they cannot remember everything that each resident did or said, or every observation they make. Documentation gives an up-to-date record of each resident's care. NAs must learn to document accurately. They must always take the time to observe and record carefully. Because documentation is so important, it should be recorded immediately and not be put off until later.

A medical chart is a legal document. What is written in the chart is considered in court to be what actually happened. If an NA gave a resident a bath and took her temperature, but never documented it, the NA could not necessarily prove that he actually performed the care. In general, if something does not appear in a resident's chart, it did not legally happen. Failing to document care could cause very serious legal problems for nursing assistants and their employers. It could also harm residents. It is important for NAs to remember that if it was not documented, it was not done.

Information found in a medical chart includes the following:

- Admission sheet (protected health information about the person, such as name, address, social security number, date of birth, and e-mail address, among other items)
- Medical history (illnesses, immunizations, medications, previous surgeries, family and social histories)
- Doctor's orders (instructions given to other members of the care team)
- Progress notes (updates from all care team members detailing changes or new information in the person's condition)
- Test results (blood tests, lab results, other tests)
- Graphic sheet (vital signs, intake and output, bladder and bowel elimination)
- Nurse's notes (the person's reported symptoms and actions taken to address them)
- Flow sheets (check-off sheets for documenting care; may also be called an ADL [activities of daily living] sheet) (Fig. 4-9)

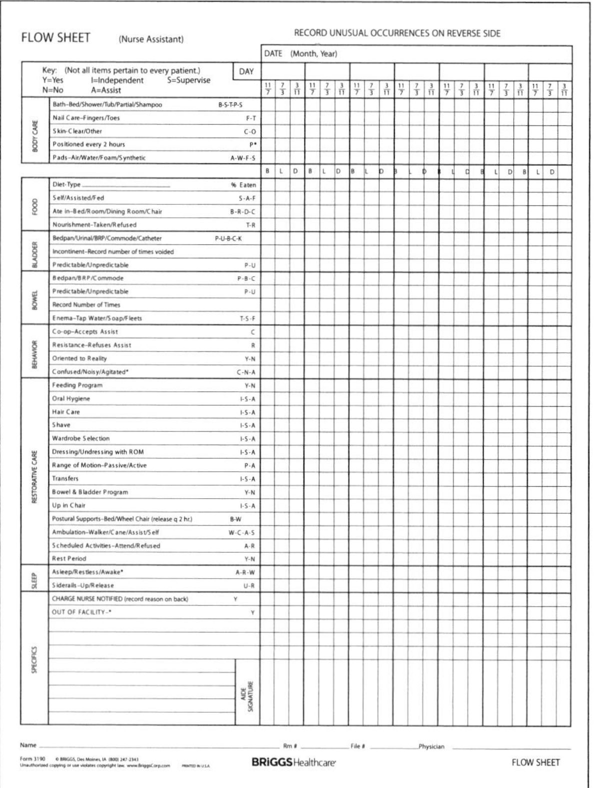

FLOW SHEET (Nurse Assistant)

RECORD UNUSUAL OCCURRENCES ON REVERSE SIDE

DATE (Month, Year)

Key: (Not all items pertain to every patient.) Y=Yes I=Independent S=Supervise N=No A=Assist

DAY

BODY CARE	Bath-Bed/Shower/Tub/Partial/Shampoo	B-S-T-P-S
	Nail Care-Fingers/Toes	F-T
	Skin-Clear/Other	C-O
	Positioned every 2 hours	P*
	Pads-Air/Water/Foam/Synthetic	A-W-F-S
FOOD	Diet-Type ______	% Eaten
	Self/Assisted/Fed	S-A-F
	Ate in-Bed/Room/Dining Room/Chair	B-R-D-C
	Nourishment-Taken/Refused	T-R
BLADDER	Bedpan/Urinal/BRP/Commode/Catheter	P-U-B-C-K
	Incontinent-Record number of times voided	
	Predictable/Unpredictable	P-U
BOWEL	Bedpan/BRP/Commode	P-B-C
	Predictable/Unpredictable	P-U
	Record Number of Times	
	Enema-Tap Water/Soap/Fleets	T-S-F
BEHAVIOR	Co-op-Accepts Assist	C
	Resistance-Refuses Assist	R
	Oriented to Reality	Y-N
	Confused/Noisy/Agitated*	C-N-A
RESTORATIVE CARE	Feeding Program	Y-N
	Oral Hygiene	I-S-A
	Hair Care	I-S-A
	Shave	I-S-A
	Wardrobe Selection	I-S-A
	Dressing/Undressing with ROM	I-S-A
	Range of Motion-Passive/Active	P-A
	Transfers	I-S-A
	Bowel & Bladder Program	Y-N
	Up in Chair	I-S-A
	Postural Supports-Bed/Wheel Chair (release q 2 hr.)	B-W
	Ambulation-Walker/Cane/Assist/Self	W-C-A-S
	Scheduled Activities-Attend/Refused	A-R
	Rest Period	Y-N
SLEEP	Asleep/Restless/Awake*	A-R-W
	Siderails-Up/Release	U-R
SPECIFICS	CHARGE NURSE NOTIFIED (record reason on back)	Y
	OUT OF FACILITY-*	Y
	AIDE SIGNATURE	

Name ______ Rm # ______ File # ______ Physician ______

Form 3190 © BRIGGS, Des Moines, IA (800) 247-2343 Unauthorized copying or use violates copyright law. www.BriggsCorp.com PRINTED IN U.S.A. BRIGGS Healthcare FLOW SHEET

Fig. 4-9. *Some facilities use an ADL flow sheet for documenting care.* (REPRINTED WITH PERMISSION OF BRIGGS CORPORATION, 800-247-2343, WWW.BRIGGSCORP.COM)

There are legal aspects to documentation that are important to remember. Careful charting is important for these reasons:

- It is the only way to guarantee clear and complete communication among all the members of the care team.
- Documentation is a legal record of every resident's treatment. Medical charts can be used in court as legal evidence.
- Documentation helps protect nursing assistants and their employers from liability by proving what they did when caring for residents.
- Documentation gives an up-to-date record of the status and care of each resident.

Guidelines: Careful Documentation

G Document care immediately after it is given. This helps to remember important details. Always wait to document until after care has been completed. Do not record any care before it has been done.

G Think about what you want to say before documenting. Be as brief and as clear as possible.

G Use facts, not opinions.

G Use black ink when documenting. Write as neatly as you can.

G If you make a mistake, draw one line through it, and write the correct information. Put your initials and the date (Fig. 4-10). Do not erase what you have written. Do not use correction fluid. Documentation done on a computer is time-stamped; it can only be changed by entering another notation.

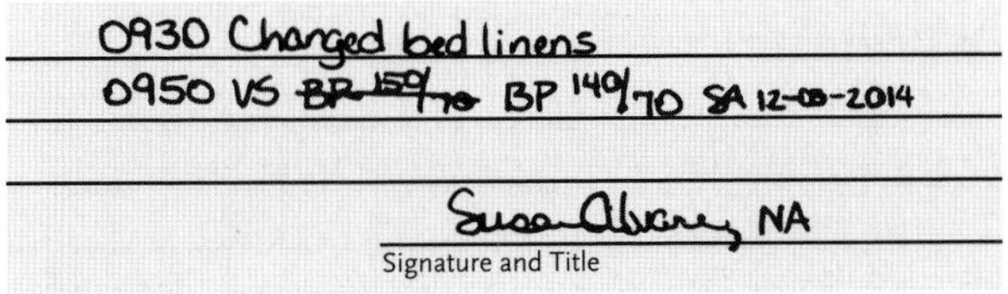

0930 Changed bed linens

0950 VS ~~BP 150/70~~ BP 140/70 SA 12-[illegible]-2014

NA

Signature and Title

Fig. 4-10. One example of how to correct a mistake.

G Sign your full name and title (for example, Sara Martinez, CNA) and write the correct date.

G Document as specified in the care plan.

G Nursing assistants may need to document using the 24-hour clock, or military time (Fig. 4-11). Regular time uses the numbers 1 to 12 to show each of the 24 hours in a day. In military time, the hours are numbered from 00 to 23. Midnight is expressed as 0000 (although it can also be written as 2400), 1:00 a.m. is 0100, 1:00 p.m. is 1300, and so on.

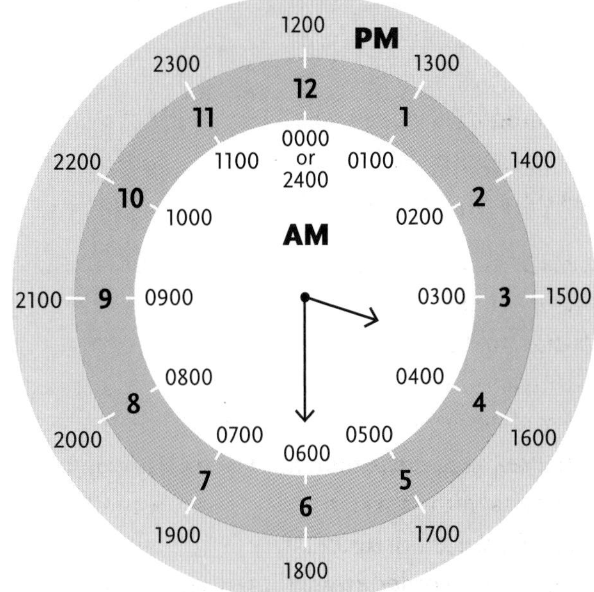

Fig. 4-11. Divisions in the 24-hour clock.

To change the regular hours between 1:00 p.m. to 11:59 p.m. to military time, add 12 to the regular time. For example, to change 3:00 p.m. to military time, add 3 + 12. The time is expressed as 1500 (fifteen hundred) hours.

To change from military time to regular time, subtract 12. For example, to change 2200 hours to standard time, subtract 12 from 22. The answer is 10:00 p.m.

Both regular and military time list minutes and seconds the same way. The minutes and seconds do not change when converting from regular to military time. The abbreviations a.m. and p.m. are used in regular time to show what time of day it is. However, these are not used in military time, since specific numbers show each hour of the day. For example, to change 4:22 p.m. to military time, add 4 + 12. The minutes do not change. The time is expressed as 1622 hours.

Midnight is the only time that differs. Midnight can be written as 0000, and it can also be written as 2400. This follows the rule of adding 12 to the regular time. Follow your facility's policy on how to express midnight.

At some facilities, computers are used to document information. Computers record and store information. It can be retrieved when it is needed. This is faster and more accurate than writing information by hand. If your facility uses computers for documentation, you will be trained to use them. HIPAA privacy guidelines apply to computer use. Make sure nobody can see private and protected health or personal information on your computer screen. Do not share confidential information with anyone except the care team.

12. Describe incident reporting and recording

An **incident** is an accident, problem, or unexpected event during the course of care. It is something that is not part of the normal routine. A mistake in care, such as feeding a resident from the wrong meal tray, is an incident. A resident falling or being injured is another type of incident. Accusations made by residents against staff and employee injuries are other types of incidents. A **sentinel event** is an accident or incident that results in grave physical or psychological injury or death. This type of event requires an immediate investigation and response. For example, a resident is given the wrong medication, which results in his death.

State and federal guidelines require that incidents be recorded in an incident report (Fig. 4-12). An incident report (also called an *occurrence* or *event* report) is a report that documents the incident and the response to it. The information in an incident report is confidential. Incident reports should be filed when any of the following occur:

- A resident falls (all falls must be reported, even if the resident says he or she is fine)
- A nursing assistant or a resident breaks or damages something
- A nursing assistant makes a mistake in care
- A resident or a family member makes a request that is outside the nursing assistant's scope of practice
- A resident or a family member makes sexual advances or remarks
- Anything happens that makes a nursing assistant feel uncomfortable, threatened, or unsafe
- A nursing assistant gets injured on the job
- A nursing assistant is exposed to blood or body fluids

Reporting and documenting incidents is done to protect everyone involved. This includes the resident, the employer, and the nursing assistant. When documenting incidents, NAs should complete the report as soon as possible and give it to the charge nurse. This is important so that they do not forget any details.

If a resident falls, and the NA did not see it, she should not write, "Mr. G fell." Instead, she should write, "Found Mr. G on the floor" or, "Mr. G states that he fell." Nursing assistants should write brief and accurate descriptions of the events as they happened without placing blame or liability within the report. Incident reports help demonstrate areas where changes can be made to avoid repeating the same incident.

Guidelines: Incident Reporting

- G Tell what happened. State the time and the mental and physical condition of the person.
- G Tell how the person tolerated the incident (his reaction).
- G State the facts; do not give opinions.
- G Do not write anything in the incident report on the medical record.

INCIDENT/ACCIDENT REPORT

PERSON INVOLVED (Last name) (First name) (Middle initial)

Adult ❑ Child ❑ Male ❑ Female ❑ Age______

Date of incident/accident | Time of incident/accident A.M. ❑ P.M. ❑ | Exact location of incident/accident Resident's room ❑ (No.______) Hallway ❑ Bathroom ❑ Other ❑ Specify ______________

RESIDENT ❑ List diagnosis if contributed to incident/accident:

Resident's condition before incident/accident

Normal ❑ Confused ❑ Disoriented ❑ Sedated ❑ (Drug__________ Dose__________ Time__________) Other ❑ (Specify) __________

Were bed rails ordered? Yes ❑ No ❑ | Were bed rails present? Yes ❑ No ❑ | If Yes, Up ❑ Down ❑ | Was height of bed adjustable? Yes ❑ No ❑ | If Yes, Up ❑ Down ❑

Was a restraint in use? Yes ❑ No ❑

Physical restraint ❑ Type______________ Chemical restraint ❑ Specify______________

EMPLOYEE ❑ Department | Job title | Length of time in this position

VISITOR ❑ OTHER ❑ Home address | Home phone

Occupation | Reason for presence at this facility

Equipment involved ❑

Property involved ❑ Describe

Was person authorized to be at location of incident/accident? Yes ❑ No ❑

Describe exactly what happened; why it happened; what the causes were. If an injury, state part of body injured. If property or equipment damaged, describe damage.

Indicate on diagram location of injury:

Temp. __________ Pulse __________ Resp. __________

B.P. __________

TYPE OF INJURY

1. Laceration ❑
2. Hematoma ❑
3. Abrasion ❑
4. Burn ❑
5. Swelling ❑
6. None apparent ❑
7. Other (specify below) ❑

LEVEL OF CONSCIOUSNESS

Name of physician notified	Time of notification __________ A.M./P.M.	Time of responded __________ A.M./P.M.
Name and relationship of family member/resident representative notified	Time of notification __________ A.M./P.M.	Time of responded __________ A.M./P.M.

Was person involved seen by a physician? Yes ❑ No ❑ If Yes, physician's name	Where	Date	Time A.M. ❑ P.M. ❑
Was first aid administered? Yes ❑ No ❑ If Yes, type of care provided and by whom	Where	Date	Time A.M. ❑ P.M. ❑
Was person involved taken to a hospital? Yes ❑ No ❑ If Yes, hospital name	By whom	Date	Time A.M. ❑ P.M. ❑

Name, title (if applicable), address & phone no. of witness(es) | Additional comments and/or steps taken to prevent recurrence:

SIGNATURE/TITLE/DATE	SIGNATURE/TITLE/DATE
Person preparing report	Medical Director
Director of Nursing	Administrator

Form 3322/2R Rev. 11/00 © 1991 BRIGGS, Des Moines, IA (800) 247-2343
Unauthorized copying or use violates copyright law. www.BriggsCorp.com PRINTED IN U.S.A.

BRiGGS Healthcare® INCIDENT/ACCIDENT REPORT

Fig. 4-12. *A sample incident report.* (REPRINTED WITH PERMISSION OF BRIGGS CORPORATION, 800-247-2343, WWW.BRIGGSCORP.COM)

- Describe the action taken to give care.
- Include suggestions for change.

13. Demonstrate effective communication on the telephone

Nursing assistants may be asked to make a call or answer the telephone at their facility. Here are guidelines that they should follow:

Guidelines: Telephone Communication

When making a call, follow these steps:

- Always identify yourself before asking to speak to someone. Never ask, "Who is this?" when someone answers your call.
- After you have identified yourself, ask for the person with whom you need to speak.
- If the person you are calling is available, identify yourself again. State why you are calling. Planning your call before you pick up the phone will help you be as efficient as possible.
- If the person is not available, ask if you can leave a message. Always leave a brief message, even if it is only to say you called. The message shows that you were trying to reach someone.
- Leave a brief and clear message. Do not give more information than necessary. A basic message includes your name, your facility's name, the phone number where you can be reached, and a brief description of the reason for your call.
- Thank the person who takes the message for you. Always be polite over the telephone, as you would be in person.

When answering calls, follow these steps:

- Always identify your facility's name, your name, and your position. Be friendly and professional.
- If you need to find the person the caller wishes to speak with, place the caller on hold after asking if it is OK to do so.
- If the caller has to leave a message, write it down and repeat it to make sure you have the correct message. Ask for proper spellings of names. Do not ask for more information than the person needs to return the call: a name, short message, and phone number is enough. Do not give out any information about staff or residents.
- Thank the person for calling and say goodbye.

14. Understand guidelines for basic office machines and computers

There are many types of machines used in various healthcare settings. Following is some brief information on office machines and computers. These machines or devices can make communication easier, faster, and more accurate.

Photocopier

A photocopier, commonly called a *copier,* is a machine that makes paper copies of documents and other images quickly. To operate a copier, a person must open the lid and place the document to be copied face-down on the glass. There may be marks on the sides of the glass to show where to place different-sized documents. Options can be selected, such as how many copies should be made. Other options may include enlarging or reducing the size of the image, making it lighter or darker, and collating the copies. Collate means to assemble or arrange in the proper order. Once the options have been selected, pressing the *Start* button produces copies.

Fax Machine

A fax machine transfers copies of documents over a telephone network. Fax machines also function as photocopiers. To send a fax, a person must place the piece of paper to be faxed in the document feeder. The machine should have instructions on whether the document must be placed face-down or face-up. The phone number of the recipient's fax should be entered, then the *Fax/Send* or *Start* button pressed. Depending on the facility, a special number may need to be dialed to reach an outside line. After the fax has been transmitted, a confirmation of the transmission may be printed.

Calculator

A calculator performs mathematical calculations. Calculators have standard symbols for performing these calculations. They include a plus sign (+) for addition problems, a minus sign (–) for subtraction, a multiplication symbol (x or *), a division sign (÷ or /), and an equal sign (=).

A person must be able to understand basic math in order to use a calculator to perform these processes. Most calculators have numbers in the middle or bottom of the device. They begin with zero and work upwards in rows of three until reaching the number 9.

Computer

Computers are electronic devices that process and store information. They are used in various ways in facilities. Some facilities and hospitals use computers to document information because it is more accurate than writing information by hand. Doctors and nurses may carry computers from room to room to review medical records; document symptoms, tests, and treatments; manage medications; and perform other functions. Computers may be used to transmit records or other patient information to other facilities and healthcare professionals. They may be used for research. Employees may use computers to clock in and out when they work so that their total hours worked are calculated for a specific time period for payment.

Computers are used to send and receive e-mail and access the Internet. E-mail, short for *electronic mail,* is a system for sending and receiving messages electronically over a computer system or network. The Internet is a worldwide communications system that links a network of computers.

Nursing assistants will be trained to use computers if their facility uses them for documentation, research, tracking employee hours, or any other reason.

15. Explain the resident call system

Long-term care facilities are required to have call systems—often called call lights—so that residents can call for help whenever they need it. They are in resident rooms and bathrooms. Some have strings for residents to pull and others have buttons to be pushed. The signal is usually both a light outside the room and a sound that can be heard in the nurses' station. This is the primary way a resident can call for help. Nursing assistants must always respond immediately when they see the light or hear the sound. They should respond in a courteous and respectful manner. It is important that they check each time before leaving a room to make sure that the call light is within the resident's reach and that the resident knows how to use it.

16. List guidelines for communicating with residents with special needs

Due to illness or impairments, some residents will need special techniques to aid communication. An **impairment** is a loss of function or ability; it can be a partial or complete loss. Special techniques for different conditions are listed below. Information on communicating with residents who have dementia, such as Alzheimer's disease, is in Chapter 19. Guidelines for communicating with residents who are mentally ill are in Chapter 20.

Hearing Impairment

There are many different kinds of hearing loss. Persons who have impaired hearing or are deaf may have lost their hearing gradually, or they may have been born with a hearing impairment. If they have a gradual hearing loss, they may not be conscious of it. Signs of hearing loss include the following:

- Speaking loudly
- Leaning forward when someone is speaking
- Cupping the ear to hear better
- Responding inappropriately
- Asking the speaker to repeat what has been said
- Speaking in a monotone
- Avoiding social gatherings or acting irritable in the presence of people who are having a conversation
- Suspecting others of talking about them or of deliberately speaking softly

People who have hearing impairment may use a hearing aid, read lips, or use sign language. People with impaired hearing also closely observe the facial expressions and body language of others to add to their knowledge of what is being said. Hearing loss may affect how well residents can express their needs.

Guidelines: Hearing Impairment

G If the person has a hearing aid, make sure he or she is wearing it and that it is turned on. Many different types of hearing aids exist (Fig. 4-13). Follow manufacturer's directions for cleaning. In general, the hearing aid needs to be cleaned daily. Wipe it with a special cleaning solution or alcohol and a soft cloth. Do not put the hearing aid in water. Handle it carefully; do not drop it. Always store it inside its case when it is not being worn. Turn it off when it is not in use. Remove it before bathing, showering, or shampooing hair. Some hearing aids need to be recharged nightly. Some have rechargeable batteries. Follow instructions in the care plan.

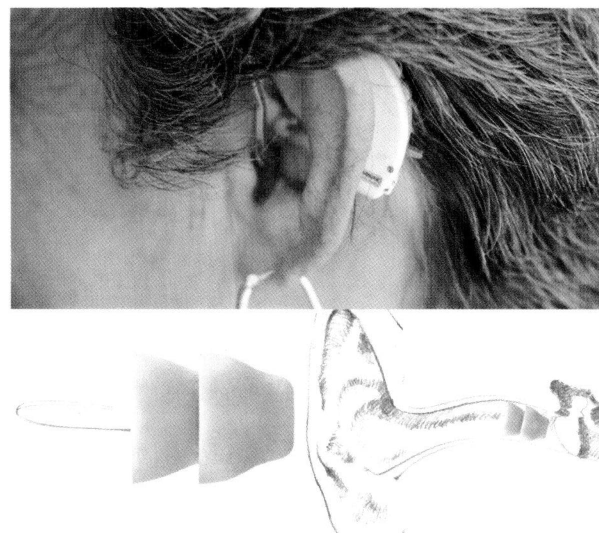

Fig. 4-13. *The top photo shows an older type of hearing aid. The bottom left photo shows a newer type of hearing aid, and the bottom right illustration shows this device placed inside the ear.* (BOTTOM PHOTOS COURTESY OF PHONAK, WWW.PHONAK-LYRIC.COM)

G Reduce or remove noise, such as TVs, radios, and loud speech. Close doors if needed.

G Get residents' attention before speaking. Do not startle them by approaching from behind. Walk in front or touch them lightly on the arm to let them know you are near.

G Speak clearly, slowly, and in good lighting. Directly face the person (Fig. 4-14). The light should be on your face, not on the resident's. Ask if she can hear what you are saying.

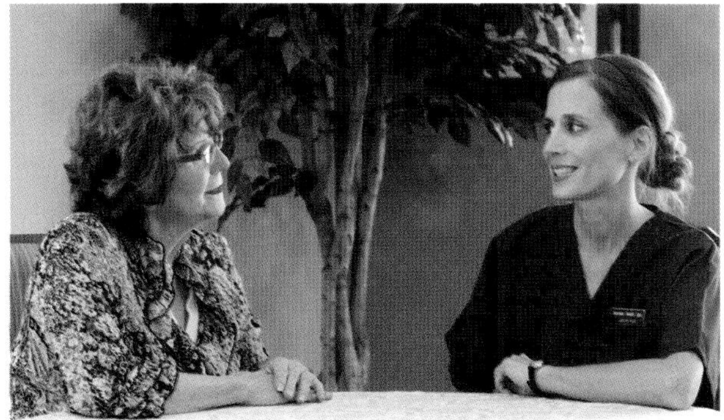

Fig. 4-14. *When communicating with residents who have hearing impairments, nursing assistants should speak face-to-face in good light.*

- G Do not shout or mouth the words in an exaggerated way.
- G Keep the pitch of your voice low.
- G Residents may read lips, so do not chew gum or eat while speaking. Keep your hands away from your face while talking.
- G If the resident hears better out of one ear, try to speak and stand on that side.
- G Use short sentences and simple words. Avoid sudden topic changes.
- G Repeat what you have said using different words when needed. Some hearing-impaired people want you to repeat exactly what you said because they miss only a few words.
- G Use picture cards or a notepad as needed.
- G Hearing-impaired residents may hear less when they are tired or ill. This is true of everyone. Be patient and empathetic. Avoid long, tiring conversations.
- G Some hearing-impaired residents have speech problems and may be difficult to understand. Do not pretend you understand if you do not. Ask the resident to repeat what was said. Observe the lips, facial expressions, and body language. Then tell the resident what you think you heard. You can also request that the resident write down words.
- G Hearing decline can be a normal aspect of aging. Be understanding and supportive.

Vision Impairment

Like hearing impairment, vision impairment can affect people of all ages. It can exist at birth or develop gradually. It can occur in one eye or in both. It can also be the result of injury, illness, or aging. Some vision impairment causes people to wear corrective lenses, such as contact lenses or eyeglasses. **Farsightedness** (hyperopia) is the ability to see objects in the distance better than objects nearby. It develops in most people as they age. **Nearsightedness** (myopia) is the ability to see things near but not far. It may occur in younger persons. Some people need to wear eyeglasses all the time. Others only need them to read or for activities that require seeing distant objects, such as driving. Surgery can also be performed to correct these eye problems. Chapter 18 has more information about vision impairment.

Guidelines: Vision Impairment

- G If the person has eyeglasses, make sure they are clean and that he or she wears them. Clean glass lenses with water and soft tissue. Clean plastic lenses with cleaning fluid and a lens cloth. Also, make sure that eyeglasses are in good condition and fit well. Report to the nurse if they do not.
- G Contact lenses are made of many types of plastic. Some can be worn and disposed of daily; others are worn for longer periods. If the resident is able, it is best to leave contact lens care to him or her.
- G Knock on the door and identify yourself immediately when you enter the room. Do not touch the resident until you have said your name. Explain why you are there and what you would like to do. Let the resident know when you are leaving the room.
- G Make sure there is proper lighting in the room. Face the resident when speaking.
- G When you enter a new room with the resident, orient him or her to where things are. Describe the things you see around you. Try not to use words such as, "see," "look," and "watch."
- G Always tell the resident what you are doing while caring for him. Give specific directions, such as, "on your right" or, "in front of you." Talk directly to the resident whom you are assisting. Do not talk to other residents or staff members.

- Use the face of an imaginary clock as a guide to explain the position of objects that are in front of resident. For example, "There is a sofa at 7 o'clock" (Fig. 4-15).

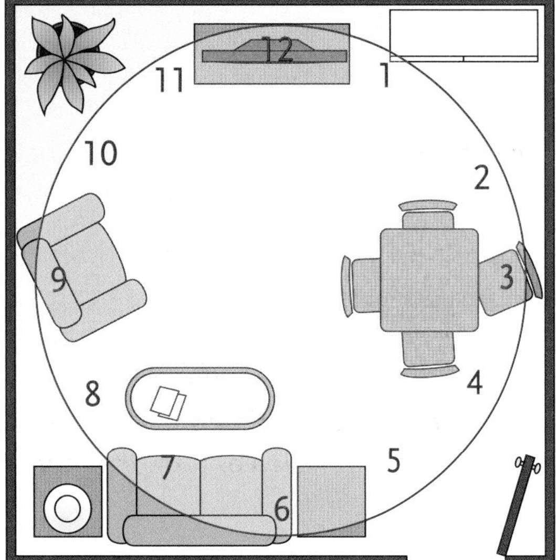

Fig. 4-15. Using the face of an imaginary clock to explain the position of objects can be helpful.

- Do not change the position of personal items or furniture. Put everything back where you found it.
- Tell the resident where the call light is.
- Leave doors completely open or completely closed, never partly open.
- If the resident needs guidance in getting around, walk slightly ahead. Let the resident touch or grasp your arm lightly.
- Encourage the use of the other senses, such as hearing, touch, and smell. Encourage the resident to feel and touch things, such as clothing, furniture, or items in the room.
- Use large clocks, clocks that chime, and radios to help keep track of time.
- Large-print books, audio books, digital books, and Braille books are available (Fig. 4-16). Learning to read Braille, however, takes a long time and requires special training.

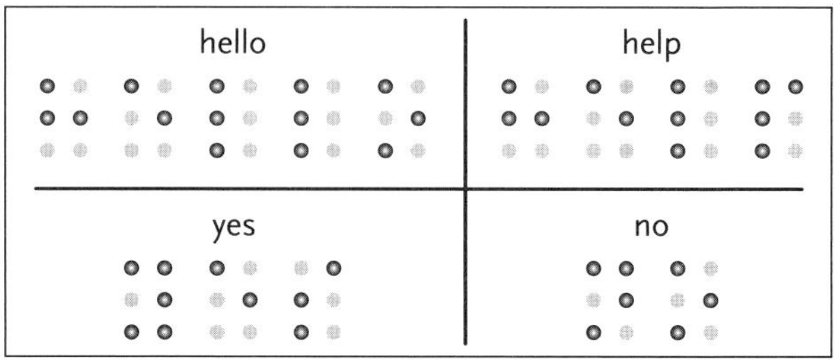

hello | help

yes | no

***Fig. 4-16.** Examples of words in Braille.*

- If the resident has a guide dog, do not play with, distract, or feed it.

CVA or Stroke

The medical term for a stroke is a **cerebrovascular accident (CVA)**. CVA, or stroke, occurs when blood supply to a part of the brain is blocked or a blood vessel leaks or ruptures within the brain. An ischemic stroke is the most common type of stroke (Fig. 4-17). With this type of stroke, the blood supply is blocked. Without blood, part of the brain does not receive oxygen. Brain cells begin to die, and additional damage can occur due to leaking blood, clots, and swelling of the tissues. Swelling can also cause pressure on other areas of the brain. Strokes can be mild or severe. After a stroke, a resident may experience any of the following:

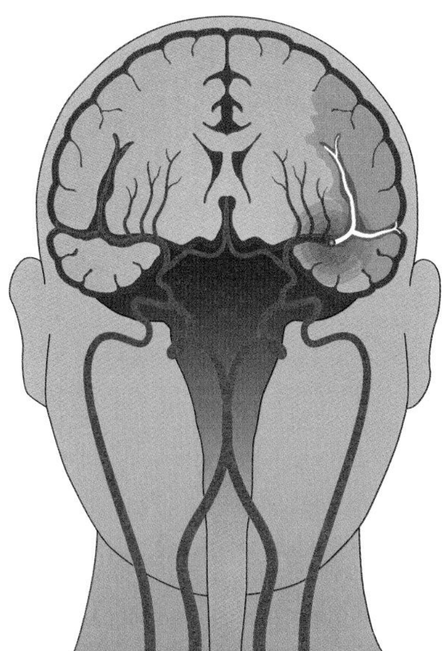

***Fig. 4-17.** An ischemic stroke is caused when the blood supply to the brain is blocked.*

- Paralysis on one side of the body, called **hemiplegia**
- Weakness on one side of the body, called **hemiparesis**
- Slurred speech or inability to speak, called **expressive aphasia**
- Inability to understand spoken or written words, called **receptive aphasia**
- Loss of sensations such as temperature or touch
- Loss of bowel or bladder control
- Confusion
- Poor judgment
- Memory loss
- Loss of cognitive abilities
- Tendency to ignore one side of the body, called one-sided neglect
- Laughing or crying without any reason, or when it is inappropriate, called **emotional lability**
- Difficulty swallowing, called **dysphagia**

Depending on the severity of the stroke and speech loss or confusion, these guidelines may be helpful:

Guidelines: Communication and Stroke

G Keep questions and directions simple. Give directions one step at a time.

G Phrase questions so they can be answered with a "yes" or "no." For example, when helping a resident with eating, ask, "Would you like to start with a drink of milk?"

G Agree on signals, such as shaking or nodding the head or raising a hand or finger for "yes" or "no."

G Give residents time to respond. Listen attentively.

G Use a pencil and paper if the resident can write. A thick handle or tape around the pencil may help the resident hold it more easily.

G Never call the weaker side the *bad side*, or talk about the *bad* leg or arm. Use the term *weaker* or *involved* to refer to the side with paralysis or weakness.

G Keep the call signal within reach of residents. They can let you know when you are needed.

G Use verbal and nonverbal communication to express your positive attitude. Let the resident know you have confidence in his or her abilities through smiles, touches, and gestures. Gestures and pointing can also help you convey information or allow the resident to speak to you.

G Use communication boards or special cards to aid communication (Fig. 4-18).

More information about strokes and related care is in Chapter 18.

Residents' Rights

Speech Impairment

Nursing assistants should never talk about residents as if they were not there. Even if residents cannot speak, it does not mean they cannot hear. All residents should be treated with respect.

Combative Behavior

Residents may display **combative**, meaning violent or hostile, behavior. Such behavior may include hitting, pushing, kicking, or verbal attacks. It may be the result of disease affecting the brain. It may also be due to frustration. Or it may just be part of someone's personality. In general, combative behavior is not a reaction to the caregiver and should not be taken personally.

Nursing assistants should always report and document combative behavior. Even if NAs do not find the behavior upsetting, the care team needs to be aware of it.

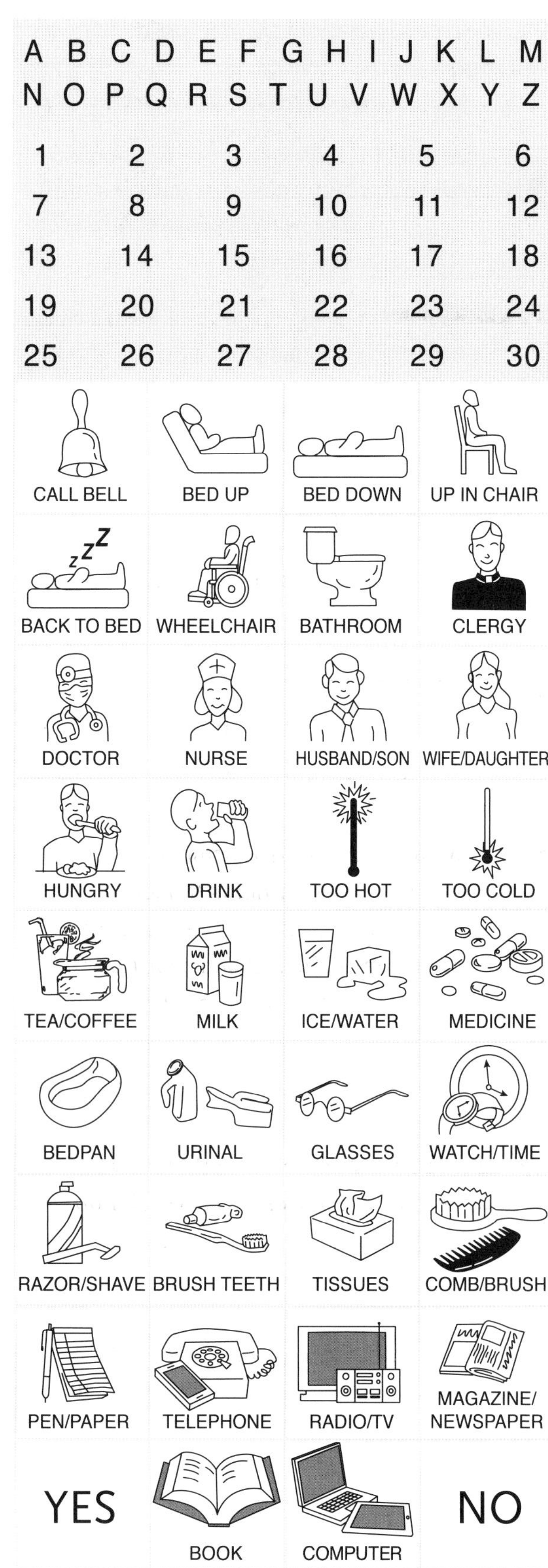

Fig. 4-18. A sample communication board.

Guidelines: Combative Behavior

- Block physical blows or step out of the way, but never hit back (Fig. 4-19). No matter how much a resident hurts you, or how angry or afraid you are, never hit or threaten a resident.

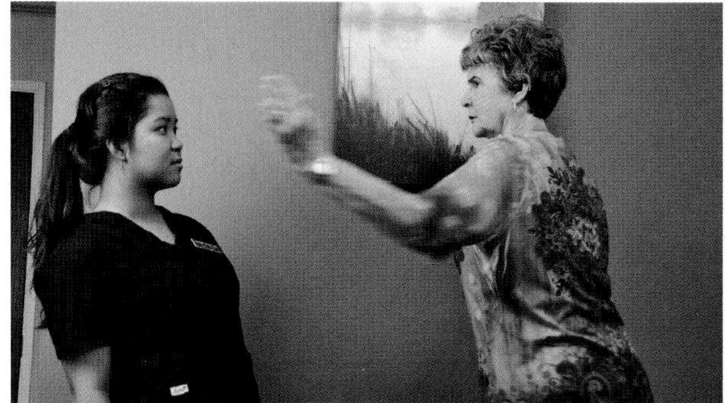

Fig. 4-19. When dealing with combative residents, nursing assistants should step out of the way, but never hit back.

- Allow the resident time to calm down before the next interaction.
- Ensure the resident is safe and give him or her space. When possible, stand at least an arm's length away.
- Remain calm. Lower the tone of your voice.
- Be flexible and patient.
- Stay neutral. Do not respond to verbal attacks. Do not argue or accuse the resident of wrongdoing. If you must respond, say something like, "I understand that you're angry and frustrated. How can I make things better?"
- Do not use gestures that could frighten or startle the resident.
- Be reassuring and supportive.
- Consider what provoked the resident. Sometimes something as simple as a change in caregiver or routine can be very upsetting to a resident. Get help to take the resident to a quieter place if needed.
- Report inappropriate behavior to the nurse.

Residents' Rights

Combative Behavior

Elderly people are sometimes abused by their caregivers. These caregivers may be family, friends, or care team members. This abuse is often the result of a stressful situation, such as the person being combative, causing the caregiver to lash out. Nursing assistants must remember that they can never hit a resident, no matter what happens. Hitting a resident is considered abuse and is grounds for termination and legal action. NAs should remain calm and professional. If an NA feels that he needs help handling stressful situations, he should talk with the charge nurse.

Anger

Anger is a natural emotion that has many causes, such as disease, fear, pain, loneliness, and loss of independence. Anger may also just be a part of someone's personality. Some people get angry more easily than others.

People express anger in different ways. Some may shout, yell, threaten, throw things, or pace. Others express their anger by withdrawing, being silent, or sulking. Angry behavior should always be reported to the nurse.

Guidelines: Angry Behavior

- G Stay calm.
- G Do not argue or respond to verbal attacks.
- G Empathize with the resident. Try to understand what he or she is feeling.
- G Try to find out what caused the resident's anger. Using silence may help the resident explain. Listen attentively as the resident speaks.
- G Treat the resident with dignity and respect. Explain what you are going to do and when you will do it.
- G Answer call lights promptly.
- G Stay at a safe distance if the resident becomes combative.

Assertive vs. Aggressive Behavior

A person is behaving assertively when he expresses thoughts, feelings, and beliefs in a direct and honest way. Being assertive involves respect for one's own needs and feelings and for those of other people. It is not the same as being aggressive, combative, or angry.

A person is behaving aggressively when he expresses thoughts, feelings, and beliefs in ways that humiliate, disgrace, or overpower the other person. Little or no respect is shown for the needs or feelings of others. Nursing assistants should report aggressive behavior when they witness it.

Inappropriate Behavior

Inappropriate behavior from a resident includes trying to establish a personal, rather than a professional, relationship with a nursing assistant. Examples include asking personal questions, requesting visits on personal time, asking for or doing favors, giving tips or gifts, and lending or borrowing money.

Inappropriate behavior also includes making sexual advances and comments to facility staff or other residents. Sexual advances include any sexual words, comments, or behavior that makes the person to whom the advances are directed feel uncomfortable.

Inappropriate behavior may include residents removing their clothes or touching themselves in public. Illness, dementia, confusion, and medication may cause this behavior. If a nursing assistant encounters a resident in any embarrassing situation, she should remain professional and not overreact, as that may actually reinforce the behavior. Trying to distract the resident may help. If it does not, the resident should be taken to a private area, and the nurse should be notified.

Confused residents may have problems that mimic inappropriate sexual behavior. They may have an uncomfortable rash, clothes that are too tight, too hot, or too scratchy, or they may need to go to the bathroom. Nursing assistants need to observe for these problems. When residents behave inappropriately, NAs should report the behavior, even if they think it was harmless.

Chapter Review

1. Briefly describe three steps in the communication process.
2. Define *nonverbal communication* and give one example that is not listed in the textbook.
3. What does the word *culture* mean?
4. What is one positive response to cultural diversity?
5. Why should "why" questions be avoided when talking with residents?
6. If a resident speaks a different language than the nursing assistant does, what can the nursing assistant do?
7. What is one way to provide feedback while listening?
8. What can silence or pauses help a resident do?
9. What is one reason that a nursing assistant should not ignore a resident's request?
10. Why should a nursing assistant sit near a resident who has started a conversation with her?
11. For each statement, decide whether it is a fact or an opinion. Write "F" for fact and "O" for opinion.

    ___ Mr. Moore looked terrible today.

    ___ Mr. Gaston had a fever of 100.7° F.

    ___ Ms. Martino needs to make some friends.

    ___ Mr. Klein has not had a visitor since last Tuesday.

    ___ The doctor says Mrs. Storey has to walk once a day.

12. What is objective information? What is subjective information?
13. With whom should NAs use medical terminology—care team members or residents and their families?
14. What does the abbreviation *ROM* stand for?
15. What does the abbreviation *NPO* stand for?
16. What does the abbreviation *DNR* stand for?
17. List ten signs and symptoms that should be reported immediately to the nurse.
18. Describe four reasons why careful documentation is important.
19. When should care be documented—before or after it is done?
20. Convert 10:00 p.m. to military time.
21. Convert 1400 hours to regular time.
22. What is considered an incident at a facility?
23. List four guidelines for incident reporting.
24. Give an example of a proper greeting when answering the phone.
25. Give two reasons why computers may be used in a facility.
26. What is the purpose of the resident call light or call system?
27. When a resident has a hearing impairment, on whose face should the light be shining while communicating—the resident's or the nursing assistant's?
28. How can a nursing assistant explain the position of objects in front of a visually-impaired resident?
29. How should questions be phrased to a resident who has had a stroke?
30. How should a nursing assistant refer to the weaker side of a resident who has had a stroke?
31. What should a nursing assistant always do after a resident behaves inappropriately?

5 Preventing Infection

1. Define *infection prevention* and discuss types of infections

Infection prevention is the set of methods practiced in healthcare facilities to prevent and control the spread of disease. Preventing the spread of infection is very important and is the responsibility of all care team members. Nursing assistants must know and follow their facility's policies relating to infection prevention; these policies help protect staff members, residents, and others from disease.

A **microorganism (MO)** is a tiny living thing that is only visible under a microscope (Fig. 5-1). A **microbe** is another name for a microorganism. Microorganisms are always present in the environment (Fig. 5-2). **Infections** occur when harmful microorganisms, called **pathogens**, invade the body and multiply.

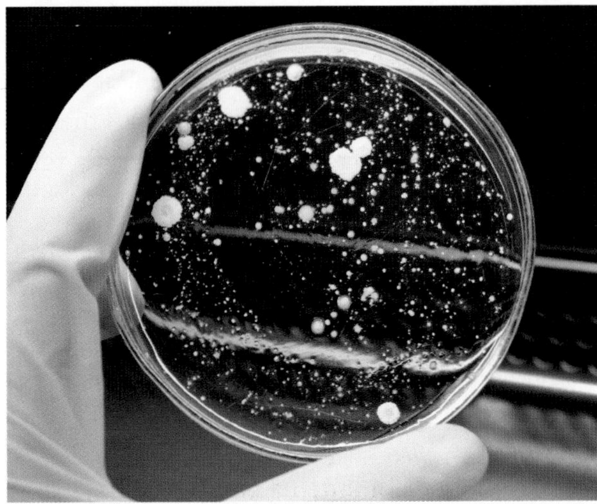

Fig. 5-1. *Microorganisms in a Petri dish.*

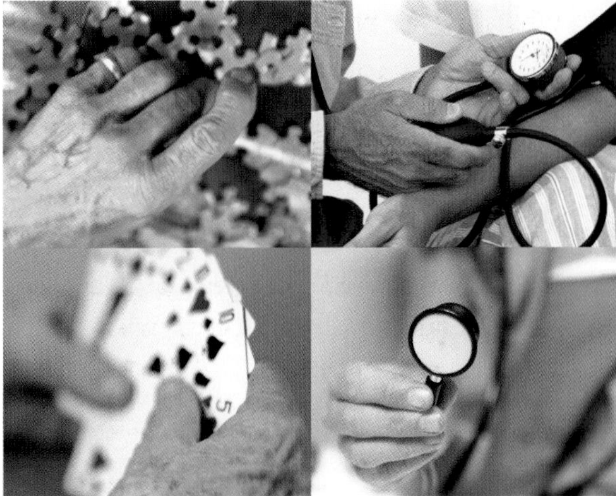

Fig. 5-2. *Microorganisms are always present in the environment. They are on almost everything a person touches.*

There are two main types of infections: localized and systemic. A **localized infection** is an infection that is limited to a specific location in the body. It has local symptoms, which means the symptoms are near the site of infection. For example, if a wound becomes infected, the area around it may become red, hot, and painful. A **systemic infection** affects the entire body. This type of infection travels through the bloodstream and is spread throughout the body. It causes general symptoms, such as fever, chills, or mental confusion.

A type of infection that can be localized or systemic is a healthcare-associated infection, formerly known as a nosocomial infection. A **healthcare-associated infection (HAI)** is an infection acquired in a healthcare setting during the delivery of medical care. Healthcare settings include hospitals, long-term care facilities, and outpatient surgery centers, among others.

Nursing assistants need to be able to recognize signs and symptoms of infections so that they can report them to the nurse promptly.

Observing and Reporting: Infections

Signs and symptoms of a localized infection include the following:

- O/R Pain
- O/R Redness
- O/R Swelling
- O/R Pus
- O/R Drainage (fluid from a wound or cavity)
- O/R Heat

Signs and symptoms of a systemic infection include the following:

- O/R Fever
- O/R Body aches
- O/R Chills
- O/R Nausea
- O/R Vomiting
- O/R Weakness
- O/R Headache
- O/R Mental confusion
- O/R Drop in person's normal blood pressure

2. Describe the chain of infection

To understand how to prevent disease, it is helpful to first understand how it is spread. The **chain of infection** is a way of describing how disease is transmitted from one being to another (Fig. 5-3). Definitions and examples of each of the six links in the chain of infection follow.

Chain Link 1: The **causative agent** is a pathogenic microorganism that causes disease. Causative agents include bacteria, viruses, fungi, and parasites.

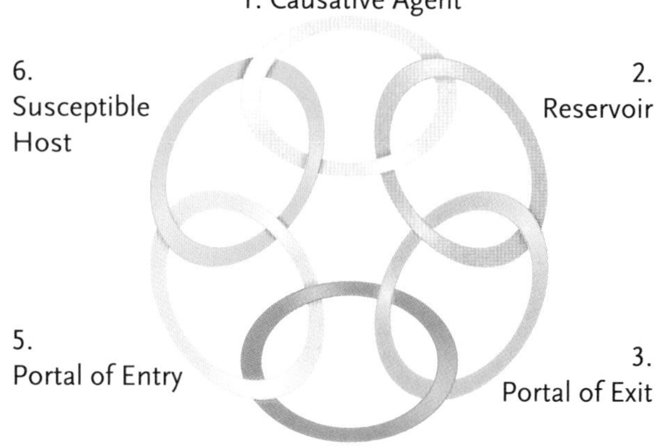

Fig. 5-3. The chain of infection.

Normal flora are the microorganisms that live in and on the body and normally do not cause harm as long as they remain in or at that particular area. When they enter a different part of the body, they may cause an infection.

Chain Link 2: A **reservoir** is where the pathogen lives and grows. A reservoir can be a human, animal, plant, soil, or a substance. Microorganisms grow best in warm, dark, and moist places where food is present. Some microorganisms need oxygen to survive while others do not. Examples of reservoirs include the lungs, blood, and the large intestine.

Chain Link 3: The **portal of exit** is any body opening on an infected person that allows pathogens to leave (Fig. 5-4). These include the nose, mouth, eyes, or a cut in the skin.

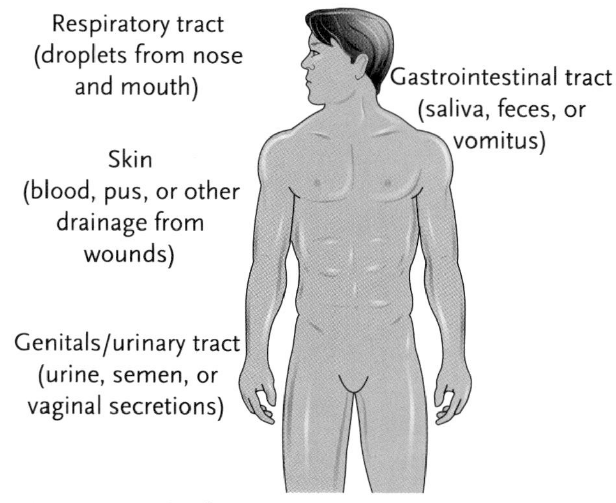

Fig. 5-4. Portals of exit.

Chain Link 4: The **mode of transmission** describes how the pathogen travels. Transmission can occur through the air or through direct or indirect contact. **Direct contact** happens by touching the infected person or his secretions. **Indirect contact** results from touching something contaminated by the infected person, such as a needle, dressing, or tissue. The primary route of disease transmission within the healthcare setting is on the hands of healthcare workers.

Chain Link 5: The **portal of entry** is any body opening on an uninfected person that allows pathogens to enter (Fig. 5-5). These include the nose, mouth, eyes, and other mucous membranes, cuts in the skin, and cracked skin. **Mucous membranes** are the membranes that line body cavities that open to the outside of the body. These include the linings of the mouth, nose, eyes, rectum, and genitals.

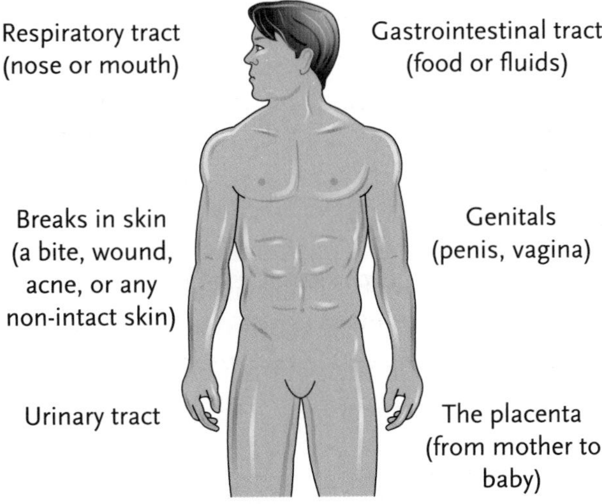

***Fig. 5-5.** Portals of entry.*

Chain Link 6: A **susceptible host** is an uninfected person who could get sick. Examples include all healthcare workers and anyone in their care who is not already infected with that particular disease.

If one of the links in the chain of infection is broken, then the spread of infection is stopped. Infection prevention practices help stop the pathogens from traveling (Link 4) and getting on a person's hands, nose, eyes, mouth, skin, etc. (Link 5). Immunizations (Link 6) reduce a person's chances of getting sick from diseases such as hepatitis B and influenza.

Transmission (passage or transfer) of most **infectious** diseases can be blocked by using proper infection prevention practices, such as handwashing. Handwashing is the most important way to stop the spread of infection. All caregivers should wash their hands often.

Handwashing is a part of medical asepsis. **Medical asepsis** refers to measures used to reduce and prevent the spread of pathogens. Medical asepsis is used in all healthcare settings. **Surgical asepsis** is the state of being free of all microorganisms, not just pathogens. Surgical asepsis, also called sterile technique, is used for many types of procedures, such as changing catheters.

3. Explain why the elderly are at a higher risk for infection

The elderly are at a higher risk for infection. This is due, in part, to weakened immune systems as a result of aging. Weakened immune systems can also result from chronic illnesses. Other physical changes of aging, such as decreased circulation and slow wound healing, may also contribute to infections in the elderly.

Older adults are at risk for **malnutrition** and dehydration. A person who is malnourished is not getting the proper nutrition. **Dehydration** is a condition that occurs when there is an inadequate amount of fluid in the body. These conditions can result from difficulty chewing and/or swallowing, lack of appetite and thirst, illnesses, weakness, and medication. Both malnutrition and dehydration are serious conditions (Chapter 15 has more information). When the body is not getting the nutrients and fluid it needs, the risk of infection greatly increases. Also, the elderly may have limited mobility, which is another risk factor for serious problems, such as pressure ulcers, skin infections, and pneumonia.

The elderly are hospitalized more often than younger people. This makes them more likely to get healthcare-associated infections. Difficulty swallowing and incontinence increase the risk of respiratory and urinary tract infections. Feeding tubes, oxygen tubes, and other types of tubing, such as catheters (Chapter 16), also increase the risk of infection.

Infection is more dangerous for the elderly because even a simple cold can turn into a life-threatening illness such as pneumonia. It also may take longer for older people to recover from an infection or illness. This is why preventing infection is so important. Nursing assistants play an important role in preventing infection.

4. Explain Standard Precautions

State and federal government agencies have guidelines and laws concerning infection prevention. The **Occupational Safety and Health Administration (OSHA)** is a federal government agency that makes rules to protect workers from hazards on the job. The **Centers for Disease Control and Prevention (CDC)** is a government agency under the Department of Health and Human Services (HHS). It issues information to protect the health of individuals and communities. It promotes public health, as well as disease, injury, and disability prevention and control through education.

In 1996, the CDC recommended a new infection prevention system to reduce the risk of contracting infectious diseases in healthcare settings. In 2007 some additions and changes were made to this system. There are two tiers of precautions within the infection prevention system: Standard Precautions and Transmission-Based, or Isolation, Precautions. To **isolate** means to keep something separate, or by itself.

Standard Precautions means treating blood, body fluids, non-intact skin (like abrasions, pimples, or open sores), and mucous membranes (linings of mouth, nose, eyes, rectum, and genitals) as if they were infected. Body fluids include saliva, sputum (mucus coughed up), urine, feces, semen, vaginal secretions, pus or other wound drainage, and vomit. They do not include sweat.

Standard Precautions must be used with every resident. Following Standard Precautions is the only safe way that nursing assistants can do their jobs. An NA cannot tell by looking at residents or even by reading their medical charts if they have a contagious disease such as tuberculosis, hepatitis, or influenza.

Standard Precautions and Transmission-Based Precautions (Learning Objective 9) are ways to stop the spread of infection by interrupting the mode of transmission. In other words, these guidelines do not stop an infected person from giving off pathogens. However, by following these guidelines, nursing assistants help prevent those pathogens from infecting them or those in their care.

- Standard Precautions must be practiced with every single person in a nursing assistant's care.
- Transmission-Based Precautions vary based on how an infection is transmitted. When indicated, these precautions are used **in addition** to Standard Precautions. More information about these precautions is located later in the chapter.

Guidelines: Standard Precautions

G **Wash your hands** before putting on gloves. Wash your hands immediately after removing your gloves. Be careful not to touch clean objects with your used gloves.

G **Wear gloves** if you may come into contact with any of the following: blood; body fluids or secretions; broken skin, such as abrasions, acne, cuts, stitches, or staples; or mucous membranes. Such contacts occur during mouth care; toilet assistance; perineal care;

helping with a bedpan or urinal; ostomy care; cleaning up spills; cleaning basins, urinals, bedpans, and other containers that have held body fluids; and disposing of wastes.

- **Remove gloves** immediately when finished with a procedure.
- **Immediately wash all skin surfaces that have been contaminated** with blood and body fluids.
- **Wear a disposable gown** that is resistant to body fluids if you may come into contact with blood or body fluids or when splashing or spraying blood or body fluids is likely.
- **Wear a mask and protective goggles** if you may come into contact with blood or body fluids or when splashing or spraying blood or body fluids is likely.
- **Wear gloves and use caution when handling razor blades, needles, and other sharps.** **Sharps** are needles or other sharp objects. Place sharps carefully in a biohazard container for sharps. Biohazard containers used for sharps are hard, leakproof containers. They are clearly labeled and warn of the danger of the contents inside (Figs. 5-6 and 5-7). There are also biohazard bags that are used for biomedical waste that is not sharp, such as soiled dressings, contaminated tubing, and other items. OSHA recommends that biomedical/biohazard waste be disposed of at the *point of origin*, or where the waste occurs.

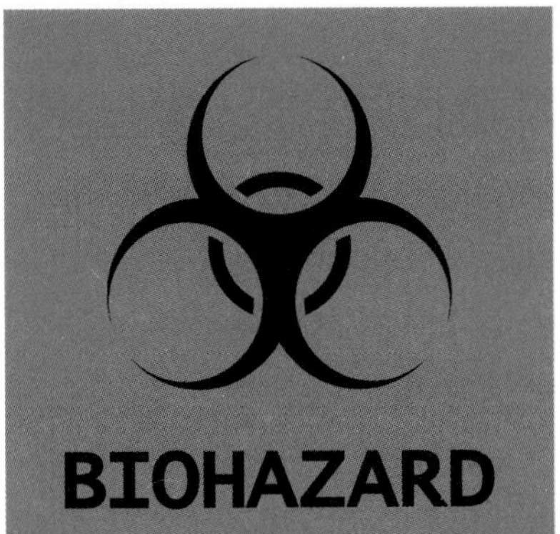

Fig. 5-6. *This label indicates that the material is potentially infectious.*

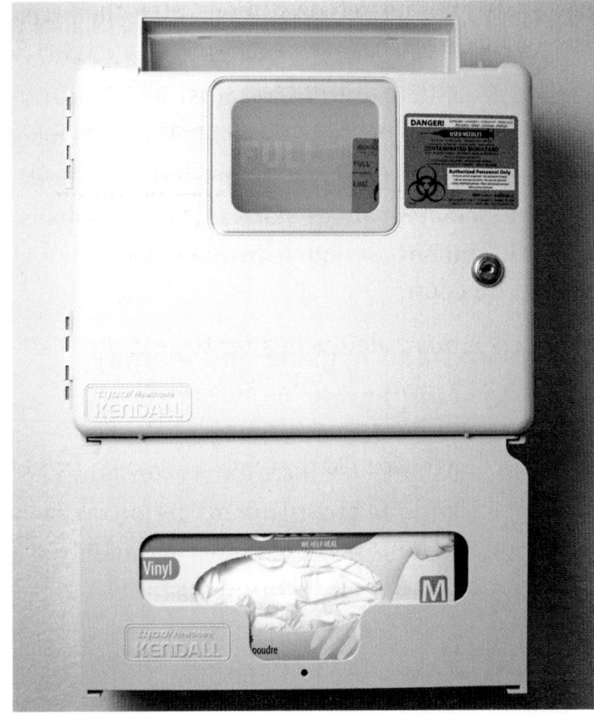

Fig. 5-7. *One type of container for sharps with an opening for gloves underneath.*

- **Never attempt to recap needles or sharps after use.** You might stick yourself. Dispose of them in a biohazard container for sharps.
- **Avoid nicks and cuts** when shaving residents.
- **Carefully bag all contaminated supplies.** Dispose of them according to your facility's policy.
- **Clearly label body fluids that are saved for a specimen** with the resident's name, date of birth, room number, and date and a biohazard label. Keep them in a container with a lid. Put in a biohazardous specimen bag for transportation if required.
- **Dispose of contaminated wastes according to your facility's policy.** Waste containing blood or body fluids is considered biohazardous waste. Liquid waste can usually be disposed through the regular sewer system as long as there is no splashing, spraying, or aerosolizing of the waste as it is being disposed. Appropriate PPE needs to be worn, followed by proper removal and handwashing. Follow instructions at your facility.

It is essential that Standard Precautions be practiced on everyone in a nursing assistant's care, regardless of their infection status. When healthcare workers practice Standard Precautions, the risk of transmitting infection is greatly reduced. More information about Standard Precautions is found in the next several learning objectives.

5. Explain hand hygiene and identify when to wash hands

Nursing assistants use their hands constantly while they work. Microorganisms are on everything they touch. The single most common way for healthcare-associated infections (HAIs) to be spread is via the hands of healthcare workers. Handwashing is the most important thing NAs can do to prevent the spread of disease (Fig. 5-8).

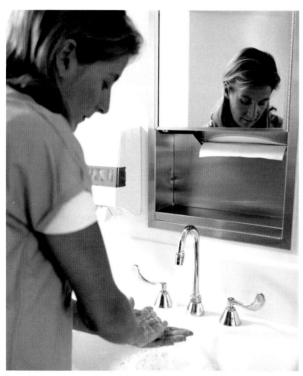

***Fig. 5-8.** All people working in health care must wash their hands often. Handwashing is the most effective measure in preventing the spread of disease.*

The CDC has defined **hand hygiene** as washing hands with either plain or antiseptic soap and water or using alcohol-based hand rubs. Alcohol-based hand rubs (often called *hand sanitizers*) include gels, rinses, and foams that do not require the use of water.

Alcohol-based hand rubs have proven effective in reducing bacteria on the skin. However, they are not a substitute for proper handwashing. When hands are visibly soiled, they should be washed using plain or antimicrobial soap and water. An **antimicrobial** agent destroys, resists, or prevents the development of pathogens. Once hands are clean, hand rubs can be used in addition to handwashing any time hands are not visibly soiled. When using a hand rub, the hands must be rubbed together until the product has completely dried. Hand lotion can help prevent dry, cracked skin.

Nursing assistants should avoid wearing rings while working. Rings may increase the risk of contamination. Fingernails should be short, smooth, and clean. Artificial nails or extenders should not be worn because they harbor bacteria and increase the risk of contamination.

Nursing assistants should wash their hands at these times:

- When first arriving at work
- Whenever hands are visibly soiled
- Before, between, and after all contact with residents
- Before putting on gloves and after removing gloves
- After contact with any body fluids, mucous membranes, non-intact skin, or wound dressings
- After handling contaminated items
- After contact with any object in the resident's room (care environment)
- Before and after touching meal trays and/or handling food
- Before and after feeding residents
- Before getting clean linen
- Before and after using the toilet

- After touching garbage or trash
- After picking up anything from the floor
- After nose-blowing or coughing or sneezing into hands
- Before and after eating
- After smoking
- After touching areas on the body, such as the mouth, face, eyes, hair, ears, or nose
- Before and after applying makeup
- After any contact with pets and after contact with pet care items
- Before leaving the facility

Washing hands (hand hygiene)

Equipment: soap, paper towels

1. Turn on water at sink. Keep your clothes dry because moisture breeds bacteria.
2. Wet hands and wrists thoroughly (Fig. 5-9).

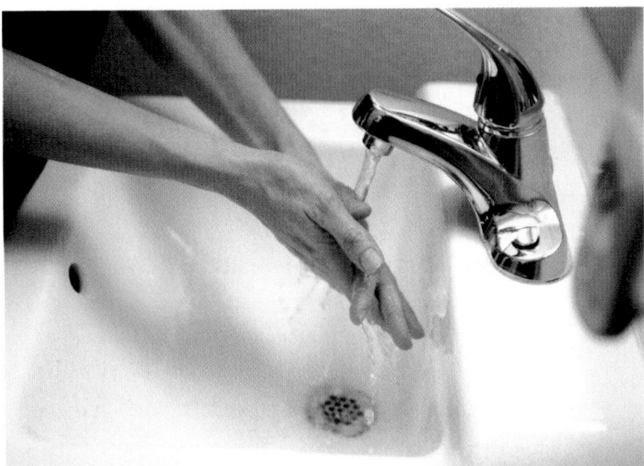

Fig. 5-9. *Keeping arms angled downward, wet hands and wrists thoroughly.*

3. Apply soap to your hands.
4. Keep your hands lower than your elbows and your fingertips down. Rub hands together and fingers between each other to create a lather. Lather all surfaces of wrists, fingers, and hands, using friction for at least 20 seconds. Friction helps clean (Fig. 5-10).

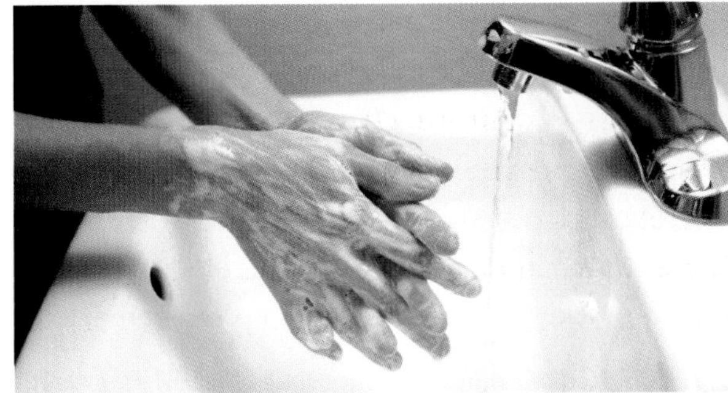

Fig. 5-10. *Using friction for at least 20 seconds, lather all surfaces of fingers and hands.*

5. Clean your nails by rubbing them in the palm of your other hand.
6. Being careful not to touch the sink, rinse thoroughly under running water. Rinse all surfaces of your hands and wrists. Run water down from wrists to fingertips (Fig. 5-11). Do not run water over unwashed arms down to clean hands.

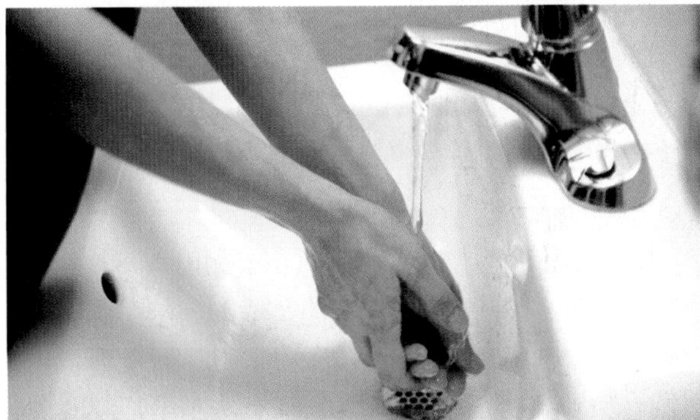

Fig. 5-11. *Rinse wrists and hands thoroughly without touching the sink. Let water run down from wrists to fingertips.*

7. Use a clean, dry paper towel to dry all surfaces of your hands, wrists, and fingers. Do not wipe towel on unwashed forearms and then wipe clean hands. Dispose of paper towel into waste container without touching the container. If your hands touch the sink or wastebasket, start over.
8. Use a clean, dry paper towel to turn off the faucet. Dispose of paper towel into waste container (Fig. 5-12). Do not contaminate your hands by touching the surface of the sink or faucet.

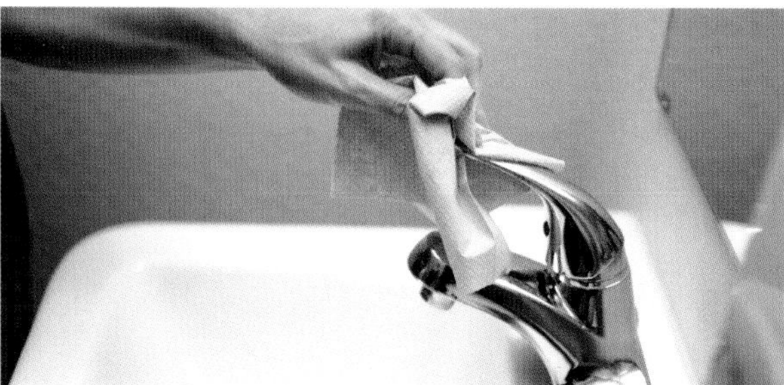

Fig. 5-12. Use a clean, dry paper towel to turn off faucet, so that you do not contaminate your hands.

6. Discuss the use of personal protective equipment (PPE) in facilities

Personal protective equipment (PPE) is equipment that helps protect employees from serious workplace injuries or illnesses resulting from contact with workplace hazards. In long-term care facilities, PPE helps protect nursing assistants from contact with potentially infectious material. Employers are responsible for providing nursing assistants with the appropriate PPE to wear.

Personal protective equipment includes gowns, masks, goggles, face shields, and gloves. Gowns protect the skin and/or clothing. Masks protect the mouth and nose. Goggles protect the eyes. Face shields protect the entire face—the eyes, nose, and mouth. Gloves protect the hands. Gloves are used most often by all caregivers.

Personal protective equipment must be worn if the caregiver could come into contact with body fluids, mucous membranes, or open wounds. Nursing assistants must wear, or **don**, gowns, masks, goggles, and face shields when splashing or spraying of body fluids or blood could occur.

Gowns

Clean, non-sterile gowns protect exposed skin. They also prevent soiling of clothing. Gowns should fully cover the torso. They should fit comfortably over the body, and have long sleeves that fit snugly at the wrists. When finished with a procedure, nursing assistants should remove, or **doff**, the gown as soon as possible and wash their hands.

Putting on (donning) and removing (doffing) gown

1. Wash your hands.
2. Open the gown. Hold it out in front of you and allow gown to open/unfold. Do not shake it (Fig. 5-13). Facing the back opening of the gown, place your arms through each sleeve.

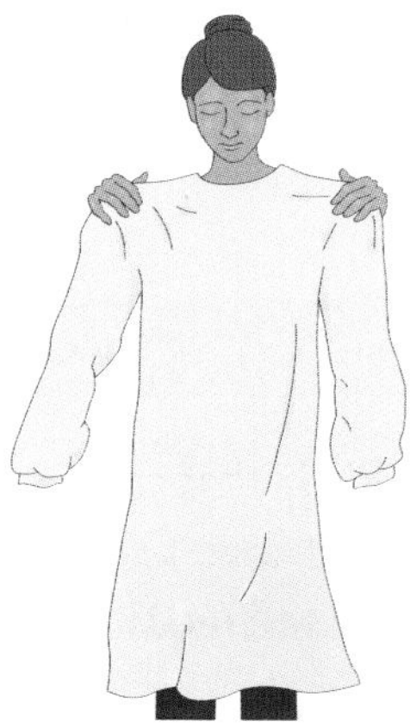

Fig. 5-13. Let the gown unfold without shaking it.

3. Fasten the neck opening.
4. Reaching behind you, pull the gown until it completely covers your clothing. Secure gown at waist (Fig. 5-14).

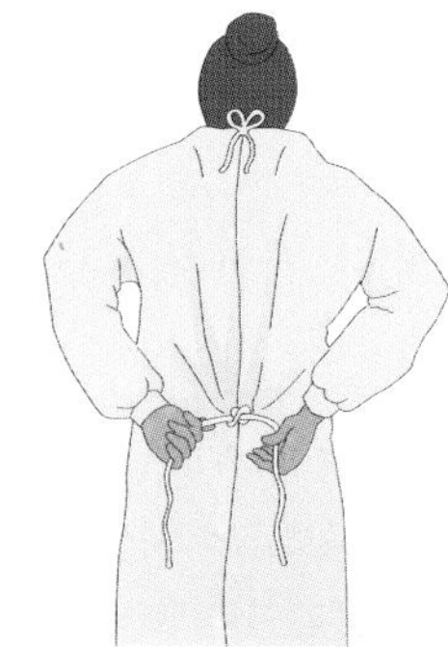

Fig. 5-14. Reaching behind you, secure the gown at the waist.

5. Use a gown only once and then remove and discard it. If gown becomes wet or soiled during care, remove it. Check your clothing, and put on a new gown. OSHA requires

non-permeable gowns—gowns that liquids cannot penetrate—when working in a bloody situation.

6. Put on your gloves after putting on gown. The cuffs of gloves should overlap the cuffs of the gown.
7. When removing a gown, remove and discard gloves properly (see procedure later in the chapter). Unfasten gown at neck and waist. Remove the gown without touching the outside of gown. Roll the dirty side in, while holding gown away from your body. Dispose of gown properly and wash your hands.

Masks and Goggles

Masks should be worn when caring for residents with respiratory illnesses. They should also be worn when it is likely that contact with blood or body fluids may occur. Sometimes special masks (respirators) are required for certain diseases, such as tuberculosis (TB). Masks should fully cover the nose and mouth and prevent fluid penetration. Masks should fit snugly over the nose and mouth. Nursing assistants must always change their masks when moving between residents; the same mask should not be worn from one resident to another. Goggles provide protection for the eyes. They are used when it is likely that blood or body fluids may be splashed or sprayed into the eye area or into the eyes. Eyeglasses alone do not provide proper eye protection. Goggles should fit snugly over and around the eyes or eyeglasses.

Putting on (donning) mask and goggles

1. Wash your hands.
2. Pick up the mask by top strings or elastic strap. Do not touch the mask where it touches your face.
3. Pull elastic strap over your head, or if mask has strings, tie top strings first, then bottom strings. Do not wear a mask hanging from only the bottom tie or strap. Masks must always be dry or they must be replaced. Never wear a mask hanging from only the bottom ties.
4. Pinch the metal strip at the top of the mask (if part of the mask) tightly around your nose so that it feels snug (Fig. 5-15).

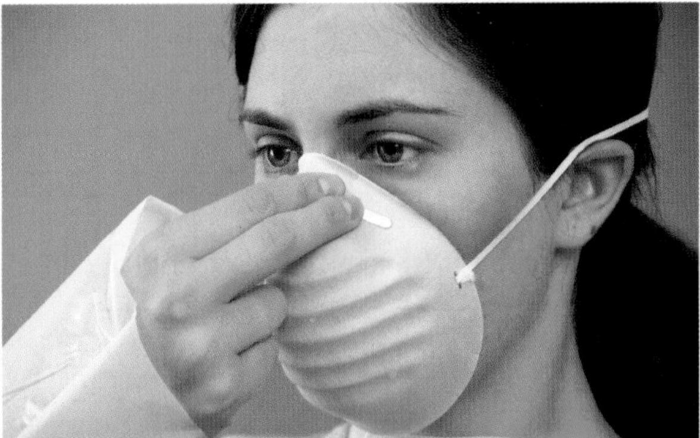

Fig. 5-15. *Adjust the metal strip until the mask fits snugly around your nose.*

5. Put on the goggles over your eyes or eyeglasses. Use the headband to secure them to your head. Make sure they are on snugly.
6. Put on gloves after putting on mask and goggles.

Face Shields

When additional skin protection is needed (if part of facility policy), a face shield can be substituted for a mask or goggles. The face shield should cover the forehead, go below the chin, and wrap around the sides of the face. The headband can secure it to the head.

Gloves

Facilities have specific policies and procedures on when to wear gloves. Nursing assistants must learn and follow these rules. Gloves must always be worn for the following tasks:

- Anytime the caregiver might come into contact with blood or any body fluid, open wounds, or mucous membranes

- When performing or helping with mouth care or care of any mucous membrane
- When performing or helping with **perineal care** (care of the genitals and anal area)
- When performing personal care on **non-intact skin**—skin that is broken by abrasions, cuts, rashes, acne, pimples, lesions, surgical incisions, or boils
- When assisting with personal care when the caregiver has open sores or cuts on her hands
- When shaving a resident
- When disposing of soiled bed linens, gowns, dressings, and pads
- When touching surfaces or equipment that is either visibly contaminated or may be contaminated

Clean, non-sterile gloves are generally adequate. They may be latex, nitrile, or vinyl; however, some people are allergic to latex. A nursing assistant should let the nurse know if he is allergic to latex. Alternative gloves will be provided. An NA should also tell the nurse if he has dry, cracked, or broken skin. Non-intact areas should be covered with bandages or gauze before putting on gloves. Gloves should fit the hands comfortably and should not be too loose or too tight.

Disposable gloves can only be worn once; they cannot be washed or reused. Gloves should be changed immediately if they become wet, worn, soiled, or torn. Gloves should also be changed before contact with mucous membranes or broken skin. After removing gloves, the NA should wash his hands before donning new gloves.

Putting on (donning) gloves

1. Wash your hands.
2. If you are right-handed, slide one glove on your left hand (reverse if left-handed).
3. Using your gloved hand, slide the other hand into the second glove.
4. Interlace fingers to smooth out folds and create a comfortable fit.
5. Carefully look for tears, holes, or discolored spots. Replace the glove if needed.
6. If wearing a gown, pull the cuff of the gloves over the sleeves of the gown (Fig. 5-16).

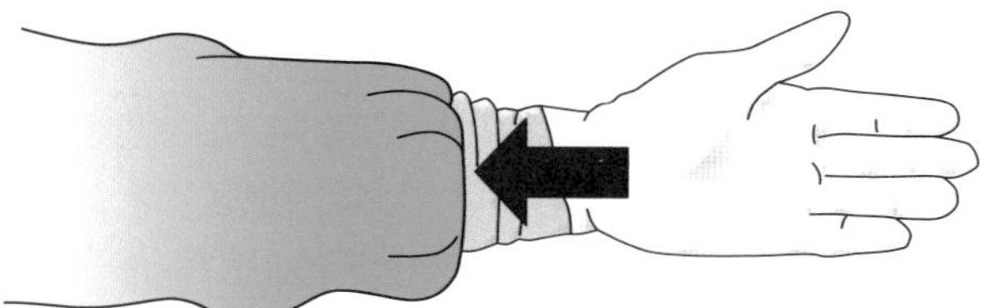

Fig. 5-16. *Adjust gloves until they are pulled up over the sleeves of the gown.*

Gloves should be removed, or doffed, promptly after use, and before caring for another resident. The NA should wash his hands. Gloves are worn to protect the skin from becoming contaminated. After giving care, gloves are contaminated. If the NA opens a door with the gloved hand, the doorknob becomes contaminated. Later, anyone who opens the door with an ungloved hand will be touching a contaminated surface. Before touching surfaces or leaving residents' rooms, the NA must remove gloves and wash his hands. Afterward, new gloves can be donned if necessary.

Removing (doffing) gloves

1. Touch only the outside of one glove. With one gloved hand, grasp the other glove at the palm and pull the glove off (Fig. 5-17).

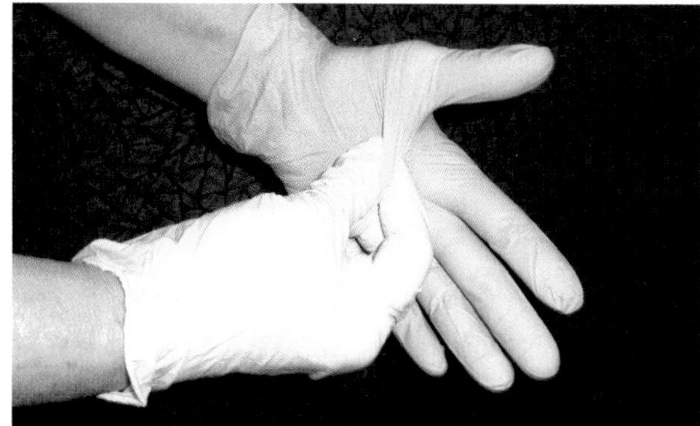

Fig. 5-17. *Grasp the glove at the palm and pull it off.*

2. With the fingertips of your gloved hand, hold the glove you just removed. With your ungloved hand, slip two fingers underneath cuff of the remaining glove at wrist. Do not touch any part of the outside of glove (Fig. 5-18).

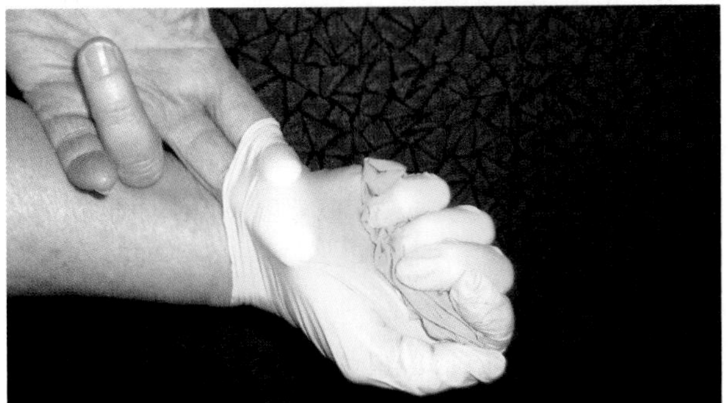

Fig. 5-18. *Reach inside glove at wrist, without touching any part of the outside of glove.*

3. Pull down, turning this glove inside out and over the first glove as you remove it.
4. You should now be holding one glove from its clean inner side and the other glove should be inside it.
5. Drop both gloves into the proper container without contaminating yourself.
6. Wash your hands.

The nursing assistant's employer will provide PPE as needed. It is the NA's responsibility to know where it is kept and how to use it (Fig. 5-19). A specific order must be followed when donning and doffing PPE. This is the correct order that the NA should follow when donning (putting on) PPE:

1. Wash hands.
2. Put on gown.
3. Put on mask.
4. Put on goggles or face shield.
5. Put on gloves.

This is the correct order that the NA should follow when doffing (removing) PPE:

1. Remove and discard gloves.
2. Remove goggles or face shield.
3. Remove and discard gown.
4. Remove and discard mask.
5. Wash hands. Washing hands is always the final step after removing and disposing of PPE.

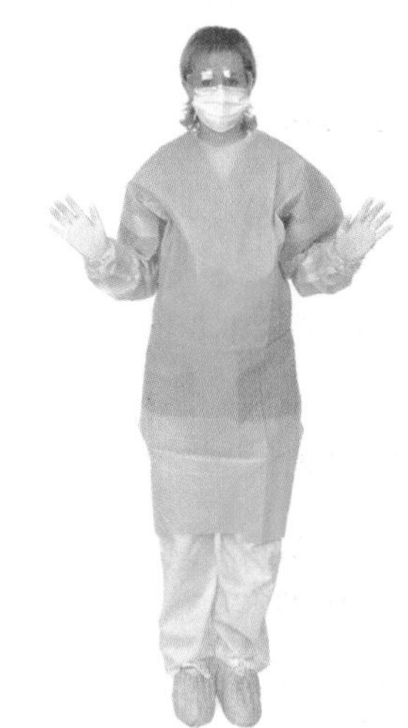

Fig. 5-19. *Using PPE is an important way to reduce the spread of infection.*

OSHA and PPE

OSHA states that it is the employer's responsibility to instruct the staff on how to properly put on (don) the PPE, how to wear the PPE effectively, and how to safely remove (doff) the PPE. This instruction needs to be given before the employee is in a situation where PPE is indicated and as an annual review.

7. List guidelines for handling equipment and linen

In health care, an object is called **clean** if it has not been contaminated with pathogens. An object that is **dirty** has been contaminated with pathogens. Measures like disinfection and sterilization decrease the spread of pathogens that could cause disease.

Disinfection is a process that kills pathogens. However, disinfection does not destroy all pathogens. It reduces the pathogen count to a level that is considered not infectious. Disinfection is carried out with pasteurization or chemical germicides. Examples of items that are usually disinfected are reusable oxygen tanks, wall mounted blood pressure cuffs, and any reusable resident care equipment.

Sterilization is a measure that destroys all microorganisms, including pathogens. This includes those that form spores. Spore-forming microorganisms are a special group of organisms that produce a protective covering that is difficult to penetrate. Sterilization is accomplished through the use of special machines and devices. An autoclave is a machine that sterilizes objects by using hot steam under pressure. Liquid or gas chemicals and dry heat are other ways to sterilize objects. Items that need to be sterilized are ones that go directly into the bloodstream or into other normally sterile areas of the body (for example, surgical instruments).

Facilities have special rooms or areas for equipment, linen, and supplies. There are separate rooms for supplies that are considered clean and for supplies that are considered dirty or contaminated (Fig. 5-20). Nursing assistants will be told where these rooms are located and what types of equipment and supplies are found in each room. NAs should perform hand hygiene before entering clean rooms and before leaving dirty rooms. This helps prevent the spread of pathogens.

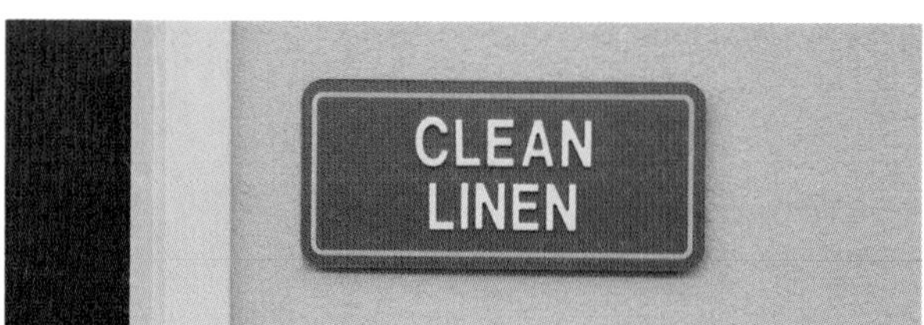

Fig. 5-20. *There are separate rooms in facilities for clean and dirty equipment, linen, and supplies.*

Guidelines: Handling Equipment, Linen, and Clothing

- Handle all equipment in a way that prevents
  - Skin/mucous membrane contact
  - Contamination of your clothing
  - Transfer of disease to other residents or areas
- Do not use reusable equipment again until it has been properly cleaned and reprocessed.
- Dispose of all single-use, or disposable, equipment properly. **Disposable** means it is discarded after one use. Disposable razors and disposable thermometers are examples of disposable equipment.
- Clean and disinfect
  - All environmental surfaces
  - Beds, bedrails, and all bedside equipment
  - All frequently touched surfaces (such as doorknobs, call lights, and handles on dressers and tables)
- Handle, transport, and process soiled linens and clothing in a way that prevents
  - Skin and mucous membrane exposure
  - Contamination of clothing (hold linen and clothing away from your uniform) (Fig. 5-21)
  - Transfer of disease to other residents and areas (do not shake linen or clothes; fold or roll linen so that the dirtiest area is inside; do not put soiled linen on floor)

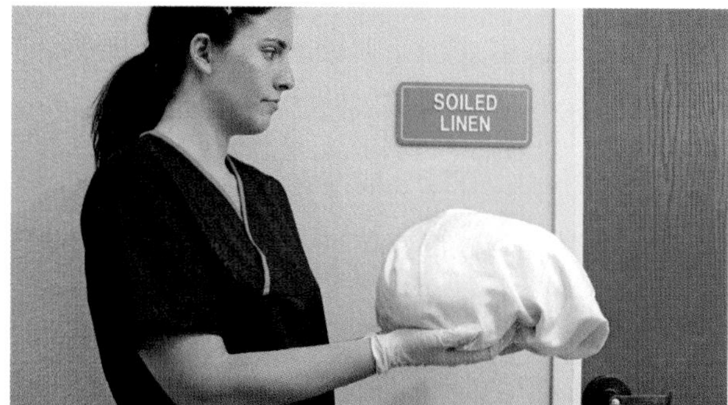

Fig. 5-21. *Hold and carry dirty linen away from your uniform.*

- Bag soiled linen at point of origin.
- Sort soiled linen away from resident care areas.
- Place wet linen in leakproof bags.

More information about cleaning equipment and supplies is in Chapter 12.

8. Explain how to handle spills

Spills, especially those involving blood or body fluids, can pose a serious risk of infection, and can put residents and staff at risk for falls.

Nursing assistants must clean spills using the proper solution and equipment.

Guidelines: Cleaning Spills Involving Blood, Body Fluids, or Glass

- G Apply gloves before starting. In some cases, industrial-strength gloves are best.
- G First, absorb the spill with whatever product is used by the facility. It may be an absorbing powder.
- G Scoop up the absorbed spill, and dispose of it in a designated container.
- G Apply the proper disinfectant to the spill area and allow it to stand wet for a minimum of 10 minutes.
- G Clean up spills immediately with the proper cleaning solution.
- G Do not pick up any pieces of broken glass, no matter how large, with your hands. Use a dustpan and broom or other tools.
- G Waste containing broken glass, blood, or body fluids should be properly bagged. Waste containing blood or body fluids may need to be placed in a special biohazard waste bag. Follow facility policy.

Cleaning Spills

Many facilities use special clean-up kits for spills. Nursing assistants should follow directions when using these kits. The CDC states that it is important to absorb and remove the fluid first. Disinfectant should not be placed directly on the spilled fluid. The spilled fluid may neutralize the disinfectant upon contact.

9. Explain Transmission-Based Precautions

The CDC set forth a second level of precautions beyond Standard Precautions. These precautions are used when caring for persons who are infected or suspected of being infected with a disease. These precautions are called **Transmission-Based Precautions**. When ordered, these precautions are used in addition to Standard Precautions. These precautions will always be listed in the resident's care plan and on the nursing assistant's assignment sheet. Following these precautions promotes the nursing assistant's safety, as well as the safety of others.

There are three categories of Transmission-Based Precautions:

- Airborne Precautions
- Droplet Precautions
- Contact Precautions

The category used depends on the disease and how it spreads to other people. They may also be used in combination for diseases that have multiple routes of transmission. Conditions that require Transmission-Based Precautions in addition to Standard Precautions include the following:

- **Multidrug-resistant organisms (MDROs)** (microorganisms, mostly bacteria, that are resistant to one or more antimicrobial agents that are commonly used for treatment), such as methicillin-resistant *Staphylococcus aureus* (MRSA) and vancomycin-resistant *enterococcus* (VRE) *
- *Clostridium difficile (C. diff or C. difficile)* *
- Scabies (a skin disease that causes itching)
- Lice
- Influenza (during an outbreak)

* There is more information about these infections later in the chapter.

Airborne Precautions

Airborne Precautions are used for diseases that are transmitted, or spread, through the air after being expelled (Fig. 5-22). The pathogens are so small that they can attach to moisture in the air and remain floating for some time. For certain care procedures, nursing assistants may be required to wear a special mask, such as N95 or HEPA masks, to avoid being infected. Airborne diseases include tuberculosis, measles, and chickenpox. More information on tuberculosis is found later in this chapter.

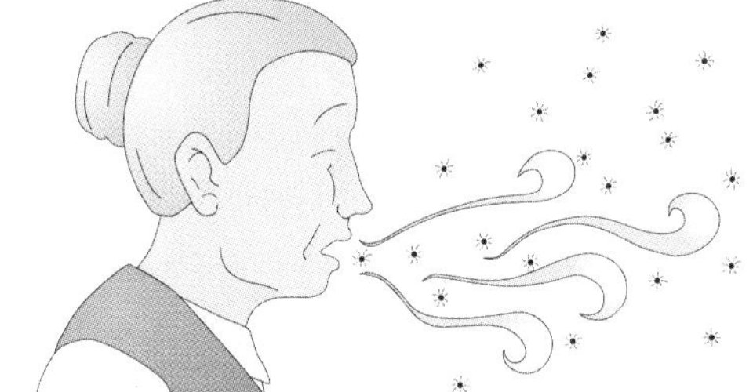

Fig. 5-22. Airborne diseases are used for diseases that can be transmitted through the air.

Droplet Precautions

Droplet Precautions are used for diseases that are spread by droplets in the air. Droplets normally do not travel more than three feet, but they may travel further. For example, the CDC recommends increasing the droplet distance from three feet to six feet for influenza. Coughing, sneezing, laughing, talking, or suctioning can spread droplets (Fig. 5-23). Droplet Precautions include wearing a face mask during care procedures and restricting visits from uninfected people. Residents should wear masks, if they are able to do so, when being moved from room to room. Nursing assistants should cover their noses and mouths with a tissue when they sneeze or cough, and ask others to do the same. Used tissues should be disposed of in the nearest waste container. Used tissues should not be placed in a pocket for later use. If a tissue is not available, NAs should cough or sneeze into their upper sleeve or elbow, not their hands. They should wash their hands immediately afterward. An example of a droplet disease is mumps.

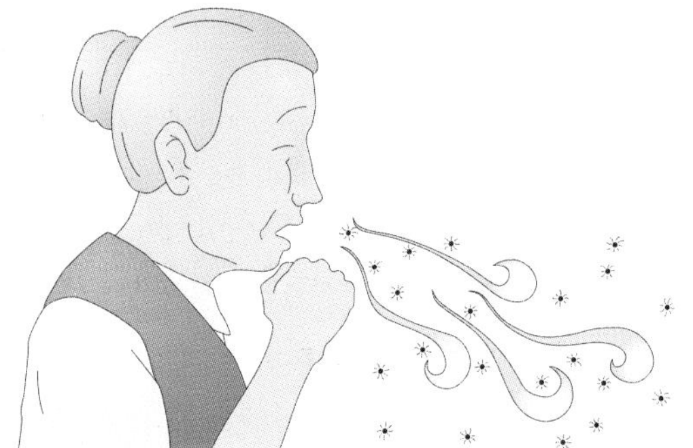

Fig. 5-23. Droplet Precautions are followed when the disease-causing microorganism does not remain in the air.

Respiratory Hygiene/Cough Etiquette

The CDC has set forth special infection prevention measures to prevent the transmission of all respiratory infections in healthcare settings. They are a part of Standard Precautions and include the following:

1. Post visual alerts at the entrances of care facilities instructing that all patients and visitors inform staff of symptoms of respiratory infections and to practice respiratory hygiene/cough etiquette.

2. All individuals with signs and symptoms of a respiratory infection must do the following:

- Cover their noses/mouths with a tissue when coughing or sneezing.
- Dispose of used tissues in the nearest waste container after use.
- Perform hand hygiene (washing hands with soap and water, using an alcohol-based hand rub or an antiseptic handwash) after contact with respiratory secretions and contaminated objects.

Healthcare facilities must make these items available to staff, patients, and visitors:

- Tissues and no-touch receptacles for used tissue disposal
- Conveniently located hand rub dispensers and handwashing supplies in areas where sinks are located

3. During times of increased respiratory infections, offer masks to anyone who is coughing, and encourage coughing people to sit at least three feet away from others in waiting areas.

4. Advise healthcare personnel to observe Droplet Precautions, in addition to Standard Precautions, when examining a patient with symptoms of a respiratory infection, particularly if fever is present.

Contact Precautions

Contact Precautions are used when there is a risk of spreading or contracting a microorganism by touching an infected object or person (Fig. 5-24). For example, bacteria could infect an open skin wound. Conjunctivitis (pink eye) and *Clostridium difficile* infection are examples of situations that require Contact Precautions. Transmission can occur with skin-to-skin contact during transfers or bathing.

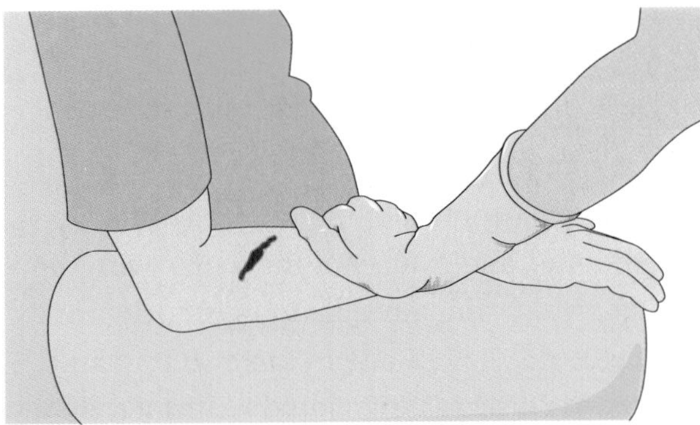

Fig. 5-24. Contact Precautions are followed when the person is at risk of transmitting a microorganism by touching an infected object or person.

Contact Precautions include wearing PPE and resident isolation. Contact Precautions require washing hands with antimicrobial soap and not touching infected surfaces with ungloved hands or uninfected surfaces with contaminated gloves.

Staff often refer to residents who need Transmission-Based Precautions as being in isolation. A sign should be on the door indicating *Isolation* or *Contact Precautions* and alerting people to see the nurse before entering the room. Other guidelines for NAs to follow include the following:

Guidelines: Isolation

- G When they are indicated, Transmission-Based Precautions are always used **in addition** to Standard Precautions.
- G Nurses will set up the isolation unit. Some facilities have a special room where isolation supplies are kept. Some facilities keep supplies within the room itself, while other facilities set up an isolation cart outside the room. Isolation supplies consist of gloves, masks, gowns or aprons, and, if indicated, goggles, face shields, respirator masks, or other forms of specialized personal protective equipment (PPE).
- G You will be told the proper PPE to wear for care of each resident in isolation. Make sure to put on the PPE properly and remove it safely. Remove PPE and place it in the appropriate container before exiting a resident's room. PPE cannot be worn outside the resident's room. Perform hand hygiene following removal of PPE and again after exiting the resident's room. In addition to handwashing areas within the resident's room, there may be an alcohol-based hand rub dispenser mounted on the wall inside the room as you exit.
- G Do not share equipment between residents. Use disposable supplies that can be discarded after use whenever possible. Use dedicated (only for use by one resident) equipment when disposable is not an option. For example, a resident in isolation has her own (dedicated) blood pressure cuff and stethoscope. Disposable thermometers are used to take her temperature. When using disposable supplies, discard them in the resident's room before leaving. Be careful not to contaminate reusable equipment by setting it on furniture or counters in the resident's room. When the resident is discharged or no longer needs the additional precautions, properly dispose of dedicated equipment if required. If the dedicated equipment is to be used for other residents, it should be cleaned and disinfected after use.
- G Wear the proper PPE, if indicated, when serving food and drink to residents in isolation. Do not leave uneaten food uncovered in the resident's room. When the meal is completed, remove the meal tray and take it to the designated area, or put it back on the food cart. When the food carts are returned to the kitchen, all soiled trays will be handled with gloves by the dietary staff, and the tray and dinnerware will be cleaned and sanitized.
- G Follow Standard Precautions when dealing with body waste removal. Wear gloves when touching or handling waste. Wear gowns and goggles when indicated. The waste must be

disposed of in such a manner as to minimize splashing and spraying.

- G If required to take a specimen from a resident in isolation, wear the proper PPE. Collect the specimen and place it in the appropriate container without the outside of the container coming into contact with the specimen. Properly remove your PPE and dispose of it in the room. Perform hand hygiene before leaving the room and take the specimen to the nurse.
- G Residents need to feel that their circumstances and feelings are appreciated and understood by members of the care team without criticism or judgment. Listen to what your resident is telling you and allow time to talk with your resident about his concerns. Reassure residents that it is the disease, not the person, that is being isolated. Explain why these steps are being taken. Relay any requests outside your scope of practice to the nurse.

Residents' Rights

Isolation

Residents' basic needs remain the same while in isolation. Basic human needs do not change, even though physical conditions may change. NAs should not avoid a resident in isolation. They should not rush through care tasks or make the resident feel that he or she should be avoided. Being professional, caring, and competent may help lessen a resident's worries or concerns and feelings about being isolated. If an NA has questions about the care he is providing, he should talk to the charge nurse.

10. Define *bloodborne pathogens* and describe two major bloodborne diseases

Bloodborne pathogens are microorganisms found in human blood that can cause infection and disease in humans. They may also be found in body fluids, draining wounds, and mucous membranes. Bloodborne diseases can be transmitted by infected blood entering the bloodstream, or if infected semen or vaginal secretions contact mucous membranes. Having sexual contact with someone carrying the disease can also transmit a bloodborne disease. Sexual contact includes sexual intercourse (vaginal and anal), contact of the mouth with the genitals or anus, and contact of the hands with the genital area. Using a needle to inject drugs and sharing needles with others can also transmit bloodborne diseases. In addition, infected mothers may transmit bloodborne diseases to their babies in the womb or at birth.

In health care, contact with infected blood or body fluids is the most common way to be infected with a bloodborne disease. Infections can be spread through contact with contaminated blood or body fluids, needles or other sharp objects, or contaminated supplies or equipment. Standard Precautions, handwashing, isolation, and using PPE are all methods of preventing transmission of bloodborne diseases. Employers are required by law to help prevent exposure to bloodborne pathogens. Following Standard Precautions and other procedures helps protect caregivers from bloodborne diseases.

Nursing assistants can safely touch, hug, and spend time talking with residents who have a bloodborne disease (Fig. 5-25). They need the same thoughtful, personal attention NAs give to all their residents. NAs need to follow Standard Precautions, but should never isolate residents emotionally because they have a bloodborne disease.

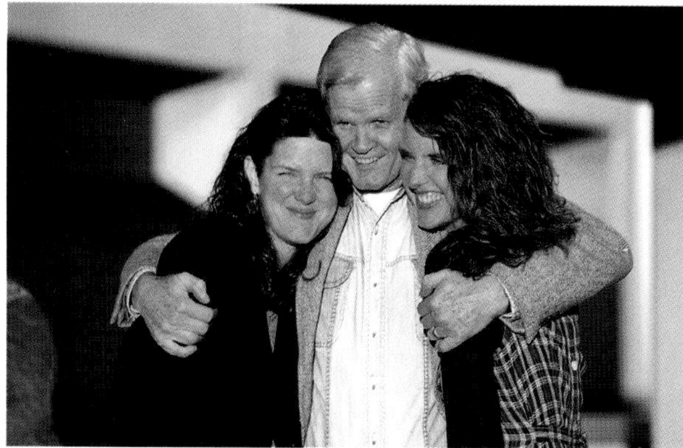

Fig. 5-25. *Hugs and touches cannot spread a bloodborne disease.*

The major bloodborne diseases in the United States are acquired immune deficiency syndrome (AIDS) and the viral hepatitis family. **HIV** stands for human immunodeficiency virus, and it is the virus that can cause AIDS. Over time, HIV weakens the immune system so that the body cannot effectively fight infections. Some HIV-infected people will develop AIDS, which is the final stage of HIV infection. People with AIDS lose all ability to fight infection. They can die from illnesses that a healthy body could handle. Chapter 18 contains more information about HIV and AIDS.

Hepatitis is inflammation of the liver caused by certain viruses and other factors, such as alcohol abuse, some medications, and trauma. Liver function can be permanently damaged by hepatitis. Several different viruses can cause hepatitis. The most common types of hepatitis are A, B, and C. Hepatitis B and C are bloodborne diseases that can cause death. Many more people have hepatitis B (HBV) than HIV. In the United States today, the risk of getting hepatitis is greater than the risk of acquiring HIV.

The virus causing hepatitis A (HAV) is spread as a result of fecal-oral contamination, which means through food or water contaminated by stool from an infected person.

Hepatitis B (HBV) is a bloodborne disease. It is spread through sexual contact, by sharing infected needles, and from a mother to her baby during delivery. It is also spread by exposure at work from accidental contact with infected needles or other sharps or from splashing blood. The hepatitis B virus can survive outside the body at least seven days and can still cause infection in others during that time. HBV may cause few symptoms or may become a severe infection. HBV can cause short-term illness that leads to

- Loss of appetite
- Diarrhea and vomiting
- Fatigue
- **Jaundice** (a condition in which the skin, whites of the eyes, and mucous membranes appear yellow)
- Pain in muscles, joints, and stomach

It can also cause long-term illness that leads to

- Liver damage (cirrhosis)
- Liver cancer
- Death

HBV is a serious threat to healthcare workers. Employers must offer nursing assistants a free vaccine to protect them from hepatitis B. The HBV vaccine can prevent hepatitis B. The hepatitis B vaccine is usually given as a series of three shots. Prevention is the best option for dealing with this disease. NAs should take the vaccine when it is offered.

Hepatitis C (HCV) is also transmitted through blood or body fluids and, possibly, sexual intercourse. Hepatitis C can lead to cirrhosis and liver cancer; it can even cause death. There is no vaccine for hepatitis C.

Less common types of hepatitis in the United States are hepatitis D (HDV) and hepatitis E (HEV). Hepatitis D is transmitted by blood. It is only found in people who carry the hepatitis B virus. Hepatitis E (HEV) is transmitted by the fecal-oral route, usually through contaminated water. Although HEV is rare in the United States, it is more common in many other parts of the world.

11. Explain OSHA's Bloodborne Pathogens Standard

OSHA has set standards for special procedures that must be followed in healthcare facilities. One of these is the **Bloodborne Pathogens Standard**. This law requires that healthcare facilities protect employees from bloodborne health hazards. By law, employers must follow these rules to reduce or eliminate the risk of exposure to infectious diseases. The standard also guides employers and employees through the steps to follow if exposed to infectious material. Significant exposures include the following:

- Exposure by injection; a needle stick
- Mucous membrane contact
- Cut from an object containing a potentially infectious body fluid (includes human bites)
- Having non-intact skin (OSHA includes acne in this category)

Guidelines employers must follow include the following:

- Employers must have a written **exposure control plan** designed to eliminate or reduce employee exposure to infectious material. This plan identifies, step by step, what to do if an employee is exposed to infectious material (for example, if an NA is stuck by a needle). This includes medical treatment and plans to prevent any similar exposures. It also includes specific work practices that must be followed. This plan must be accessible to all employees, and they must receive training on the plan.
- Employers must give all employees, visitors, and residents proper personal protective equipment (PPE) to wear when needed at no cost. Employers must make sure the PPE is available in the appropriate sizes and is readily accessible.
- Employers must make biohazard containers available for disposal of sharps and other infectious waste. These containers must be puncture-resistant, labeled or color-coded, and leakproof.
- Employers must provide a free hepatitis B vaccine to all employees after hire.
- Warning labels must be affixed to waste containers and refrigerators and freezers that contain blood or any other potentially infectious material.
- Employers must keep a log of injuries from contaminated sharps. The information recorded must protect the confidentiality of the injured employee. Employers are also required to select safer needle devices and to involve employees in choosing these devices.
- Employers must provide training for employees to explain the Bloodborne Pathogens Standard and its contents.

When an employee is exposed to blood or other potentially infectious material, an incident report or a special exposure report form must be completed. Tests and follow-up care may be needed. The employer will take steps to help keep the employee from becoming sick. Steps will also be taken to help keep similar incidents from occurring again. Nursing assistants must report any potential exposures immediately. Doing this helps protect their health and that of others. OSHA's website has more information at osha.gov.

12. Define *tuberculosis* and list infection prevention guidelines

Tuberculosis, or **TB**, is a highly contagious lung disease caused by a bacterium that is carried on mucous droplets suspended in the air. TB is an airborne disease. When a person infected with TB talks, coughs, breathes, sings, laughs, or sneezes, he may release mucous droplets carrying the disease. TB usually infects the lungs, causing coughing, trouble breathing, fever, weight loss, and fatigue (Fig. 5-26). Usually TB can be cured by taking all prescribed medication. However, if left untreated, TB may cause death.

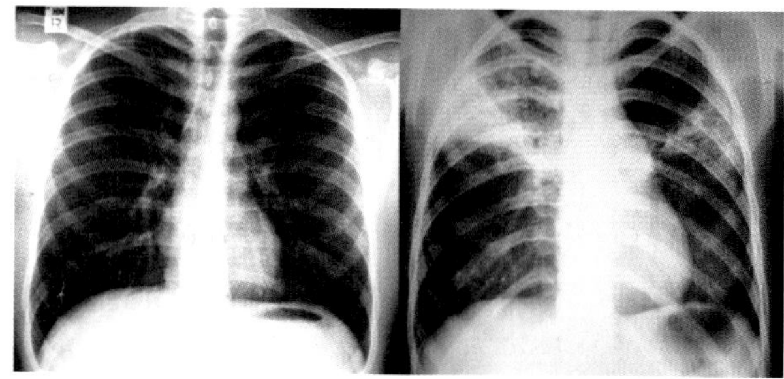

Fig. 5-26. *A normal lung X-ray on the left, and an X-ray of a lung with TB on the right.*

There are two types of TB: **latent TB infection** and **TB disease**. Someone with latent TB infection carries the disease but does not show symptoms and cannot infect others. However, if TB bacteria become active and multiply in the body, latent TB infection progresses to TB disease. A person with TB disease shows symptoms of the disease and can spread TB to others. The signs and symptoms of TB disease include the following:

- Fatigue
- Loss of appetite
- Weight loss
- Slight fever and chills
- Night sweats
- Prolonged coughing
- Coughing up blood
- Chest pain
- Shortness of breath
- Trouble breathing

Tuberculosis is more likely to be spread in small, confined, or poorly ventilated places. TB is more likely to develop in people whose immune systems are weakened by illness, malnutrition, alcoholism, or drug abuse. People with cancer or HIV/AIDS are more susceptible to developing TB disease. This is due to their weakened immune systems.

Multidrug-resistant TB (MDR-TB) is a type of TB that can develop when a person with TB disease does not take all the prescribed medication. **Resistant** means drugs no longer work to kill the specific bacteria. When the full course of medication is not taken, bacteria remain in the body and are less likely to be killed by the TB medication. If the TB bacilli develop a resistance to the drugs that treat TB, fighting the disease becomes more difficult. Surgery may be the only option for treatment. However, if the disease is widespread throughout both lungs, surgery may not be possible.

Guidelines: Tuberculosis

G Follow Standard Precautions and Airborne Precautions.

G Wear personal protective equipment as instructed. Special masks, such as N95, high efficiency particulate air (HEPA), or other masks, must be used. These masks filter out very small particles, such as the bacteria that cause TB. You must be fit-tested for these special masks. You will also be trained on how to use the masks.

G Use special care when handling sputum or phlegm. **Phlegm** is thick mucus from the respiratory passage.

G Residents with TB will be placed in a special airborne infection isolation room (AIIR). Other names for the isolation room may be *Negative Air Pressure Room* or *Acid-Fast Bacillus (AFB) isolation room*. In this type of room, the flow of air is carefully controlled. Airborne particles are not trapped in the room. The air is changed often through a special air system. The air is exhausted directly outside or forced through filters to remove particles. The room will be marked with a sign identifying it as a special respiratory isolation room. When entering this room, do not open or close the door quickly. This pulls contaminated room air into the hallway. The door should remain closed as much as possible.

G Follow isolation procedures for airborne diseases if directed.

G Help the resident remember to take all medication prescribed. Failure to take all medication is a major factor in the spread of TB.

13. Discuss MRSA, VRE, and C. *Difficile*

Multidrug-resistant organisms (MDROs) are microorganisms, mostly bacteria, that are resistant to one or more antimicrobial agents that are commonly used for treatment. MDROs are increasing, and this is a serious problem. Two common types of MDROs are methicillin-resistant *Staphylococcus aureus*, commonly called MRSA, and vancomycin-resistant *enterococcus*, called VRE.

Staphylococcus aureus is a common type of bacteria that can cause illness. Methicillin is a powerful antibiotic drug. **MRSA** is an antibiotic-resistant infection often acquired in healthcare facilities. This type of MRSA is also known as *HA-MRSA*, which stands for *hospital-associated MRSA*.

Community-associated methicillin-resistant *Staphylococcus aureus* (CA-MRSA) is a type of MRSA infection that occurs in people who have not recently been admitted to healthcare facilities and who have no past diagnosis of MRSA. Often CA-MRSA manifests as skin infections, such as boils or pimples. This type of infection is becoming more common.

MRSA is almost always spread by direct physical contact with infected people. This means if a person has MRSA on his skin, especially on the hands, and touches another person, he may spread MRSA. Spread also occurs through indirect contact by touching equipment or supplies (for example, towels, sheets, wound dressings, or clothes) contaminated by a person with MRSA.

Nursing assistants can help prevent MRSA by practicing good hygiene. Handwashing, using soap and warm water, is the single most important measure to control the spread of MRSA. NAs must always follow Standard Precautions, along with Transmission-Based Precautions, as ordered. Cuts and abrasions should be kept clean and covered with a proper dressing (e.g., bandage) until healed. Contact with other people's wounds or material that is contaminated from wounds should be avoided.

VRE stands for vancomycin-resistant *enterococcus. Enterococci* are bacteria that live in the digestive and genital tracts. They normally do not cause problems in healthy people. Vancomycin is a powerful antibiotic used to treat bacterial infections. Vancomycin-resistant *enterococci* are bacteria that have developed resistance to antibiotics as a result of being exposed to vancomycin. VRE is spread through direct and indirect contact.

Symptoms of VRE infection include fever, fatigue, chills, and drainage. VRE infections are often difficult to treat and may require the use of several medications. VRE infections can cause life-threatening infections in those with compromised immune systems—the very young, the very old, and the very ill.

Preventing VRE is much easier than trying to treat it. Proper hand hygiene can help prevent the spread of VRE. Nursing assistants should wash their hands often and wear PPE as directed. NAs must always follow Standard Precautions, along with Transmission-Based Precautions, as ordered. Items may need to be disinfected, and that information should be listed in the care plan.

Clostridium difficile infection is commonly known as ***C. diff*** or ***C. difficile.*** It is a spore-forming bacterium which can be part of the normal intestinal flora. When the normal intestinal flora is altered, *C. difficile* can flourish in the intestinal tract. It produces a toxin that causes a watery diarrhea. Enemas, nasogastric tube insertion, and GI tract surgery increase a person's risk of developing the disease. The elderly are at a higher risk of getting *C. difficile* infection. The overuse of antibiotics may also alter the normal intestinal flora and increase the risk of developing *C. difficile.* It can also cause colitis, a more serious intestinal condition.

When released in the environment, *C. difficile* can form a spore that makes it difficult to kill. These spores can be carried on the hands of people who have direct contact with infected residents or with environmental surfaces (floors, bedpans, toilets, etc.) contaminated with *C.*

difficile. Touching an object contaminated with *C. difficile* can transmit *C. difficile*. Alcohol-based hand sanitizers are not considered effective on *C. difficile*. Soap and water must be used each time hand hygiene is performed.

Symptoms of *C. difficile* include frequent, foul-smelling, watery stools. Other symptoms include diarrhea that contains blood and mucus, nausea, lack of appetite, and abdominal cramps. Proper handwashing with soap and water is vital in preventing the spread of the disease. Handling contaminated wastes properly can help prevent the spread of the disease. Cleaning surfaces with an appropriate disinfectant, such as bleach, can also help. Limiting the use of antibiotics helps lower the risk of developing *C. difficile* diarrhea.

14. List employer and employee responsibilities for infection prevention

Several state and federal government agencies have guidelines and laws concerning infection prevention. OSHA requires employers to provide for the safety of their employees through rules and suggested guidelines. The CDC issues guidelines for healthcare workers to follow on the job. Some states have additional requirements. Facilities consider these rules very carefully when writing their policies and procedures. It is important that nursing assistants learn these policies and procedures and follow them. They exist to protect all staff members and residents. Some infection prevention requirements for NAs and their employers are listed below.

Employers' responsibilities for infection prevention include the following:

- Establish infection prevention procedures and an exposure control plan to protect workers
- Provide continuing in-service education on infection prevention, including education on bloodborne and airborne pathogens and updates on any new safety standards
- Have written procedures to follow should an exposure occur, including medical treatment and plans to prevent similar exposures
- Provide personal protective equipment (PPE) for employees to use and teach them when and how to properly use it
- Provide free hepatitis B vaccinations for all employees

Employees' responsibilities for infection prevention include the following:

- Follow Standard Precautions
- Follow all of the facility's policies and procedures
- Follow care plans and assignments
- Use provided personal protective equipment as indicated or as appropriate
- Take advantage of the free hepatitis B vaccination
- Immediately report any exposure to infection
- Participate in annual education programs covering the prevention of infection

Chapter Review

1. What does *infection prevention* mean?
2. How does infection occur?
3. What is the chain of infection?
4. Which link in the chain of infection is broken by wearing gloves, and why?
5. Define the term *mucous membranes*.
6. Why are elderly people at a higher risk for infection?
7. Under Standard Precautions, what does body fluids include?
8. On whom should Standard Precautions be practiced?
9. What is the single most important thing a nursing assistant can do to prevent the spread of disease?

10. What is hand hygiene? It is the process of properly washing hands with plain or anticeptic soap. (Also alchol-based handrubs)
11. For how long should a nursing assistant use friction when washing her hands? For at least 20 seconds.
12. How many times can disposable gloves be worn? Only once!
13. In what order should PPE be donned? In what order should it be doffed? Wash hands, put on gown, put on mask, put on goggles or face shield. Last put on gloves
14. What is always the final step after removing PPE? The final step is to wash your hands again
15. Define *sterilization*. Define *disinfection*. sterilization is also sergical asepsis – free of all microorganisms. disinfection is also medical asepsis – reduced microorganisms that could contribute to disease
16. How should soiled linen be carried? Away from your uniform & any exposed body part.
17. When blood or body fluids are spilled, what should an NA do first, before starting to clean the spill? Always apply gloves. The absorb spill as facility instructs Us disinfect on area " " " Dispose of contaminated materials as facility instructs.
18. What are Transmission-Based Precautions?
19. If an NA sneezes and does not have a tissue, into what area of the body should she sneeze? Where her elbow bends or her upper sleeve
20. What are bloodborne pathogens? Microorganisms found in human blood that can cause infection & disease in humans.
21. How are bloodborne diseases transmitted? What is the most common way to be infected with a bloodborne disease in a healthcare setting? By infected blood entering the bloodstream If infected persons body fluids contact mucus membranes Sexual contact. Hands with cuts etc. contacting mucus areas. By coming in contact with infected blood or body fluids / needles & sharp objects & containated equipment
22. What does HIV do to a person's immune system? It weakens the immune system so the person connot fight infections which leads to aids (Aquired immune deficiency syndrome)
23. What is hepatitis? It is an inflammation of the liver caused by viruses or maybe med's, trauma, alcohol etc. The liver function can be permanently damaged by hepatitus.
24. How is hepatitis B (HBV) contracted? You can be vaccinated for this virus. It is contracted by contact with blood or sharp needle pricks By sexual contact. Same as any blood borne disease
25. Describe what an exposure control plan is. It is designed to eliminate or reduce exposure to infectious materials for employees. It has a step by step plan of what to do if they are exposed. Employers must provide PPE free. Employees receive training on the plan.
26. List four guidelines employers must follow under the Bloodborne Pathogen Standard. Warning labels have to be fixed on waste containers, refrigerators & freezers contain blood samples. The employer has to keep a log of injuries from sharp objects used by employees. A Hepatitis B vaccination must be provided free to employees Employers must provide training for Bloodborne precautions
27. In which people is tuberculosis more likely to develop? People whose immune systems are weakened, drug abuse, malnutrition & alcoholism.
28. What is a major factor in the spread of TB? Breathing in air droplets from a person coughing, sneezing, laughing etc. People who have TB and don't take their medications can spread disease more easily too.
29. What are multidrug-resistant organisms (MDROs)? Are microorganisms (usually bacteria) that are resistant to one or more antimicrobial agents.
30. What is one of the best ways to prevent the spread of MRSA and VRE? NA can help prevent the spread by using good hygeine especially good handwashing and following the OSHA standard precautions along with Transmission-Based precautions.
31. What are two ways that an NA can help prevent the spread of *C. difficile*? Proper handwashing! Cleaning surfaces & equipment with a disifectant Properly disposing of contaminated waste.
32. List five employer responsibilities for infection prevention. List five employee responsibilities for infection prevention.

Employers

1) Free hepititus B vaccination
2) Infection prevention procedures
3) & what to do if an employee is exposed
4) Provide continuing education on preventing blood-borne & air born diseases
5) Provide free personal protective equipment for employees & visitors Etc

Employees

1) Follow Standard precautions by OSHA
2) Follow all the facilities policies & procedures
3) Follow care plans & assignments
4) Use personal protective equipment & follow policies on how to use it.
5) Participate in yearly education programs
6) Get Hepatitus B vaccination
7) Immediately report any exposure to infection

6 Safety and Body Mechanics

1. Identify the persons at greatest risk for accidents and describe accident prevention guidelines

All staff members, including nursing assistants, are responsible for safety in a facility. Elderly people have more safety concerns due to issues like dementia, confusion, illness, disability, and diminished senses. Walking aids, such as crutches, walkers, canes, or boots for foot or leg injuries, put people at risk for falling. Residents who take medications that cause dizziness and light-headedness are likely to have accidents.

The senses of sight, hearing, touch, smell, and taste relay information about surroundings and help keep people safe. As people grow older, however, they suffer sensory losses. The senses of vision, hearing, taste, and smell decrease. Sensitivity to heat and cold decreases. And in addition to normal aging changes, diseases can cause diminished senses. Diseases of the circulatory and integumentary (skin) systems and paralysis can reduce the skin's ability to feel. **Paralysis** is the loss of ability to move all or part of the body. It often includes loss of feeling in the affected area. Strokes and brain or spinal injuries affect sensation and awareness of surroundings. A loss of sensation can lead to burns or other accidents. Drowsiness due to illness, lack of sleep, medications, or even feeling depressed can also cause a lack of awareness. Being in pain may reduce awareness. Individuals who are less aware may not know the positions of their body parts. Reflexes slow, making it more difficult to react in time to avoid accidents such as falls. Visual or hearing problems can also cause falls. Residents with vision problems may not see hazards, such as an object or water on the floor. Those who cannot hear well may not understand directions.

There are many factors that put residents at risk for serious injury. This is why it is very important to try to prevent accidents *before* they occur. Prevention is the key to safety. As nursing assistants work, they should observe for safety hazards and report unsafe conditions to the supervisor promptly.

Falls

A fall is any sudden, uncontrollable descent from a higher to a lower level, with or without injury resulting. Falls make up the majority of accidents that occur in long-term care facilities. They can be caused by an unsafe environment, loss of abilities, diseases, and medications. Problems resulting from falls range from minor bruises to fractures and life-threatening injuries. A **fracture** is a broken bone. Falls are particularly common among the elderly. Older people are often more seriously injured by falls because their bones are more fragile. Hip fractures are one of the most common types of fractures from falls. Hip fractures cause the greatest number of deaths and can lead to severe health problems. Nursing assistants should be especially alert to the risk of falls. All falls must be reported to the supervisor.

Factors that increase the risk of falls include the following:

- Clutter
- Throw rugs
- Exposed electrical cords
- Slippery or wet floors
- Uneven floors or stairs
- Poor lighting
- Call lights that are out of reach or not promptly answered

Personal conditions that increase the risk of falls include medications, loss of vision, gait (walking) or balance problems, weakness, paralysis, and disorientation. **Disorientation** means confusion about person, place, or time.

Guidelines: Preventing Falls

- G Clear all walkways of clutter, trash, throw rugs, and cords.
- G Use rugs with a non-slip backing.
- G Have residents wear non-skid, sturdy shoes. Make sure shoelaces are tied.
- G Residents should avoid wearing clothing that is too long or drags on the floor.
- G Keep frequently-used personal items close to residents, including call lights (Fig. 6-1).

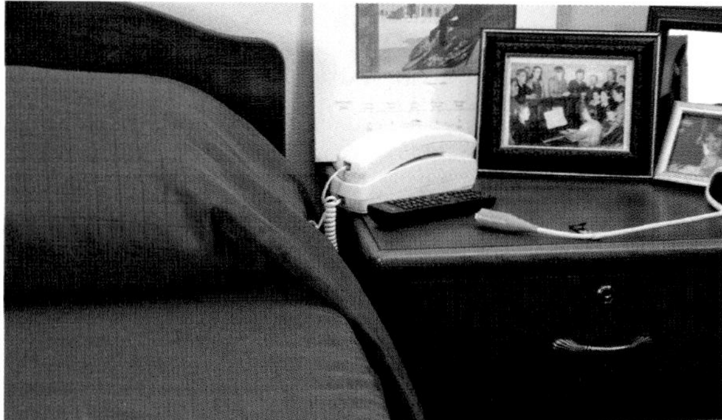

Fig. 6-1. *Keep call lights within reach of residents so they can use them when needed. Respond to call lights promptly.*

- G Answer call lights right away.
- G Immediately clean up spills on the floor.
- G Report loose hand rails immediately.
- G Mark uneven flooring or stairs with tape of a contrasting color to indicate a hazard.
- G Improve lighting where needed.
- G Lock wheels before helping residents into or out of wheelchairs (Fig. 6-2).

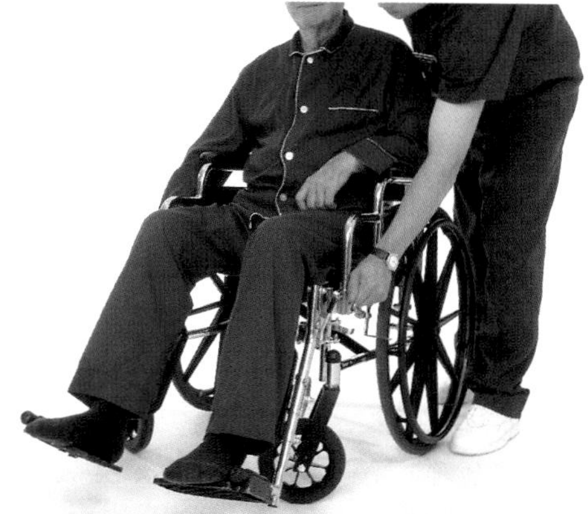

Fig. 6-2. *Always lock a wheelchair before transferring a resident into or out of it.*

- G Lock bed wheels before helping a resident into and out of bed or when giving care (Fig. 6-3).

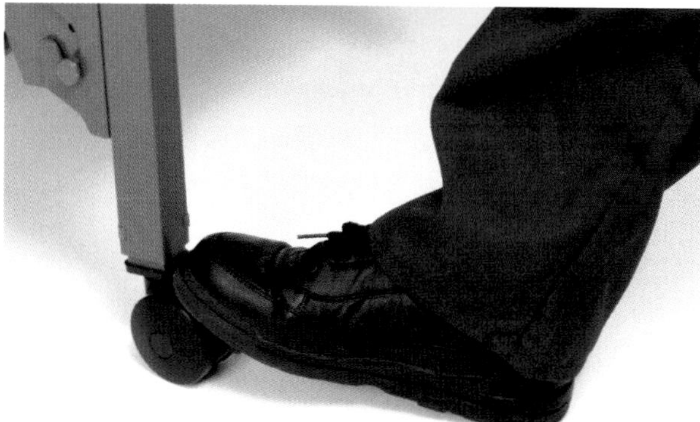

Fig. 6-3. *Always lock the bed wheels before helping a resident into or out of bed and before giving care.*

- G Before giving care, there are many times that you will need to raise beds to make your job easier and safer. After completing care, return beds to their lowest positions.
- G Get help when moving a resident; do not assume you can do it alone. When in doubt,

ask for help. Keep residents' walking aids, such as canes or walkers, within their reach.

- G Offer help with toileting regularly. Respond to residents' requests for bathroom assistance immediately. Think about how you would feel if you had to wait for help to go to the bathroom.
- G Leave furniture in the same place as you found it.
- G Know which residents are at risk for falls and pay close attention so that you can give help often.
- G If a resident starts to fall, be in a good position to help support her. Never try to catch a falling resident. Use your body to slide her to the floor. If you try to reverse a fall, you may hurt yourself and/or the resident.
- G Whenever a resident falls, it must be reported to the nurse. Always complete an incident report, even if the resident says he or she feels fine.

Burns/Scalds

Burns can be caused by dry heat (e.g., a hot iron, stove, other electrical appliances), wet heat (e.g., hot water or other liquids, steam), or chemicals (e.g., lye, acids). Small children, older adults, or people with loss of sensation (such as from paralysis or diabetes) are at the greatest risk of burns.

Scalds are burns caused by hot liquids. It takes five seconds or less for a serious burn to occur when the temperature of a liquid is 140°F. Coffee, tea, and other hot drinks are usually served at 160°F to 180°F. These temperatures can cause almost instant burns that require surgery. Preventing burns is very important.

Guidelines: Preventing Burns and Scalds

- G Always check water temperature with a water thermometer or on your wrist before using.
- G Report frayed electrical cords or unsafe-looking appliances immediately, and do not use them. Remove them from the room.
- G Let residents know you are about to pour or set down a hot liquid.
- G Pour hot drinks away from residents. Keep hot drinks and liquids away from edges of tables. Put lids on them.
- G Make sure residents are sitting down before serving hot drinks.
- G If plate warmers or other equipment that produces heat are used, monitor them carefully.

Resident Identification

Residents must always be identified before giving care or serving food. Failure to identify residents can cause serious problems, even death. Facilities have different methods of identification. Some have pictures to identify residents. Others have signs outside residents' doors (Fig. 6-4). Nursing assistants must identify each resident before beginning any procedure or giving any care. They should identify residents before placing meal trays or helping with feeding. The diet card should be checked against the resident's identification to make sure they match. The resident should be called by name.

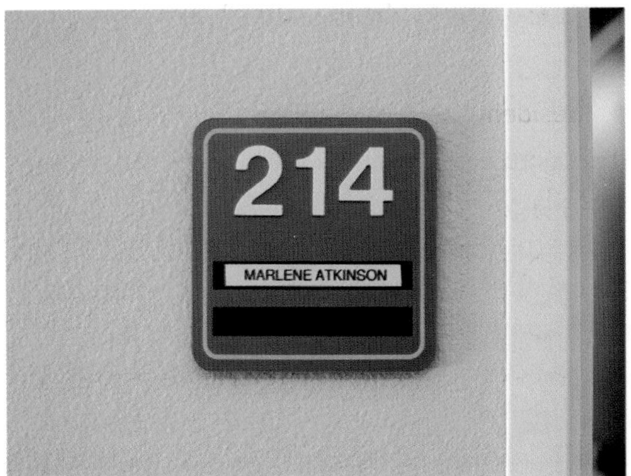

Fig. 6-4. *A resident's name may be displayed outside the room to identify who is living in that room. Before giving any care, nursing assistants must always identify residents.*

Choking

Choking can occur when eating, drinking, or swallowing medication. Babies and young children who put objects in their mouths are at great risk of choking. People who are weak, ill, or unconscious can choke on their own saliva. A person's tongue can also become swollen and obstruct the airway. To guard against choking, residents should eat in as upright a position as possible (Fig. 6-5). Residents with swallowing problems may have special diets with liquids thickened to the consistency of honey or syrup. Thickened liquids are easier to swallow. More information about helping with feeding and thickened liquids is found in Chapter 15.

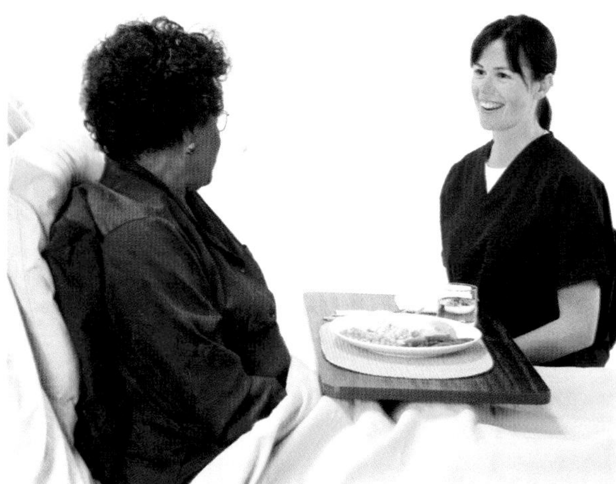

Fig. 6-5. *Residents must be sitting upright when eating, whether in a bed or a chair.*

Poisoning

There are many harmful substances in facilities that should not be swallowed. These include cleaners, paints, medicines, toiletries, and glues. These products should be stored or locked away from confused residents or those with limited vision. Cleaning products should not be left in residents' rooms. Residents with dementia may hide food and let it spoil in closets, drawers, or other places. Nursing assistants should investigate any odors they notice. The number for the Poison Control Center should be posted near all telephones.

Cuts/Abrasions

Cuts or abrasions typically occur in the bathroom at a facility or in the kitchen or bathroom when at home. An **abrasion** is an injury that rubs off the surface of the skin. Sharp objects, such as scissors, nail clippers, and razors, should be put away after use. Nursing assistants should take care when transferring residents into and out of beds, chairs, and wheelchairs. When moving residents in wheelchairs, NAs should push the wheelchair forward. Wheelchairs should not be pulled from behind. When using elevators, wheelchairs should be turned around before entering, so that residents are facing forward.

Nursing assistants should also follow these additional guidelines for working safely in facilities:

- NAs should not run in halls, on stairs, or in the dining room.
- They should keep paths clear and free of clutter.
- NAs must wipe up spilled liquids right away.
- Trash should be discarded properly.
- NAs should follow instructions and ask about anything they do not understand.
- Injuries must be reported immediately.

Promoting safety is part of nursing assistants' responsibilities. Reporting hazards immediately helps make workplaces safer for everyone.

Residents' Rights

Safety

One requirement of OBRA is that residents in long-term care facilities have the right to a safe environment. Nursing assistants should observe the environment carefully to identify safety hazards. If any safety hazard exists, such as a frayed electrical cord on a resident's radio, it should be reported immediately. Residents have the right to have personal items and to have these items treated with respect. However, if a resident's possession is a potential safety hazard, it should be reported to the nurse. The safety of all residents and staff members is most important.

2. List safety guidelines for oxygen use

Residents with breathing problems may receive oxygen that is more concentrated than what is in the air. Oxygen is prescribed by a doctor. Nursing assistants never stop, adjust, or administer oxygen. Oxygen may be piped into a resident's room through a central system. It may be in tanks or produced by an oxygen concentrator. An oxygen concentrator is a box-like device that changes air in the room into air with more oxygen. Chapter 14 contains more information about oxygen therapy.

Combustion means the process of burning. Oxygen is a very dangerous fire hazard because it supports combustion (makes other things burn). Working around oxygen requires special safety precautions.

Guidelines: Working Safely Around Oxygen

- G Post *No Smoking* and *Oxygen in Use* signs. Never allow smoking where oxygen is used or stored.
- G Remove all fire hazards from the room or area. Fire hazards include electrical equipment, such as electric razors and hair dryers. Other fire hazards are cigarettes, matches, and flammable liquids. **Flammable** means easily ignited and capable of burning quickly. Examples of flammable liquids are alcohol and nail polish remover. Read the labels on liquids if you are unsure. If a label has the word *flammable* on it, remove it from the area. Notify the nurse if a resident does not want a fire hazard removed.
- G Do not burn candles, light matches, or use lighters around oxygen. Any type of open flame that is present around oxygen is a dangerous fire hazard.
- G Do not use an extension cord with an oxygen concentrator.
- G Do not place electrical cords or oxygen tubing under rugs or furniture.
- G Avoid using fabrics such as nylon and wool that can cause static electricity discharges.
- G Report if the nasal cannula or face mask is causing skin irritation. Check the nasal area and behind the ears for signs of irritation. (Fig. 6-6).

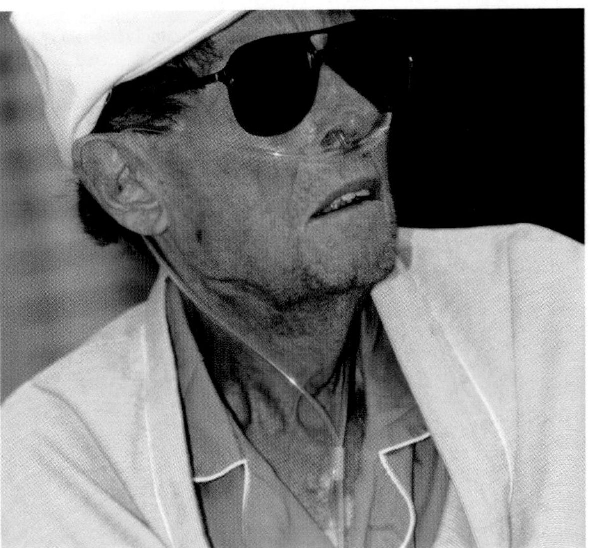

Fig. 6-6. *A resident with a nasal cannula.*

- G Do not use any petroleum-based products, such as Vaseline or Chapstick, on the resident or on any part of the cannula or mask.
- G Learn how to turn oxygen off in case of fire. Never adjust the oxygen setting or dose.

3. Explain the Material Safety Data Sheet (MSDS)

The Occupational Safety and Health Administration (OSHA) requires that all hazardous chemicals have a Material Safety Data Sheet (MSDS) (Fig. 6-7). This sheet details the chemical ingredients, chemical dangers, emergency response actions to be taken, and safe handling procedures for the product. Some facilities use a toll-free number to access MSDS information. Material Safety Data Sheets must be accessible in work areas for all employees.

Material Safety Data Sheet
May be used to comply with OSHA's Hazard Communication Standard, 29 CFR 1910 1200. Standard must be consulted for specific requirements.

U.S. Department of Labor
Occupational Safety and Health Administration
(Non-Mandatory Form)
Form Approved
OMB No. 1218-0072

IDENTITY *(as Used on Label and List)*	*Note: Blank spaces are not permitted. If any item is not applicable or no information is available, the space must be marked to indicate that.*

Section I

Manufacturer's name	Emergency Telephone Number
Address *(Number, Street, City, State and ZIP Code)*	Telephone Number for Information
	Date Prepared
	Signature of Preparer *(optional)*

Section II—Hazardous Ingredients/Identity Information

Hazardous Components (Specific Chemical Identity, Common Name(s))	OSHA PEL	ACGIH TLV	Other Limits Recommended	% (optional)

Section III—Physical/Chemical Characteristics

Boiling Point		Specific Gravity ($H_20 = 1$)	
Vapor Pressure (mm Hg)		Melting Point	
Vapor Density (AIR = 1)		Evaporation Rate (Butyl Acetate = 1)	

Solubility in Water

Appearance and Odor

Section IV—Fire and Explosion Hazard Data

Flash Point (Method Used)	Flammable Limits	LEL	UEL

Extinguishing Media

Special Fire Fighting Procedures

Unusual Fire and Explosion Hazards

OSHA 174 Sept. 1985

Fig. 6-7. *A Material Safety Data Sheet.*

Important information about the MSDS includes the following:

- Employers must have an MSDS for every chemical used.
- Employers must provide easy access to the MSDS.
- Staff members must know where these sheets are kept and how to read them. If they do not know how to read them, they should ask for help.

The list of hazardous chemicals that have to have an MSDS will be updated as new chemicals are purchased.

Emergency Eyewash Stations

OSHA requires that emergency eyewash stations be placed in all hazardous areas in case an eye injury occurs (Fig. 6-8). Employees must know where the closest eyewash station is and how to get there with restricted vision.

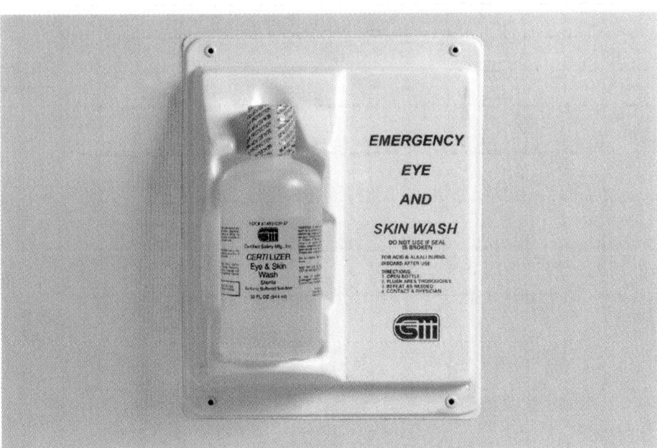

Fig. 6-8. *One type of wall-mounted emergency eye and skin wash.* (REPRINTED WITH PERMISSION OF BRIGGS CORPORATION, 800-247-2343, WWW.BRIGGSCORP.COM)

4. Define the term *restraint* and give reasons why restraints were used

A **restraint** is a physical or chemical way to restrict voluntary movement or behavior. Examples of physical restraints are vests and jacket restraints, belt restraints, wrist/ankle restraints, and mitt restraints. Raised side rails on beds and geriatric chairs with tray tables attached are also considered physical restraints (Figs. 6-9 and 6-10). Chemical restraints are medications given to control a person's behavior.

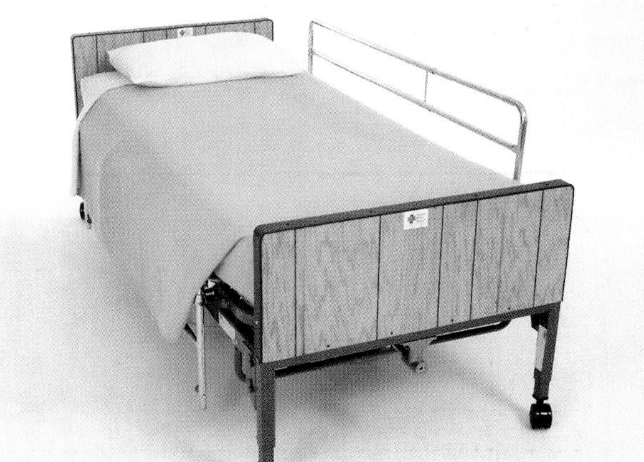

Fig. 6-9. *Raised side rails are considered restraints because they restrict movement.*

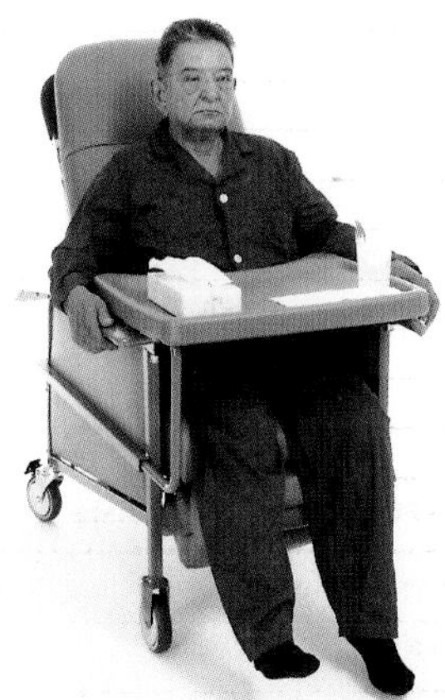

Fig. 6-10. *When the tray table is attached or locked, a geriatric chair, or geri-chair, is considered a restraint.*

In the past, restraints were commonly used to prevent confused people from wandering, to prevent falls, to keep people from injuring themselves or others, or to prevent people from pulling out tubing needed for treatment. Restraint use was sometimes abused by caregivers, and residents were injured. This led to new laws restricting the use of restraints.

Today, long-term care facilities are prohibited from using restraints unless they are medically necessary. They are only used as a last resort and only after less restrictive measures have been tried. If a restraint is needed, a doctor must order it. Very specific guidelines apply to carrying out a restraint order, including frequent monitoring of the resident. Nursing assistants cannot use physical restraints unless a doctor has ordered it in the care plan and they have been trained in the restraint's use. It is against the law for staff to apply a restraint for convenience or to discipline a resident. Nursing assistants can check with their supervisor for policies regarding restraints.

5. List physical and psychological problems associated with restraints

There are many serious problems associated with restraint use, including the following:

- Pressure ulcers
- Pneumonia
- Risk of suffocation (**suffocation** is the stoppage of breathing from a lack of oxygen or excess of carbon dioxide in the body that may result in unconsciousness or death)
- Reduced blood circulation
- Stress on the heart
- Incontinence
- Constipation
- Muscle **atrophy** (weakening or wasting away of the muscle)
- Loss of bone mass
- Poor appetite and malnutrition
- Depression and/or withdrawal
- Sleep disorders
- Loss of dignity
- Loss of independence
- Stress and anxiety
- Increased agitation (anxiety, restlessness)
- Loss of self-esteem
- Severe injury
- Death

Nursing assistants must never use restraints unless their supervisor has told them to do so and they have been instructed in the proper use of the restraint. They must follow the care plan. The care plan will include instructions on frequent monitoring and repositioning.

6. Discuss restraint alternatives

Restraint usage has significantly decreased in facilities. State and federal agencies encourage facilities to take steps to create restraint-free environments. **Restraint-free care** means that restraints are not kept or used for any reason. Creative ideas that help avoid the need for restraints are being used instead. **Restraint alternatives** are any interventions used in place of a restraint or that reduces the need for a restraint. Many scientific studies have shown that restraints are not needed. People tend to respond better to the use of creative ways to reduce tension, pulling at tubes, wandering, and boredom. Examples of restraint alternatives include the following:

- Improve safety measures to prevent accidents and falls. Improve lighting.
- Make sure the call lights are within reach, and respond to call lights promptly.
- Ambulate the resident when he is restless. The doctor or nurse may add exercise into the care plan.
- Provide activities for those who wander at night.
- Encourage activities and independence. Escort the resident to social activities. Increase visits and social interaction.
- Give frequent help with toileting. Help with cleaning immediately after an episode of incontinence.
- Offer food or drink. Offer reading materials.
- Distract or redirect interest. Give the resident a repetitive task.

- Decrease the noise level. Listen to soothing music. Offer back massages or use relaxation techniques.
- Reduce pain levels through medication. The resident should be monitored closely and complaints of pain should be reported immediately.
- Provide familiar caregivers, and increase the number of caregivers with family and volunteers.
- Use a team approach to meeting the resident's needs. Offer training to teach gentle approaches to difficult people.

There are also several types of pads, belts, special chairs, and alarms that can be used instead of restraints. Bed or body alarms can be used in place of side rails. They can also be used with wheelchairs or chairs (Fig. 6-11). They help prevent falls by alerting staff when residents attempt to leave the bed or chair. Alarms can also be used for confused residents who wander. If a resident is ordered to have a body alarm (bed or chair), the nursing assistant should make sure it is on the person and is turned on.

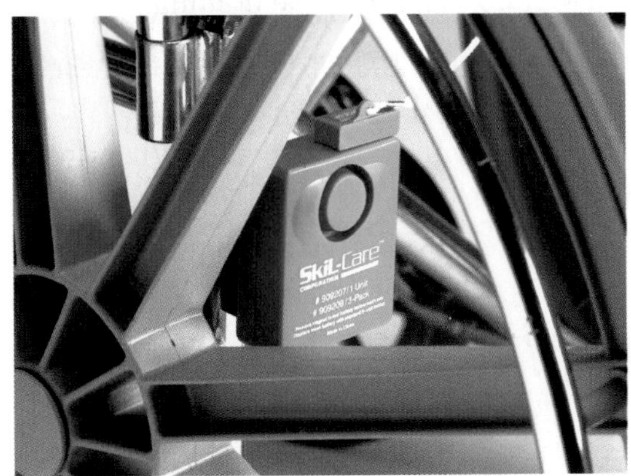

Fig. 6-11. *A chair alarm warns caregiver of chair exits.* (REPRINTED WITH PERMISSION OF BRIGGS CORPORATION, 800-247-2343, WWW.BRIGGSCORP.COM)

7. Describe guidelines for what must be done if a restraint is ordered

OBRA sets specific rules for restraint use. Restraints can only be applied with a doctor's order. A nursing assistant cannot use a restraint unless the charge nurse has approved its use and the NA has been trained to use it properly.

Guidelines: Restraints

- Know your state's laws and facility rules regarding applying restraints. Check to make sure there is a doctor's order for restraint use and that it is in the care plan before applying one.
- Follow manufacturer's instructions when applying restraints.
- Restraints can only be tied to the movable part of a bed frame, not to the side rails or other areas on the bed.
- Check to make sure that the restraint is not too tight. You should be able to place your hand in a flat position between the resident and the restraint. This helps to ensure that the device fits properly and is comfortable.
- Make sure that the breasts or skin are not caught in the restraint.
- Place the call light within the resident's reach. Answer call lights immediately.
- Document restraint use according to facility policy.

A restrained resident must be monitored constantly; the resident must be checked at least every 15 minutes. At regular, ordered intervals, the following must be done:

- Release the restraint (or discontinue use). Follow facility policy and the care plan's instructions.
- Offer help with toileting. Check for episodes of incontinence. Provide incontinence care.
- Offer fluids and food.
- Check the skin for signs of irritation. Report any red, purple, blue, gray, or pale skin or any discolored areas to the nurse immediately.

- Check for swelling of the body part and report any swelling to the nurse immediately.
- Reposition the resident.
- Ambulate the resident if he is able.

If any problems occur with the restraint, especially resident injury, notify the nurse and complete an incident report as soon as possible.

8. Explain the principles of body mechanics

Back strain or injury can be a serious problem for nursing assistants. In fact, an increasing injury rate is one reason why many long-term care facilities have *lift-free* or *zero-lift* policies. These policies set strict guidelines on the use of lifts and transfers of residents in order to reduce injuries. Using proper body mechanics is an important step in preventing back strain and injury.

Body mechanics is the way the parts of the body work together when a person moves. Using proper body mechanics helps save energy and prevent injury. Nursing assistants can keep themselves and their residents safer if they understand the basic principles of body mechanics.

Alignment: Alignment is based on the word *line.* When a person stands up straight, a vertical line could be drawn through the center of his body and his center of gravity (Fig. 6-12). When the line is straight, the body is in alignment. Whether standing, sitting, or lying down, the body should be in alignment and should have good posture. This means that the two sides of the body are mirror images of each other, with body parts lined up naturally. **Posture** is the way a person holds and positions his body. A person can maintain correct body alignment when lifting or carrying an object by keeping it close to his body. His feet and body should be pointed in the direction he is moving. He should avoid twisting at the waist.

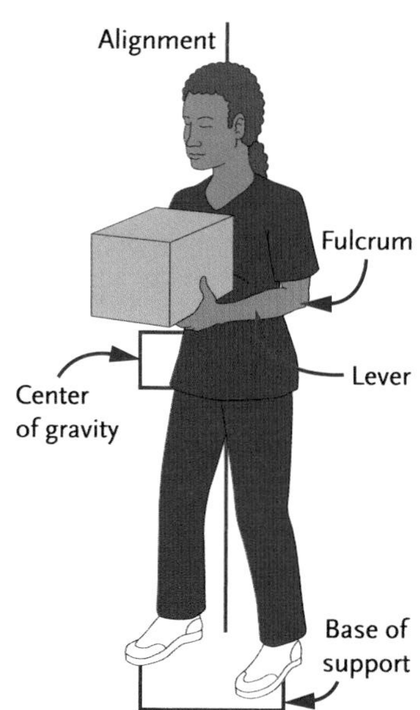

Fig. 6-12. *Proper body alignment is important when standing and sitting.*

Base of support: The base of support is the foundation that supports an object. The feet are the body's base of support. The wider the support, the more stable a person will be. Standing with legs apart allows for a greater base of support. This is more stable than standing with feet together.

Fulcrum and lever: A **lever** moves an object by resting on a base of support, called a fulcrum. For example, on a seesaw, the flat board a person sits on is the lever. The triangular base that the board rests on is the fulcrum. When two children sit on opposite sides of the seesaw, they easily move each other up and down. This is because the fulcrum and lever of the seesaw are doing the work.

Thinking of the body as a set of fulcrums and levers can be helpful when trying to find smart ways to lift without working as hard. For example, an arm is a lever and the elbow is the fulcrum. When a person lifts something, he can rest it against his forearm. This will shorten the lever and make the item easier to lift than it would be if he was holding it in his hands.

Center of gravity: The center of gravity in the body is the point where the most weight is concentrated (Fig. 6-13). This point will depend on the position of the body. When a person stands, weight is centered in the pelvis. A low center of gravity gives a more stable base of support. Bending the knees when lifting an object lowers the pelvis and, therefore, lowers a person's center of gravity. This gives the person more stability. It makes him less likely to fall or strain the working muscles.

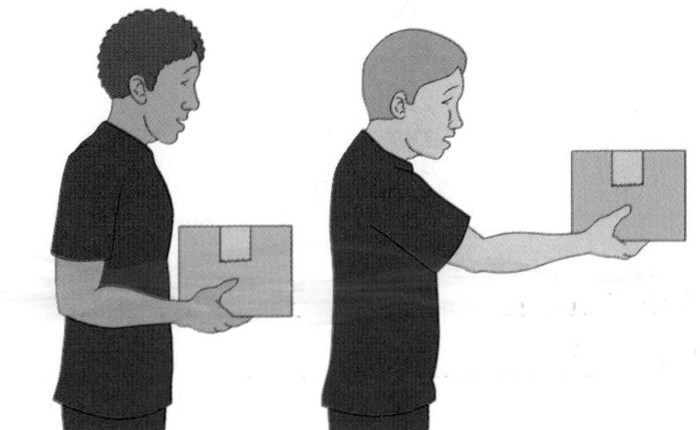

Fig. 6-13. Holding things close to the body moves weight toward the center of gravity. In this illustration, who is more likely to strain his back muscles?

9. Apply principles of body mechanics to daily activities

By applying the principles of body mechanics to daily activities, injury can be avoided and less energy is used. Procedures for properly transferring, positioning, and ambulating residents are located throughout this textbook. These procedures include instructions for maintaining proper body mechanics. In addition, nursing assistants should keep the following guidelines in mind:

Guidelines: Using Proper Body Mechanics

G Use both arms and hands to lift, push, or carry objects.

G When lifting a heavy object from the floor, spread your feet shoulder-width apart. Bend your knees. Use the strong, large muscles in your thighs, upper arms, and shoulders to lift the object. Raise your body and the object together (Fig. 6-14).

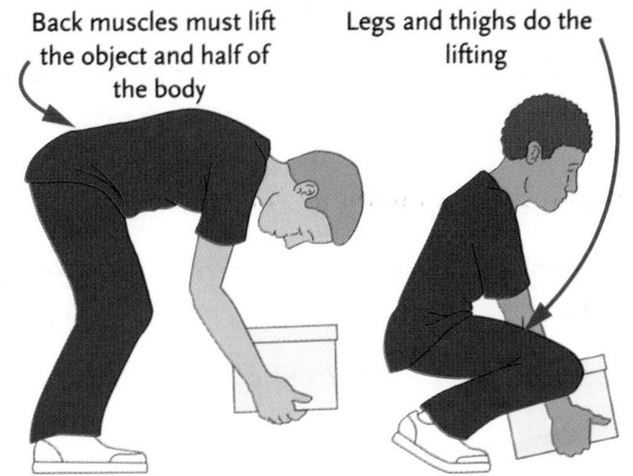

Fig. 6-14. In this illustration, which person is lifting correctly?

G Hold objects close to you when you are lifting or carrying them. This keeps the object closer to your center of gravity and base of support.

G Push or slide objects rather than lifting them.

G Avoid bending and reaching as much as possible. Move or position furniture so that you do not have to bend or reach.

G If you are making an adjustable bed, adjust the height to a safe working level, usually waist high. If you are making a regular bed, lean or kneel to support yourself at working level. Avoid bending at the waist.

G When a task requires bending, use a good stance. Bend your knees to lower yourself, rather than bending from the waist. This allows you to use the big muscles in your legs and hips rather than the smaller muscles in your back.

G Avoid twisting at the waist when you are lifting or moving something. Instead, turn your whole body, pivoting with your feet instead of twisting at the waist. Your feet should point toward what you are lifting or moving.

G Get help from coworkers when possible for lifting or helping residents.

G Talk to residents before moving them. Let them know what you will do so they can help if possible. Agree on a signal, such as counting to three. Lift or move on three so that everyone moves together.

- To help a resident sit up, stand up, or walk, place your feet 12 inches, or shoulder-width, apart. Place one foot in front of the other, and bend your knees. Your upper body should stay upright and in alignment. Do this whenever you have to support a resident's weight.
- Never try to catch a falling resident. If the resident falls, assist her to the floor (Fig. 6-15). If you try to reverse a fall in progress, you could injure yourself and/or the resident.
- Report to the nurse any task you feel that you cannot safely do. Never try to lift an object or a resident that you feel you cannot handle.

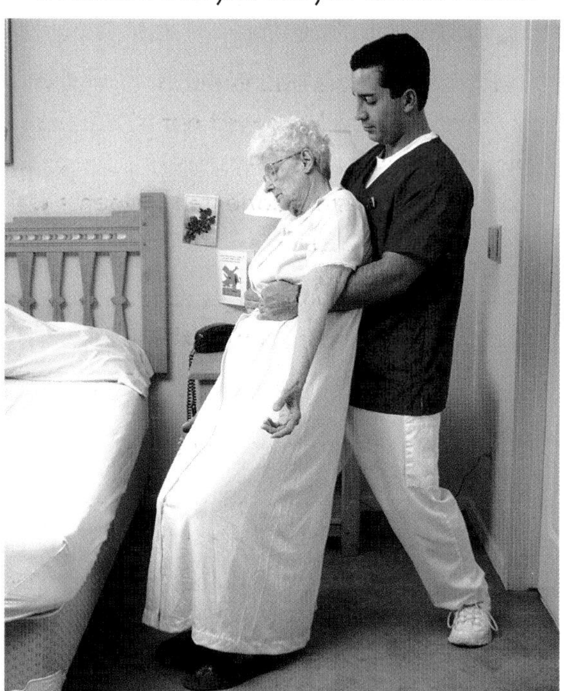

Fig. 6-15. *Maintaining a wide base of support and low center of gravity will enable you to help a falling resident.*

10. Identify major causes of fire and list fire safety guidelines

In order for a fire to occur, three elements must be present: heat, fuel, and oxygen. A fire can be prevented or extinguished by removing any one of these elements.

Nursing assistants must be able to recognize and report any fire hazards they observe. There are many potential fire hazards in facilities, including the following:

- Smoking
- Frayed or exposed electrical wires
- Damaged electrical equipment
- Oxygen use
- Flammable liquids or rags with oils on them
- Overloaded electrical sockets

All facilities have a fire safety plan, and all workers need to know this plan. Guidelines regarding fires and evacuations will be explained to all employees. Evacuation routes are posted in facilities. Nursing assistants should read and review them often and should attend fire and disaster in-service trainings when they are offered. These in-services will explain what NAs must do in an emergency. A fast, calm, and confident response by the staff saves lives.

Guidelines: Reducing Fire Hazards and Responding to Fires

- Never leave smokers unattended. If residents smoke, make sure they are in the proper area for smoking. Be sure that cigarettes are extinguished. Empty ashtrays often. Before emptying ashtrays, make sure there are no hot ashes or hot matches in ashtray.
- Report frayed or damaged electrical cords immediately. Report electrical equipment in need of repair immediately.
- Fire alarms and exit doors should not be blocked. If they are, report this to the nurse.
- Every facility will have fire extinguishers (Fig. 6-16). The PASS acronym will help you understand how to use it:

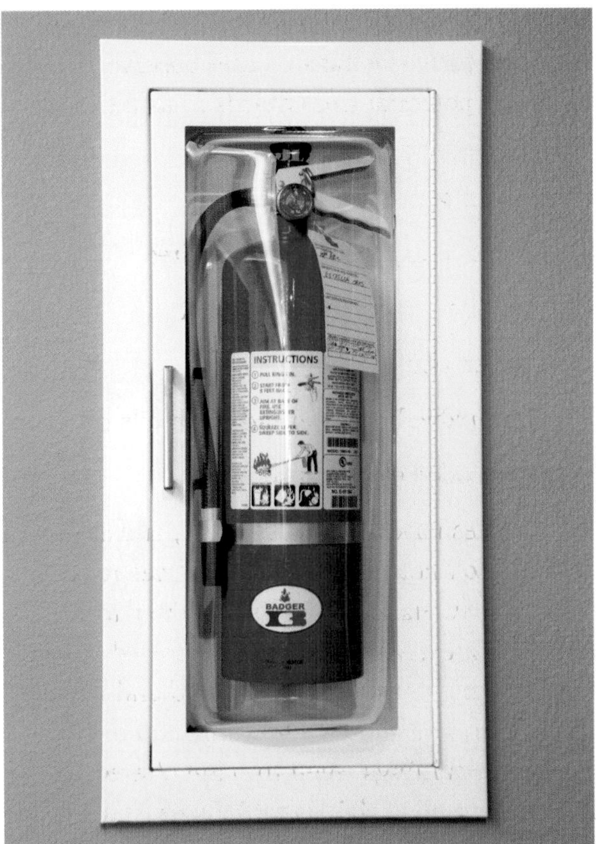

Fig. 6-16. *Know where the extinguisher is stored in your facility and how to use it.*

- **P**ull the pin.
- **A**im at the base of fire when spraying.
- **S**queeze the handle.
- **S**weep back and forth at the base of the fire.

G In case of fire, the RACE acronym is a good rule to follow:

- **R**emove residents from danger.
- **A**ctivate alarm or call 911.
- **C**ontain fire if possible.
- **E**xtinguish, or fire department will extinguish.

Follow these guidelines for helping residents exit the building safely:

G Know the facility's fire evacuation plan.

G Stay calm.

G Follow the directions of the fire department.

G Know which residents need one-on-one help or assistive devices. Immobile residents can be moved in several ways. If they have a wheelchair, help them into it. You can also use other wheeled transporters, such as carts, bath chairs, stretchers, or beds. A blanket can be used as a stretcher or even pulled across the floor with someone on it.

G Residents who can walk will also need assistance getting out of the building. Those who are hearing impaired may not hear the warnings and instructions. Staff will need to tell them directly what to do while guiding them to the nearest safe exit. People with visual problems should be moved out of the way of the wheelchairs, carts, etc., and helped to the exit. Confused and disoriented residents will also need guidance.

G Remove anything blocking a window or door that could be used as a fire exit.

G Do not use elevators.

G Stay low in a room to escape a fire.

G If the door of the room you are in is closed, check for heat coming from it before opening it. If the door or doorknob feels hot, stay in the room if there is no safe exit. Plug the doorway (use wet towels or clothing) to prevent smoke from entering. Stay in the room until help arrives.

G Use the *stop, drop, and roll* fire safety technique to extinguish a fire on clothing or hair. Stop running or stay still. Drop to the ground, lying down if possible. Roll on the ground to try to extinguish the flames.

G Use a damp covering over the mouth and nose to reduce smoke inhalation.

G After leaving the building, move away from it.

Remove residents
Activate 911 call
Contain fire if possible
Extinguis fire

Working a fire extingusher
Pull pin
Aim at base of fire
Squeeze handle
Sweep back & forth across base of fire

Chapter Review

1. List five reasons that elderly people have more safety concerns than others do.

Disabilities, confusion, illness, everythings slower, all senses have diminished. Walking devices for even be hazards. Med's can cause dizziness. Paralysis can cause problems. Many have loss of feeling.

2. What type of accident occurs most frequently in long-term care facilities?

Falls like A broken hip

3. List eleven guidelines to prevent falls.

1) Clear clutter from walk areas
2) Use non-slip rugs
3) Have residents wear non-slip sturdy shoes
4) No long clothing
5) Keep call light & personal items close.
6) answer call lights right away
7) Clean up spills immediately!
8) Watch for disfunctional equipment like loose handrails
9) Mark uneven flooring with bright colored tape
10) Improving lighting could help
11) Lock wheelchairs when transferring & beds too.
12) lower raised beds to safe levels when finished making them.
13) Ask for help when moving a resident
14) Offer help to a resident when they need to use the restroom
15) Dont switch furniture around.

4. Describe five ways to guard against burns/scalds.

1) check temp. of water or hot drinks 2) Report any frayed electrial wiring 3) Pour hot drinks away from residents 4) Make sure residents sit down before serving a hot drink 5) Keep an eye out for any hot plates, toasters & stoves used by a resident.

5. What should nursing assistants always do before giving care or serving meal trays?

identify the resident by name. Match tray.

6. In what position should residents eat to avoid choking? Sitting up

7. What are three guidelines for working safely around oxygen?

1) absolutely no smoking 2) No flammable liquids like alcohol 3) No use of fabrics that create static electricity.

8. What is the purpose of the Material Safety Data Sheet (MSDS)?

It details the chemical ingredients & dangers. It tells you safe emergency response actions & safe handling procedures for the product.

9. When can a restraint be used?

Only if a doctor orders it!

10. List ten problems associated with restraint use.

1) pressure ulcers 2) pnemonia 3) possible suffocation 4) ↓ Blood circ. 5) Constipation & incontinence 6) muscle atrophy 7) Loss of bone mass 8) poor appetite or depression 9) Sleep disorders 10) Loss of Dignity 11) anxiety etc.

11. Define *restraint-free care* and *restraint alternatives*.

not used at all. Activities for residents. Walk patient when restless, distract him. Make safe environment. Call lights handy. Help with toileting. Music. Back massages. Reduce pain. Use more caregivers.

12. List six things that must be done if a resident is restrained.

1) Dr. orders. 2) follow manufactures guidlines 4) Make sure they are not too tight 5) Check skin for irritations 6) call light handy.

13. What is body mechanics?

The way the parts of body work together.

14. What is the name for the point in the body where most weight is concentrated?

The center of gravity

15. When lifting a heavy object from the floor, how should the feet be placed? How should the knees be positioned?

The feet should be shoulder-width apart. Bent

16. When a task requires bending, which of the following demonstrates proper body mechanics: bending the knees or bending from the waist?

17. Is it better to push an object or to lift an object? Push an object

18. What three elements are needed for a fire to occur?

Oxygen
fuel
heat

19. Identify what the acronyms *PASS* and *RACE* stand for.

20. If a fire has started, what should the nursing assistant do before opening a closed door?

Touch door knob & do not open if hot. Put something damp under door to prevent smoke from entering room.

7 Emergency Care and Disaster Preparation

1. Demonstrate how to recognize and respond to medical emergencies

Medical emergencies may be the result of accidents or sudden illnesses. This chapter discusses how to respond appropriately to medical emergencies. Heart attacks, strokes, diabetic emergencies, choking, automobile accidents, and gunshot wounds are all medical emergencies. Falls, burns, and cuts can also be emergencies when they are severe.

In an emergency situation, it is important for responders to remain calm, act quickly, and communicate clearly. The following steps illustrate the correct response to emergencies:

Assess the situation. The responder should try to determine what has happened. She must make sure she is not in danger and notice the time.

Assess the victim. The responder should ask the injured or ill person what has happened. If the person is unable to respond, he may be unconscious. Being **conscious** means being mentally alert and having awareness of surroundings, sensations, and thoughts. Tapping the person and asking if he is all right helps to determine if a person is conscious. The responder should speak loudly and use the person's name if she knows it. If there is no response, she should assume the person is unconscious and that an emergency situation exists. She should call for help right away or send someone else to call.

If a person is conscious and able to speak, then he is breathing and has a pulse. The responder should talk with the person about what happened. She should get the person's permission to touch him. (Anyone who is unable to give consent for treatment, e.g., a child with no parent near or an unconscious or seriously injured person, may be treated with *implied consent*. This means that if the person were able or the parent were present, they would have given consent.) The person should be checked for the following:

- Severe bleeding
- Changes in consciousness
- Irregular breathing
- Unusual color or feel to the skin
- Swollen places on the body
- Medical alert tags
- Anything the person says is painful

If any of these conditions exists, professional medical help may be needed. When a nursing assistant is responding to an emergency, she should always get help and call the nurse before doing anything else.

If an injured or ill person is conscious, he may be frightened. Whoever responds to the emergency should listen to the person and tell him what actions are being taken to help him. A calm and confident response will help reassure him that he is being taken care of.

In the case of an emergency in an long-term care facility, the NA will need to document the emergency in her notes and complete an incident or accident report once the emergency is over. It is important to include as many details as possible and report only facts. If the NA thinks a resident had a heart attack, she should only document the signs and symptoms she observed and the actions she took. Knowing the kind of information the NA will have to document will help her remember the important facts during the emergency. For instance, it is especially important to remember the time at which a resident became unconscious.

Reporting Emergencies

If a resident needs emergency help, the nurse may ask a nursing assistant to call emergency services. The NA should know the procedure for dialing an outside line. Emergency medical services can be reached by dialing 911. The NA should be prepared to give the following information when calling emergency services:

- The phone number and address of the emergency, including exact directions or landmarks, and the location within the building, if necessary
- The person's condition, including any known medical background
- The NA's name and position
- Details of any first aid being given

The dispatcher may need other information or may want to give the person calling other instructions. The NA should not hang up the phone until the dispatcher hangs up or tells her to hang up.

2. Demonstrate knowledge of first aid procedures

First aid is emergency care given immediately to an injured person. **Cardiopulmonary resuscitation (CPR)** refers to medical procedures used when a person's heart or lungs have stopped working. CPR is used until medical help arrives.

Quick action is necessary. CPR must be started immediately to help prevent or minimize brain damage. Brain damage can occur within four to six minutes after the heart stops beating and breathing stops. The person can die within ten minutes.

Only properly trained people should administer CPR. Facilities often arrange for nursing assistants to be trained in CPR. If a nursing assistant's facility does not provide training, the NA can contact the American Heart Association (heart.org) or Red Cross (redcross.org) for more information. CPR is an important skill to learn. If a person is not trained, he should not attempt to perform CPR.

Nursing assistants need to know their facility's policies on initiating CPR if they have been trained to do so. Some facilities do not allow nursing assistants to begin CPR without direction of the nurse. This is due, in part, to residents' advance directives. Some people have made the decision that they do not want CPR. The nurse should be notified immediately if an emergency occurs.

Residents' Rights

CPR

Nursing assistants can protect the privacy of residents who need CPR by pulling the privacy curtain around the bed and closing the door. Anyone who is not directly involved in giving care should leave the room. NAs should remain calm and be professional. They should remember that a resident receiving CPR may be able to hear what is being said. Some residents have do-not-resuscitate (DNR) orders in place, which means that no CPR may be given. This is a legal order; the resident's decision for a DNR order and other advance directives must be honored. NAs should not judge these very personal decisions.

Choking

When something is blocking the tube through which air enters the lungs, the person has an **obstructed airway**. When people are choking, they usually put their hands to their throats (Fig. 7-1). Nursing assistants may encounter residents who are choking or seem to be choking. As long as the resident can speak, breathe, or cough, the NA should only encourage her to cough as forcefully as possible to get the object out. The NA should stay with the resident at all times, until she stops choking or can no longer speak, cough, or breathe.

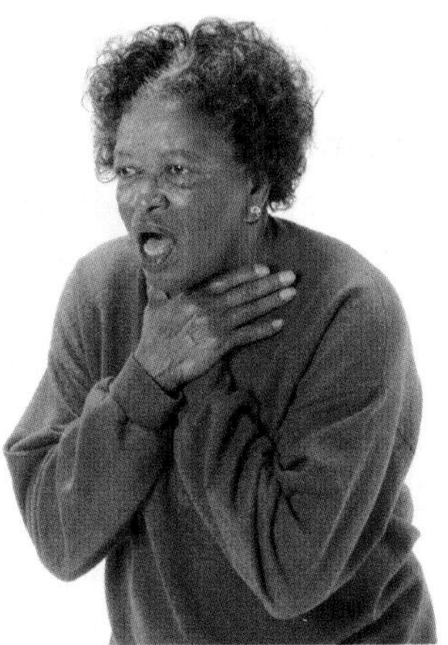

Fig. 7-1. *People who are choking usually put their hands to their throats.*

If a resident can no longer speak, cough, or breathe, the NA should call for help immediately by using the call light or emergency cord. The choking victim should not be left alone. **Abdominal thrusts** are a method of attempting to remove an object from the airway of someone who is choking. These thrusts work to remove the blockage upward, out of the throat.

The NA should make sure the resident needs help before starting to give abdominal thrusts. She must show signs of a severely obstructed airway. These signs include poor air exchange, an increase in trouble breathing, silent coughing, blue-tinged skin (cyanosis), or inability to speak, breathe, or cough. The NA should ask, "Are you choking?" If the resident nods her head, "Yes," she has a severe airway obstruction and needs immediate help. The NA should begin giving abdominal thrusts. This procedure should never be performed on a person who is not choking. Abdominal thrusts risk injury to the ribs or internal organs.

Performing abdominal thrusts for the conscious person

1. Stand behind the person and bring your arms under her arms. Wrap your arms around the person's waist.
2. Make a fist with one hand. Place the flat, thumb side of the fist against the person's abdomen, above the navel but below the breastbone.
3. Grasp the fist with your other hand. Pull both hands toward you and up, quickly and forcefully (Fig. 7-2).

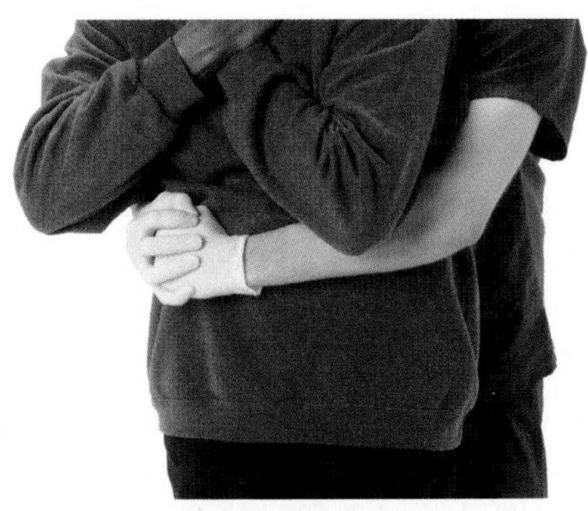

Fig. 7-2. *When giving abdominal thrusts, pull both hands toward you and up (inward and upward), quickly and forcefully.*

4. Repeat until the object is pushed out or the person loses consciousness.
5. Report and document the incident properly.

If the resident becomes unconscious while choking, she should be helped to the floor gently so she is lying on her back with her face up. The NA should begin CPR for an unconscious person if trained and allowed to do so. The NA should make sure help is on the way. The resident may have a completely blocked airway and need professional medical help immediately. The NA should stay with the victim until help arrives.

Emergency Codes

Facilities often use codes to inform staff of emergencies while preventing panic and stress among residents and visitors. These codes are frequently described by color. For example, *Code Red* usually means fire. *Code Blue* usually means cardiac arrest. However, the meanings of these codes vary from facility to facility. It is important for nursing assistants to know the codes for their facility. NAs should not panic when codes are announced; they should respond calmly and professionally.

Shock

Shock occurs when organs and tissues in the body do not receive an adequate blood supply. Bleeding, heart attack, severe infection, and falling blood pressure can lead to shock. Shock can become worse when the person is extremely frightened or in severe pain.

Shock is a dangerous, life-threatening situation. Signs of shock include pale or bluish skin, staring, increased pulse and respiration rates, low blood pressure, and extreme thirst. A nursing assistant should always call for help if she suspects a resident is experiencing shock.

Responding to shock

1. Notify the nurse immediately. Victims of shock should always receive medical care as soon as possible.
2. If controlling bleeding, put on gloves first. The procedure for controlling bleeding is described later in the chapter.
3. Have the person lie down on her back. If the person is bleeding from the mouth or vomiting, place her on her side (unless you suspect that the neck, back, or spinal cord is injured).
4. Check pulse and respirations if possible (Chapter 14). Begin CPR if breathing and pulse are absent and if you are trained to do so.
5. Keep the person as calm and comfortable as possible.
6. Maintain normal body temperature. If the weather is cold, place a blanket around the person. If the weather is hot, provide shade.
7. Elevate the legs approximately eight to 12 inches unless the person has a head, neck, back, spinal, or abdominal injury, breathing difficulties, or fractures (Fig. 7-3). Elevating the legs allows blood to flow from the lower extremities back to the brain (and other vital areas.) Elevate the head and shoulders if a head wound or breathing difficulties are present. Never elevate a body part if the person has a broken bone or if it causes pain.

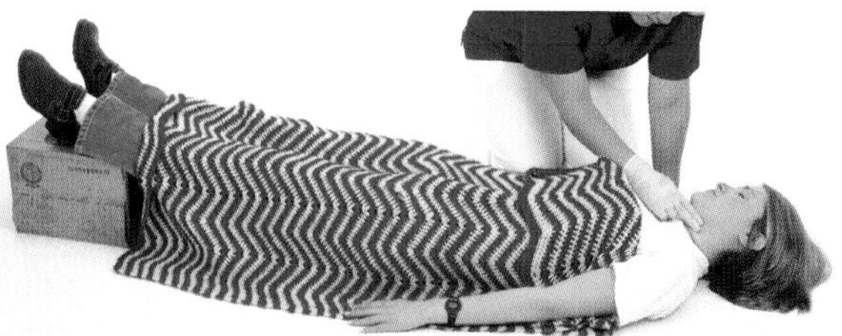

Fig. 7-3. *If a person is in shock, elevate the legs eight to 12 inches unless she has a head, neck, back, spinal, or abdominal injury, breathing difficulties, or fractures.*

8. Do not give the person anything to eat or drink.
9. Report and document the incident properly.

Myocardial Infarction or Heart Attack

Myocardial infarction (MI), or heart attack, occurs when the heart muscle itself does not receive enough oxygen because blood vessels are blocked. More information about MIs is found in Chapter 18. A myocardial infarction is an emergency that can result in serious heart damage or death. The following are signs and symptoms of MI:

- Sudden, severe pain in the chest, usually on the left side or in the center, behind the sternum (breastbone)
- Pain or discomfort in other areas of the body, such as one or both arms, the back, neck, jaw, or stomach
- Indigestion or heartburn
- Nausea and vomiting
- **Dyspnea** or difficulty breathing
- Dizziness
- Bluish or gray (cyanotic) skin color, indicating lack of oxygen
- Perspiration
- Cold and clammy skin
- Weak and irregular pulse rate

- Low blood pressure
- Anxiety and a sense of doom
- Denial of a heart problem

The pain of a heart attack is commonly described as a crushing, pressing, squeezing, stabbing, piercing pain, or, "like someone is sitting on my chest." The pain may go down the inside of the left arm. A person may also feel it in the neck and/or in the jaw. The pain usually does not go away.

As with men, women may experience chest pain or pressure. However, women can have heart attacks without chest pressure. Women are more likely to have shortness of breath, pressure or pain in the lower chest or upper abdomen, dizziness, lightheadedness, fainting, pressure in the upper back, or extreme fatigue. Some women's symptoms seem more flu-like, and women are more likely to deny that they are having a heart attack. Nursing assistants must take immediate action if a resident experiences any of these symptoms.

Responding to a heart attack

1. Notify the nurse immediately.
2. Place the person in a comfortable position. Encourage him to rest and reassure him that you will not leave him alone.
3. Loosen clothing around the person's neck (Fig. 7-4).

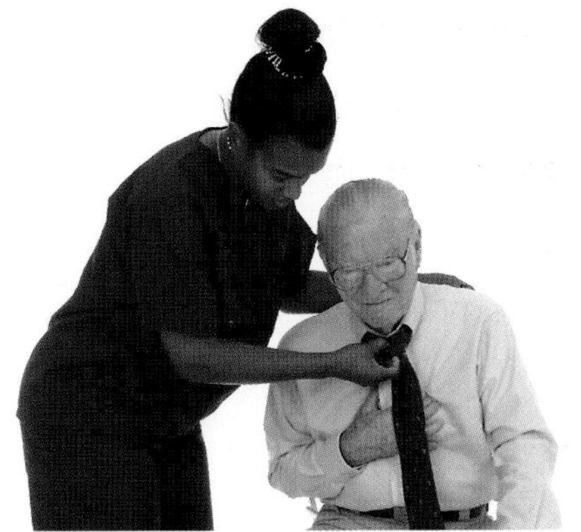

Fig. 7-4. *Loosen clothing around the person's neck if you suspect he is having an MI.*

4. Do not give the person liquids or food.
5. Monitor the person's breathing and pulse. If the person stops breathing or has no pulse, begin CPR if trained and allowed to do so.
6. Stay with the person until help arrives.
7. Report and document the incident properly.

Some states allow nursing assistants to offer heart medication, such as nitroglycerin, to a resident having a heart attack. If allowed to do this, NAs can only offer the medication; they cannot place it in the resident's mouth.

Bleeding

Severe bleeding can cause death quickly and must be controlled.

Controlling bleeding

1. Notify the nurse immediately.
2. Put on gloves. Take time to do this. If the resident is able, he can hold his bare hand over the wound until you can put on gloves.
3. Hold a thick sterile pad, clean cloth, handkerchief, or towel against the wound.
4. Press down hard directly on the bleeding wound until help arrives. Do not decrease pressure (Fig. 7-5). Put additional pads over the first pad if blood seeps through. Do not remove the first pad.

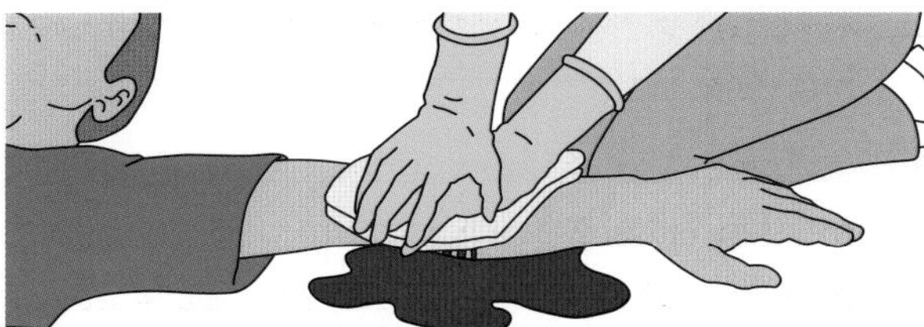

Fig. 7-5. *Press down hard directly on the bleeding wound; do not decrease pressure.*

5. If you can, raise the wound above the level of the heart to slow down the bleeding. If the wound is on an arm, leg, hand, or foot, and there are no broken bones, prop up the limb. Use towels or other absorbent material.

6. When bleeding is under control, secure the dressing to keep it in place. Check for symptoms of shock (pale skin, staring, increased pulse and respiration rates, low blood pressure, and extreme thirst). Stay with the person until help arrives.
7. Remove and discard gloves. Wash hands thoroughly.
8. Report and document the incident properly.

Poisoning

Facilities contain many harmful substances that should not be swallowed. Signs and symptoms of poisoning vary widely, depending on the substance that the person ingested.

Responding to poisoning

1. Notify the nurse immediately.
2. Put on gloves. Look for a container that will help you find out what the resident has taken or eaten. With your gloves on, check the mouth for chemical burns and note the breath odor.
3. The nurse may have you call the local or state Poison Control Center. Follow their instructions.
4. Remove and discard gloves. Wash your hands.
5. Report and document the incident properly.

Burns

Care of a burn depends on its depth, size, and location. There are three types of burns: first-degree (superficial), second-degree (partial-thickness), and third-degree (full-thickness) burns (Fig. 7-6). First-degree burns involve just the outer layer of skin. The skin becomes red, painful, and swollen, but no blisters appear. Second-degree burns extend from the outer layer of skin to the next deeper layer of skin. The skin is red, painful, swollen, and blisters appear. Third-degree burns involve all three layers of the skin and may extend to the bone. If the nerves are destroyed, no pain occurs. The skin is shiny and appears hard. It may be white in color.

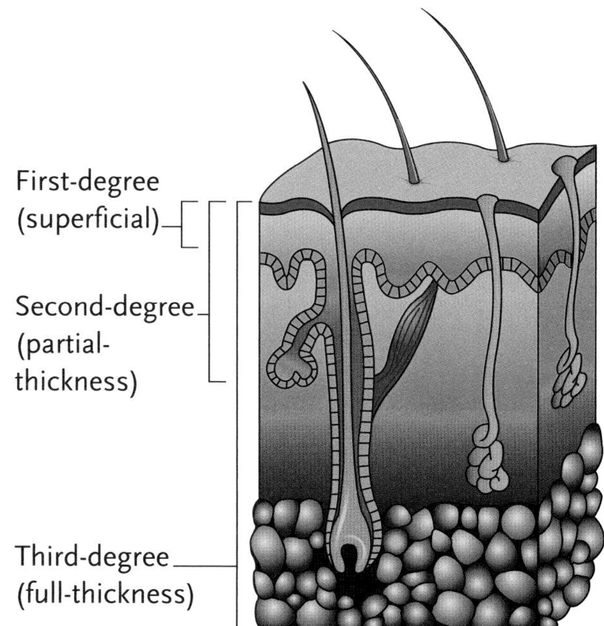

Fig. 7-6. *Different degrees of burns.*

Treating burns

To treat a minor burn:

1. Notify the nurse immediately. Put on gloves.
2. Use cool, clean water to decrease the skin temperature and prevent further injury (Fig. 7-7). Do not use ice or ice water, as ice may cause further skin damage. Dampen a clean cloth with cool water and place it over the burn.

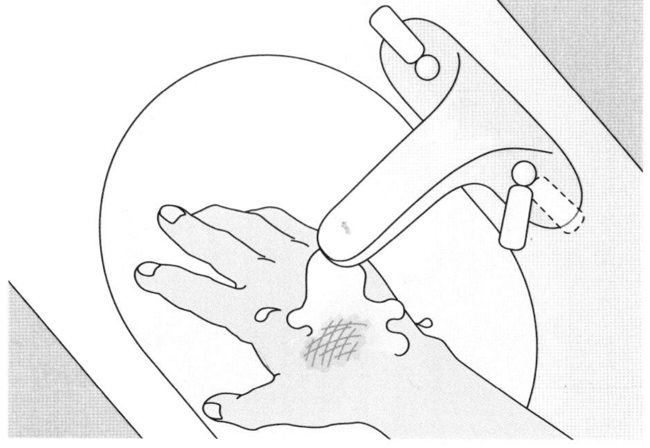

Fig. 7-7. *Use cool, clean water, not ice, on burned skin.*

3. Once the pain has eased, you may cover the area with dry, sterile gauze or clean dressing.
4. Remove and discard gloves. Wash your hands.
5. Never use any kind of ointment, salve, or grease on a burn.

For more serious burns:

1. Remove the person from the source of the burn. If clothing has caught fire, have the person stop, drop, and roll, or smother the fire with a blanket or towel to put out flames. Protect yourself from the source of the burn.
2. Notify the nurse immediately. Put on gloves.
3. Check for breathing, pulse, and severe bleeding. If the person is not breathing and has no pulse, begin CPR if trained and allowed to do so.
4. Do not use any type of ointment, water, salve, or grease on the burn.
5. Do not try to pull away any clothing from burned areas. Cover the burn with thick, dry, sterile gauze, a clean cloth, or a clean white sheet. A dry, insulated cool pack may be used over the dressing (Fig. 7-8). Take care not to rub the burned area.

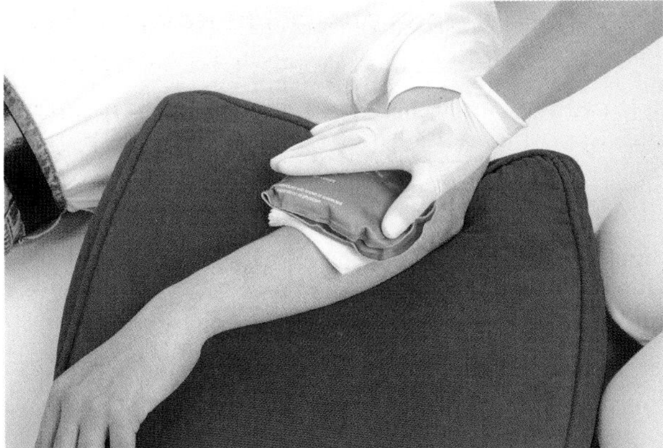

Fig. 7-8. *A dry cool pack may be used over a dressing to treat a serious burn.*

6. Ask the person to lie down and elevate the affected part if this does not cause greater pain.
7. Wait for emergency medical help.
8. Remove and discard gloves. Wash your hands.
9. Report and document the incident properly.

Chemical burns require special care. Call for help immediately. The chemical must be washed away thoroughly. A shower or a hose may be needed when the burns cover a large area.

Fainting

Fainting, also called **syncope**, occurs as a result of decreased blood flow to the brain, causing a loss of consciousness. Fainting may be the result of hunger, fear, pain, fatigue, standing for a long time, poor ventilation, certain medications, pregnancy, or overheating. Signs and symptoms of fainting include dizziness, nausea, perspiration, pale skin, weak pulse, shallow respirations, and blackness in the visual field. If someone appears likely to faint, the nursing assistant should follow these steps:

Responding to fainting

1. Notify the nurse immediately.
2. Have the person lie down or sit down before fainting occurs.
3. If the person is in a sitting position, have him bend forward (Fig. 7-9). He can place his head between his knees if he is able. If the person is lying flat on his back, elevate the legs.
4. Loosen any tight clothing.
5. Have the person stay in position for at least five minutes after symptoms disappear.
6. Help the person get up slowly. Continue to observe him for symptoms of fainting. Stay with him until he feels better. If you need help but cannot leave the person, use the call light.

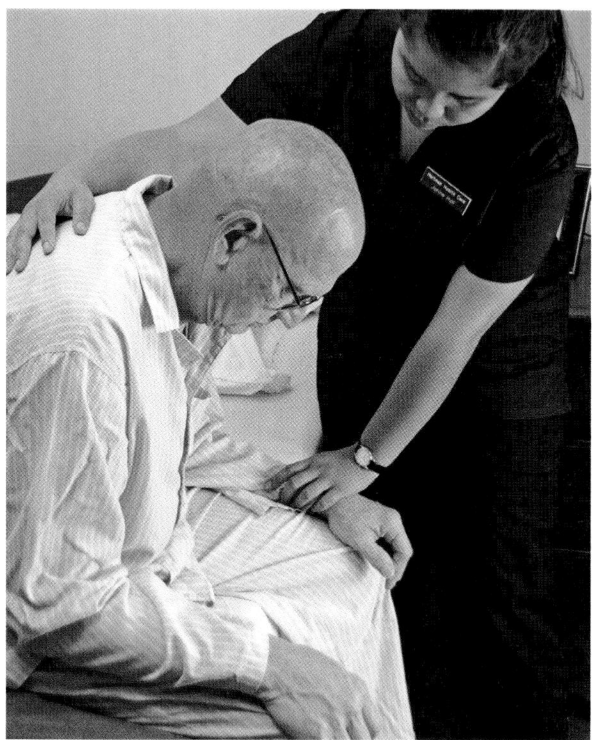

Fig. 7-9. Have the person bend forward if he is sitting.

7. If a person does faint, lower him to the floor or other flat surface. Position him on his back. Elevate his legs eight to 12 inches. Loosen any tight clothing. Check to make sure the person is breathing. He should recover quickly, but keep him lying down for several minutes. Report the incident to the nurse immediately.
8. Report and document the incident properly. Fainting may be a sign of a more serious medical condition.

Nosebleed

A nosebleed can occur suddenly when the air is dry, when injury has occurred, or when a person has taken certain medications. The medical term for a nosebleed is **epistaxis**.

Responding to a nosebleed

1. Notify the nurse immediately.
2. Elevate the head of the bed, or tell the person to remain in a sitting position, leaning forward slightly. Offer tissues or a clean cloth to catch the blood. Do not touch blood or bloody clothes, tissues, or cloths without gloves.
3. Put on gloves. Apply firm pressure over the bridge of the nose. Squeeze the bridge of the nose with your thumb and forefinger (Fig. 7-10). Have the resident do this until you are able to put on gloves.

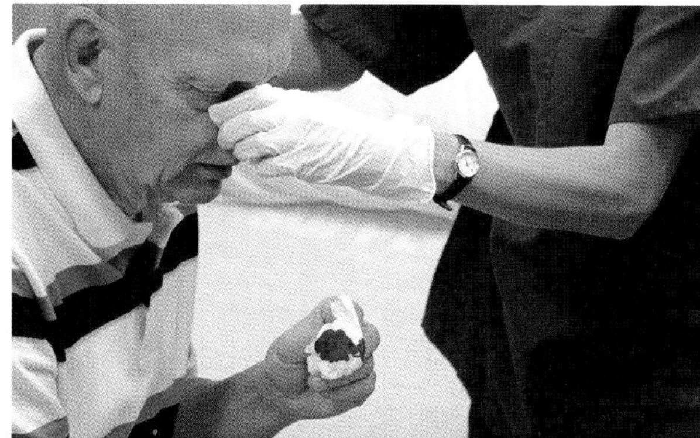

Fig. 7-10. With gloves on, squeeze the bridge of the nose with your thumb and forefinger.

4. Apply the pressure until the bleeding stops.
5. Use a cool cloth or ice wrapped in a cloth on the back of the neck, forehead, or upper lip to slow the flow of blood. Never apply ice directly to skin.
6. Remove and discard gloves. Wash your hands.
7. Report and document the incident properly.

Insulin Reaction and Diabetic Ketoacidosis

Insulin reaction and diabetic ketoacidosis are complications of diabetes that can be life-threatening. More information about diabetes and related care is in Chapter 18.

Insulin reaction, or **hypoglycemia**, can result from either too much insulin or too little food. It occurs when a dose of insulin is given and the person skips a meal or does not eat all the food required. Even when a regular amount of food is eaten, physical activity may rapidly metabolize the food. This causes too much insulin to be in the body. Vomiting and diarrhea may also lead to insulin reaction in people who have diabetes.

The first signs of insulin reaction include feeling weak or different, nervousness, dizziness, and perspiration. These signal that the resident needs food in a form that can be rapidly absorbed. A lump of sugar, a hard candy, or a glass of orange juice should be consumed right away. A diabetic should always have a quick source of sugar handy. The nurse should be notified if a resident has shown signs of insulin reaction. Signs and symptoms of insulin reaction include the following:

- Hunger
- Weakness
- Rapid pulse
- Headache
- Low blood pressure
- Perspiration
- Cold, clammy skin
- Confusion
- Trembling
- Nervousness
- Blurred vision
- Numbness of the lips and tongue
- Unconsciousness

Diabetic ketoacidosis (DKA), also called **hyperglycemia**, is caused by having too little insulin. It can result from undiagnosed diabetes, going without insulin or not taking enough, eating too much, not getting enough exercise, infection, or physical or emotional stress. The signs of the onset of diabetic ketoacidosis include increased thirst or urination, abdominal pain, deep or labored breathing, and breath that smells sweet or fruity. The nurse should be notified immediately if a resident has shown signs of diabetic ketoacidosis. Other signs and symptoms include the following:

- Hunger
- Headache
- Weakness
- Rapid, weak pulse
- Low blood pressure
- Dry skin
- Flushed cheeks
- Drowsiness
- Nausea and vomiting
- Abdominal pain
- Air hunger, or resident gasping for air and being unable to catch his breath
- Unconsciousness

Seizures

Seizures are involuntary, often violent, contractions of muscles. They can involve a small area or the entire body. Seizures are caused by an abnormality in the brain. They can occur in a young child who has a high fever. Older children and adults who have a serious illness, fever, head injury, or a seizure disorder such as **epilepsy** may also have seizures.

The main goal during a seizure is to make sure the resident is safe. During a seizure, a person may shake severely and thrust arms and legs uncontrollably. He may clench his jaw, drool, and be unable to swallow. Most seizures only last a short time.

Responding to a seizure

1. Note the time. Put on gloves.
2. Lower the person to the floor. Loosen clothing to help with breathing. Try to turn the person's head to one side to help lower the risk of choking. This may not be possible during a violent seizure.
3. Have someone call the nurse immediately or use the call light. Do not leave a person dur-

ing a seizure unless you must do so to get medical help.

4. Move furniture away to prevent injury. If a pillow is nearby, place it under his head.
5. Do not try to restrain the person or stop the seizure.
6. Do not force anything between the person's teeth. Do not place your hands in the person's mouth for any reason. You could be bitten.
7. Do not give the person liquids or food.
8. When the seizure is over, note the time. Gently turn the person to his left side if you do not suspect a head, neck, or spinal injury. This reduces the risk of choking on vomit or saliva. If the person begins to choke, get help immediately. Check for adequate breathing and pulse. Begin CPR if breathing and pulse are absent and if you are allowed and trained to do so. Do not begin CPR during a seizure.
9. Remove and discard gloves. Wash your hands.
10. Report and document the incident properly, including how long the seizure lasted.

CVA or Stroke

Cerebrovascular accident (CVA), or stroke, was first discussed in Chapter 4. A quick response to a suspected stroke is critical. Tests and treatment need to be given within a short time of the stroke's onset. Early treatment may be able to reduce the severity of the stroke.

A **transient ischemic attack** (**TIA**) is a warning sign of a CVA. It is the result of a temporary lack of oxygen in the brain. Symptoms may last up to 24 hours. They include difficulty speaking, weakness on one side of the body, temporary loss of vision, and numbness or tingling. These symptoms should not be ignored; they should be reported to the nurse immediately. These are signs that a CVA is occurring:

- Facial numbness, weakness, or drooping, especially on one side (hemiparesis)
- Arm numbness or weakness, especially on one side
- Slurred speech or inability to speak (expressive aphasia)
- Use of inappropriate words
- Inability to understand spoken or written words (receptive aphasia)
- Redness in the face
- Noisy breathing
- Dizziness
- Blurred vision
- Ringing in the ears
- Headache
- Nausea/vomiting
- Seizures
- Loss of bowel and bladder control
- Paralysis on one side of the body (hemiplegia)
- Elevated blood pressure
- Slow pulse rate
- Loss of consciousness

Chapter 18 contains more information on CVA and related care.

Vomiting

Vomiting, or **emesis**, is the act of ejecting stomach contents through the mouth and/or nose. It can be a sign of a serious illness or injury. Some residents, such as those with cancer who are undergoing chemotherapy, may vomit frequently as a result of treatment. Because a nursing assistant may not know when a resident is going to vomit, she may not have time to explain what she will do and assemble supplies ahead of time. The NA should talk to the resident soothingly as she helps him clean up. She should tell the resident what she is doing to help him.

Responding to vomiting

1. Notify the nurse immediately.
2. Put on gloves.
3. Make sure the head is up or turned to one side. Place an emesis basin under the chin. Remove it when vomiting has stopped.
4. Remove soiled linens or clothes and set aside. Replace with fresh linens or clothes.
5. If resident's intake and output (I&O) is being monitored (Chapter 15), measure and note amount of vomitus.
6. Flush vomit down the toilet unless vomit is red, has blood in it, or looks like wet coffee grounds. If these symptoms are observed, show this to the nurse before discarding the vomit. After disposing of vomit, wash and store basin.
7. Remove and discard gloves.
8. Wash your hands.
9. Put on fresh gloves.
10. Provide comfort to resident. Wipe face and mouth (Fig. 7-11). Position comfortably, and offer a drink of water. Provide oral care (Chapter 13). It helps get rid of the taste of vomit in the mouth.

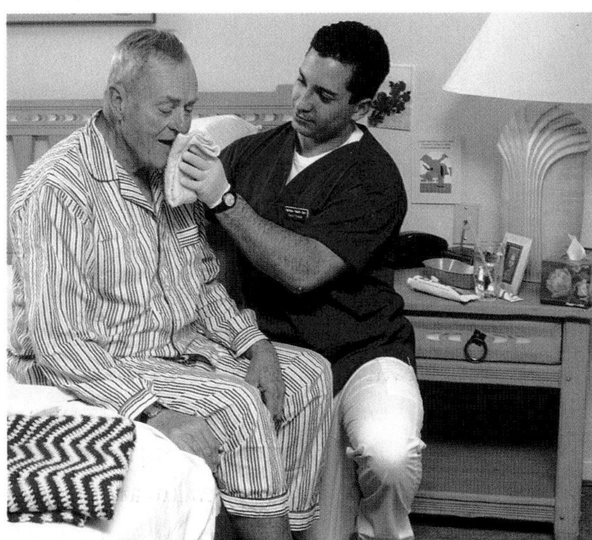

***Fig. 7-11.** Be calm and comforting when helping a resident who has vomited.*

11. Put soiled linen in proper containers.
12. Remove and discard gloves.
13. Wash your hands again.
14. Document time, amount, color, odor, and consistency of vomitus.

Falls

Falls can be minor or severe. All falls should be reported to the nurse immediately, even if the resident says he feels fine. The nursing assistant will need to complete an incident report. In the case of a severe fall, the nurse may ask the NA to call emergency medical services. To help a resident who is falling, the nursing assistant should do the following:

- Widen her stance. Bring the resident's body close to the NA's body to break the fall. The NA should bend her knees and support the resident as she lowers the resident to the floor.
- The nursing assistant should not try to reverse or stop a fall. Doing this can cause more injury.
- The NA should notify the nurse immediately. She should not attempt to get the resident up or move the resident after the fall.

Chapter 6 has more information about falls and fall prevention.

3. Describe disaster guidelines

Disasters can include fire, flood, earthquake, hurricane, tornado, or severe weather. Manmade dangers, such as acts of terrorism or bomb threats, are also considered disasters.

Nursing assistants need to be competent and professional when a disaster occurs. Facilities have disaster plans, and NAs will be trained on these plans. Annual in-services and disaster drills are often held at facilities. NAs should take advantage of these sessions when offered and pay close attention to instructions.

During natural disasters, a nurse or the administrator will give directions. Nursing assistants should listen carefully to all directions and follow instructions. Facilities may rely on local or state management groups and the American Red Cross to assume overall responsibility for the ill and disabled.

Guidelines: Disasters

The following guidelines apply in any disaster situation:

- Remain calm.
- Know the locations of all exits and stairways.
- Know where the fire alarms and extinguishers are located.
- Know the appropriate action to take in any situation.
- Use the Internet to stay informed, or keep the radio or television tuned to a local station to get the latest information.

In addition, you will be required to apply specific guidelines for the area in which you work. For example, an NA working where hurricanes are prevalent, such as Florida, needs to know the guidelines for hurricane preparedness as well as for storms and fires. The following general guidelines are separated by the type of disaster and can be applied to any particular geographical area that applies to your specific job and location.

Tornadoes

- Seek shelter inside, ideally in a steel-framed or concrete building.
- Stay away from windows.
- Stand in the hallway or in a basement, or take cover under heavy furniture.
- Do not stay in a mobile home or trailer.
- Lie as flat as possible.

Lightning

If outdoors, follow these guidelines:

- Avoid the largest objects, such as trees, and avoid open spaces.
- Stay out of the water.
- Seek shelter in buildings.
- Stay away from metal fences, doors, or other objects.
- Avoid holding metal objects, such as golf clubs, in your hands.
- Stay in automobiles.
- It is safe to perform CPR on lightning victims; they carry no electricity.

If indoors, follow these guidelines:

- Stay inside and away from open doors and windows.
- Avoid the use of electrical equipment, such as hair dryers and televisions.
- Do not use the telephone.

Floods

- Fill the bathtub with fresh water.
- Board up windows.
- Evacuate if advised to do so.
- Check the fuel level in automobiles.
- Have a portable battery-operated radio, flashlight, and cooking equipment available.
- Do not drink water or eat food that has been contaminated with flood water.
- Do not handle electrical equipment.
- Do not turn off gas yourself. Ask the gas company to turn off the gas.

Blackouts

- Get a flashlight. Take prompt action to keep calm and provide light.

- Use a backup pack for electrical medical equipment, such as an IV pump. Backup packs do not last more than 24 hours, so contact emergency personnel when instructed.

Hurricanes

- Know what category the hurricane is and track the expected path.
- Know which residents must go to shelters, hospitals, or other facilities, and which need assistance. Be aware of people with special needs. High-risk people include the elderly and those unable to evacuate on their own. High-risk areas include mobile homes or trailers.
- Call your employer for instructions.
- Fill the bathtub with fresh water.
- Board up windows.
- Evacuate if advised to do so.
- Check the fuel level in automobiles.
- Have a portable battery-operated radio, flashlight, and cooking equipment available.

Earthquakes

If indoors, follow these guidelines:

- Drop to the ground.
- If possible, get under a sturdy piece of furniture, such as a heavy table, and hold on until the shaking stops.
- If no table or desk is available, stay crouched down in the inside corner of a building, and cover your face and head with your arms.
- Stay away from windows, outside walls, and anything that might fall over or fall down.
- Do not exit a building during the shaking.
- Do not use elevators.

If outdoors, follow these guidelines:

- Move away from buildings, electric poles and wires, and streetlights. Falling or flying debris is a far greater danger than ground movement.
- If driving, stop as quickly as is safely possible and stay in the vehicle. Avoid stopping under overpasses or near buildings or wires if possible.
- If trapped under debris after an earthquake, do not light a match or ignite a lighter, and avoid kicking up dust. Breathe through a handkerchief or clothing and make tapping noises or use a whistle, if available, to get rescuers' attention. Do not shout. Shouting could cause you to inhale dangerous amounts of dust.

In addition to the above, when working in the home, follow these guidelines for disasters:

- If a disaster is forecast (for example, a tornado or hurricane), be ready. Wear appropriate clothing and shoes. Have family members dressed and ready in case evacuation is necessary.
- Stay in contact with your supervisor or others if possible. Let someone know where you are, what conditions are, and where you will go if you must evacuate.
- Locate disaster supplies. Ideally, a disaster supply kit should meet your needs for at least three days. It should be assembled before disaster strikes and should include the following:
    - A three-day supply of water (one gallon per person per day) and food that will not spoil
    - One change of clothing and footwear per person and one blanket or sleeping bag per person

- A first aid kit that includes your family's prescription medications
- Emergency tools, including a battery-powered radio, flashlight, and plenty of extra batteries
- An extra set of car keys and a credit card, cash, or debit card
- Sanitation supplies
- Special items for infant, elderly, or disabled family members
- An extra pair of eyeglasses
- Important family documents in a waterproof container

Chapter Review

1. List two steps to follow when encountering an emergency situation. 1) Stay calm 2) act quickly
2. What kind of information should a nursing assistant be prepared to give when calling emergency services? The phone number and address of the emergency. Location within the building. The persons condition and medical background. The NA name and background. Details of any 1st aid being given.
3. Why should a nursing assistant not perform CPR if she is not trained to do so? The NA could do more damage if she does not have this skill.
4. How are abdominal thrusts used to help someone who is choking? The thrusts work to remove the blockage upward and out of the throat
5. If the person becomes unconscious while choking, what should the nursing assistant do? Lay the resident gently on the floor on his back face up. Then make sure help is on the way & stay with resident until help arrives.
6. List the signs of shock. Pale or bluish skin. Staring into space, increased pulse & respiration rates low BP. extreme thirst.
7. List seven signs that a person is having a heart attack. 1) Sudden, severe pain in the chest, Usually in left side. 2) Pain in other parts of the body like one or both arms, neck or jaw or stomach. 3) Indigestion or heartburn 4) Nausea & vomiting 5) Difficulty breathing 6) Dizziness 7) Bluish or grey skin color, 8) Perspiration 9) Cold, clammy skin. 10) weak & irregular pulse 11) Low blood pressure 12) Anxiety and a sense of doom
8. What can be done to a wound to slow bleeding? Put pressure on the wound and don't let up. Raise the wounded area above the heart if possible.
9. Why should ice not be applied to burns? It can cause further skin damage.
10. If a person feels like he is going to faint, in what position should he be placed? Lying down or sitting down. If he is sitting down, he can place his head between his knees. Lying down the NA can elevate his legs. Loosen tight clothing
11. Why should a nursing assistant put on gloves if a resident has a nosebleed? Because of coming in contact with blood & any blood pathogens you are not aware that the person has.
12. What causes insulin reaction? What causes diabetic ketoacidosis? insulin reaction happens when there is too much insulin or too little food. Too little insulin. Eating too much & little exercise.
13. Why should a nursing assistant not force anything into the mouth of a person who is having a seizure? The person could bite them.
14. List signs that a CVA/stroke is occurring. Facial numbness or drooping especially on one side. Arm numbness especially on one side, or arm weakness. Slurred speech or inability to speak (aphasia). Inability to understand spoken or written words. Redness in the face. Noisy breathing. Dizziness. Blurred vision. Ringing in the ears. Headache, Nausea & vomiting. Seizures. Paralysis on one side of the body (hemiplegia). ↑ BP. Slow pulse rate.
15. What should a nursing assistant do if a resident starts to fall? Widen her stance, bring resident close to her body and gently lower resident to the floor
16. What are three things that a nursing assistant should observe for in a resident's vomit? red vomit. Blood in vomit. Blood in vomit like wet coffee grounds.
17. What are four guidelines that apply in any disaster situation? Remain calm. Know locations of all exits & stairways. Know where fire alarms & all extinguishers are. Stay informed by internet & radio

8
Human Needs and Human Development

1. Identify basic human needs

People have different genes, physical appearances, cultural backgrounds, ages, and social or financial positions. But all human beings have the same basic physical needs:

- Food and water
- Protection and shelter
- Activity
- Sleep and rest
- Comfort, especially freedom from pain

Activities of daily living (ADLs), such as eating, toileting, bathing, and grooming, are the ways humans meet their most basic physical needs. By assisting with ADLs or helping residents learn to perform them independently, nursing assistants help residents meet their basic needs.

Human beings also have **psychosocial needs**, which involve social interaction, emotions, intellect, and spirituality. Although they are not as easy to define as physical needs, psychosocial needs include the following:

- Love and affection
- Acceptance by others
- Safety and security
- Self-reliance and independence in daily living
- Contact with others (Fig. 8-1)
- Success and self-esteem

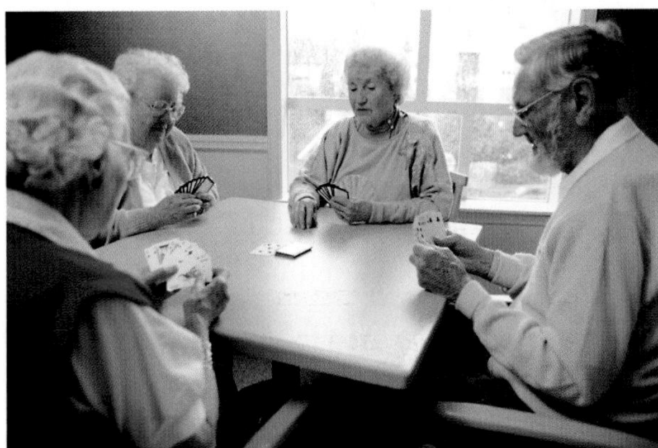

Fig. 8-1. *Interaction with other people is a basic psychosocial need. Nursing assistants can encourage residents to be with friends or relatives. Social contact is important.*

Health and well-being affect how well psychosocial needs are met. Stress and frustration occur when basic needs are not met. This can lead to fear, anxiety, anger, aggression, withdrawal, indifference, and depression. Stress can also cause physical problems that may eventually lead to illness.

Abraham Maslow, a researcher of human behavior, wrote about human physical and psychosocial needs. He arranged these needs into an order of importance. He thought that physical needs must be met before psychosocial needs can be met. His theory is called *Maslow's Hierarchy of Needs* (Fig. 8-2).

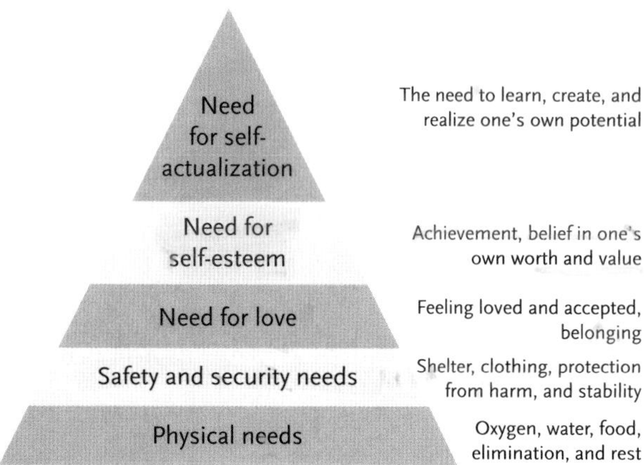

***Fig. 8-2.** Maslow's Hierarchy of Needs is a model developed by Abraham Maslow to show how physical and psychosocial needs are arranged in order of importance. Maslow believed that physical needs must be met before psychosocial needs can be met.*

After meeting physical needs, safety and security needs must be met. Feeling safe means not feeling afraid and unstable. Residents need to feel safe in facilities. Many things can cause a person to feel unsafe. An illness or disability can be frightening and make a person feel fearful and insecure. Losing some independence and needing help from caregivers, such as NAs, may cause some uncertainty or discomfort. Residents need to feel safe with all care team members; they need to know that they and their personal possessions will be protected.

After physical and safety needs are met, the need for love and belonging is important. This level involves feeling accepted, needed, and cared for. Regardless of their condition, residents need to know that their contributions are meaningful.

The need for self-esteem is the next level. This need involves respecting and valuing oneself, which comes from within, as well as from other people. Achievements that make a person feel valued are important. For residents, being able to do a task they were not able to do previously may satisfy this need. Hearing praise from NAs about this new achievement may also help meet this need.

Self-actualization is the highest level. It means that a person tries to be the best person he can be; he tries to reach his full potential. This may mean different things for each person. The quest to reach this need continues throughout a person's life and may change as a person enters different stages of life.

2. Define *holistic care* and explain its importance in health care

Holistic means considering a whole system, such as a whole person, rather than dividing the system up into parts. **Holistic care** means caring for the whole person—the mind as well as the body (Fig. 8-3). This is the approach nursing assistants should use when caring for residents. A simple example of holistic care is an NA talking with residents while helping them bathe. She is meeting the physical need with the bath and meeting the psychosocial need for interaction with others at the same time.

Another way of practicing holistic care is considering psychosocial factors in illness, as well as physical factors. For example, Mr. Hartman looks thin and tired. The cause might be depression rather than an infection. An NA does not need to determine the cause of his condition. However, by talking with him, the NA might learn something that would help the rest of the care team. For example, the NA may learn that last year at this time Mr. Hartman's wife died, and he is still coping with that loss. The NA can and should share this information with the care team and document it.

3. Explain why independence and self-care are important

Any big change in lifestyle, such as moving into a long-term care facility, requires a huge emotional adjustment. Residents may be experiencing fear, loss, and uncertainty, along with a decline in health and independence. Other common reactions to illness are denial, withdrawal, anger, hostility, and depression. All of these feelings may cause residents to behave differently

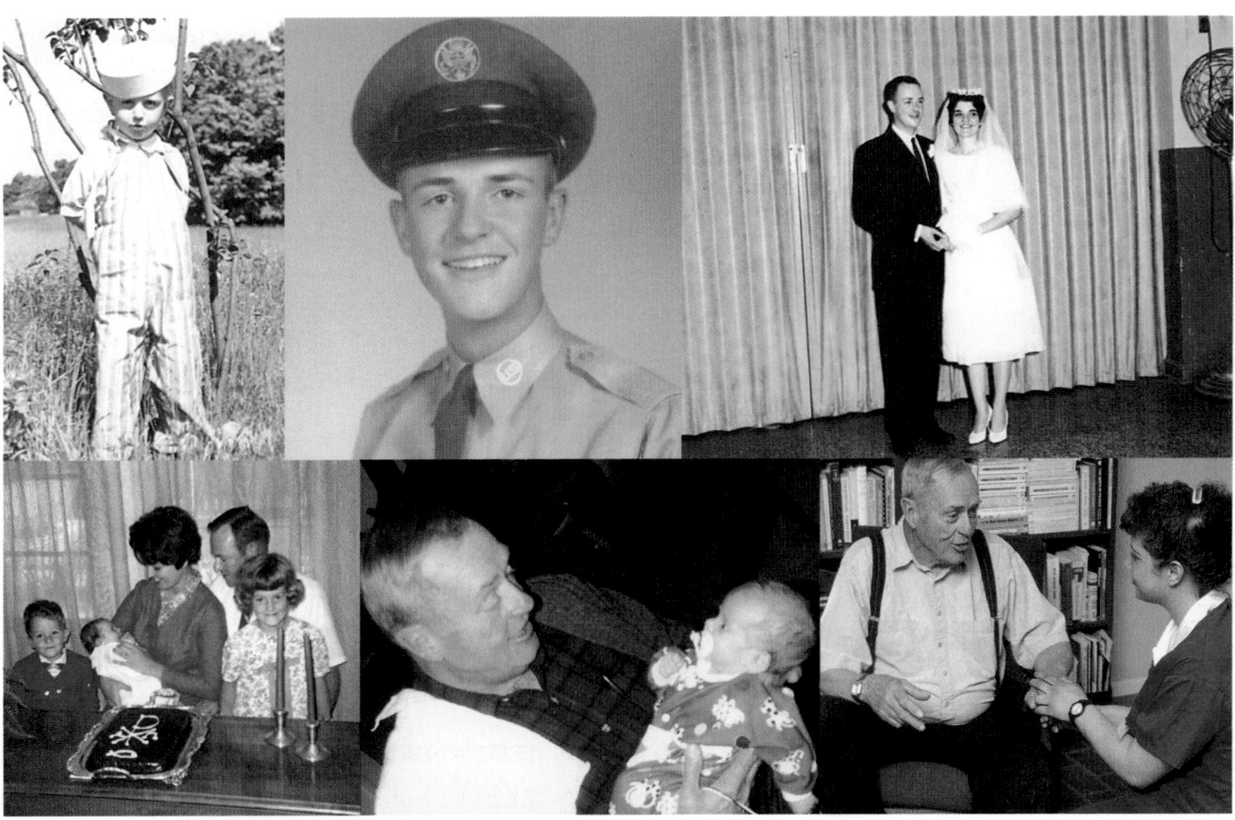

Fig. 8-3. Residents are people, not just lists of illnesses and disabilities. They have many needs, like any other person. Many have had rich and wonderful lives. NAs should take time to know and care for each resident as a whole person.

than they have before. Each person adjusts to illness and change in his or her own way and in his or her own time. It is important for nursing assistants to remain supportive and encouraging. NAs should be patient, understanding, and empathetic.

Moving to a care facility represents a tremendous loss of independence for a resident, and loss of independence can be very difficult. Somebody else must now do what residents did for themselves all of their lives. NAs should try to imagine what it would be like to have to call someone to help every time they had to go to the bathroom. The loss of independence is also difficult for residents' friends and family members. For example, a resident may have been the main provider for his or her family. A resident may have been the person who did all of the cooking for the family. Other losses residents may be experiencing include the following:

- Loss of spouse, family members, or friends due to death
- Loss of workplace and its relationships due to retirement
- Loss of ability to go to favorite places
- Loss of ability to attend services and meetings at their faith communities
- Loss of home and personal possessions (Fig. 8-4)
- Loss of health and the ability to care for themselves
- Loss of ability to move freely
- Loss of pets
- Lesbian, gay, bisexual, or transgender (LGBT) residents may fear the loss of a comfortable and accepting environment.

Independence often means not having to rely on others for money, daily care, or participation in social activities. Activities of daily living (ADLs) are the personal care tasks a person does every day to care for himself. People may take these activities for granted until they can no longer do them for themselves. ADLs include bathing or showering, dressing, caring for teeth and hair, toileting, eating and drinking, and moving from place to place.

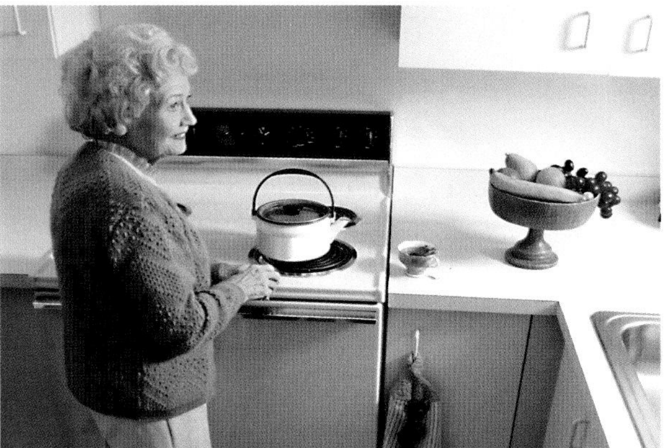

Fig. 8-4. Nursing assistants should understand and be sympathetic to the fact that many residents had to leave familiar places.

A loss of independence can cause the following problems:

- Poor self-image
- Anger toward caregivers, others, and self
- Feelings of helplessness, sadness, and hopelessness
- Feelings of being useless
- Increased dependence
- Depression

To prevent these feelings, NAs should encourage residents to do as much as possible for themselves. Even if it seems easier for the NA to do a task for a resident, the resident should be allowed to do it independently. NAs must encourage self-care, regardless of how long it takes or how poorly residents are able to do it. NAs should be patient (Fig. 8-5).

Allowing residents to make choices is another way to promote independence. For example, residents can choose where to sit while they eat. They can choose what they eat and in what order. Respect a resident's right to make choices.

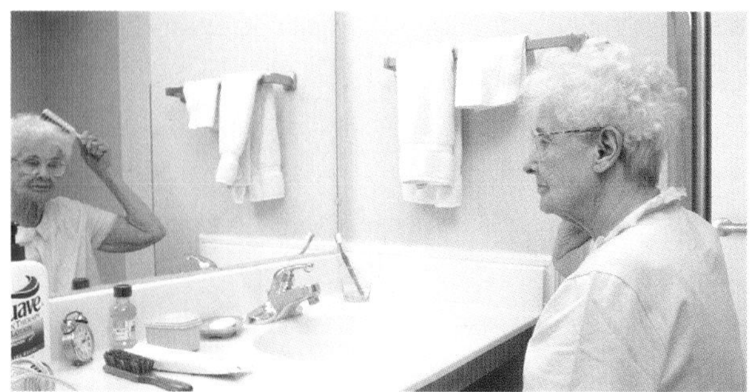

Fig. 8-5. Even if personal care tasks take a long time, residents should be encouraged to do what they can for themselves.

Residents' Rights

Dignity and Independence

Residents are adults; they should not be treated as if they were children. Nursing assistants should encourage residents to do self-care without rushing them. Residents have the right to refuse care and to make their own choices. Promoting dignity and independence is part of protecting their legal rights. It is also the proper and ethical way for NAs to work.

4. Respect different forms of sexual identity and explain ways to accommodate sexual needs

In addition to the needs discussed earlier, people also have sexual needs. These needs continue throughout their lives (Fig. 8-6). The ability to engage in sexual activity, such as intercourse and masturbation, continues unless a disease or injury occurs. **Masturbation** means to touch or rub sexual organs in order to give oneself or another person sexual pleasure.

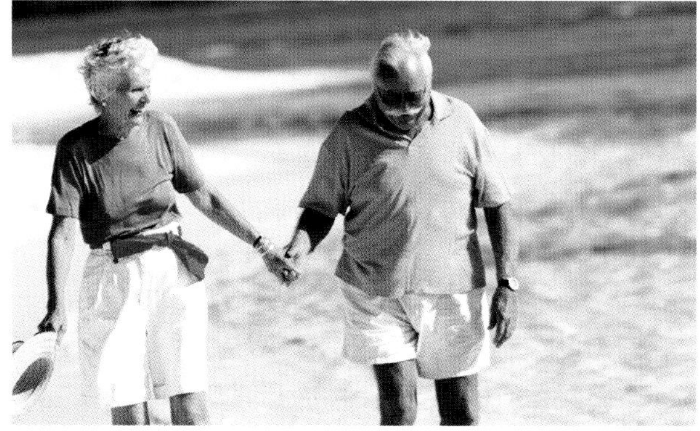

Fig. 8-6. Human beings continue to have sexual needs throughout their lives.

Residents have the right to choose how they express their sexuality. In all age groups, there is a variety of sexual behavior. This is true of residents, also. Sexual orientation is a person's preference for one gender (male or female) or the other, or both. Terms defining sexual identity include the following:

- **Gay**: 1. A person whose sexual preference is for people of the same sex. 2. A man whose sexual preference is for men.
- **Heterosexual**: A person whose sexual preference is for people of the opposite sex; also known as *straight*.
- **Homosexual**: A person whose sexual preference is for people of the same sex; terms *gay* and *lesbian* are usually preferred.
- **Lesbian**: A woman whose sexual preference is for women.
- **Bisexual**: A person who is sexually attracted to both men and women.
- **Transsexual**: 1. One who wishes to be accepted by society as a member of the opposite sex. 2. One who has undergone a sex change operation.
- **Transgender**: A person whose gender identity conflicts with his or her birth sex (sex assigned at birth due to anatomy).
- **Transitioning**: The process of changing genders.

The abbreviation *LGBT* stands for lesbian, gay, bisexual, transsexual/transgender. The National Resource Center on LGBT Aging estimates that more than 1.5 million U.S. adults over 65 are LGBT (Fig. 8-7).

Many states have laws making it illegal for LTC facilities to discriminate in any way against residents due to sexual identity or orientation. In some states, LTC staff must be trained specifically to understand and respect different forms of sexual identity. One part of respecting residents' sexual identity is not making the automatic assumption that a resident is heterosexual.

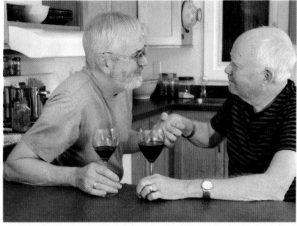

Fig. 8-7. *The number of lesbian, gay, bisexual, and transgender older adults continues to increase.*

No matter what a nursing assistant's personal or religious feelings regarding sexuality may be, he or she must always treat residents with respect. NAs must use terms and pronouns residents prefer (using "she," for example, to refer to a resident who is physically male but identifies as female), and must not gossip or break confidentiality regarding residents' sexual behavior or orientation/identity. It is also important for NAs to remember that every resident is a human being, first and foremost, and sexual identity is only one aspect of the resident's experience.

To meet and respect residents' sexual needs, nursing assistants can do the following:

Guidelines: Respecting Sexual Needs

- G Always knock or announce yourself before entering residents' rooms. Listen and wait for a response before entering.
- G If you encounter a sexual situation between consenting adult residents, provide privacy and leave the room. However, if you see sexual abuse occurring, take the resident to a safe place and notify the nurse immediately.
- G Be open and nonjudgmental about residents' sexual attitudes. Do not judge residents' sexual orientation or sexual behavior.
- G Honor *Do Not Disturb* signs.

- G Do not view any expression of sexuality by the elderly as disgusting or cute. That attitude is inappropriate and deprives residents of their right to dignity and respect.

Illness and disability can affect sexual desires, needs, and abilities. Residents may be sensitive about this. Sexual desire may not be lessened by a disability, although ability to meet sexual needs may be limited. Many people confined to wheelchairs can have sexual and intimate relationships, though adjustments may have to be made. Nursing assistants should not assume they know what impact a physical disability has had on sexuality.

Sexual needs may also be affected by residents' living environments. A lack of privacy and no available partner are often reasons for a lack of sexual expression in care facilities. NAs should always be sensitive to privacy needs.

Residents' Rights

Sexual Abuse

Residents must be protected from unwanted sexual advances. If an NA sees sexual abuse occurring, he should remove the resident from the situation and take the resident to a safe place. The NA should then report to the nurse immediately.

5. Identify ways to help residents meet their spiritual needs

Residents may have spiritual needs, and nursing assistants can help with these needs. **Spiritual** means of, or relating to, the spirit or soul. Helping residents meet their spiritual needs can help them cope with illness or disability. Spirituality is a sensitive area. NAs must not offend residents by making judgments or imposing their beliefs.

Residents may have strong beliefs in God, or very little or no belief in God. Residents may consider themselves spiritual, but may not believe in God. The important thing for nursing assistants to remember is to respect all residents' beliefs, whatever they are. NAs should not make judgments about residents' spiritual beliefs or lack of beliefs. They should not try to push their beliefs on residents. Here are some ways NAs can help residents meet their spiritual needs:

Guidelines: Assisting with Spiritual Beliefs

- G Learn about residents' religions or beliefs. Listen carefully to what residents say.
- G Respect residents' decisions to participate in, or refrain from, food-related rituals. Accommodate practices such as dietary restrictions. Never make judgments about them.
- G If residents are religious, encourage participation in religious services.
- G Respect all religious items.
- G Report to the nurse (or social worker) if a resident expresses the desire to see clergy.
- G Get to know the priest, rabbi, or minister who visits or calls a resident.
- G Allow privacy for clergy visits (Fig. 8-8).

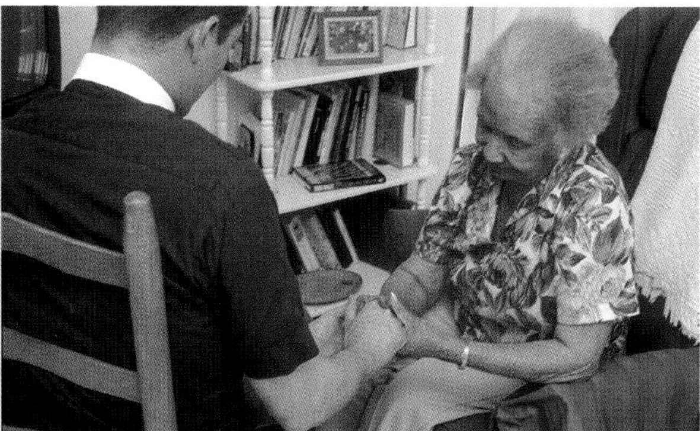

Fig. 8-8. *Be open to your residents' spiritual needs. Be welcoming and provide privacy when they receive visits from a spiritual leader.*

- G If asked, read religious materials aloud.
- G If a resident asks you, help find spiritual resources available in the area. Check the Internet or phone book for churches, synagogues, and other houses of worship. You can also refer this request to the nurse or social worker.

G You should never do any of the following:

- Try to change someone's religion
- Tell residents their belief or religion is wrong
- Express judgments about a religious group
- Insist residents join religious activities
- Interfere with religious practices

6. Identify ways to accommodate cultural and religious differences

Culture and cultural diversity were first discussed in Chapter 4. Cultural diversity has to do with the wide variety of people living throughout the world. Nursing assistants will take care of residents with backgrounds and traditions different from their own. It is important that NAs respect and value each person as an individual. They should respond to differences and new experiences with acceptance, not prejudice.

There are so many different cultures that they cannot all be listed here. One might talk about American culture being different from Japanese culture. But within American culture there are thousands of different groups with their own cultures: Japanese-Americans, African-Americans, and Native Americans are just a few. Even people from a particular region, state, or city can be said to have a different culture (Fig. 8-9). The culture of the South is not the same as the culture of New York City.

Cultural background affects how friendly people are to strangers. It can affect how close they want others to stand to them when talking. It can affect how they feel about NAs performing care for them or discussing their health with them. For example, a care team member asks a resident when he last had a bowel movement. One resident may freely answer this, while another may be embarrassed to have this discussion. One resident may be fine with an NA undressing him to help him bathe, while another may be uncomfortable with this. These reactions may also just be a part of a person's personality. Nursing assistants should be sensitive to residents' backgrounds. They may have to adjust their behavior around some residents. Regardless of their backgrounds, all residents must be treated with respect and professionalism. NAs should expect to be treated respectfully as well.

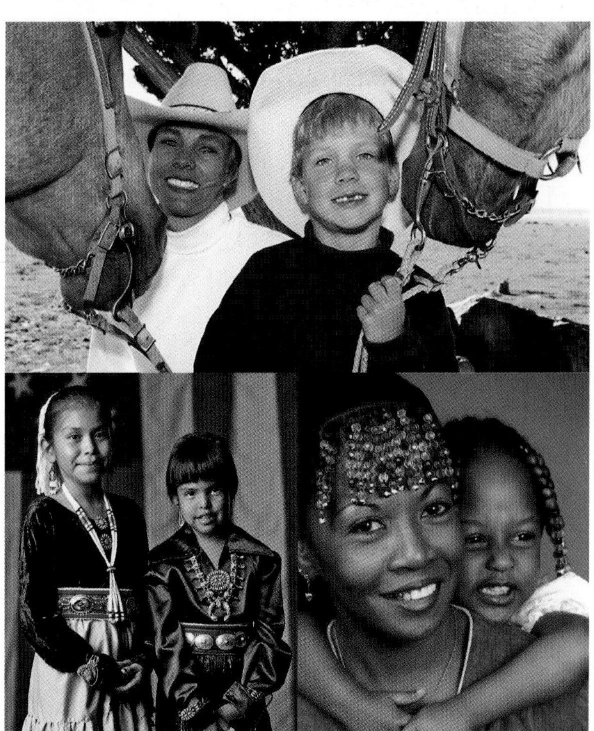

Fig. 8-9. *There are many different cultures in the United States.*

A resident's primary language may not be English. If he or she speaks a different language, an interpreter may be necessary. It can be helpful if staff members make an effort to learn a few common phrases in a resident's language. Picture cards and flash cards can assist with communication.

Religious differences also influence the way people behave. Religion can be very important in people's lives, particularly when they are ill or dying. Some people belong to a religious group, but do not practice everything that religion teaches. Some people consider themselves spiritual but not religious. Others do not believe in any religion or God, and do not consider themselves spiritual. Nursing assistants must respect the religious beliefs and practices of their residents, even if they are different from their own. Common religions, listed alphabetically, follow:

Buddhism: Buddhism started in Asia but has many followers in other parts of the world. Buddhism is based on the teachings of Siddhartha Gautama, called Buddha. Buddhists believe that life is filled with suffering that is caused by desire and that suffering ends when desire ends. Buddhism emphasizes meditation. Proper conduct and wisdom release a person from desire, suffering, and a repeating sequence of births and deaths (reincarnation). Nirvana is the highest spiritual plane a person can reach. It is the state of peace and freedom from worry and pain. The Dalai Lama is considered to be the highest spiritual leader.

Christianity: Christians believe Jesus Christ was the son of God and that he died so their sins would be forgiven. Christians may be Catholic or Protestant. There are many subgroups or denominations (such as Baptist, Episcopalian, Evangelical, Lutheran, Methodist, Mormon, Presbyterian, and Roman Catholic). Christians may go to church on Saturdays or Sundays; read the Bible, including the Old and New Testaments; receive communion; and be baptized. Some Christians may try to share their beliefs and convert others to their faith. Religious leaders may be called priests, ministers, pastors, preachers, or deacons.

Hinduism: Hinduism is the dominant faith of India, but it is practiced in other places as well. Hindus follow the teachings of ancient scriptures like the Vedas and Upanishads, as well as other major scriptures. Hindu beliefs vary widely; there may be a belief in only one God or in multiple gods. Worship can occur at a temple or at home. Hindus believe in **reincarnation**, which is a belief that some part of a living being survives death to be reborn in a new body. Hindus also believe in **karma**, which is the belief that all past and present deeds affect one's future and future lives. Hindus advocate respect for all life, and some Hindus are vegetarians. Vegetarians do not eat any meat. Hindus who do eat meat almost always refrain from eating beef. Holy men are called Sadhus.

Islam: Muslims, or followers of Mohammed, believe that Allah (God) wants people to follow the teachings of the prophet Mohammed as recorded in the Koran, the sacred text. Many Muslims pray five times a day facing Mecca, the holy city for their religion. Muslims also fast during a month-long observation called Ramadan. Muslims worship at mosques and do not drink alcohol or eat pork. There are other dietary restrictions, too. Islamic religious leaders may be called ayatollah, caliph, imam, mufti, and mullah, among other titles.

Judaism: Judaism is divided into Reform, Conservative, and Orthodox movements. Jewish people believe that God gave them laws through Moses and in Jewish scriptures, and that these laws should order their lives. Jewish services are held in synagogues or temples on Friday evenings and sometimes on Saturdays. Jewish men may wear a **yarmulke**, or small skullcap, as a sign of their faith. Some Jewish people observe dietary restrictions. They may not do certain things, such as work or drive, on the Sabbath, which lasts from Friday sundown to Saturday sundown. Religious leaders are called **rabbis**.

Spirituality concerns a person's beliefs about the spirit or the soul. It may center on how a person relates to his community, to nature, or to the divine. It may involve reflection and contemplation and a search for inner peace. Spiritual practices can include meditation or prayer, but spirituality does not have to encompass religious beliefs. Many people consider themselves to be spiritual but not religious.

Native Americans follow many different spiritual traditions and practices. An emphasis is placed on the personal and the communal, rather than the institutional, and there is a deep connection with nature. There are many varied practices and rituals.

As mentioned earlier, people have varying beliefs in religion, spirituality, and God. Some people may not believe in God or a higher power and identify themselves as agnostic. **Agnostics** believe that they do not know or cannot know if God exists. They do not deny that God might exist, but they feel there is no true knowledge of God's existence.

Atheists are people who believe that there is no God. This is different from what agnostics believe. Atheists actively deny the existence of God. For many atheists, this belief is as strongly held as any religious belief.

In addition to showing respect for different cultural and religious traditions, there may be specific practices that affect nursing assistants' work. Many religious beliefs include **dietary restrictions**. These are rules about what and when followers can eat. Some examples are listed below:

- Many Buddhists are vegetarians, though some include fish in their diet.
- Some Christians, particularly Roman Catholics, do not eat meat on Fridays during Lent.
- Many Jewish people eat kosher foods, do not eat pork, and do not eat lobster, shrimp, and clams (shellfish). Kosher food is food prepared in accordance with Jewish dietary laws. Kosher and non-kosher foods cannot come into contact with the same plates. Jewish people who observe dietary laws may not eat meat products at the same meal with dairy products.
- Mormons may not drink alcohol, coffee, or tea. They may not use tobacco in any form.
- Muslims do not eat pork. Certain birds may need to be avoided, too. They may not drink alcohol. Muslims may have regular periods of fasting. **Fasting** means not eating food or eating very little food.
- Some people are **vegetarians** and do not eat any meat for religious, moral, or health reasons.
- Some people are vegans. **Vegans** do not eat any animals or animal products, such as eggs or dairy products. In addition, some vegans do not use or wear any animal products, including wool and leather.

7. Describe the need for activity

Activity is an essential part of a person's life; it improves and maintains physical and mental health. Meaningful activities help promote independence, memory, self-esteem, and quality of life. In addition, physical activity can help manage illnesses, such as diabetes, high blood pressure, or high cholesterol. Regular physical activity can also help by doing the following:

- Lessening the risk of heart disease, colon cancer, diabetes, and obesity
- Relieving symptoms of depression
- Improving mood and concentration
- Improving body function
- Lowering the risk of falls
- Improving sleep quality
- Improving the ability to cope with stress
- Increasing energy
- Increasing appetite and promoting better eating habits

Just as activity aids physical and mental health, inactivity and immobility can result in physical and mental problems, such as the following:

- Loss of self-esteem
- Depression
- Boredom
- Pneumonia
- Urinary tract infection
- Constipation

- Blood clots
- Dulling of the senses

OBRA requires that facilities provide an activities program that is designed to meet the interests and the physical, mental, and psychosocial well-being of each resident. The activities are created to help residents socialize and to keep them physically and mentally active. Daily schedules are normally posted with activities for that particular day. Activities include exercise, arts and crafts, board games, newspapers, magazines, music, books, TV and radio, pet therapy, gardening, and group religious events. When activities are scheduled, nursing assistants should help residents with grooming beforehand, as needed and requested. They should assist with any personal care that residents require. NAs may need to help residents with walking and wheelchairs as well.

8. Discuss family roles and their significance in health care

Families play an important part in most people's lives. The concept of family is always changing. Often the support people give each other defines the family more than the particular people involved. There are many different kinds of families (Fig. 8-10):

- Nuclear families (two parents and one or more children)
- Single-parent families (one parent and one or more children)
- Married or committed couples of the same sex or opposite sex, with or without children
- Extended families (parents, children, grandparents, aunts, uncles, cousins, other relatives, and even friends)
- Blended families (divorced or widowed parents who have remarried and have children from previous relationships and/or the current marriage)

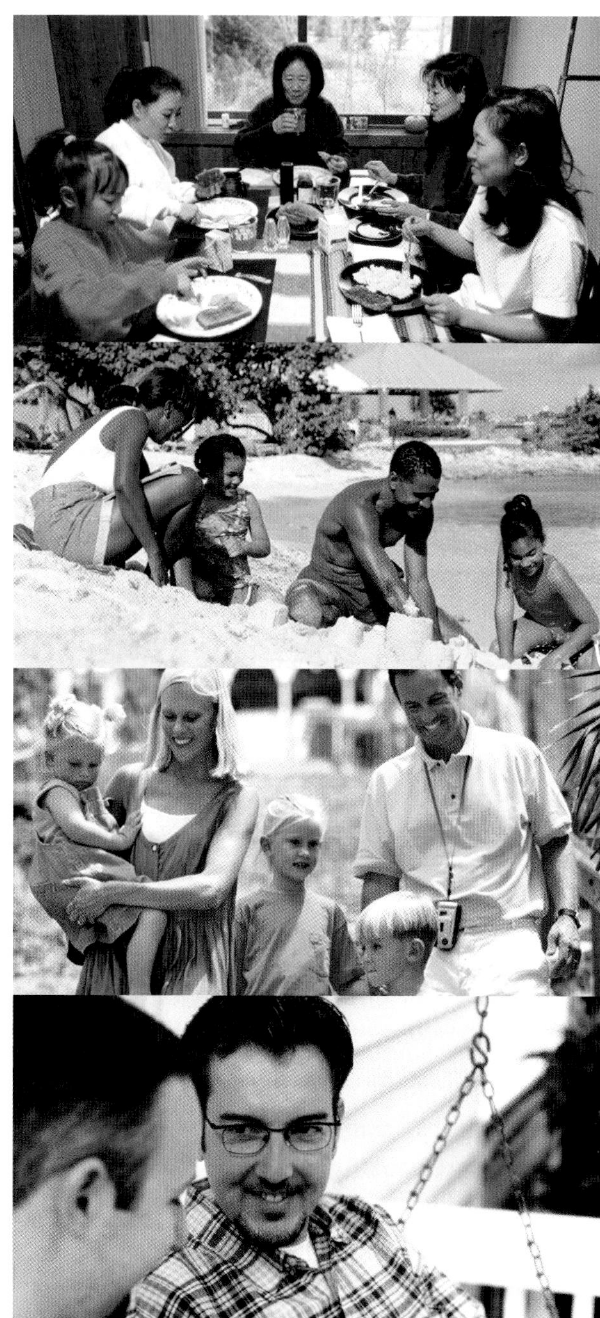

Fig. 8-10. *Families come in all shapes and sizes.*

Residents' families may not look like the kind of family that nursing assistants are used to. Residents with no living relatives may have friends or neighbors who function as a family. Whatever kinds of families residents have, they have an important role to play. Family members help in many ways:

- Helping residents make care decisions
- Communicating with the care team

- Giving support and encouragement
- Connecting the resident to the outside world
- Offering assurance to dying residents that family memories and traditions will be valued and carried on

Residents' Rights

Families

No matter whether a nursing assistant has the same understanding of family as a resident or not, no resident should ever be denied the right to have the people he loves around him. Families of all descriptions make residents' lives more meaningful. Staff should always make residents' families feel welcome and make it clear that the resident's right to spend time with them is being honored.

Illness or disability requires residents and families to make adjustments. Making these adjustments may be difficult (Fig. 8-11). It depends on the family's emotional, spiritual, and financial resources. Some personal adjustments include the following:

- Accepting the illness or disability and its long-term consequences or results
- Finding money needed to pay the expenses of hospitalization or long-term or home care
- Dealing with paperwork involved in insurance, Medicaid, or Medicare benefits
- Taking care of tasks the resident can no longer handle
- Understanding medical information and making difficult care decisions
- Caring for their children while caring for an elderly loved one (called the *sandwich generation*—being "sandwiched" between two generations)

Nursing assistants should be sensitive to the big adjustments residents and their families may be making. NAs can help them by doing their job well. NAs should be respectful and pleasant to friends and family members and allow privacy for visits. After any visitor leaves, the NA should observe the effect the visit had on the resident. Any noticeable effects should be reported to the nurse. Some residents have good relationships with their families; others do not. NAs must immediately report any abusive behavior from a visitor toward a resident to the charge nurse.

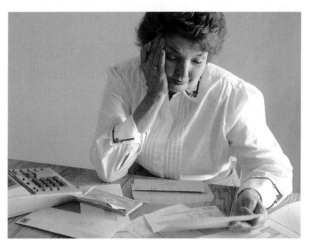

Fig. 8-11. *Family members may have a hard time adjusting to the additional responsibilities when a loved one becomes ill or disabled.*

9. List ways to respond to emotional needs of residents and their families

Residents or family members may come to nursing assistants with problems or needs. Changes in residents' health status can cause fear, uncertainty, stress, and anger. An NA's response will depend on many factors. These include how comfortable he feels with emotions in general, how well he knows the person, and what the need or problem is. NAs should try to empathize, or understand how the person feels. In addition, the following are good ways for NAs to respond to this situation:

Listen. Often just talking about a problem or concern can make it easier to handle. Sitting quietly and letting someone talk or cry may be the best help a nursing assistant can give (Fig. 8-12). Families often seek out nursing assistants because they are closest to the residents. This is an important responsibility. NAs should show families that they have time for them.

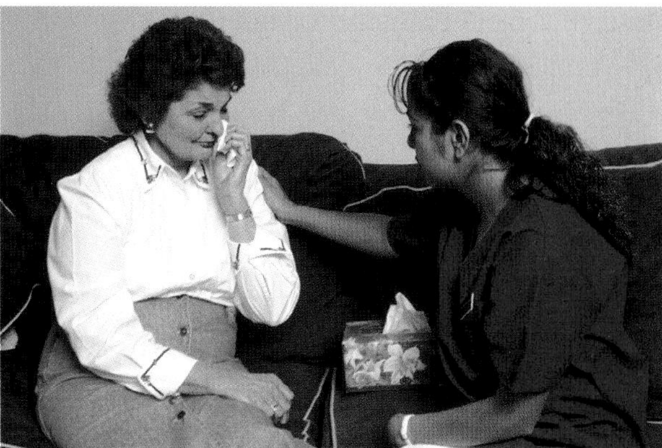

Fig. 8-12. Sometimes listening to someone is the best way to provide emotional support.

Offer support and encouragement. Saying things like "You have really been under a lot of stress, haven't you?" or "I can imagine that really is scary" can provide a lot of comfort. NAs should avoid using clichés (common phrases that really do not mean anything), like "It'll all work out." Things may not all work out. It is more comforting to the resident if the NA acknowledges how hard the situation is. Feelings should not be simply dismissed with a cliché.

Refer the problem to a nurse or social worker. When an NA feels that he cannot help the resident, he should get someone else on the care team to handle the situation. He can say something like "Mrs. Pfeiffer, I think my supervisor would be better at getting you the help you need."

10. Describe the stages of human growth and development and identify common disorders for each stage

Throughout their lives, people change physically and psychologically. Physical changes occur in the body. Psychological changes occur in the mind and also in the person's behavior. These changes are called human growth and development.

Everyone will go through the same stages of development during their lives. However, no two people will follow the exact same pattern or rate of development. The age ranges given in this learning objective provide a general idea of developmental stages rather than an exact description. Each resident must be treated as an individual and as a whole person who is growing and developing. He or she should not be treated as someone who is merely ill or disabled.

Infancy (Birth to 12 Months)

Infants grow and develop very quickly. In one year a baby moves from total dependence to the relative independence of moving around, communicating basic needs, and feeding himself. Physical development in infancy moves from the head down. For example, infants gain control over the muscles of the neck before the muscles in their shoulders. Control over muscles in the trunk area, such as the shoulders, develops before control of arms and legs (Fig. 8-13). This head-to-toe sequence should be respected when caring for infants. For example, newborns must be supported at the shoulders, head, and neck. Babies who cannot sit or crawl should not be encouraged to stand or walk.

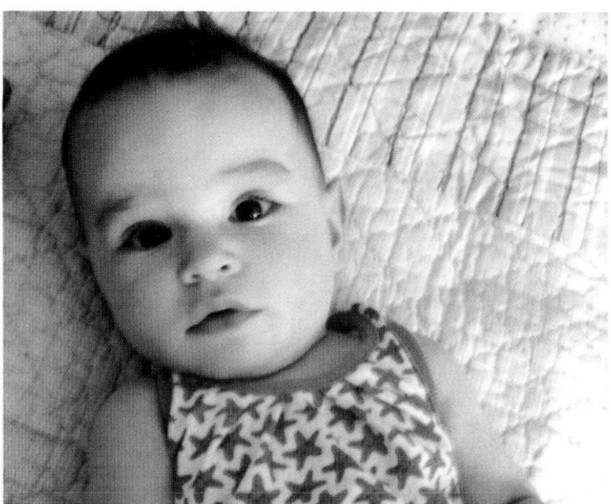

Fig. 8-13. An infant's physical development moves from the head down.

Common Disorders: Infancy

CD Babies who are born before 37 weeks gestation (more than three weeks before the due date) are considered **premature**. These babies may weigh from one to six pounds, depending on how early they are born. Often, premature babies will remain in the hospital for some time after birth. At home, premature babies may need special care. This includes medication, heart monitoring, and frequent feedings to ensure weight gain.

CD Babies born at full term but weighing less than five pounds are called low-birth-weight babies. Low-birth-weight babies can have many of the same problems premature babies have. They are cared for in much the same way as premature babies.

CD The term *birth defects* is very general. It includes many different conditions that affect an infant from birth. Some birth defects are inherited from parents. Injury or disease during pregnancy causes others. Some of the conditions include cerebral palsy, Down syndrome, and cystic fibrosis.

CD Viral or bacterial infections can cause fever, runny nose, coughing, rash, vomiting, diarrhea, or secondary infections of the sinuses or ears. Bacterial infections can be treated with antibiotics. Viral infections are treated with extra rest and fluids.

CD **Sudden infant death syndrome** (**SIDS**) is a condition in which babies stop breathing and die for no known reason while asleep. Doctors do not know how to prevent SIDS. However, studies have shown that putting the baby to sleep on its back can reduce the chances of SIDS. Because SIDS is more common among premature or low-birth-weight babies, these infants often wear apnea monitors to alert parents if breathing stops. Another factor that may contribute to SIDS is second-hand smoke. Parents and caregivers should never smoke around infants or children.

Toddler (Ages 1 to 3)

During the toddler years, children gain independence. One part of this independence is new control over their bodies. Toddlers learn to speak, gain coordination of their limbs, and gain control over their bladders and bowels (Fig. 8-14). Toddlers assert their new independence by exploring. Poisons and other hazards, such as sharp objects, must be locked away. Psychologically, toddlers learn that they are individuals, separate from their parents. Children of this age may try to control their parents. They may try to get what they want by throwing tantrums, whining, or refusing to cooperate. This is a key time for parents to set rules and standards.

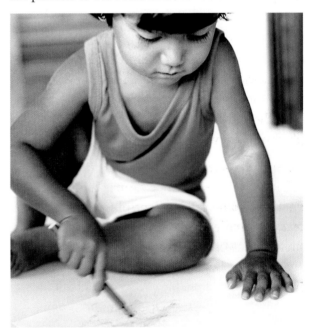

Fig. 8-14. *Toddlers gain coordination of their limbs.*

Preschool (Ages 3 to 6)

Children in their preschool years develop skills that help them become more independent and have social relationships (Fig. 8-15). They develop a vocabulary and language skills. They learn to play in groups. They become more physically coordinated and learn to care for themselves. Preschoolers also develop ways of relating to family members. They begin to learn right from wrong.

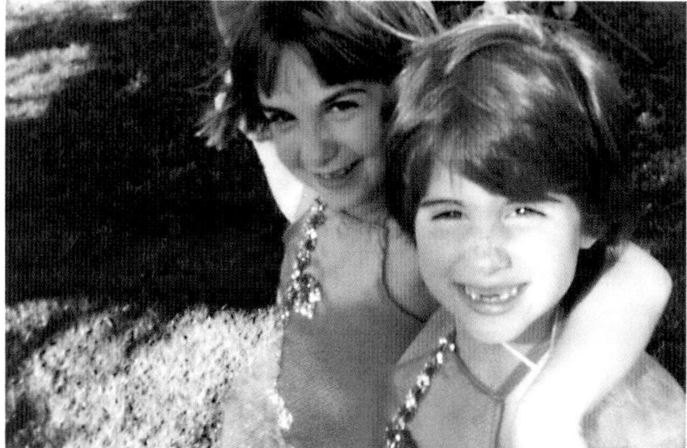

Fig. 8-15. Children in their preschool years develop social relationships.

School-Age (Ages 6 to 10)

From ages 6 to about 10 years, children's development is centered on **cognitive** (related to thinking and learning) and social development. As children enter school, they also explore the world around them. They relate to other children through games, peer groups, and classroom activities. In these years, children learn to get along with each other. They also begin to behave in ways common to their gender. They begin to develop a conscience, morals, and self-esteem.

Common Disorders: Childhood

- CD **Chickenpox** is a highly contagious, viral illness. It generally has no serious effects for healthy children. However, in adults or in anyone with a weakened immune system, it can have more serious effects. Taking the varicella-zoster vaccine, commonly called the chickenpox vaccine, can prevent chickenpox.
- CD Children, as well as infants, may be susceptible to infections caused by viruses or bacteria. Bacterial infections can be treated with antibiotics. Viral infections are treated with extra rest, fluids, and over-the-counter medications for cough or congestion.
- CD **Leukemia** is a form of cancer. It refers to the inability of the body's white blood cells to fight disease. Children with leukemia may be susceptible to infections and other disorders. Chemotherapy can be used to fight this disease. Chapter 18 has more information on cancer.
- CD Child abuse refers to physical, emotional, and sexual mistreatment of children. Physical abuse includes hitting, kicking, burning, or intentionally causing injury to a child. Psychological abuse includes withholding affection, constantly criticizing, or ridiculing a child. Sexual abuse includes engaging in or allowing another person to engage in a sexual act with a child. Abuse also includes allowing children to use alcohol or drugs, leaving children alone, or exposing them to danger. Child neglect includes not providing adequate food, clothing, or support.
- CD Measles, mumps, rubella, diphtheria, smallpox, whooping cough, and polio are diseases that were once common during childhood. They can all be prevented now with vaccinations.

Preadolescence (Ages 10 to 13)

During the years between 10 and 13, children enjoy a growing sense of self-identity and a strong sense of identity with their peers. They tend to be very social. Friends are generally of the same gender, but relationships with children of the opposite sex may become more complicated as puberty approaches. This is usually a relatively calm period, and preadolescents are often easy to get along with and able to handle more responsibility at home and school. Childhood fears of ghosts or monsters will give way to fears based in the real world, and it is important that preadolescents feel able to trust in the attention and care of parents or other adults.

Adolescence (Ages 13 to 19)

Puberty is the stage of growth when secondary sex characteristics, such as body hair, appear. Reproductive organs begin to function due to the secretion of reproductive hormones. The onset of puberty marks the beginning of adolescence and although it varies, it generally occurs between the ages of 10 and 14 for girls and 12 and 16 for boys.

Many teenagers have a hard time adapting to changes that occur in their bodies during puberty. Peer acceptance is important to them. Adolescents may be afraid that they are unattractive or abnormal. This concern for body image and peer acceptance, combined with changing hormones that influence moods, can cause rapid mood swings. Conflicting pressures develop as they remain dependent on their parents and yet need to express themselves socially and sexually (Fig. 8-16). This causes conflict and stress.

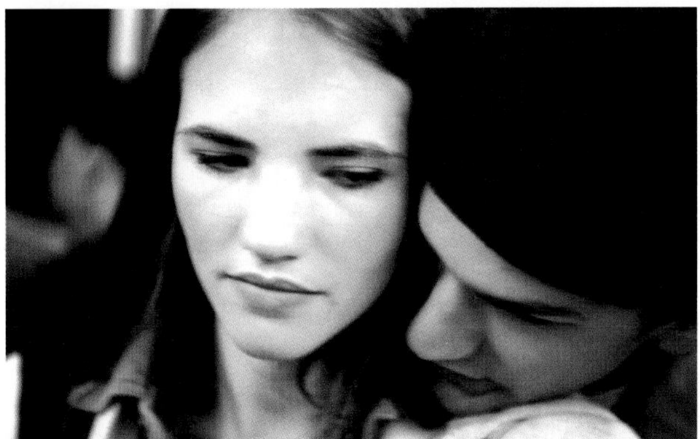

Fig. 8-16. *Adolescence is a time of adapting to change.*

Common Disorders: Adolescence

CD As their bodies change, adolescents, especially girls, may develop eating disorders. **Anorexia** is a disease in which a person does not eat or exercises excessively to lose weight. A person with **bulimia** binges, eating huge amounts of foods or very fattening foods, and then purges, or eliminates the food by vomiting, using laxatives, or exercising excessively. Eating disorders can be serious and even life-threatening. These disorders must be treated with therapy and, in some cases, hospitalization.

CD Teenagers can contract sexually-transmitted infections (STIs), such as chlamydia, herpes, and AIDS, if they are sexually active. If teenagers are sexually active, only condoms offer some protection from sexually-transmitted infections. Chapter 18 has more information on STIs.

CD Girls who are sexually active and do not use birth control, or who do not use it properly, can become pregnant. Teenage pregnancy can have terrible consequences for adolescents, their families, and for the babies born to teenage parents. Teenagers should understand that they can avoid pregnancy by using birth control or by not having sexual intercourse. Teenagers who choose to be sexually active should know what birth control methods are available and how to use them. Pregnancy puts a great deal of stress on teenage bodies. Their bodies are still developing. In most cases, they are not physically ready to bear a child. It is common for teenage mothers to give birth to premature or low-birth-weight babies.

CD Because of the many physical and emotional changes they are experiencing, adolescents may become depressed and even attempt suicide. Parents, teachers, and friends should watch for the signs of depression. These include withdrawal, loss of appetite, weight gain or loss, sleep problems, moodiness, and apathy. Teenagers who are depressed should see a doctor, counselor, therapist, minister, or other trusted adult who can get them the help they need.

CD Adolescents can sustain **trauma**, or severe injury, to the head or spinal cord in car accidents or sports injuries. These injuries can be temporarily or permanently disabling or even fatal.

Young Adulthood (Ages 19 to 40)

Physical growth has usually been completed by this time. Adopting a healthy lifestyle in these years can make life better now and prevent health problems in later adulthood. Psychological and social development continues, however. The developmental tasks of these years include the following:

- Selecting an appropriate education
- Selecting an occupation or career
- Selecting a mate (Fig. 8-17)
- Learning to live with a mate or others
- Raising children
- Developing a satisfying sex life

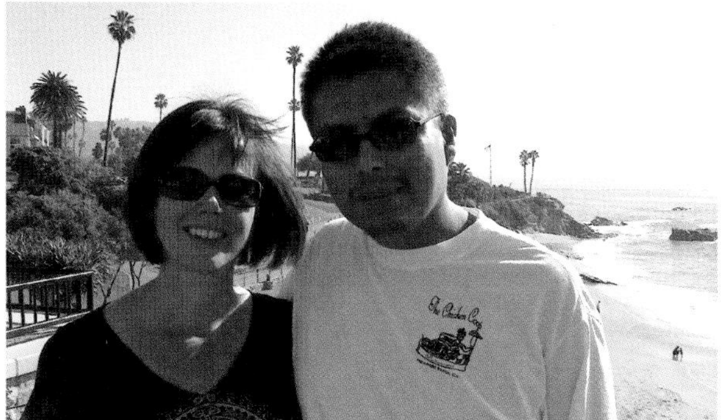

Fig. 8-17. Young adulthood often involves finding mates.

Middle Adulthood (Ages 40 to 65)

In general, people in middle adulthood are more comfortable and stable than they were in previous stages. Many of their major life decisions have already been made. In the early years of middle adulthood people sometimes experience a "mid-life crisis." This is a period of unrest centered on a subconscious desire for change and fulfillment of unmet goals.

Physical changes related to aging also occur in middle adulthood. Adults in this age group may notice that they have difficulty maintaining their weight or notice a decrease in strength and energy. Metabolism and other body functions slow down. Wrinkles and gray hair appear. Vision and hearing loss may begin. Women experience **menopause**, the end of menstruation. This occurs when the ovaries stop secreting hormones. Many diseases and illnesses can develop in these years. These disorders can become chronic and life-threatening.

Late Adulthood (65 years and older)

Persons in late adulthood must adjust to the effects of aging. These changes can include the loss of strength and health, the death of loved ones, retirement, and preparation for their own death. Although the developmental tasks of this age appear to deal entirely with loss, solutions often involve new relationships, friendships, and interests. Common disorders of this age group (arthritis, Alzheimer's disease, cancer, diabetes, and stroke) are covered in Chapters 18 and 19.

11. Distinguish between what is true and what is not true about the aging process

Geriatrics is the study of health, wellness, and disease later in life. It includes the health care of older people and the well-being of their caregivers. **Gerontology** is the study of the aging process in people from mid-life through old age. Gerontologists look at the impact of the aging population on society.

Because later adulthood covers an age range of as many as 25 to 35 years, people in this age category can have very different abilities, depending on their health. Some 70-year-old people enjoy active sports, while others are not active. Many 85-year-old people can still live alone, though others may live with family members or in skilled care facilities.

Ideas and stereotypes about older people are often false. They create prejudices against the elderly that are as unfair as prejudices against racial, ethnic, or religious groups. On television or in movies, older people are often shown as helpless, lonely, disabled, slow, forgetful, dependent, or inactive. However, research indicates that most older people are active and engaged in work, volunteer activities, learning programs, and exercise regimens. Aging is a normal process, not a disease. Most older people live independent lives and do not need assistance (Fig. 8-18). Prejudice toward, stereotyping of, and/or discrimination against older persons or the elderly is called **ageism**.

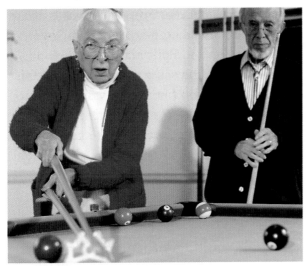

Fig. 8-18. Most older people lead active lives.

Nursing assistants are likely to spend much of their time working with elderly residents. They must be able to know what is true about aging and what is not true. Aging causes many physical, psychological, and social changes. However, normal changes of aging do not mean an older person must become dependent, ill, or inactive. Knowing normal changes of aging from signs of illness or disability will allow nursing assistants to better help residents. Normal changes of aging include the following:

- Skin is thinner, drier, more fragile, and less elastic.
- Muscles weaken and lose tone.
- Bones lose density and become more brittle.
- Sensitivity of nerve endings in the skin decreases.
- Responses and reflexes slow.
- Short-term memory loss occurs.
- Senses of vision, hearing, taste, touch, and smell weaken.
- Heart works less efficiently.
- Oxygen in the blood decreases.
- Appetite decreases.
- Urinary elimination is more frequent.
- Digestion takes longer and is less efficient.
- Levels of hormones decrease.
- Immunity weakens.
- Lifestyle changes occur.

There are also changes that are NOT considered normal changes of aging and should be reported to the nurse. These include the following:

- Signs of depression
- Loss of ability to think logically
- Poor nutrition
- Shortness of breath
- Incontinence

This is not a complete list. A nursing assistant's job includes reporting any change, normal or not. More information about normal changes of aging is found in Chapter 9.

12. Explain developmental disabilities and list care guidelines

Developmental disabilities refer to disabilities that are present at birth or emerge during childhood. A developmental disability is a chronic condition that restricts physical and/or mental ability. These disabilities prevent a child from developing physically or mentally at a "normal" rate. Language, mobility, learning, and the ability to perform self-care may be affected. These disabilities include intellectual disabilities, Down syndrome, cerebral palsy, spina bifida, and autism.

Intellectual Disability

According to the Centers for Disease Control, an intellectual disability, formerly called *mental retardation*, is the most common developmental disorder. Approximately one percent of the general population has an intellectual disability.

An intellectual disability is neither a disease nor a mental illness. People with an intellectual disability develop at a below-average rate. They have below-average mental functioning. They experience difficulty with learning, communicating, moving, and may have problems adjusting socially. The ability to care for themselves may be affected. The potential for living independently and for achieving financial independence may be limited.

Despite their special needs, people who have an intellectual disability have the same emotional and physical needs that others have (Fig. 8-19). They experience the same emotions, such as anger, sadness, love, and joy, as others do, but their ability to express their emotions may be limited.

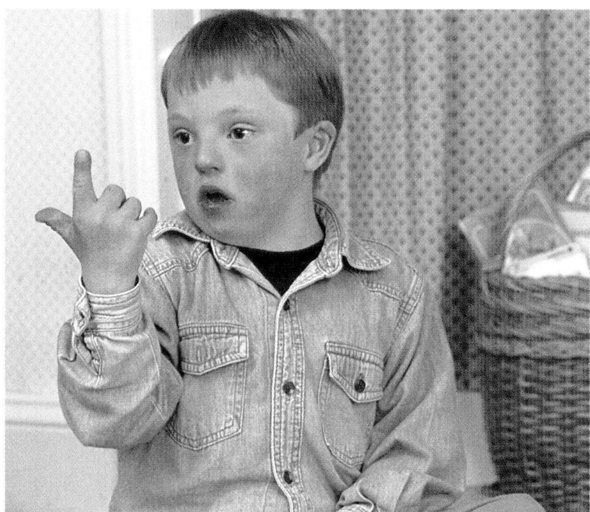

Fig. 8-19. *People who have an intellectual disability have the same emotional and physical needs that others do.*

A diagnosis of an intellectual disability can be made by testing intellectual functioning level (IQ, or intelligence quotient). There are four different degrees of intellectual disability: mild, moderate, severe, and profound. Each degree is related to specific IQ ranges: 50–69 is mild; 35–49 is moderate; 20–34 is severe; and below 20 is profound. However, focus is usually on the person's specific abilities and needs, rather than on IQ measurement:

- Mild intellectual disability usually causes a delay in walking and talking. With special support and education, the person can acquire academic skills up to the sixth grade level. With some assistance, he can become fairly independent and have some social skills and the ability to work.
- Moderate intellectual disability causes delays in speech and motor development. Simple communication skills may be acquired in childhood. With some support and supervision, the person can usually work and function successfully. He may be able to live alone or may live in a facility or group home.
- Severe intellectual disability causes noticeable delays in motor development, and the person has few communication skills. Very basic self-care skills, such as self-feeding, toileting, and dressing may be mastered. The person may live in a facility or group home.
- Profound intellectual disability causes obvious delays in most areas of development. The person may not respond to his environment, and often there are physical problems as well. Walking may be mastered; communication skills are extremely basic. The person may need nursing care and require help in self-care. He will need a high level of support and supervision.

For residents who have an intellectual disability, the main goal of care is to help the person have as normal a life as possible. For a person with an intellectual disability, this means recognizing her individuality, basic human rights, and physical and emotional needs, as well as her special needs.

Some residents and/or their families will use the term *intellectually disabled,* while others may use *developmentally delayed, special,* or *challenged.* Nursing assistants should respect the resident's wishes about which term or terms to use.

Guidelines: Intellectual Disability

- G Treat adult residents as adults, regardless of their behavior.
- G Praise and encourage often, especially positive behavior.

- G Help teach the resident to perform ADLs by dividing a task into smaller units.
- G Promote independence, but also assist residents with activities and motor functions that are difficult.
- G Encourage social interaction.
- G Repeat what you say to make sure they understand.
- G Be patient.

Down Syndrome

Down syndrome is most often caused by an abnormal cell division, resulting in an extra number 21 chromosome (three copies of chromosome 21, instead of the usual two copies). People who are born with Down syndrome experience different degrees of an intellectual disability, along with physical symptoms. A person with Down syndrome typically has a small skull, a flattened nose, short fingers, and a wider space between the first two fingers and the first two toes. As with some of the types of intellectual disabilities, a person with Down syndrome can become fairly independent.

Guidelines: Down Syndrome

- G Give the same type of care and instruction that you would for any other person with an intellectual disability.
- G Praise and encourage often, especially positive behavior.
- G Help teach the resident to perform ADLs by dividing a task into smaller units.

Cerebral Palsy

People who have cerebral palsy have suffered brain damage either while in the uterus or during birth. They may have both physical and mental disabilities. Damage to the brain stops the development of the child. It can cause disorganized or abnormal development. Muscle coordination and nerves are affected. People with cerebral palsy may lack control of their head, have trouble using the arms and hands, and have poor balance or posture. They may be either stiff and spastic or limp and flaccid and may have impaired speech. Gait and mobility may be affected. Intelligence may also be affected. With or without assistance, a person with cerebral palsy may be able to live independently.

Guidelines: Cerebral Palsy

- G Allow the resident to move slowly. People with cerebral palsy take longer to adjust their body positions. They may repeat movements several times.
- G Keep the resident's body in as normal an alignment as possible.
- G Talk to the resident, even if he or she cannot speak. Be patient and listen.
- G Use touch as a form of communication.
- G Avoid activities that are tiring or frustrating.
- G Be gentle when handling parts of the body that may be painful (Fig. 8-20).

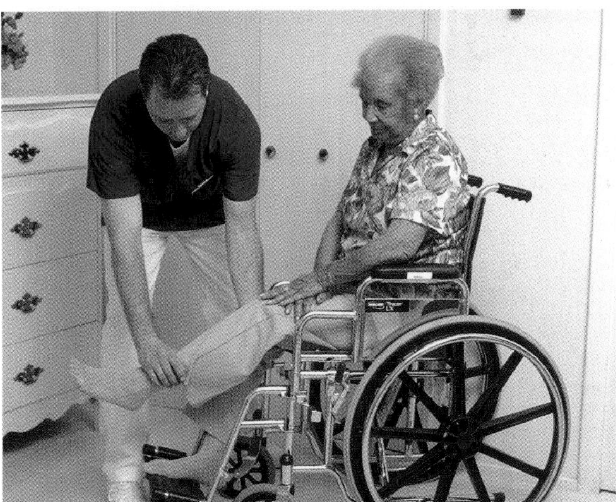

Fig. 8-20. *Be gentle when moving body parts of a resident who has cerebral palsy.*

- G Promote independence and encourage socialization.

Spina Bifida

Spina bifida literally means *split spine.* When part of the backbone is not well-developed at birth, the spinal cord may bulge out of the back. Spina bifida can cause a range of disabilities. Some babies born with spina bifida will be able to walk and will experience no lasting disabilities. Others may be in a wheelchair and/or may have little or no bladder or bowel control. In some cases, complications of spina bifida may cause brain damage.

Guidelines: Spina Bifida

G Provide assistance with range of motion exercises and ADLs.

G Be a positive role model for the resident and family in learning to deal with the resident's disabilities.

Autism

Autism is part of a group of developmental disorders called autism spectrum disorders (ASDs). They are also called pervasive developmental disorders (PDDs). Autism appears in early childhood, usually by age 3. Parents may notice that a child does not engage in pretend play or has problems with communication and social interaction. A diagnosis of autism may be made after comprehensive testing, including physical and neurological examinations, among other screening tests.

Autism continues throughout the person's life. It causes problems with communication and social skills. For example, a person with autism may be unable to communicate using words. He or she may be withdrawn and unable to make eye contact. Autism can cause a wide range of problems, including intense tantrums, repetitive body movements, aggression, a short attention span, and an inability to be empathetic.

The exact cause of autism is unknown, but genetics may be a factor. Autism affects boys three to four times more often than girls.

Treatment for autism includes many types of therapies, including behavior, speech, and occupational therapies. Having familiar caregivers and keeping a routine may be helpful. Medications are also used to treat autism. Ideally, treatment should be started early and must be tailored to the individual.

13. Identify community resources available to help the elderly and the developmentally disabled

Government and private agencies exist in most areas to serve the needs of the elderly. These agencies may have counselors to work with victims of abuse or neglect and other programs to protect senior citizens' rights and contribute to their quality of life. The Internet or phone book lists these organizations under community services, senior citizens, aging, or elder services. Local churches or synagogues may also have programs for seniors. Resources include the following:

- Eldercare Locator, a public service of the U.S. Administration on Aging (eldercare.gov or 800-677-1116)
- Ombudsman program (ltcombudsman.org or 202-332-2275)
- Alzheimer's Association (alz.org or 800-272-3900)
- The National Hospice and Palliative Care Organization (NHPCO) (nhpco.org or 800-658-8898)
- The National Resource Center on LGBT Aging (lgbtagingcenter.org or 212-741-2247)
- Social workers
- Resident advocacy organizations
- Support groups
- Meal or transportation services (Fig. 8-21)

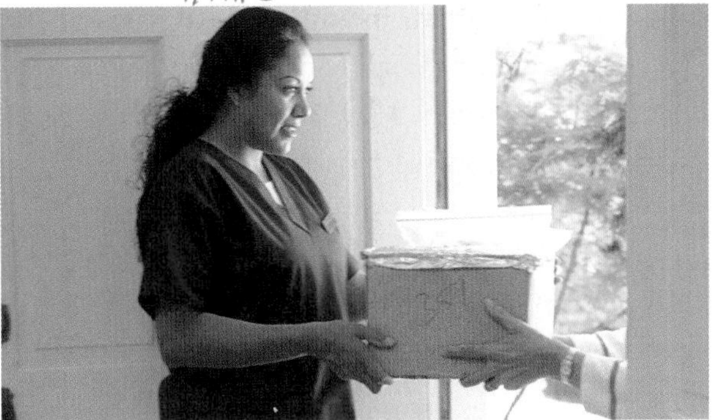

Fig. 8-21. Meals on Wheels and similar services provide nutritious meals to people unable to cook for themselves.

There are many services available to help people who have developmental disabilities, including the following resources:

- American Association on Intellectual and Developmental Disabilities (AAIDD) (aamr.org or 800-424-3688)
- Autism Science Foundation (autismsciencefoundation.org or 646-723-3977)
- National Down Syndrome Congress (ndsccenter.org or 800-232-6372)
- Special Olympics (specialolympics.org or 800-700-8585)
- Spina Bifida Association (spinabifidaassociation.org or 800-621-3141)
- United Cerebral Palsy (ucp.org or 800-872-5827)

If residents ask a nursing assistant for help, the NA should refer them to the nurse or social worker. If no one asks, but the NA thinks help is needed, she should speak to her supervisor.

Chapter Review

1. List six basic human needs.
2. What psychosocial needs do humans have?
3. According to Maslow, which needs must be met first, physical or emotional?
4. What does giving holistic care mean?
5. List six examples of losses that residents may be experiencing.
6. What are six problems that a lack of independence can cause?
7. List four ways that nursing assistants can accommodate residents' sexual needs.
8. What is one way that NAs can show respect for residents' sexual identity?
9. List five ways that NAs can help residents meet their spiritual needs.
10. What can NAs never do regarding residents' spiritual or religious needs?
11. Pick three religions listed in Learning Objective 6 and briefly describe them. Feel free to add information that is not included in the Learning Objective.
12. If a resident is an atheist, but her NA believes in God, is it okay for the NA to ask the resident to pray with her?
13. List seven ways that regular physical activity can help a person.
14. List seven ways that inactivity and immobility can cause problems for a person.
15. List four ways that families can help residents.
16. Name three ways nursing assistants can meet emotional needs of residents and their families.
17. Name at least two common disorders for each stage of human development.
18. What is ageism?
19. In movies, elderly people are often shown as helpless, lonely, disabled, slow, forgetful, dependent, or inactive. What is actually true of most older adults?
20. List ten normal changes of aging.
21. What are developmental disabilities?
22. What is the most common developmental disorder?
23. List four community resources that can help residents meet their needs.

9 The Healthy Human Body

1. Describe body systems and define key anatomical terms

Bodies are organized into body systems. Each system in the body has a condition under which it works best. **Homeostasis** is the name for the condition in which all of the body's systems are working at their best. To be in homeostasis, the body's **metabolism**, or physical and chemical processes, must be working at a steady level. When disease or injury occurs, the body's metabolism is disturbed, and homeostasis is lost.

Changes in metabolic processes are called signs and symptoms. For instance, changes in body temperature could indicate that the body is fighting an infection. Noticing and reporting changes in residents is a very important part of a nursing assistant's job. The changes the NA notices could be signs of significant problems.

Each system in the body has its own unique structure and function. There are also normal, age-related changes for each body system. Knowing normal changes of aging will help nursing assistants be able to recognize any abnormal changes in residents. This chapter also includes tips on how NAs can help residents with their normal changes of aging.

The body's systems can be broken down in different ways. In this book we divide the human body into ten systems:

1. Integumentary (skin)
2. Musculoskeletal
3. Nervous
4. Circulatory or cardiovascular
5. Respiratory
6. Urinary
7. Gastrointestinal
8. Endocrine
9. Reproductive
10. Immune and Lymphatic

Body systems are made up of **organs**. An organ has a specific function. Organs are made up of **tissues**. Tissues are made up of groups of cells that perform a similar task. For example, in the circulatory system, the heart is one of the organs. It is made up of tissues and cells. **Cells** are the building blocks of the body. Living cells divide, grow, and die, renewing the tissues and organs of the body systems.

Anatomical Terms of Location

Anatomical terms of location are descriptive terms to help identify positions or directions of the body. Here are some anatomical terms used to describe location in the human body:

- Anterior or ventral: the front of the body or body part
- Posterior or dorsal: the back of the body or body part
- Superior: toward the head
- Inferior: away from the head
- Medial: toward the midline of the body
- Lateral: to the side, away from the midline of the body
- Proximal: closer to the torso
- Distal: farther away from the torso

This chapter discusses the structure and function of each body system, as well as age-related changes and what is important to observe and report about each system. The bulk of information on diseases and disorders of each system and related care will be discussed in Chapter 18. Chapters 16, 17, and 19 also have information on diseases.

2. Describe the integumentary system

The largest organ and system in the body is the skin, a natural protective covering, or **integument**. Skin prevents injury to internal organs. It also protects the body against entry of bacteria. Skin also prevents the loss of too much water, which is essential to life. Skin is made up of layers of tissues. Within these layers are sweat glands, which secrete sweat to help cool the body when needed, and sebaceous glands, which secrete oil (sebum) to keep the skin lubricated. There are also hair follicles, many tiny blood vessels (capillaries), and tiny nerve endings (Fig. 9-1).

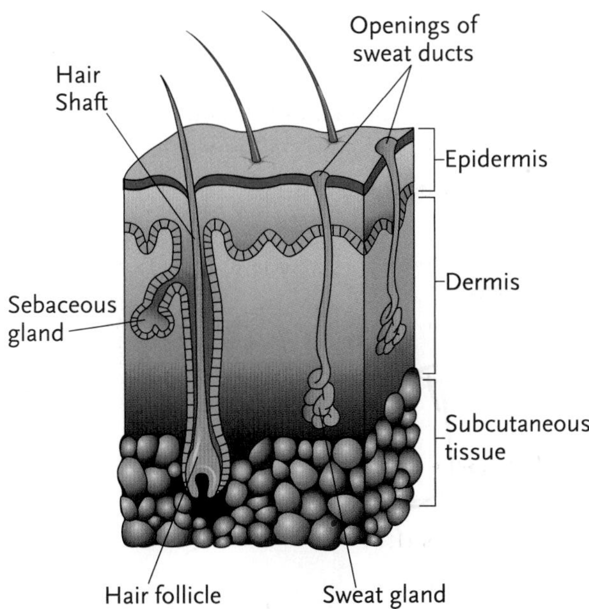

Fig. 9-1. *Cross-section showing details of the integumentary system.*

The skin is also a *sense organ* that feels heat, cold, pain, touch, and pressure. It then tells the brain what it is feeling. Body temperature is regulated in the skin. Blood vessels **dilate** or widen, when the outside temperature is too high. This brings more blood to the body surface to cool it off. The same blood vessels **constrict**, or narrow, when the outside temperature is too cold. By restricting the amount of blood reaching the skin, the blood vessels help the body retain heat.

The blood vessels, called capillaries, are located in the dermis, which is the inner layer of skin. The dermis also contains nerves, sweat glands, sebaceous (oil) glands, and hair roots. Sweat glands help control body temperature by secreting sweat. Sweat is made up mostly of water, but it also contains salt and a small amount of waste products. Sweat comes to the body's surface through pores, or tiny openings in the skin. It cools the body as it evaporates. Sebaceous glands in the dermis secrete sebum (oil). Sebum comes to the skin surface through hair follicles, or roots. Sebum keeps the skin and hair lubricated.

No blood vessels and only a few nerve endings are located in the epidermis, which is the outer layer of skin. Thinner than the dermis, the epidermis contains both dead and living cells. The dead cells begin deeper in the epidermis. They are pushed to the surface as other cells divide. They are eventually worn off. The epidermis also contains pigment cells that give the skin its color.

Hair grows from roots located in the dermis. It grows through hair follicles that extend through the epidermis to the outside of the body. Hair protects the body from heat and cold. Hair inside the nose and ears keeps out particles and bacteria trying to enter the body.

The functions of the integumentary system are to protect internal organs from injury, protect the body against bacteria, and prevent the loss of too much water. It also responds to heat, cold, pain, touch, and pressure, and it regulates body temperature.

Normal changes of aging include the following:

- Skin is thinner, drier, and more fragile. It is more easily damaged.

- Skin is less elastic.
- Protective fatty tissue is lost, so person may feel colder.
- Hair thins and may turn gray.
- Wrinkles and brown spots, or "liver spots," appear.
- Nails are harder and more brittle.
- Dry, itchy skin may result from lack of oil from the sebaceous glands.

How The NA Can Help

Older adults perspire less and do not need to bathe as often. Most elderly people generally need a complete bath only twice a week, with sponge baths every day. Hair also becomes drier and needs to be shampooed less often. Using lotions as ordered helps to relieve dry skin. Gently brushing dry hair stimulates and distributes the natural oils. The NA should be gentle because elderly skin may be fragile and can tear easily. Clothing and bed covers can be layered for additional warmth. Bed linens should be kept wrinkle-free. The NA should be careful when providing nail care; toenails should not cut. Fluid intake should be encouraged.

Observing and Reporting: Integumentary System

During daily care, a resident's skin should be observed for changes that may indicate injury or disease. Observe and report these signs and symptoms:

- O/R Pale, white or reddened, or purple areas
- O/R Blisters or bruises
- O/R Complaints of tingling, warmth, or burning
- O/R Dry or flaking skin
- O/R Itching or scratching
- O/R Rash or any skin discoloration
- O/R Swelling
- O/R Cuts, boils, sores, wounds, or abrasions
- O/R Fluid or blood draining from the skin
- O/R Broken skin
- O/R Changes in moistness/dryness
- O/R Changes in wound or ulcer (size, depth, drainage, color, odor)
- O/R Redness or broken skin between toes or around toenails
- O/R Scalp or hair changes
- O/R Skin that appears different from normal or that has changed
- O/R In darker complexions, look for any change in the feel of the tissue; any change in the appearance of the skin, such as an "orange-peel" look or a purplish hue; and extremely dry, crust-like areas that might be covering a tissue break.

3. Describe the musculoskeletal system

Muscles, bones, ligaments, tendons, and cartilage give the body shape and structure. They work together to move the body. The skeleton, or framework, of the human body has 206 bones (Fig. 9-2). Besides allowing the body to move, **bones** also protect organs. For example, the skull protects the brain and the vertebrae protect the spinal cord. Bones are hard and rigid, but are made up of living cells. Blood vessels supply oxygen and nutrients to the bones, as well as to other tissues of the body.

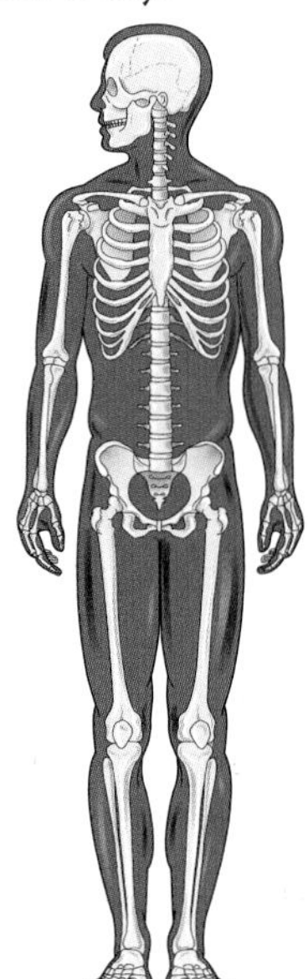

Fig. 9-2. *The skeleton is composed of 206 bones that aid movement and protect organs.*

Two bones meet at a **joint**. Some joints, such as the ball and socket joint, make movement possible in all directions. This joint is a type of synovial joint. In this joint, the round end of one bone fits into the hollow end of the other bone, which allows it to move in all directions. The hip and shoulder joints are examples.

Other joints permit movement in one direction only. The hinge joint is another example of a synovial joint. Like the hinge of a door, a hinge joint permits movement in one direction only. The elbow and knee are hinge joints. They only bend in one direction (Fig. 9-3).

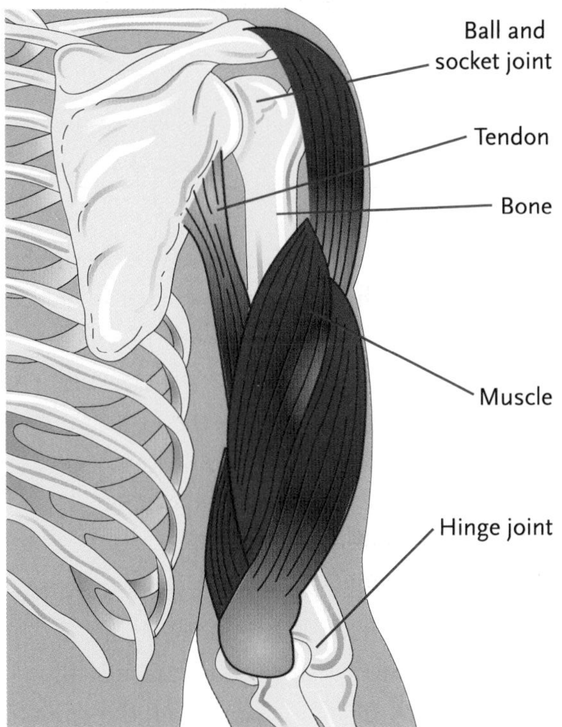

Fig. 9-3. *Muscles are connected to bones by tendons. Bones meet at different types of joints. The ball and socket joint and the hinge joint are shown here.*

Muscles provide movement of body parts to maintain posture and to produce heat. Muscles can be voluntary or involuntary. Voluntary muscles are also called skeletal muscles. They are attached to bones and can be moved when a person wants them to move. Examples of voluntary muscles are the arm and leg muscles, which are consciously controlled. Involuntary muscles cannot be consciously controlled. They automatically regulate the movement of organs and blood vessels. Examples of involuntary muscles are the heart and the diaphragm. The diaphragm is the muscle that makes humans breathe.

Exercise is important for improving and maintaining physical and mental health. Inactivity and immobility can result in a loss of self-esteem, depression, pneumonia, and urinary tract infections. They can also lead to constipation, blood clots, dulling of the senses, and muscle atrophy or contractures. When **atrophy** occurs, the muscle wastes away, decreases in size, and becomes weak. When a **contracture** develops, the muscle shortens, becomes inflexible, and "freezes" in position. This causes permanent disability of the limb.

Range of motion (ROM) exercises can help prevent these conditions. With ROM exercises, the joints are extended and flexed in the measured degrees of a circle. Exercise increases circulation of blood, oxygen, and nutrients and improves muscle tone. Chapter 21 contains more information on ROM exercises.

The functions of the musculoskeletal system are to give the body shape and structure, to allow the body to move, to protect body organs, to maintain posture, and to produce heat.

Normal changes of aging include the following:

- Muscles weaken and lose tone.
- Body movement slows.
- Bones lose density. They become more brittle, making them more susceptible to breaks.
- Joints may stiffen and become painful.
- Height is gradually lost.

How The NA Can Help

Falls can cause life-threatening complications, including fractures. The NA can help prevent falls by doing the following:

- Keep items out of residents' paths
- Keep furniture in the same place
- Place walkers or canes where residents can easily reach them

- Answer call lights immediately.
- Make sure residents are wearing non-skid shoes with the laces tied.
- Immediately clean up spills.

In addition the NA should promote self-care and encourage regular movement.

Residents should perform as many ADLs as possible. To prevent or slow osteoporosis, the condition that is responsible for fragile bones, residents should be encouraged to walk and do other light exercise. Exercise can strengthen bones as well as muscles. The NA should help with range of motion (ROM) exercises as needed.

Observing and Reporting: Musculoskeletal System

Observe and report these signs and symptoms:

O/R Changes in ability to perform routine movements and activities

O/R Any changes in residents' abilities to perform ROM exercises

O/R Pain during movement

O/R Any new or increased swelling of joints

O/R White, shiny, red, or warm areas over a joint

O/R Bruising

O/R Aches and pains reported

4. Describe the nervous system

The nervous system is the control and message center of the body. It controls and coordinates all body functions. The nervous system also senses and interprets information from outside the human body.

The neuron, or nerve cell, is the basic unit of the nervous system. Neurons send messages or sensations from the receptors in different parts of the body, through the spinal cord, to the brain.

The nervous system has two main parts: the **central nervous system (CNS)** and the **peripheral nervous system (PNS)**. The central nervous system is composed of the brain and spinal cord. The peripheral nervous system deals with the periphery, or outer part, of the body via the nerves that extend throughout the body (Fig. 9-4).

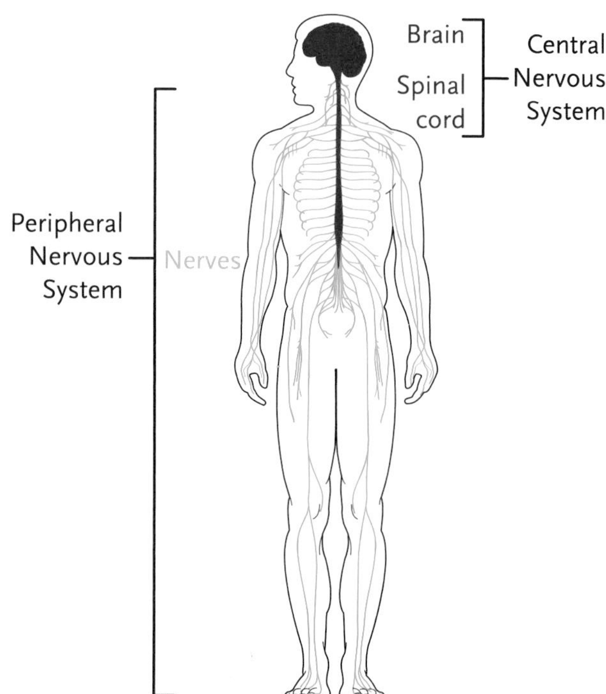

Fig. 9-4. The nervous system includes the brain, spinal cord, and nerves throughout the body.

The Central Nervous System

The brain is housed within the skull. The spinal cord is housed within the spinal column. The spinal column extends from the brain into the trunk of the body. Both the brain and the spinal cord are covered by a protective membrane made up of three layers. Between two of these layers is the cerebrospinal fluid. This fluid circulates around the brain and spinal cord. It provides a cushion against injuries.

The brain has three main sections: the cerebrum, the cerebellum, and the brainstem (Fig. 9-5). The largest section of the human brain is the cerebrum. The outside layer of the cerebrum is the cerebral cortex. The cerebral cortex is the part of the brain in which thinking, analysis, association of ideas, judgment, emotions, and memory occur. The cerebral cortex also

- Directs speech and emotions
- Interprets messages from the eyes, ears, nose, tongue, and skin
- Controls voluntary muscle movement

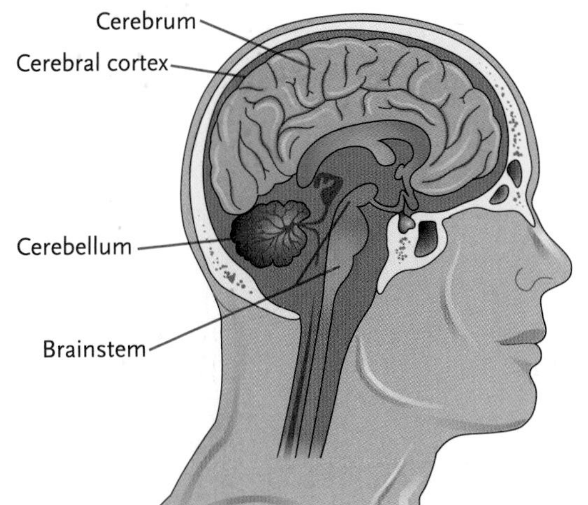

Fig. 9-5. The three main sections of the brain are the cerebrum, cerebellum, and brainstem.

The cerebrum is divided into right and left hemispheres. The right hemisphere controls movement and function in the left side of the body. The left hemisphere controls movement and function in the right side of the body (Fig. 9-6). Any illness or injury to the right hemisphere affects functions on the left side of the body. Illness or injury to the left hemisphere disrupts function on the right side.

The cerebellum controls balance and regulates the body's voluntary muscles. It produces and coordinates smooth movements. Someone who has a problem in the cerebellum will be uncoordinated and have jerky movements and muscle weakness.

The cerebrum and cerebellum are connected to the spinal cord by the brainstem. The brainstem contains a kind of regulatory center. It controls heart rate, breathing, swallowing, coughing, vomiting, and closing or opening of blood vessels.

The spinal cord is connected to the brain. It is protected by the bones of the spinal column. Nerve pathways run through the spinal cord. They conduct messages between the brain and the body. Cranial nerves attach to the brain and brainstem. Some of these nerves bring information from the sense organs to the brain. Some control muscles and others are connected to glands or organs, such as the lungs. There are 12 pairs of cranial nerves. Nerves that are attached to the spinal cord and connect the spinal cord with other parts of the body are called spinal nerves. The brain communicates with most of the body through the spinal nerves. There are 31 pairs of spinal nerves.

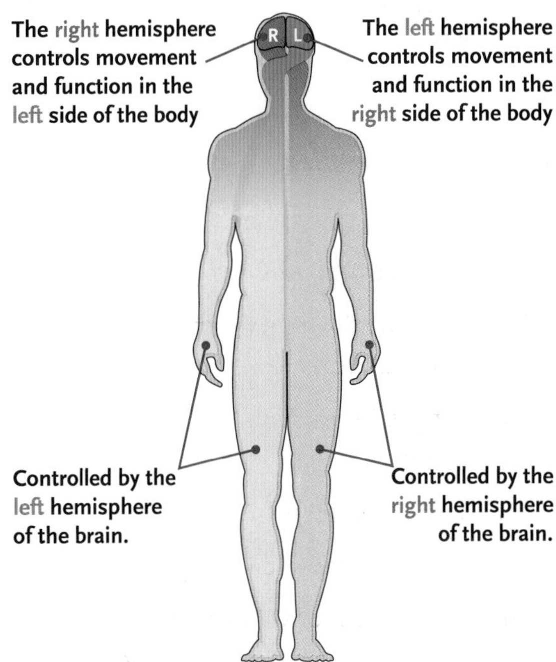

***Fig. 9-6.** The right hemisphere controls movement and function in the left side of the body. The left hemisphere controls movement and function in the right side of the body.*

The functions of the nervous system are to control and coordinate all body functions and to sense, interpret, and respond to changes occurring both inside and outside the human body.

Normal changes of aging include the following:

- Responses and reflexes slow.
- Sensitivity of nerve endings in skin decreases.
- Person may show some memory loss, more often with short-term memory. Long-term memory, or memory of past events, usually remains sharp.

How The NA Can Help

Suggesting residents make lists or write notes about things they want to remember can help with memory loss. Placing a calendar nearby may also help. If residents enjoy reminiscing, the NA can take an interest in their past by asking to see photos or hear stories. The NA should allow time for decision-making and avoid sudden changes in schedule. Plenty of time should be allowed for movement; the NA should not rush the resident. Reading, thinking, and other mental activities should be encouraged.

Observing and Reporting: Central Nervous System

Observe and report these signs and symptoms:

- O/R Fatigue or pain with movement or exercise
- O/R Shaking or trembling
- O/R Inability to move one side of body
- O/R Difficulty speaking or slurring of speech
- O/R Numbness or tingling
- O/R Disturbance or changes in vision or hearing
- O/R Dizziness or loss of balance
- O/R Changes in eating patterns and/or fluid intake
- O/R Difficulty swallowing
- O/R Bowel and bladder changes
- O/R Depression or mood changes
- O/R Memory loss or confusion
- O/R Violent behavior
- O/R Any unusual or unexplained change in behavior
- O/R Decreased ability to perform ADLs

The Nervous System: Sense Organs

The eyes, ears, nose, tongue, and skin are the body's major sense organs. They are considered part of the central nervous system because they contain receptors that receive impulses from the environment. They relay these impulses to the nerves.

The eye, which is about an inch in diameter, is located in a bony socket in the skull (Fig. 9-7). The bony socket protects the eye, which is surrounded by muscles that control its movements.

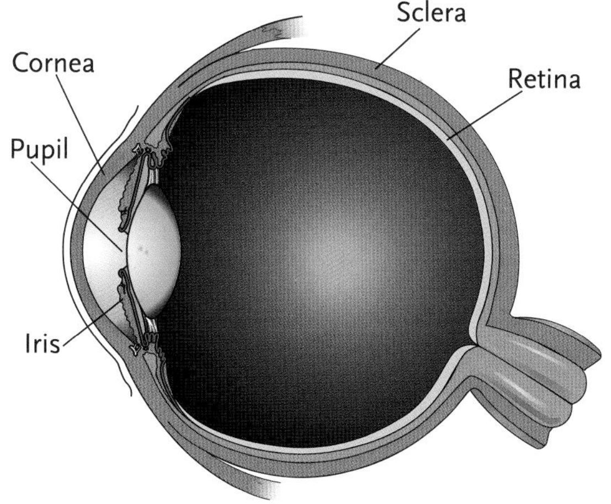

Fig. 9-7. *The parts of the eye.*

The outer part of the eye is called the sclera. The sclera appears white, except in front, where it is called the cornea. The cornea is actually clear, but it appears colored because it lies over the iris, or the colored part of the eye. The pupil, or black circle in the center of the iris, widens or narrows to adjust the amount of light that enters the eye. Inside the back of the eye is the retina. The retina contains cells that respond to light and send a message to the brain, where the picture is interpreted so a person can see.

The ear is a sense organ that provides balance and hearing. It is divided into three parts: the outer, middle, and inner ear (Fig. 9-8). The outer ear is the funnel-shaped outer part, sometimes called the auricle or pinna. It guides sound waves into the auditory canal. This canal is about one inch long and contains many glands that secrete earwax. Earwax and hair in the ear protect the ear from foreign objects. The eardrum, or tympanic membrane, separates the outer ear from the middle ear.

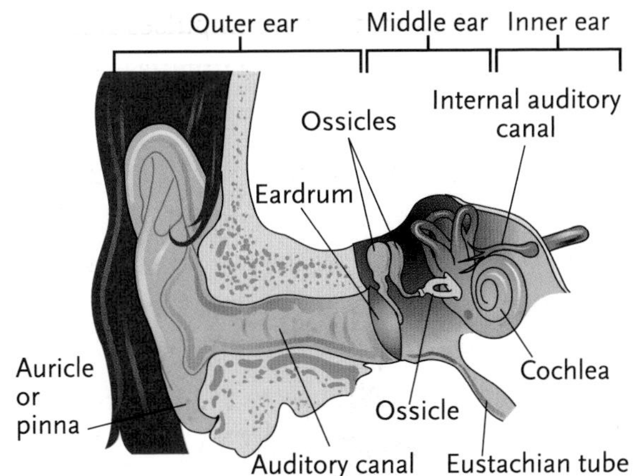

Fig. 9-8. *The outer ear, middle ear, and inner ear are the three main divisions of the ear.*

The middle ear consists of the eustachian tube and three ossicles, small bones that amplify sound. The ossicles transmit sound to the inner ear. The eustachian tube connects the middle ear to the throat. It functions to allow air into the middle ear to equalize pressure on the tympanic membrane. The inner ear contains fluid that carries sound waves from the middle ear to the auditory nerve. The auditory nerve then transmits the impulse to the brain. The inner ear also contains structures that help in maintaining balance.

Normal changes of aging include the following:

- Vision and hearing decrease. Sense of balance may be affected.
- Senses of taste, smell, and touch decrease.
- Sensitivity to heat and cold decreases.

How The NA Can Help

Residents should use their eyeglasses. The NA can help by keeping eyeglasses clean. Bright colors and proper lighting will also help. The use of hearing aids should be encouraged, and hearing aids should be kept clean. In addition, the NA should face the resident when speaking and should speak slowly and clearly in a low-pitched voice. Shouting should be avoided. The NA should repeat words when necessary. The loss of senses of taste and smell may lead to decreased appetite. Providing regular oral care and offering foods with a variety of tastes and textures may help. The loss of smell may make resident unaware of increased body odor. The NA should assist as needed with regular bathing. Due to decreased sense of touch, residents may not be able to tell if something is too hot for them. The NA should be careful with hot drinks and hot bath water.

Observing and Reporting: Eyes and Ears

Observe and report these signs and symptoms:

- O/R Changes in vision or hearing
- O/R Signs of infection
- O/R Dizziness
- O/R Complaints of pain in eyes or ears

5. Describe the circulatory system

The circulatory, or cardiovascular, system is made up of the heart, blood vessels, and blood (Fig. 9-9). The heart pumps blood through the blood vessels to the cells. The blood carries food, oxygen, and other substances cells need to function properly. A healthy circulatory system is essential for life. Cells, tissues, and organs need proper circulation to function well. If circulation is reduced, cells do not receive enough oxygen and nutrients. Waste products of cell metabolism are not removed, and organs become diseased.

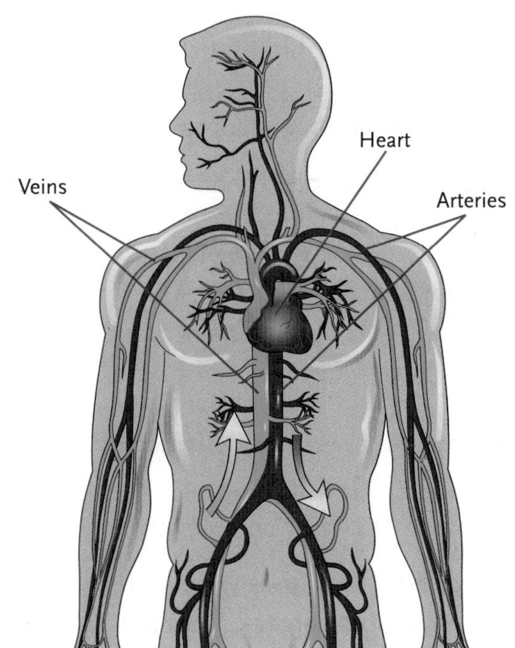

Fig. 9-9. *The heart, blood vessels, and blood are the main parts of the circulatory system.*

The heart is the pump of the circulatory system (Fig. 9-10). The heart is a muscle. It is located in the middle lower chest, on the left side. The heart muscle is made up of three layers: the pericardium, the myocardium, and the endocardium.

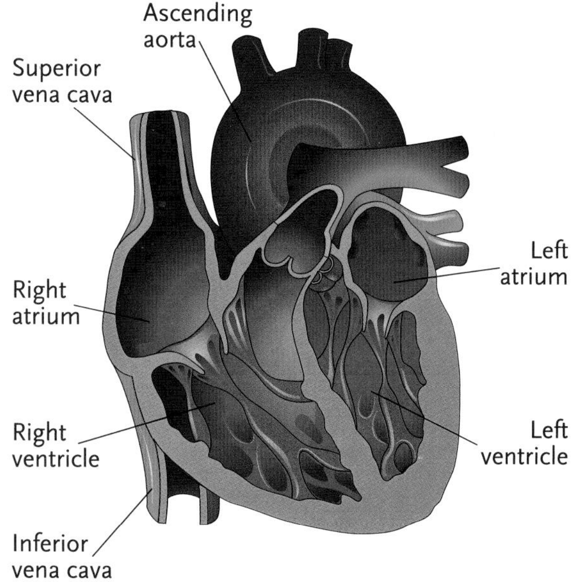

Fig. 9-10. The four chambers of the heart connect to the body's largest blood vessels.

The interior of the heart is divided into four chambers. The two upper chambers are called the left atrium and right atrium. They receive blood. The two lower chambers, or ventricles, pump blood. The right atrium receives blood from the veins. This blood, containing carbon dioxide, then flows into the right ventricle. It is pumped to the blood vessels in the lungs. Carbon dioxide is exchanged for oxygen. The heart's left atrium receives the oxygen-saturated blood. It then flows into the left ventricle. There it is pumped through the arteries to all parts of the body. Two valves, one located between the right atrium and right ventricle and the other between the left atrium and left ventricle, allow the blood to flow in only one direction (Fig. 9-11).

The heart functions in two phases: the contracting phase, or **systole**, when the ventricles pump blood through the blood vessels, and the resting phase, or **diastole**, when the chambers fill with blood. When a person's blood pressure is taken, the numbers measure these two phases. Chapter 14 has more information on how to take blood pressure.

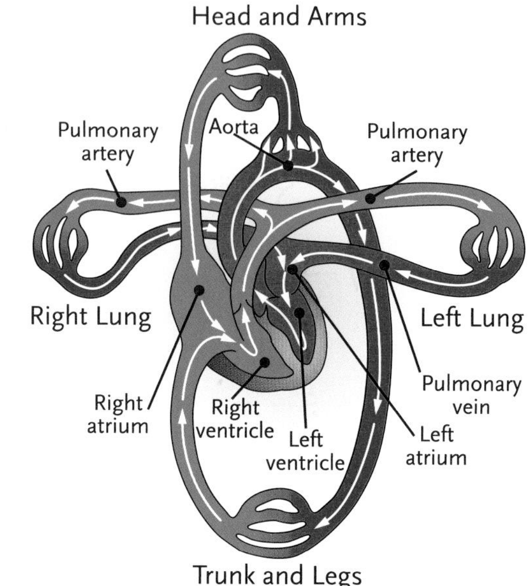

Fig. 9-11. The flow of blood through the heart.

Three types of blood vessels are found in the body: arteries, capillaries, and veins. Arteries carry oxygen-rich blood away from the heart. The blood is pumped from the left ventricle, through the aorta, the largest artery. Blood is then pumped through other arteries that branch off from it. The coronary arteries carry blood to the heart itself.

Capillaries are tiny blood vessels that receive blood from the arteries. Nutrients, oxygen, and other substances in the blood pass from the capillaries to the cells. Waste products, including carbon dioxide, pass from the cells into the capillaries.

Veins carry the blood containing waste products from the capillaries back to the heart. Near the heart, the veins come together to form the two largest veins, the inferior vena cava and the superior vena cava. These empty into the right atrium. The inferior vena cava carries blood from the legs and trunk. The superior vena cava carries blood from the arms, head, and neck.

Blood is made up of blood cells and plasma. There are three different types of blood cells: red blood cells, or erythrocytes; white blood cells, or leukocytes; and platelets, or thrombocytes.

Red blood cells (erythrocytes) carry oxygen from the lungs to all parts of the body. Red blood cells are produced by bone marrow, a substance found inside hollow bones. Iron, found in bone marrow and red blood cells, is essential to blood. It gives it its red color. Red blood cells function for a short time, then die. They are filtered out of the blood by the liver and spleen. Iron in diets allows bodies to produce new red blood cells.

White blood cells (leukocytes) defend the body against foreign substances, such as bacteria and viruses. When the body becomes aware of these invaders, white blood cells rush to the site of infection. They multiply rapidly. The bone marrow, spleen, and thymus gland produce white blood cells.

Platelets (thrombocytes) are also carried by the blood. They cause the blood to clot, preventing excess bleeding. Platelets are also produced by the bone marrow.

Plasma is the liquid portion of the blood. It is made up of mostly water and carries many substances, including blood cells, nutrients, and waste products.

The functions of the circulatory system are to supply food, oxygen, and hormones to cells and to supply the body with infection-fighting blood cells. The circulatory system removes waste products from cells and also helps control body temperature.

Normal changes of aging include the following:

- Heart pumps less efficiently.
- Blood flow decreases.
- Blood vessels narrow.

How The NA Can Help

Movement and exercise to improve circulation should be encouraged. Walking, stretching, and even lifting light weights can help maintain strength and promote circulation. Range of motion exercises are important for residents who cannot get out of bed. The NA should allow enough time to complete activities and try to prevent residents from tiring. Layering clothing will help keep residents warm. Socks, slippers, or shoes help keep the feet warm.

Observing and Reporting: Circulatory System

Observe and report these signs and symptoms:

- O/R Changes in pulse rate
- O/R Weakness, fatigue
- O/R Loss of ability to perform activities of daily living (ADLs)
- O/R Swelling of hands and feet
- O/R Pale or bluish hands, feet, or lips
- O/R Chest pain
- O/R Weight gain
- O/R Shortness of breath, changes in breathing patterns, inability to catch breath
- O/R Severe headache
- O/R Inactivity (which can lead to circulatory problems)

6. Describe the respiratory system

Respiration, the body taking in oxygen and removing carbon dioxide, involves breathing in, **inspiration**, and breathing out, **expiration**. The lungs accomplish this process (Fig. 9-12).

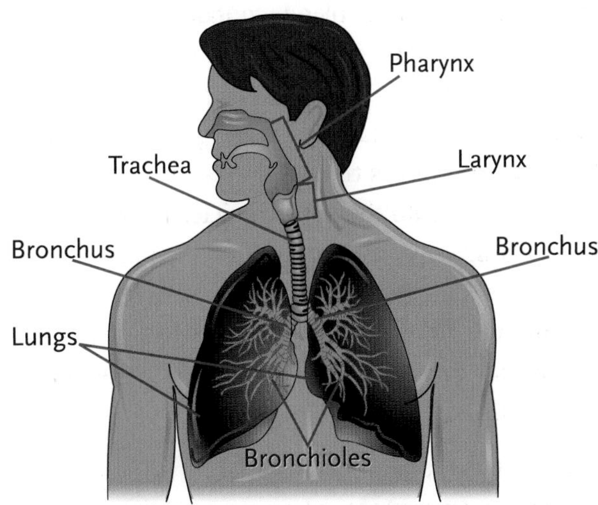

Fig. 9-12. The respiratory process begins with inspiration through the nose or mouth. The air travels through the trachea and into the lungs via the bronchi, which then branch into bronchioles.

As the lungs inhale, the air is pulled in through the nose and into the pharynx, a tubular passageway for both food and air. From the pharynx, air passes into the larynx, or voice box. The larynx is located at the beginning of the trachea, or windpipe. The trachea divides into two branches at its lower portion, the right bronchus and the left bronchus, or bronchi. Each bronchus leads into a lung and then subdivides into bronchioles. These smaller airways subdivide further. They end in alveoli: tiny sacs that appear in grape-like clusters. Blood is supplied to the alveoli by capillaries. Oxygen and carbon dioxide are exchanged between the alveoli and capillaries.

Oxygen-saturated blood then circulates through the capillaries and venules (small veins) of the lungs, into the pulmonary vein and left side of the heart. The carbon dioxide is exhaled through the alveoli into the bronchioles and bronchi of the lungs, the trachea, through the larynx, the pharynx, and out the nose and mouth.

Each lung is covered by the pleura, a membrane with two layers. One is attached to the chest wall. The other is attached to the surface of the lung. The space between the layers is filled with a thin fluid that lubricates the layers, preventing them from rubbing together during breathing.

The functions of the respiratory system are to bring oxygen into the body and to eliminate carbon dioxide produced as the body uses oxygen.

Normal changes of aging include the following:

- Lung strength decreases.
- Lung capacity decreases.
- Oxygen in the blood decreases.
- Voice weakens.

How The NA Can Help

Residents with acute or chronic upper respiratory conditions should not be exposed to cigarette smoke or polluted air. The NA should provide rest periods as needed and encourage exercise and regular movement. The NA should assist with deep breathing exercises as ordered. Residents who have difficulty breathing will usually be more comfortable sitting up, rather than lying down.

Observing and Reporting: Respiratory System

Observe and report these signs and symptoms:

- O/R Change in respiratory rate
- O/R Shallow breathing or breathing through pursed lips
- O/R Coughing or wheezing
- O/R Nasal congestion or discharge
- O/R Sore throat, difficulty swallowing, or swollen tonsils
- O/R The need to sit after mild exertion
- O/R Pale, bluish, or gray color of the lips, arms, and/or legs
- O/R Pain in the chest area
- O/R Discolored **sputum**, or mucus a person coughs up from the lungs (green, yellow, blood-tinged, or gray)

7. Describe the urinary system

The urinary system is composed of two kidneys, two ureters, one urinary bladder, a single urethra, and a meatus (Figs. 9-13 and 9-14).

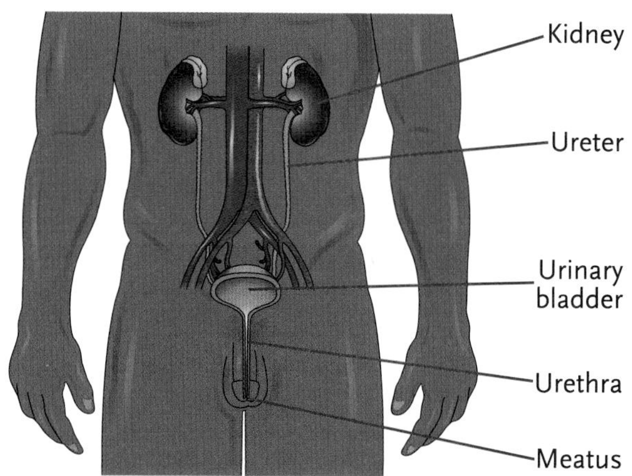

***Fig. 9-13.** The urinary system consists of two kidneys and their ureters, the bladder, the urethra, and the meatus. This is an illustration of the male urinary system.*

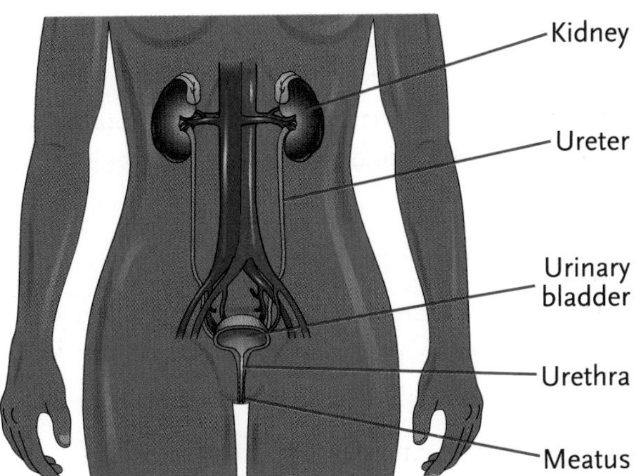

Fig. 9-14. *The female urethra is shorter than the male urethra. Because of this, the female bladder is more likely to become infected by bacteria traveling up the urethra. To help prevent infection, females should wipe from front to back after elimination.*

The kidneys are located in the upper part of the abdominal cavity on each side of the spine. These two bean-shaped organs are protected by the muscles of the back and the lower part of the rib cage. When blood flows through the kidneys, waste products and excess water are filtered out. Necessary water and substances are reabsorbed into the bloodstream. Waste and the remaining fluid form urine. The body must maintain a proper balance between water absorbed in the body and waste fluids that are released from the body. Chapter 15 contains information about fluid intake and output.

Each kidney has a ureter, which is attached to the bladder. Urine flows through the ureters to the bladder, a muscular sac in the lower part of the abdomen. Urine flows from the bladder through the urethra. It then passes out of the body through the meatus, the opening at the end of the urethra. In the female, the meatus is located in the genital area just in front of the opening of the vagina. In the male, the meatus is located at the end of the penis.

The urinary system has two important functions. Through urine, the urinary system eliminates waste products created by the cells. The urinary system also maintains the water balance in the body.

Normal changes of aging include the following:

- The ability of kidneys to filter blood decreases.
- Bladder muscle tone weakens.
- Bladder holds less urine, which causes more frequent urination.
- Bladder may not empty completely, causing a greater chance of infection.

How The NA Can Help

The NA should encourage fluids and offer frequent trips to the bathroom. If residents are incontinent, the NA should never show frustration or anger. **Urinary incontinence** is the inability to control the bladder, which leads to an involuntary loss of urine. Residents should be kept clean and dry.

Observing and Reporting: Urinary System

Observe and report these signs and symptoms:

- O/R Weight loss or gain
- O/R Swelling in the upper or lower extremities
- O/R Pain or burning during urination
- O/R Changes in urine, such as cloudiness, odor, or color
- O/R Changes in frequency and amount of urination
- O/R Swelling in the abdominal/bladder area
- O/R Complaints that bladder feels full or painful
- O/R Urinary incontinence/dribbling
- O/R Pain in the kidney or back/flank region
- O/R Inadequate fluid intake

8. Describe the gastrointestinal system

The gastrointestinal (GI) system, also called the digestive system, is made up of the gastrointestinal tract and the accessory digestive organs (Fig. 9-15). The gastrointestinal tract is a long passageway extending from the mouth to the anus, the opening of the rectum. Food passes from the mouth through the pharynx, esophagus, stomach, small intestine, large intestine, and out of the body as solid waste. The teeth, tongue, salivary glands, liver, gall bladder, and pancreas are the accessory organs to digestion. They help prepare the food so that it can be absorbed.

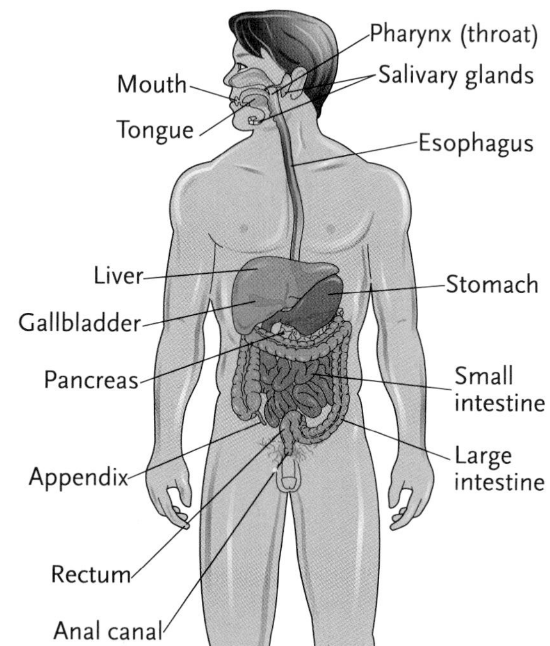

***Fig. 9-15.** The GI system consists of all the organs needed to digest food and process waste.*

Food is first placed in the mouth. The teeth chew it by cutting it, then chopping and grinding it into smaller pieces that can be swallowed. Saliva moistens the food and begins chemical digestion. The tongue helps with chewing and swallowing by pushing the food around between the teeth and then into the pharynx.

The pharynx is a muscular structure located at the back of the mouth. It extends into the throat. It contracts with swallowing and pushes food into the esophagus. The muscles of the esophagus then move food into the stomach through involuntary contractions called **peristalsis**.

The stomach is a muscular pouch located in the upper left part of the abdominal cavity. It provides physical digestion by stirring and churning the food to break it down into smaller particles. The glands in the stomach lining aid in digestion. They secrete gastric juices that chemically break down food. This process turns food into a semi-liquid substance called chyme. Peristalsis continues in the stomach, pushing the chyme into the small intestine.

The small intestine is about twenty feet long. Here enzymes secreted by the liver and the pancreas finish digesting the chyme. Bile, a green liquid produced by the liver, is stored in the gallbladder and released into the small intestine. Bile helps break down dietary fat. The liver converts fats and sugars into glucose, a sugar that can be carried to cells by the blood. The liver also stores glucose. The pancreas produces insulin, a hormone that regulates the body's conversion of sugar into glucose.

The chyme is moved by peristalsis through the small intestine. There villi, tiny projections lining the small intestine, absorb the digested food into the capillaries.

Peristalsis moves the chyme that has not already been digested through the large intestine. In the large intestine, most of the water in the chyme is absorbed. What remains is feces, a semi-solid material of water, solid waste material, bacteria, and mucus. Feces passes by peristalsis through the rectum, the lower end of the colon. It moves out of the body through the anus, the rectal opening.

The gastrointestinal system has two functions: digestion and elimination. **Digestion** is the process of preparing food physically and chemically so that it can be absorbed into the cells. **Elimination** is the process of expelling solid wastes (made up of the waste products of food) that are not absorbed into the cells.

Normal changes of aging include the following:

- Decreased saliva production affects the ability to chew and swallow.
- Dulled sense of taste may result in poor appetite.

- Absorption of vitamins and minerals decreases.
- Process of digestion takes longer and is less efficient.
- Body waste moves more slowly through the intestines, causing more frequent constipation.

How The NA Can Help

Fluids and nutritious, appealing meals should be encouraged. The NA should allow time to eat and make mealtime enjoyable. Regular oral care should be provided. Dentures must fit properly and should be cleaned regularly. Residents who have trouble chewing and swallowing are at risk of choking. The NA should offer fluids during mealtime. Residents should eat a diet that contains fiber and drink plenty of fluids to help prevent constipation. Residents should be given the opportunity to have a bowel movement around the same time each day.

Observing and Reporting: Gastrointestinal System

Observe and report these signs and symptoms:

- O/R Difficulty swallowing or chewing (including denture problems, tooth pain, or mouth sores)
- O/R **Fecal incontinence** (inability to control the bowels, leading to involuntary passage of stool)
- O/R Weight gain/weight loss
- O/R Loss of appetite
- O/R Abdominal pain and cramping
- O/R Diarrhea
- O/R Nausea and vomiting (especially vomitus that looks like coffee grounds)
- O/R Constipation
- O/R Flatulence
- O/R Hiccups, belching
- O/R Bloody, black, or hard stools
- O/R Heartburn
- O/R Poor nutritional intake

9. Describe the endocrine system

The endocrine system is made up of glands in different areas of the body (Fig. 9-16). **Glands** are organs that produce and secrete chemicals called hormones. **Hormones** are chemical substances created by the body that control numerous body functions.

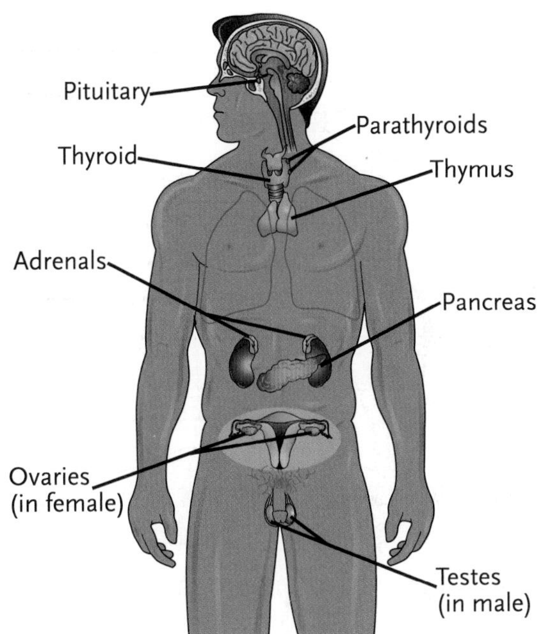

Fig. 9-16. The endocrine system includes organs that produce hormones that regulate body processes.

The pituitary gland, called the *master gland,* is located behind the eyes at the base of the brain. It secretes key hormones that cause other glands to produce other hormones. Following are some hormones secreted by the pituitary gland:

- Growth hormone, which regulates growth and development
- Antidiuretic hormone (ADH), which controls the balance of fluids in the body
- Oxytocin, which causes the uterus to contract during and after childbirth

The pituitary gland also produces hormones that regulate the thyroid gland and the adrenal glands. The thyroid gland is located in the neck in front of the larynx. It produces thyroid hormone, which regulates metabolism, the burning of food for heat and energy.

The parathyroid glands secrete a hormone that regulates the body's use of calcium. Nerves and muscles require calcium to function smoothly. A deficiency of this hormone can cause severe muscle contractions and spasms. It can be fatal if untreated.

The pancreas, a gland located in the upper midsection of the abdomen, secretes insulin. Insulin is a hormone that regulates the amount of glucose (sugar) available to the cells for metabolism. The cells cannot absorb glucose without insulin.

Two adrenal glands are located at the tops of the kidneys. They produce hormones that are essential to life. These hormones are important because they help the body regulate carbohydrate metabolism. They also control the body's reaction to stress and regulate salt and water absorption in the kidneys. Adrenal glands also produce the hormone adrenaline, which regulates muscle power, heart rate, blood pressure, and energy levels during stressful situations or emergencies.

Gonads, or sex glands, produce hormones that regulate the body's ability to reproduce. The testes in the male secrete testosterone. The ovaries in the female secrete estrogen and progesterone.

The functions of the endocrine system are to maintain homeostasis, influence growth and development, regulate levels of sugar in the blood and levels of calcium in the bones. The endocrine system also regulates the body's ability to reproduce and determines how fast cells burn food for energy.

Normal changes of aging include the following:

- Levels of hormones, such as estrogen and progesterone, decrease.
- Insulin production lessens.
- Body is less able to handle stress.

How The NA Can Help

The NA should encourage proper nutrition and try to eliminate or reduce stressors. Stressors are anything that causes stress. The NA can help by offering encouragement and listening to residents.

Observing and Reporting: Endocrine System

Observe and report these signs and symptoms:

- O/R Headache
- O/R Weakness
- O/R Blurred vision
- O/R Dizziness
- O/R Irritability
- O/R Sweating/excessive perspiration
- O/R Change in "normal" behavior
- O/R Confusion
- O/R Change in mobility
- O/R Change in sensation
- O/R Numbness or tingling in arms or legs
- O/R Weight gain/weight loss
- O/R Loss of appetite/increased appetite
- O/R Increased thirst
- O/R Frequent urination or any change in urine output
- O/R Hunger
- O/R Dry skin
- O/R Skin breakdown
- O/R Sweet or fruity breath
- O/R Sluggishness or fatigue
- O/R Hyperactivity

10. Describe the reproductive system

The reproductive system is made up of the reproductive organs, which are different in men and women. The reproductive system allows human beings to **reproduce**, or create new human life. Reproduction begins when a male's and female's sex cells (sperm and ovum) join. These sex cells are formed in the male and female sex glands. These sex glands are called the **gonads**.

The Male Reproductive System

In the male, the sex glands or gonads are the testes or testicles. The two oval glands are located outside the body in the scrotum. The scrotum is a sac made of skin and muscle, and it is suspended between the thighs. The testes produce the male sex cells, called sperm, and testosterone (Fig. 9-17). Testosterone is the male hormone needed for the reproductive organs to function properly. Testosterone also promotes development of male secondary sex characteristics, which include the following:

- Facial hair
- Pubic and underarm hair
- Hair on the chest, legs, and arms
- Deepening of the voice
- Development of muscle mass

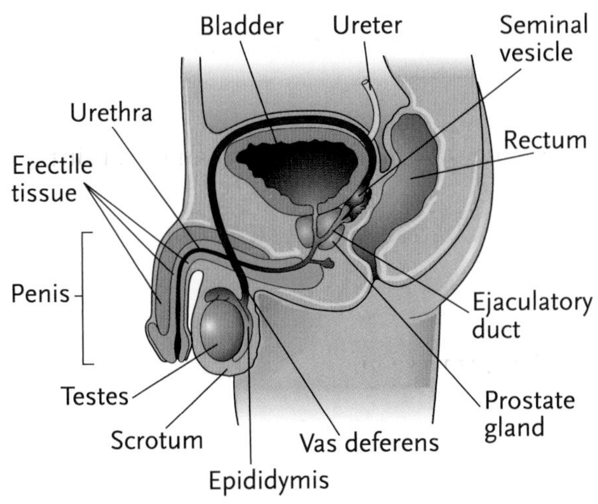

Fig. 9-17. The male reproductive system.

Sperm travel from the testes through a coiled tube, the epididymis, and another tube called the vas deferens. Sperm then pass into the seminal vesicle where semen is produced. Semen carries sperm out of the body.

The ducts coming from each seminal vesicle unite to form the ejaculatory ducts. They pass through the prostate gland, where more fluid is added to the semen. In the prostate, the ejaculatory ducts join the urethra, the tube through which both urine and semen pass. The urethra continues through the penis, the sex organ located outside the body, in front of the scrotum. The penis is composed of erectile tissue that becomes filled with blood during sexual excitement. As the penis fills with blood, it becomes enlarged and erect. It then can enter the vagina, the female reproductive tract, where it releases semen containing sperm.

The Female Reproductive System

In the human female, the gonads are two oval glands called the ovaries. There is one ovary on each side of the uterus (Fig. 9-18). The ovaries make the female sex cells or eggs (ova). They release the female hormones, estrogen and progesterone. Each month, from puberty to menopause, an egg is released from an ovary. This cycle is maintained by estrogen and progesterone. These hormones control development of female secondary sex characteristics, which include the following:

- Increased breast size
- Wider and rounder hips
- Axillary and pubic hair
- A slightly deeper voice

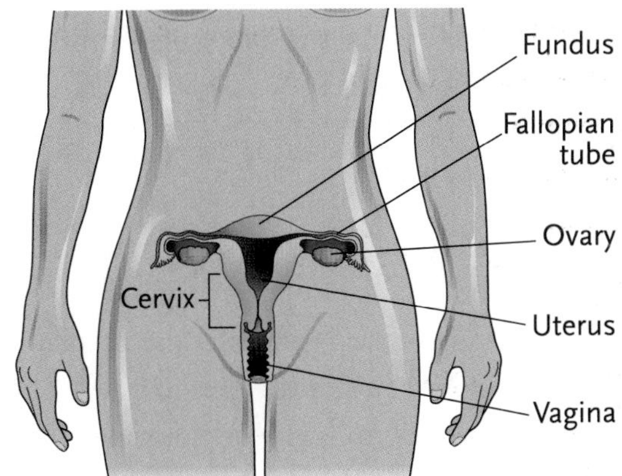

Fig. 9-18. The female reproductive system.

Once an egg is released from an ovary, it travels through the fallopian tube to the uterus. The uterus is a hollow, pear-shaped, muscular organ that is located within the pelvis. It lies behind the bladder and in front of the rectum. If sexual intercourse takes place while the egg is in the fallopian tube, the egg may be fertilized by sperm in the fallopian tube. The fertilized egg then travels down into the uterus. It implants in the endometrium, the lining of the uterus. Stimulated by hormones, the endometrium builds up during the menstrual cycle. It has many blood vessels supplying it for the growth and feeding of an embryo. If the egg is not fertilized, the hormones decrease. The blood supply to the endometrium decreases. The endometrium then breaks up in a process called menstruation.

The main section of the uterus is the fundus. This is where the fetus develops after the fertilized egg is implanted. The narrow neck of the uterus extending into the vagina is the cervix. The cervix has an opening through which menstrual fluid can pass and semen can enter the vagina.

The vagina is the muscular canal that opens to the outside of the body. The external vaginal opening is partially closed by the hymen membrane. The vagina is kept moist by secretions from glands in the vaginal walls. The vagina receives the penis during sexual intercourse. It also serves as the birth canal. The baby passes through the cervix, which is made thin by pressure from the baby's head during contractions. Once the cervix opens, the baby can then move out through the vagina.

For males, the function of the reproductive system is to manufacture sperm and the male hormone testosterone. For females, the reproductive system manufactures ova (eggs) and the female hormones estrogen and progesterone. It also provides an environment for the development of a fetus and produces milk for the nourishment of a baby after birth.

Normal changes of aging for males include the following:

- Sperm production decreases.
- Prostate gland enlarges, which can interfere with urination.

Normal changes of aging for females include the following:

- Menstruation ends. Menopause is when a female stops having menstrual periods.
- Decrease in estrogen may lead to a loss of calcium. This can cause brittle bones and, potentially, osteoporosis.
- Vaginal walls become drier and thinner.

How The NA Can Help

Sexual needs and desires continue as people age. The NA should provide privacy when necessary for sexual activity. The NA must respect residents' sexual needs and never make fun of or judge any sexual behavior. However, any behavior that makes the NA uncomfortable or seems inappropriate should be reported. Inappropriate behavior is not a normal sign of aging and could be a sign of illness.

Observing and Reporting: Reproductive System

Observe and report these signs and symptoms:

- O/R Discomfort or difficulty with urination
- O/R Discharge from the penis or vagina
- O/R Swelling of the genitals
- O/R Blood in urine or stool
- O/R Breast changes, including size, shape, lumps, or discharge from the nipple
- O/R Sores on the genitals
- O/R Resident reports of erectile dysfunction (ED), or trouble getting or keeping an erection
- O/R Resident reports of painful intercourse

Residents' Rights

Sexual Expression and Privacy

Residents have the right to sexual freedom and expression. Residents have the right to privacy and to meet their sexual needs.

11. Describe the immune and lymphatic systems

The immune system protects the body from disease-causing bacteria, viruses, and microorganisms in two ways. **Nonspecific immunity** protects the body from disease in general. **Specific immunity** protects against a particular disease that is invading the body at a given time.

Nonspecific Immunity

To protect itself against disease in general, the body has several defenses:

- Anatomic barriers include the skin and the mucous membranes. They provide a physical barrier to keep foreign materials—bacteria, viruses, or microorganisms—from invading the body. Saliva, tears, and mucous secretions also help protect the body by washing away substances.
- Physiologic barriers include body temperature and acidity of certain organs. Most organisms that cause disease cannot survive high temperatures or high acidity. When the body senses foreign organisms, it can raise its temperature (by running a fever) to kill off the invaders. The acidity of organs like the stomach keeps harmful bacteria from growing there.
- Inflammatory response refers to the body's ability to fight infection through inflammation or swelling of an infected area. When inflammation occurs, it indicates that the body has sent extra disease-fighting cells and extra blood to the infected area to fight the infection.

Specific Immunity

To protect itself against specific diseases, the body makes different types of cells that will fight a range of different invaders. Once it has successfully eliminated an invader, the immune system records the invasion in the form of antibodies. Antibodies are carried within cells. They prevent a disease from threatening the body a second time.

Acquired immunity is a kind of specific immunity. The body acquires it either by fighting an infection or by vaccination. For example, a person can acquire immunity to a disease like the measles in two ways:

1. The person gets measles. His body forms antibodies to the disease to make sure he will not get it again; or
2. He gets a vaccine for the measles. This causes his body to produce the same antibodies to protect him from the disease.

The lymphatic system removes excess fluids and waste products from the body's tissues. It also helps the immune system fight infection. It is closely related to both the immune and the circulatory systems. The lymphatic system consists of lymph vessels and lymph capillaries in which a fluid called lymph circulates (Fig. 9-19). **Lymph** is a clear yellowish fluid that carries disease-fighting cells called lymphocytes.

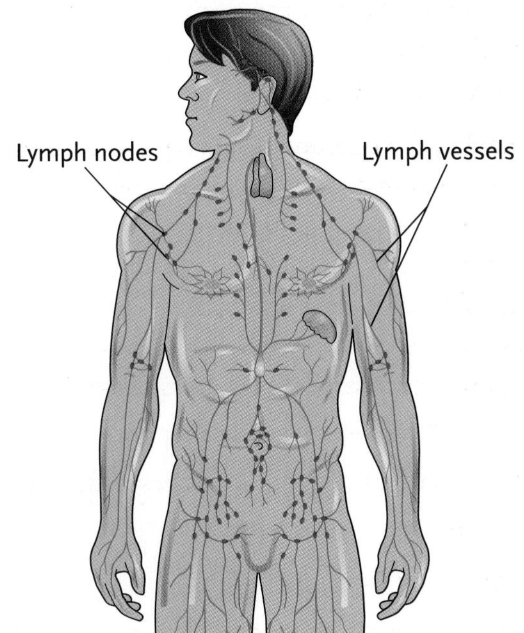

Fig. 9-19. *Lymph nodes work to fight infection and are located throughout the body.*

When the body is fighting an infection, swelling may occur in the lymph nodes. These are oval-shaped bodies that can be as small as a pinhead or as large as an almond. Located in the neck, groin, and armpits, the lymph nodes filter out germs and waste products carried from the tissues by the lymph fluid. After lymph fluid has been purified in the lymph nodes, it flows into the bloodstream.

Unlike the circulatory system, in which the heart functions as a pump to move the blood, the lymph system has no pump. Lymph fluid is circulated by muscle activity, massage, and breathing. A sore muscle may feel better if it is rubbed. The rubbing action helps the lymph fluid circulate, carrying waste products away from the tired muscle.

The functions of the immune and lymphatic systems are to protect the body against disease-causing bacteria, viruses, and microorganisms and to remove excess fluids and waste products from the body's tissues.

Normal changes of aging include the following:

- Immune system weakens, increasing the risk of all types of infections.
- It may take longer for a person to recover from an illness.
- Number and size of lymph nodes decrease, which results in body being less able to contract a fever to fight infection.
- Response to vaccines decreases.

How The NA Can Help

Factors that weaken the immune system include not enough sleep, poor nutrition, chronic illness, and stress. Preventing infection is important. The NA can help by washing her hands often and keeping the resident's environment clean. She can help with personal hygiene as needed. Proper nutrition and fluid intake should be encouraged to help residents stay healthy. A slight temperature increase may indicate that a resident is fighting an infection. The NA should take accurate vital sign measurements.

Observing and Reporting: Immune and Lymphatic Systems

Observe and report these signs and symptoms:

- O/R Recurring infections (such as fevers and diarrhea)
- O/R Swelling of the lymph nodes
- O/R Increased fatigue

Chapter Review

1. What is homeostasis?
2. What are three functions of the skin, or integument?
3. List ten signs and symptoms to observe and report about the integumentary system.
4. How many bones make up the skeleton of the human body?
5. What type of exercises can help prevent contractures and muscle atrophy?
6. List five signs and symptoms to observe and report about the musculoskeletal system.
7. What are two functions of the nervous system?
8. List ten signs and symptoms to observe and report about the central nervous system.
9. List three signs and symptoms to observe and report about the eyes and ears.
10. What are four functions of the circulatory system?
11. List seven signs and symptoms to observe and report about the circulatory system.
12. What does respiration mean? What are the two parts involved in respiration?
13. List seven signs and symptoms to observe and report about the respiratory system.
14. What are two functions of the urinary system?

→ Signs & Symptons about the respiratory system
1) Change in rate of respirations
2) Shallow breathing & breathing through pursed lips.
3) coughing or wheezing 4) Nasal congestion or dischage
5) The need to sit after mild exertion 6) Pale blue or gray lips, arms or legs 7) sputum - green, yellow blood-colored or grey.

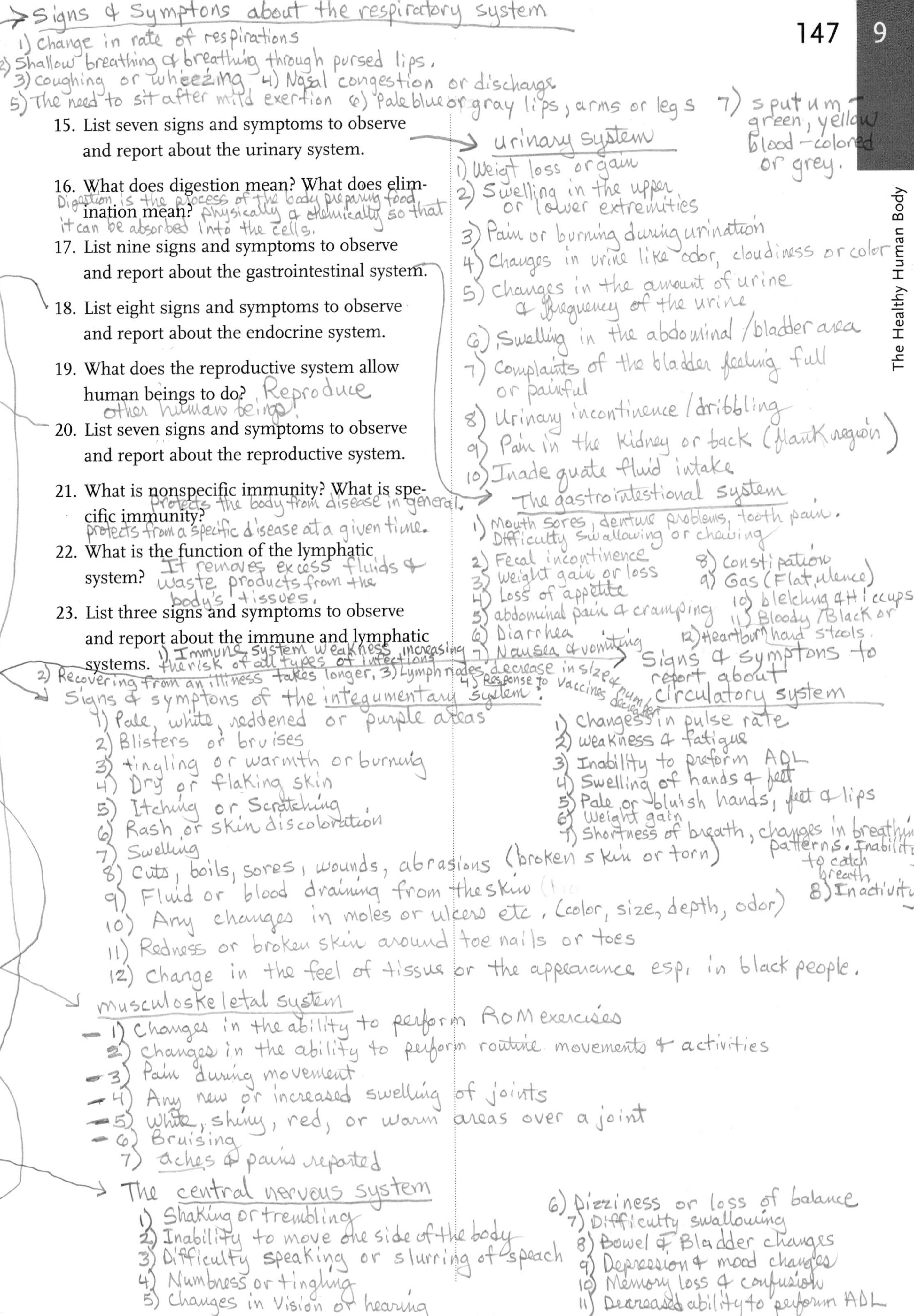

15. List seven signs and symptoms to observe and report about the urinary system.

→ urinary system
1) Weigt loss or gain
2) Swelling in the upper or lower extremities
3) Pain or burning during urination
4) Changes in urine like odor, cloudiness or color
5) changes in the amount of urine & frequency of the urine
6) Swelling in the abdominal /bladder area
7) Complaints of the bladder feeling full or painful
8) Urinary incontinence / dribbling
9) Pain in the kidney or back (flank region)
10) Inadequate fluid intake

16. What does digestion mean? What does elimination mean?

Digestion is the process of the body preparing food physically & chemically so that it can be absorbed into the cells.

17. List nine signs and symptoms to observe and report about the gastrointestinal system.

→ The gastrointestional system
1) Mouth sores, denture problems, tooth pain. Difficulty swallowing or chewing
2) Fecal incontinence
3) weight gain or loss
4) Loss of appetite
5) abdominal pain & cramping
6) Diarrhea
7) Nausea & vomiting
8) constipation
9) Gas (Flatulence)
10) belching & Hiccups
11) Bloody / Black or hard stools.
12) Heartburn

18. List eight signs and symptoms to observe and report about the endocrine system.

19. What does the reproductive system allow human beings to do?

Reproduce other human beings.

20. List seven signs and symptoms to observe and report about the reproductive system.

21. What is nonspecific immunity? What is specific immunity?

Protects the body from disease in general.
protects from a specific disease at a given time.

22. What is the function of the lymphatic system?

It removes excess fluids & waste products from the body's tissues.

23. List three signs and symptoms to observe and report about the immune and lymphatic systems.

1) Immune system weakness increasing the risk of all types of infections
2) Recovering from an illness takes longer. 3) Lymph nodes decrease in size & number
4) Response to Vaccines decreases

→ Signs & symptons of the integumentary system:
1) Pale, white, reddened or purple areas
2) Blisters or bruises
3) tingling or warmth or burning
4) Dry or flaking skin
5) Itching or Scratching
6) Rash or skin discoloration
7) Swelling
8) Cuts, boils, sores, wounds, abrasions (broken skin or torn)
9) Fluid or blood draining from the skin
10) Any changes in moles or ulcers etc. (color, size, depth, odor)
11) Redness or broken skin around toe nails or toes
12) Change in the feel of tissue or the appearance esp. in black people.

→ Signs & symptons to report about circulatory system
1) Changes in pulse rate
2) weakness & fatigue
3) Inability to preform ADL
4) Swelling of hands & feet
5) Pale or bluish hands, feet & lips
6) Weight gain
7) Shortness of breath, changes in breathing patterns. Inability to catch breath
8) Inactivity

→ musculoskeletal system
1) Changes in the ability to perform ROM exercises
2) changes in the ability to perform routine movements & activities
3) Pain during movement
4) Any new or increased swelling of joints
5) White, shiny, red, or warm areas over a joint
6) Bruising
7) aches & pains reported

→ The central nervous system
1) Shaking or trembling
2) Inability to move one side of the body
3) Difficulty speaking or slurring of speach
4) Numbness or tingling
5) Changes in Vision or hearing
6) Dizziness or loss of balance
7) Difficulty swallowing
8) Bowel & Bladder changes
9) Depression & mood changes
10) Memory loss & confusion
11) Decreased ability to perform ADL

10 Positioning, Transfers, and Ambulation

1. Review the principles of body mechanics

This chapter deals with how nursing assistants can safely position and move residents. Using proper body mechanics when assisting with positioning or moving helps prevent injury to both staff and residents. The following guidelines are a brief review of how to use proper body mechanics. Chapter 6 has more information.

Guidelines: Proper Body Mechanics

- G Assess the load. Before lifting, assess the weight of the load. Determine if you can safely move the object without help. Know the lift policies at your facility. Never attempt to lift someone you are not sure you can lift.
- G Think ahead, plan, and communicate the move. Check for any objects in your path. Look for any potential risks, such as a wet floor. Make sure the path is clear. Watch for hazards, such as high-traffic areas, combative residents, or a loose toilet seat or hand rail. Decide exactly what you and the resident are going to do together. Agree on the verbal cues you will use before attempting to transfer.
- G Check your base of support and be sure you have firm footing. Use a wide but balanced stance to increase support. Keep this stance when walking. Make sure you and the resident are wearing non-skid shoes with the laces tied.
- G Face what you are lifting. Your feet should always face the direction you are moving. Do not twist; twisting at the waist increases the likelihood of injury. Twisting should always be avoided. Turn and face the area you are moving the object to, then set the object down.
- G Keep your back straight. Keeping your head up and shoulders back will keep the back in the proper position. Taking a deep breath will help you regain correct posture.
- G Begin in a squatting position and lift with your legs. Bend at the hips and knees. Use the strength of your leg muscles to stand and lift the object. You will need to push your buttocks out to do this. Before you stand with the object you are lifting, remember that your legs, not your back, will enable you to lift. You should be able to feel your leg muscles as they work. Lift with the large leg muscles to decrease stress on the back.
- G Tighten your stomach muscles when beginning the lift. This will help to take weight off the spine and maintain alignment.
- G Keep the object close to your body. This decreases stress to your back. Lift objects only to your waist. Carrying them any higher can affect your balance.
- G Push when possible, rather than lifting. When you lift an object, you must overcome grav-

ity to balance the load. When you push an object, you only need to overcome the friction between the surface and the object. Use your body weight to move the object, rather than your lifting muscles. Stay close to the object. Use both arms and tighten your stomach muscles.

2. Explain positioning and describe how to safely position residents

Residents who spend a lot of time in bed often need help getting into comfortable positions. They also need to change positions periodically to avoid muscle stiffness and skin breakdown or pressure ulcers. Too much pressure on one area for too long can cause a decrease in circulation, which can lead to the formation of pressure ulcers, a serious condition. Chapter 13 contains information about pressure ulcers and prevention guidelines.

Positioning means helping residents into positions that promote comfort and good health. Bedbound residents should be repositioned at least every two hours. Residents in wheelchairs or chairs should be repositioned at least every hour. Each time there is a change of position, nursing assistants should document the position and the time. Which positions a resident uses will depend on the diagnosis, the condition, and the resident's preference. The care plan will give specific positioning instructions. Nursing assistants must always keep principles of body mechanics and alignment in mind when positioning residents. NAs should also check skin for whiteness or redness, especially around bony areas, each time they reposition residents.

The following are guidelines for positioning residents in the five basic body positions:

Supine: In this position, the resident lies flat on his back. To maintain correct body position, the head and shoulders should be supported with a pillow (Fig. 10-1). Pillows, rolled towels, or washcloths can also be used to support the arms (especially a weak or immobilized arm) or hands. A firm pillow should be placed under the calves so the heels do not touch the bed. Pillows or a footboard (padded board placed against the resident's feet) can keep the feet properly positioned.

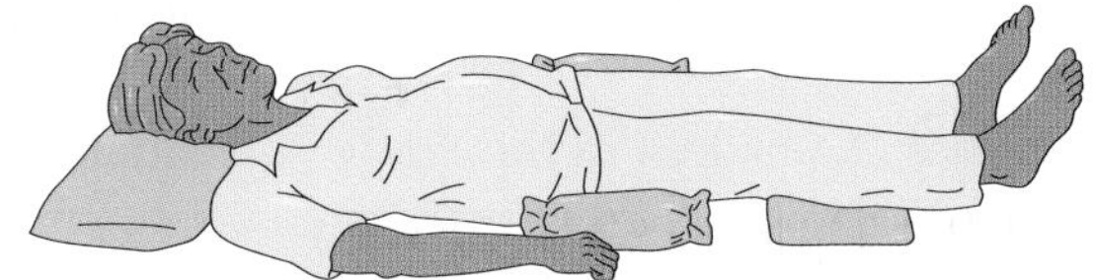

Fig. 10-1. *A person in the supine position is lying flat on his or her back.*

Lateral: A resident in the lateral position is lying on either side (Fig. 10-2). There are many variations on this position. Pillows can support the arm and leg on the upper side, the back, and the head. Ideally, the knee on the upper side of the body should be flexed. The leg is brought in front of the body and supported on a pillow. There should be a pillow under the bottom foot so that the toes are not touching the bed. If the top leg cannot be brought forward, it should be placed slightly behind the bottom leg, not resting directly on it. Pillows should be used between the two legs to relieve pressure and avoid skin breakdown.

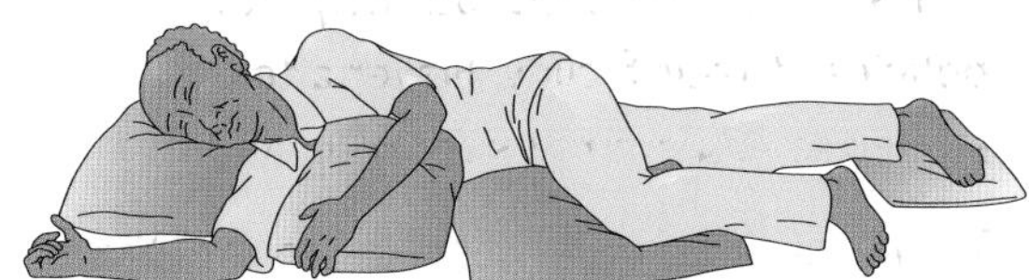

Fig. 10-2. *A person in the lateral position is lying on his or her side.*

Prone: A resident in the prone position is lying on the stomach, or front side of the body (Fig. 10-3). This is not comfortable for many people, especially elderly people. Nursing assistants should not leave residents in a prone position for very long. In this position, the arms are either at the sides or raised above the head. The head is turned to one side. A small pillow may be used under the head and legs. This keeps the feet from touching the bed.

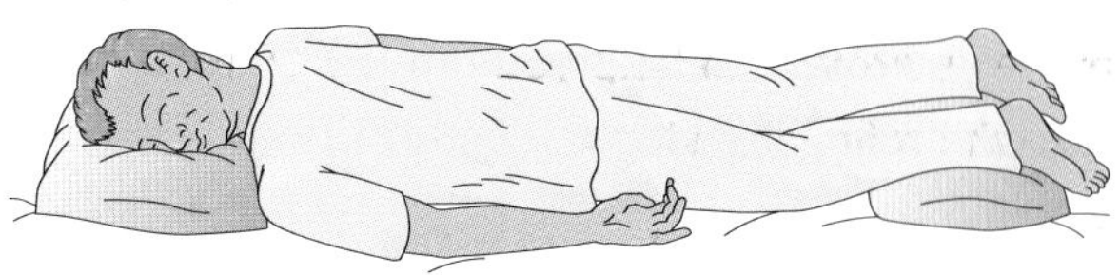

Fig. 10-3. A person lying in the prone position is lying on his or her stomach.

Fowler's: A resident in the Fowler's position is in a semi-sitting position (45 to 60 degrees). The head and shoulders are elevated. The resident's knees may be flexed and elevated using a pillow or rolled blanket as a support (Fig. 10-4). The feet may be supported using a footboard or other support. The spine should be straight. In a high-Fowler's position, the upper body is sitting nearly straight up (60 to 90 degrees). In a semi-Fowler's position, the upper body is not raised as high (30 to 45 degrees).

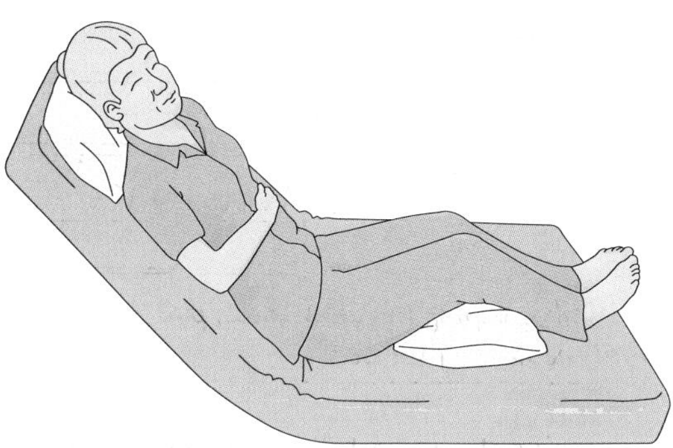

Fig. 10-4. A person in the Fowler's position is partially reclined.

Sims': The Sims' position is a left side-lying position. The lower arm is behind the back, and the upper knee is flexed and raised toward the chest, using a pillow as support. There should be a pillow under the bottom foot so that the toes do not touch the bed (Fig. 10-5).

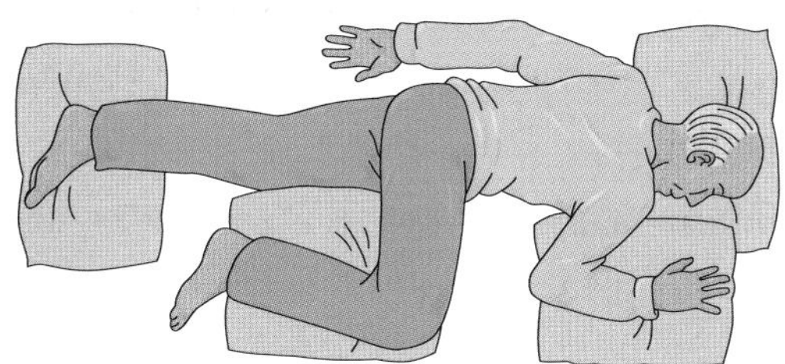

Fig. 10-5. A person in the Sims' position is lying on his or her left side with one leg drawn up.

Helping a resident move up in bed helps prevent skin irritation that can lead to pressure ulcers. A nursing assistant should get help if she thinks it is not safe to move the resident by herself. A draw sheet or turning sheet should be used if the resident cannot help with moving. A **draw sheet** is an extra sheet placed on top of the bottom sheet when the bed is made (Fig. 10-6). It allows a caregiver to reposition the resident without causing shearing. **Shearing** is rubbing or friction that results from the skin moving one way and the bone underneath it remaining fixed or moving in the opposite direction.

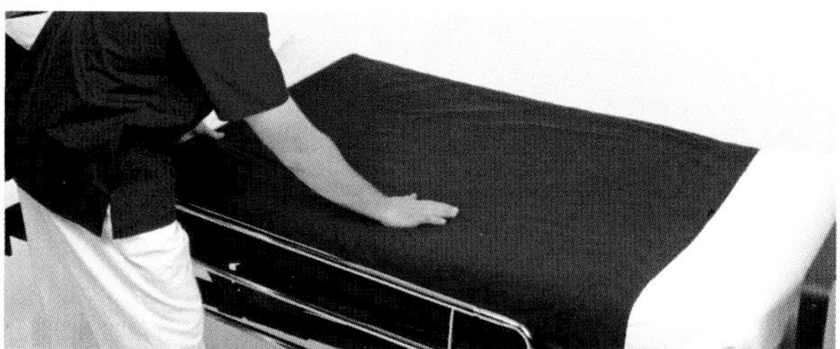

Fig. 10-6. A draw sheet is a special sheet (or a regular bed sheet folded in half) that is used to help move residents in bed without causing shearing.

Moving a resident up in bed

Equipment: draw sheet

When the resident can help you move her up in bed, take the following steps:

1. Identify yourself by name. Identify the resident by name.
2. Wash your hands.
3. Explain procedure to the resident. Speak clearly, slowly, and directly. Maintain face-to-face contact whenever possible.
4. Provide for the resident's privacy with curtain, screen, or door.
5. Adjust bed to a safe level, usually waist high. Lock bed wheels.
6. Lower the head of bed to make it flat. Move the pillow to the head of the bed.
7. If the bed has side rails, raise the rail on the far side of the bed.

8. Stand by bed with your feet shoulder-width apart, facing the resident.
9. Place one arm under resident's shoulder blades. Place the other arm under resident's thighs. Use proper body mechanics.
10. Ask resident to bend her knees, place her feet firmly on the mattress, and push her feet and hands on the count of three.
11. On the count of three, shift your body weight, and help move resident while she pushes with her feet (Fig. 10-7). As always, allow the resident to do all she can for herself.

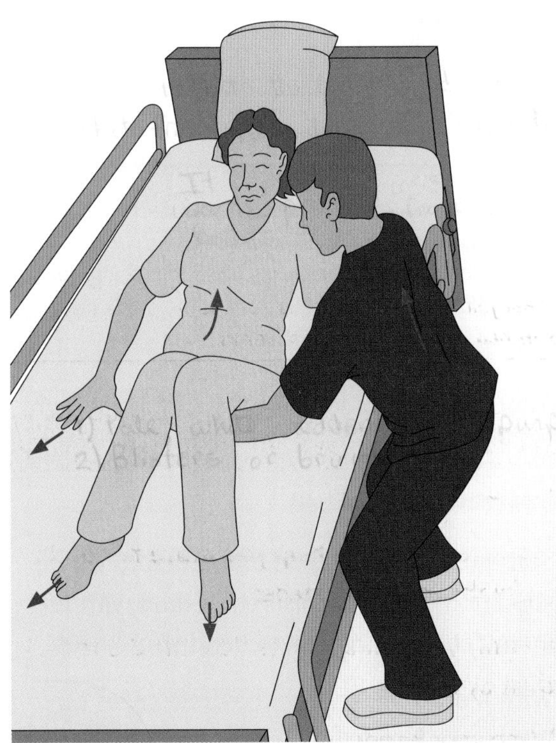

Fig. 10-7. *Keep your back straight and your knees bent.*

12. Make resident comfortable. Put pillow back under resident's head and arrange the blankets for her.
13. Return bed to lowest position. Remove privacy measures.
14. Place call light within resident's reach.
15. Wash your hands.
16. Report any changes in resident to the nurse. Document procedure using facility guidelines.

When the resident cannot assist and there is no one else around to help you move her up in bed, take the following steps:

1. Follow steps 1 through 6 above.
2. Stand behind the head of the bed with your feet shoulder-width apart and one foot slightly in front of the other.
3. Roll and grasp the top edge of the draw sheet.
4. Bend your knees and keep your back straight. Rock your weight from the front foot to the back foot in one smooth motion, while pulling the draw sheet and resident toward the head of the bed (Fig. 10-8).

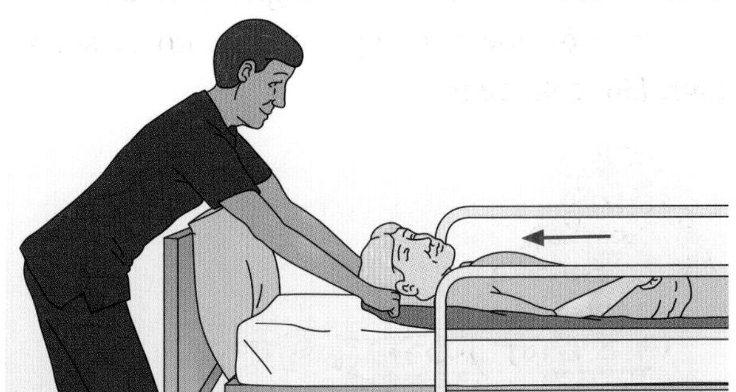

Fig. 10-8. *While grasping the draw sheet, pull the resident toward the head of the bed.*

5. Make resident comfortable. Put pillow back under resident's head and arrange the blankets for her. Unroll the draw sheet and leave it in place for the next repositioning.
6. Return bed to lowest position. Remove privacy measures.
7. Place call light within resident's reach.
8. Wash your hands.
9. Report any changes in resident to the nurse. Document procedure using facility guidelines.

When you have help from another person, you can modify the procedure as follows:

1. Follow steps 1 through 6 above.
2. Stand on the opposite side of the bed from your helper. Each of you should be turned

slightly toward the head of the bed. For each of you, the foot that is closest to the head of the bed should be pointed in that direction. Stand with your feet about shoulder-width apart. Bend your knees. Keep your back straight.

3. Roll the draw sheet up to the resident's side and have your helper do the same on her side of the bed. Grasp the sheet with your palms up, and have your helper do the same.
4. Shift your weight to your back foot (the foot closer to the foot of the bed), and have your helper do the same (Fig. 10-9). On the count of three, you and your helper both shift your weight to the forward foot. Slide the draw sheet and resident toward the head of the bed.

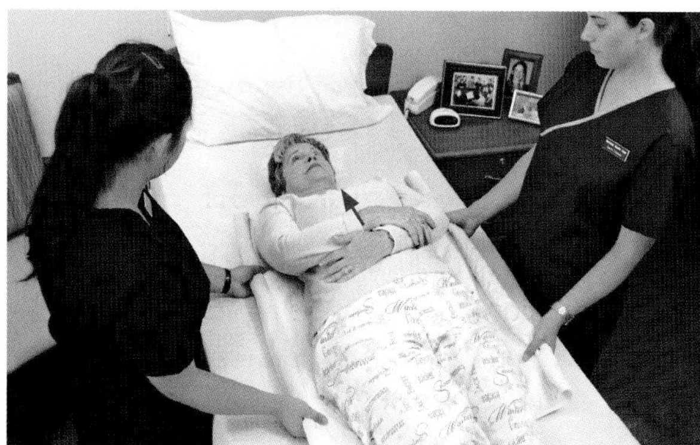

Fig. 10-9. *Both people shift their weight to their back foot and prepare to move.*

5. Make resident comfortable. Put pillow back under resident's head and arrange the blankets for her. Unroll the draw sheet and leave it in place for the next repositioning (Fig. 10-10).

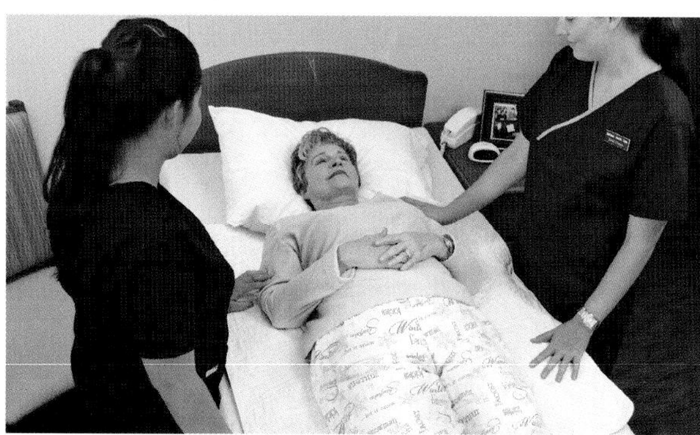

Fig. 10-10. *Unroll the draw sheet and leave it in place.*

6. Return bed to lowest position. Remove privacy measures.
7. Place call light within resident's reach.
8. Wash your hands.
9. Report any changes in resident to the nurse. Document procedure using facility guidelines.

Moving a resident to the side of the bed

Equipment: draw sheet

1. Identify yourself by name. Identify the resident by name.
2. Wash your hands.
3. Explain procedure to the resident. Speak clearly, slowly, and directly. Maintain face-to-face contact whenever possible.
4. Provide for the resident's privacy with curtain, screen, or door.
5. Adjust bed to a safe level, usually waist high. Lock bed wheels.
6. Lower the head of bed.
7. Stand on the same side of the bed to where you are moving the resident. Stand with feet shoulder-width apart and bend your knees.
8. **With a draw sheet**: Roll the draw sheet up to the resident's side and grasp the sheet with your palms up. One hand should be at the resident's shoulders, the other about level with the resident's hips. Apply one knee against the side of the bed and lean back with your body. On the count of three, slowly pull the draw sheet and resident toward you.

   Without a draw sheet: Gently slide your hands under the resident's head and shoulders and move toward you (Fig. 10-11). Gently slide your hands under her midsection and move it toward you. Gently slide your hands under the hips and legs and move them toward you (Fig. 10-12).

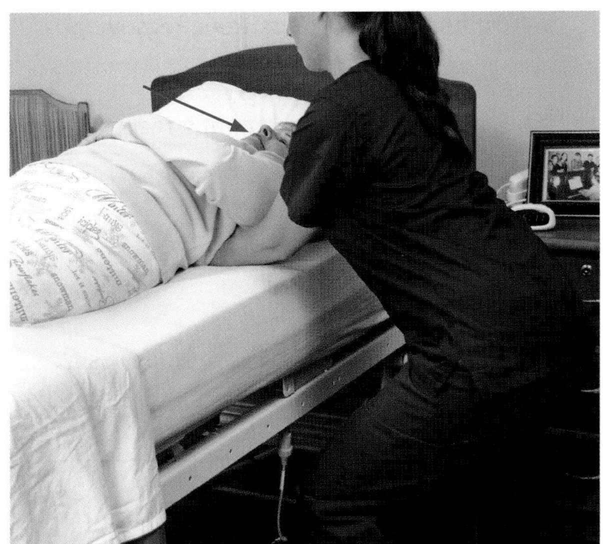

Fig. 10-11. Gently move the resident's head and shoulders toward you.

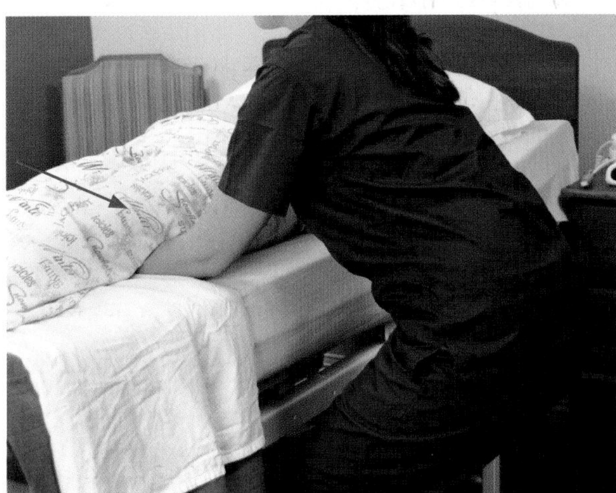

Fig. 10-12. Gently move the hips and legs toward you.

9. Make resident comfortable.
10. Return bed to lowest position. Remove privacy measures.
11. Place call light within resident's reach.
12. Wash your hands.
13. Report any changes in resident to the nurse. Document procedure using facility guidelines.

Residents may be turned on their sides in preparation for sitting up or to change position and take pressure off their backs. This helps prevent skin irritation and pressure ulcers.

Turning a resident

1. Identify yourself by name. Identify the resident by name.
2. Wash your hands.
3. Explain procedure to the resident. Speak clearly, slowly, and directly. Maintain face-to-face contact whenever possible.
4. Provide for the resident's privacy with curtain, screen, or door.
5. Adjust bed to a safe level, usually waist high. Lock bed wheels.
6. Lower the head of bed.
7. Stand on side of bed opposite to where resident will be turned. If the bed has side rails, raise the far side rail. Lower side rail nearest you if it is up.
8. Move resident to side of bed nearest you using previous procedure.
9. **Turning resident away from you:**

a. Cross resident's arm over her chest. Move arm on side resident is being turned to out of the way. Cross the leg nearest you over the far leg (Fig. 10-13).

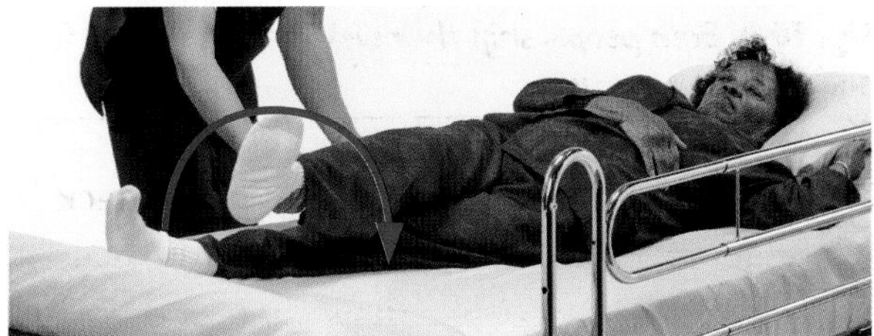

Fig. 10-13. Cross leg nearest you over far leg.

b. Stand with feet shoulder-width apart. Bend your knees.

c. Place one hand on the resident's shoulder. Place the other hand on the resident's nearest hip.

d. Gently push the resident onto side as one unit, toward the other side of bed (toward raised side rail if present). Shift your weight from your back leg to your front leg (Fig. 10-14).

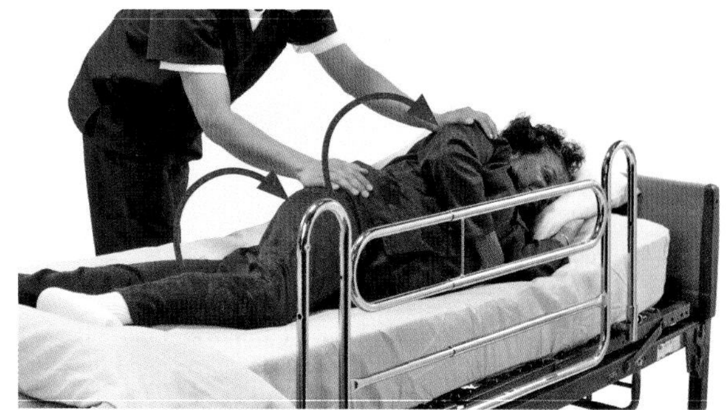

Fig. 10-14. *Gently push resident as you shift your weight from your back leg to your front leg.*

Turning resident toward you:

a. Cross resident's arm over his chest. Move arm on side resident is being turned to out of the way. Cross the leg furthest from you over the near leg.

b. Stand with feet shoulder-width apart. Bend your knees.

c. Place one hand on the resident's far shoulder. Place the other hand on the far hip.

d. Gently roll the resident toward you (Fig. 10-15). Your body will block resident and prevent him from rolling out of bed.

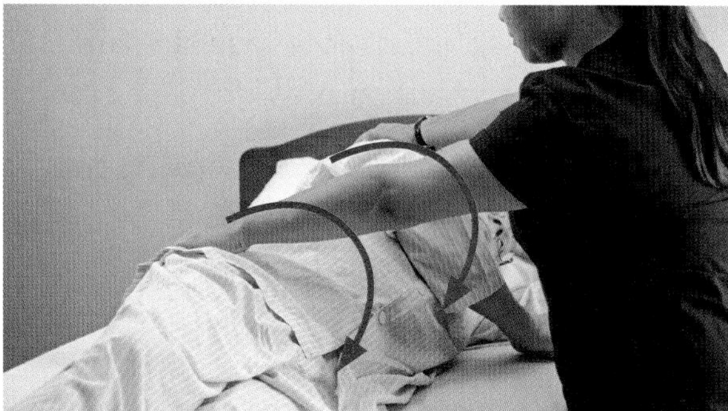

Fig. 10-15. *Gently roll resident toward you.*

10. Position the resident properly, comfortably, and in good alignment. Proper positioning includes the following:
    - Head supported by pillow
    - Shoulder adjusted so resident is not lying on arm
    - Top arm supported by pillow
    - Back supported by supportive device
    - Top knee flexed
    - Supportive device between legs with top knee flexed; knee and ankle supported
11. Return bed to lowest position. Remove privacy measures.
12. Place call light within resident's reach.
13. Wash your hands.
14. Report any changes in resident to the nurse. Document procedure using facility guidelines.

Some residents' spinal columns must be kept in alignment. To turn these residents in bed, nursing assistants will use a procedure called logrolling. **Logrolling** means moving a resident as a unit, without disturbing the alignment of the body. The head, back, and legs must be kept in a straight line. This is necessary in cases of neck or back problems, spinal cord injuries, or back or hip surgeries. It is safer for two people to perform this procedure together. A draw sheet assists with moving.

Logrolling a resident

Equipment: draw sheet, coworker

1. Identify yourself by name. Identify the resident by name.
2. Wash your hands.
3. Explain procedure to the resident. Speak clearly, slowly, and directly. Maintain face-to-face contact whenever possible.
4. Provide for the resident's privacy with curtain, screen, or door.
5. Adjust bed to a safe level, usually waist high. Lock bed wheels.
6. Lower the head of the bed.
7. Both people stand on the same side of the bed. One person stands at the resident's head and shoulders. The other stands near the resident's midsection.

8. Place the resident's arms across his chest. Place a pillow between the knees.
9. Stand with your feet shoulder-width apart. Bend your knees.
10. Grasp the draw sheet on the far side (Fig. 10-16).

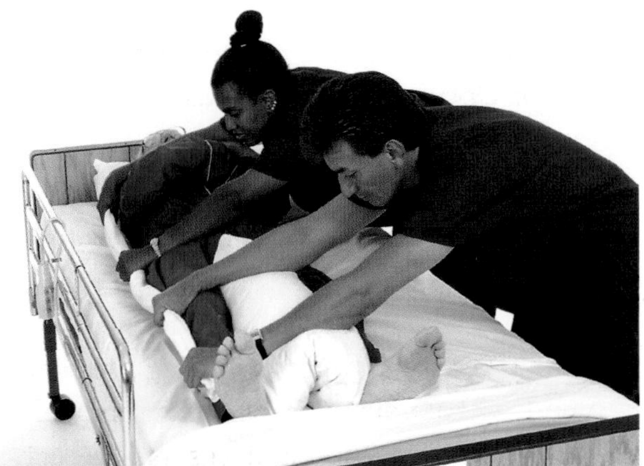

Fig. 10-16. *Both workers should grasp the draw sheet on the far side.*

11. On the count of three, gently roll the resident toward you. Turn the resident as a unit (Fig. 10-17). Your bodies will block the resident and prevent him from rolling out of bed.

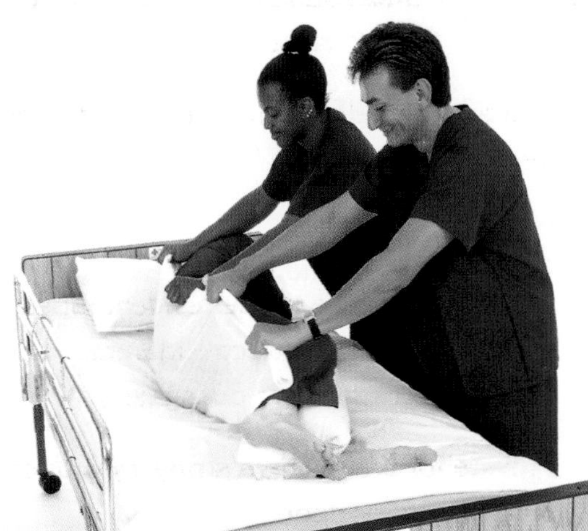

Fig. 10-17. *On the count of three, both workers should roll the resident toward them, turning the person as a unit.*

12. Make resident comfortable. Arrange pillows and covers for comfort.
13. Return bed to lowest position. Remove privacy measures.
14. Place call light within resident's reach.
15. Wash your hands.
16. Report any changes in resident to the nurse. Document procedure using facility guidelines.

Before a resident who has been lying down moves to a standing position, he should dangle. To **dangle** means to sit up on the side of the bed with the legs hanging over the side. This helps residents regain balance before standing up and allows blood pressure to stabilize. For some residents who are unable to walk, sitting up and dangling the legs for a few minutes may be ordered in the care plan.

Assisting a resident to sit up on side of bed: dangling

1. Identify yourself by name. Identify the resident by name.
2. Wash your hands.
3. Explain procedure to the resident. Speak clearly, slowly, and directly. Maintain face-to-face contact whenever possible.
4. Provide for the resident's privacy with curtain, screen, or door.
5. Adjust bed to lowest position. Lock bed wheels.
6. Raise the head of bed to sitting position. Fanfold (fold into pleats) the top covers to the foot of the bed. Ask the resident to turn onto his side, facing you. Assist as needed (see earlier procedure).
7. Tell the resident to reach across his chest with his top arm and place his hand on the edge of the bed near his opposite shoulder. Ask him to push down on that hand to raise his shoulders up while swinging his legs over the side of the bed (Fig. 10-18).

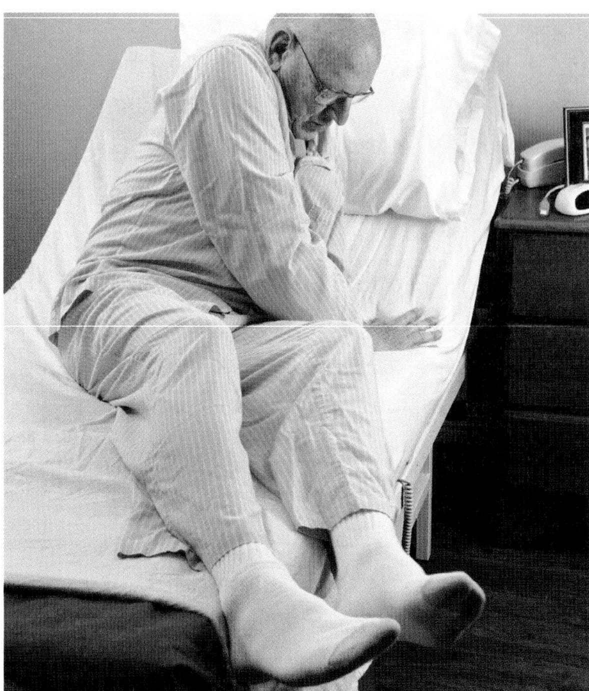

Fig. 10-18. Have the resident push himself up while swinging his legs over the side of the bed.

8. Always allow the resident to do all he can for himself. However, if the resident needs assistance, follow these steps:

a. Stand with your legs shoulder-width apart. Bend your knees.

b. Place one arm under the resident's shoulder blades. Place the other arm under the resident's thighs (Fig. 10-19).

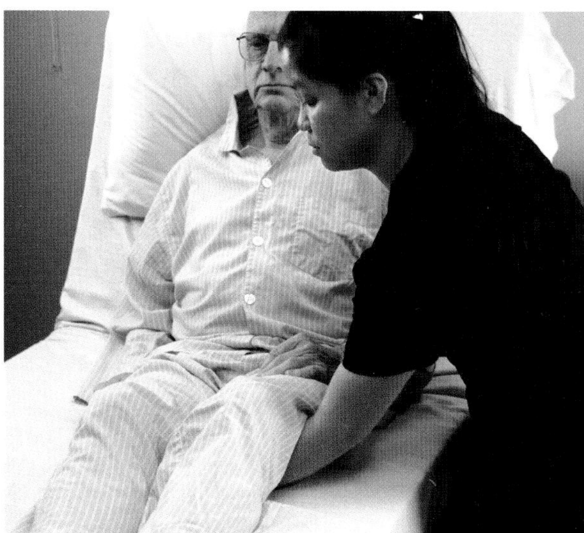

Fig. 10-19. One arm should be under the resident's shoulder blades and the other arm should be under the thighs.

c. On the count of three, slowly turn resident into sitting position with legs dangling over side of bed. The weight of the resident's legs hanging down from the bed helps the resident sit up (Fig. 10-20).

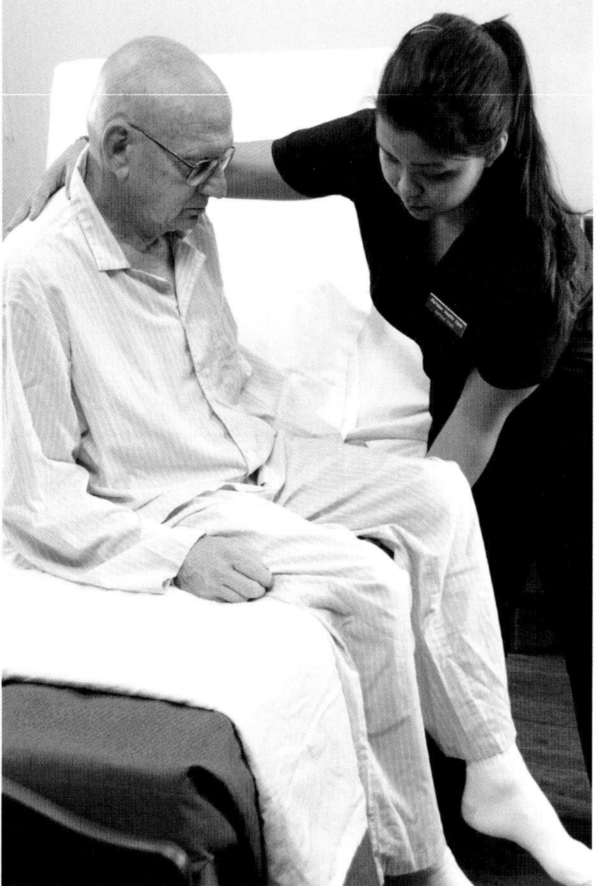

Fig. 10-20. The weight of the resident's legs hanging down from the bed helps the resident sit up.

9. Ask resident to hold onto the edge of mattress with both hands. Assist resident to put on non-skid shoes or slippers.

10. Have resident dangle as long as ordered. The care plan may direct you to allow the resident to dangle for several minutes and then return him to lying down, or it may direct you to allow the resident to dangle in preparation for walking or a transfer. Follow the care plan. Do not leave the resident alone. If the resident is dizzy for more than a minute, have him lie down again and report to the nurse.

11. Take vital signs as ordered (vital signs information is located in Chapter 14).

12. Remove slippers or shoes.
13. Gently assist resident back into bed. Place one arm around resident's shoulders and the other arm under the resident's knees. Slowly swing resident's legs onto bed.
14. Make resident comfortable.
15. Leave bed in lowest position. Remove privacy measures.
16. Place call light within resident's reach.
17. Wash your hands.
18. Report any changes in resident to the nurse. Document procedure using facility guidelines.

Residents' Rights

Positioning and Moving

When positioning and moving residents, nursing assistants should make sure residents are not unnecessarily exposed. They should be kept properly covered, dressed, or draped to protect their privacy and to promote dignity. NAs should pull the privacy curtain around the bed when moving residents in bed.

3. Describe how to safely transfer residents

Transferring a resident means that a nursing assistant is moving him from one place to another. Transfers can move residents from a bed to a chair or wheelchair, from a wheelchair to a shower or toilet, and so on.

Safety is one of the most important factors to consider during transfers. The Occupational Safety and Health Administration (OSHA) set specific ergonomic guidelines to help avoid injuries during transfers. **Ergonomics** is the science of designing equipment, areas, and work tasks to make them safer and to suit the worker's abilities. OSHA states that manual lifting and transferring of residents should be reduced and eliminated when possible. Manual lifting, transferring, and repositioning of residents may increase risks of injury.

To reduce the risk of injury, many facilities have adopted *no-lift, zero-lift,* or *lift-free* policies. These policies set strict guidelines for lifting and transferring of residents. Lift-free polices vary; facilities decide how they want to address the goal of reducing lifting and transferring of residents. Some do not allow any lifting at all and require that equipment always be used when lifting and moving residents.

The more restrictions placed on lifting, the less chance there is of injury. The amount and type of equipment available also factor into reducing workplace injuries. This learning objective teaches procedures for manual lifting and transferring of residents. It is important for nursing assistants to carefully follow facility policies on lifting and to use equipment properly. If NAs are unsure how to use equipment, they should ask for help and always get help when they need it.

A **transfer belt** is a safety device used to transfer residents who are weak, unsteady, or uncoordinated. It is called a **gait belt** when it is used to help residents walk. The belt is made of canvas or other heavy material. It has a buckle and sometimes has handles. It fits around the resident's waist outside the clothing. The transfer belt is a safety device that gives NAs something firm to hold on to when assisting with transfers. Transfer belts cannot be used if a resident has fragile bones or recent fractures.

Residents' Rights

Communicate!

Any time an NA helps a resident transfer, she should talk to the resident about what she would like to do. The NA can promote residents' independence by letting them do what they can. Both NA and resident must work together, especially during transfers.

Applying a transfer belt

Equipment: transfer belt, non-skid footwear

1. Identify yourself by name. Identify the resident by name.
2. Wash your hands.
3. Explain procedure to the resident. Speak clearly, slowly, and directly. Maintain face-to-face contact whenever possible.
4. Provide for the resident's privacy with curtain, screen, or door.
5. Adjust bed to lowest position. Lock bed wheels.
6. Assist the resident to a sitting position with feet flat on the floor.
7. Put non-skid footwear on resident and make sure laces are tied.
8. Place the transfer belt over the resident's clothing and around the waist. Do not put it over bare skin.
9. Tighten the buckle until it is snug. Leave enough room to insert flat fingers/hand comfortably under the belt.
10. Check to make sure that skin or skin folds (for example, breasts) are not caught under the belt.
11. Position the buckle slightly off-center in the front or back for comfort.

A **slide board**, or transfer board, may be used to help transfer residents who are unable to bear weight on their legs. Slide boards can be used for almost any transfer that involves moving from one sitting position to another (for example, from bed to chair) (Fig. 10-21). Slide boards should not be used against bare skin. The nursing assistant must make sure that the resident's fingers are not under the board before beginning the transfer.

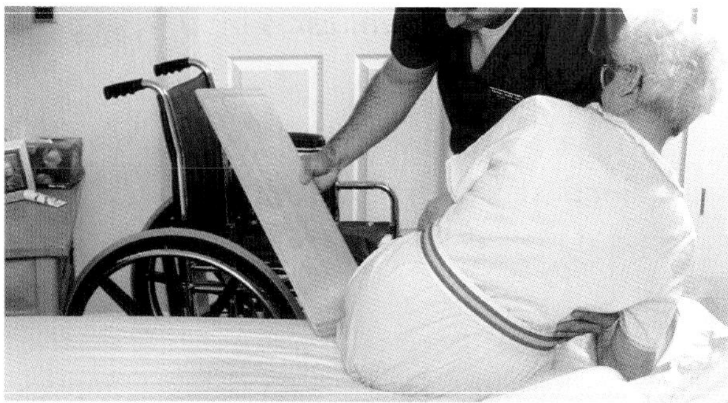

Fig. 10-21. *A slide board can help with bed-to-chair transfers.*

Guidelines: Wheelchairs

- G Learn how each wheelchair works. Residents may use manual (require human power to move) or electric wheelchairs. Know how to apply and release the brake and how to operate the armrests and footrests. Always lock a wheelchair before helping a resident into or out of it (Fig. 10-22). After a transfer, unlock the wheelchair.

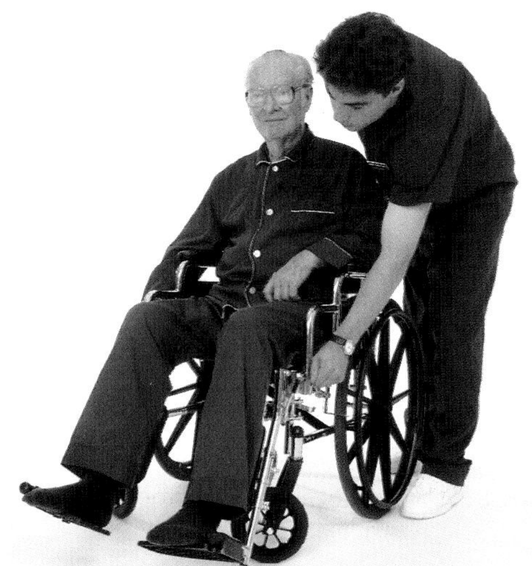

Fig. 10-22. *You must always lock the wheelchair before a resident gets into or out of it.*

- G To unfold a standard wheelchair, tilt the chair slightly to raise the wheels on the opposite side. Press down on one or both seat rails until the chair opens and the seat is flat. To fold a standard wheelchair, lift up under the center edge of the seat.
- G To remove an armrest, release the arm lock by the armrest, and lift the arm from the cen-

ter. To replace the armrest, simply reverse the procedure.

- G To move a footrest out of the way, press or pull the release lever. Swing the footrest out toward the side of the wheelchair. To remove the footrest, lift it off when it is toward the side of the wheelchair (Fig. 10-23). To replace a footrest, simply put it back in the side position, then swing it back to the front position. It should lock into place.

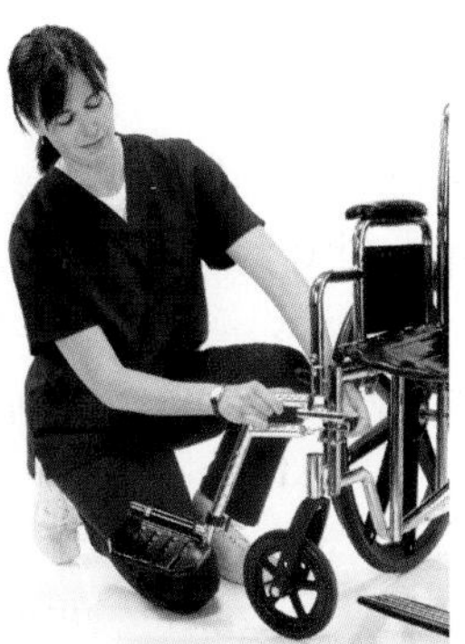
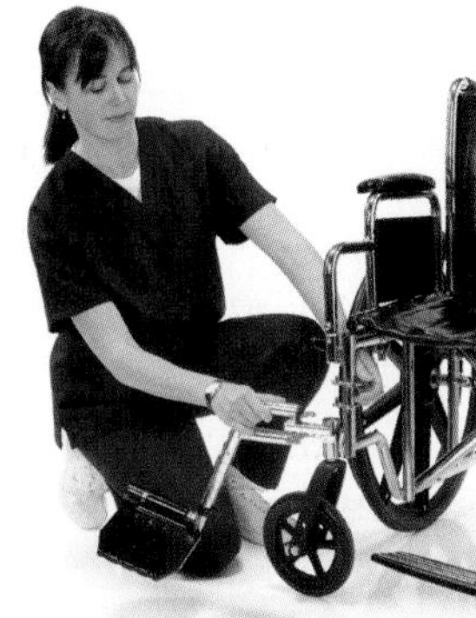

Fig. 10-23. *To remove a footrest, swing the footrest toward the side of the wheelchair and lift it off.*

- G To lift or lower a footrest, support the leg or foot. Squeeze the lever and pull up or push down.
- G To transfer to or from a wheelchair, the resident must use the side of the body that can bear weight to support and lift the side that cannot bear weight. Residents who can bear no weight with their legs may use leg braces or an overhead trapeze to support themselves.
- G Before any transfer, make sure the resident is wearing non-skid footwear that is securely fastened. This promotes residents' safety and reduces the risk of falls.
- G During wheelchair transfers, make sure the resident is safe and comfortable. Ask the resident how you can help. Some may only want you to bring the chair to the bedside. Others may want you to be more involved. Always be sure the chair is as close as possible to the resident and is locked in place. Use a transfer belt if you are going to assist with the transfer. Be sure the transfer is done slowly, allowing time for the resident to rest. Check the resident's alignment in the chair when the transfer is complete.
- G Keep the resident's body in proper alignment while in a wheelchair or chair. Special cushions and pillows can be used for support. The hips should be well-positioned back in the chair. If the resident needs to be moved back in the wheelchair, lock wheelchair wheels. Go to the back of the chair. Gently reach forward and down under the resident's arms. Ask the resident to place his feet on the ground and push up. Gently pull the resident up in the chair while the resident pushes.
- G When a resident is in a wheelchair or any chair, he or she should be repositioned at least every hour. The reasons for doing this are as follows:
    - It promotes comfort.
    - It reduces pressure.
    - It increases circulation.
    - It exercises the joints.
    - It improves muscle tone.

Falls

If a resident starts to fall during a transfer or while walking, the NA should do the following:

- Widen her stance
- Bring the resident's body close to her to break the fall
- Bend her knees and support the resident as she lowers the resident to the floor
- If necessary, the NA can drop to the floor with the resident to avoid injury to herself or the resident

The NA should not try to reverse or stop a fall because she or the resident can suffer worse injuries if she tries to stop, rather than break, a fall. If a resident has fallen, the NA should call for help. She should not try to get the resident up after the fall.

Some residents have one-sided weakness due to paralysis or stroke. When transferring these residents, NAs should move the stronger side first. The weaker (also called *involved* or *affected*) side follows.

Transferring a resident from bed to wheelchair

Equipment: wheelchair, transfer belt, non-skid footwear, and lap robe or folded blanket

1. Identify yourself by name. Identify the resident by name.
2. Wash your hands.
3. Explain procedure to the resident. Speak clearly, slowly, and directly. Maintain face-to-face contact whenever possible.
4. Provide for the resident's privacy with curtain, screen, or door. Check the area to be certain it is uncluttered and safe.
5. Remove both wheelchair footrests close to the bed.
6. Place wheelchair near the head of the bed with arm of the wheelchair almost touching the bed. Wheelchair should be facing the foot of the bed. The wheelchair should be placed on resident's stronger, or unaffected, side.
7. Lock wheelchair wheels.
8. Raise the head of the bed. Adjust bed to lowest position. Lock bed wheels.
9. Assist resident to sitting position with feet flat on the floor. Let resident sit for a few minutes to adjust to the change in position.
10. Put non-skid footwear on resident and fasten securely.
11. Stand in front of resident with your feet about shoulder-width apart. Bend your knees.
12. Place the transfer belt around resident's waist over clothing (not on bare skin). Grasp belt securely on both sides.
13. Provide instructions to allow resident to help with transfer. Instructions may include: "When you start to stand, push with your hands against the bed." "Once standing, if you're able, you can take small steps in the direction of the chair." "Once standing, reach for the chair with your stronger hand."
14. With your legs, brace (support) resident's lower legs to prevent slipping (Fig. 10-24). This can be done by placing one or both of your knees in front of the resident's knees.

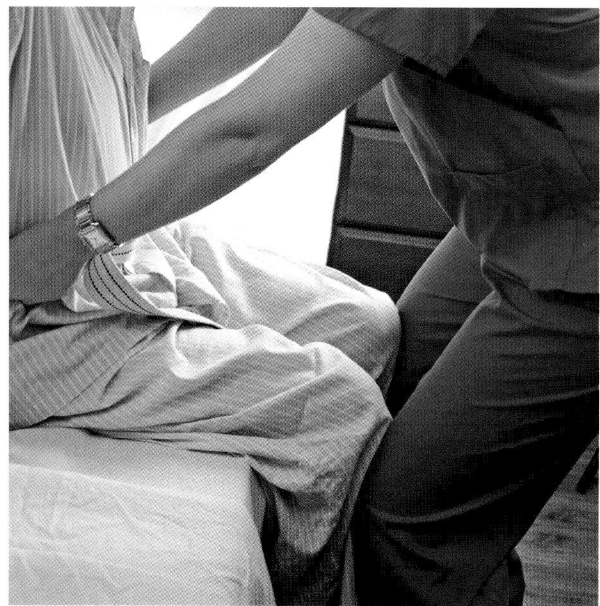

Fig. 10-24. *Brace the resident's lower legs to prevent slipping.*

15. Count to three to alert resident. On three, with hands still grasping the transfer belt on both sides and moving upward, slowly help resident to stand.
16. Tell the resident to take small steps in the direction of the wheelchair while turning his back toward it. Or, if more assistance is needed, help the resident pivot (turn) to stand in front of wheelchair with back of resident's legs against wheelchair (Fig. 10-25).
17. Ask the resident to put hands on wheelchair armrests if able. When the chair is touching the back of the resident's legs, help the resident lower himself into the chair.

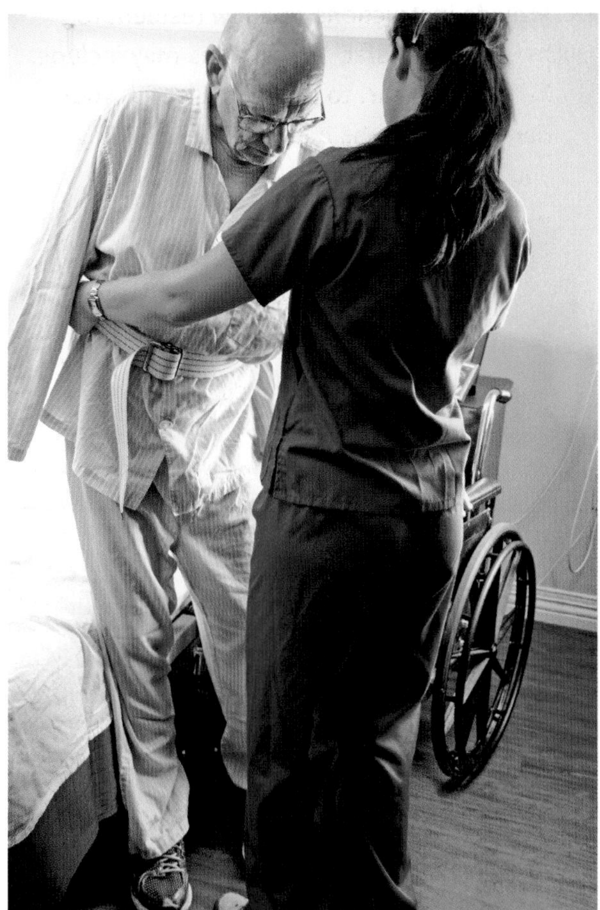

Fig. 10-25. Help him pivot to the front of the wheelchair. Pivoting is safer than twisting.

18. Reposition resident so that his hips touch the back of the wheelchair seat. Remove transfer belt if used.
19. Attach footrests and place the resident's feet on the footrests. Check that the resident is in proper alignment. Make resident comfortable. Place a lap robe or folded blanket over the resident's lap as appropriate.
20. Remove privacy measures.
21. Place call light within resident's reach.
22. Wash your hands.
23. Report any changes in resident to the nurse. Document procedure using facility guidelines.

When transferring back to bed from a wheelchair, the height of the bed should be equal to or slightly lower than the chair. Help the resident pivot to the bed. When the resident feels the bed with the back of his legs, help him sit down slowly.

Stretchers

A stretcher, also called a gurney, is a medical device used to move injured or ill persons from one place to another. Stretchers may be used for serious injuries and illnesses and/or when a person cannot or should not walk but needs to be transported somewhere. Stretchers transfer residents within facilities or to other facilities.

Guidelines: Safe Use of a Stretcher

- **G** Lock the stretcher wheels before transferring a resident onto or off of a stretcher.
- **G** Secure resident with the safety belts while in the stretcher.
- **G** Raise the safety rails.
- **G** Cover the resident with a sheet. Hands, feet, fingers, etc., should remain inside the sheet during transport.
- **G** Keep the wheels locked at all times except when moving the stretcher.
- **G** Get help if you cannot move the stretcher alone.
- **G** Move slowly and carefully.
- **G** Push the stretcher from the head end.
- **G** Go through doorways by opening the door, entering first, and pulling the stretcher through.
- **G** Avoid hitting walls or doorways.
- **G** Be cautious going down sloping areas.
- **G** Stay with the resident at all times.

A draw sheet is used to transfer a resident to a stretcher. The procedure below shows how to transfer a resident to a stretcher from a bed using four staff members. At least three people are necessary to safely transfer a resident to a stretcher.

Transferring a resident from bed to stretcher

Equipment: stretcher, blanket, draw sheet

1. Identify yourself by name. Identify the resident by name.
2. Wash your hands.
3. Explain procedure to the resident. Speak clearly, slowly, and directly. Maintain face-to-face contact whenever possible.
4. Provide for the resident's privacy with curtain, screen, or door.
5. Lower the head of bed so that it is flat. Lock bed wheels.
6. Fold linens to the foot of the bed. Cover resident with a blanket.
7. Move the resident to the side of the bed. Have your coworkers help you do this. Refer to the procedure *Moving a resident to the side of the bed* earlier in this chapter.
8. Place stretcher solidly against the bed, and lock stretcher wheels. Bed height should be equal to or slightly above the height of the stretcher. Move stretcher safety belts out of the way.
9. Two workers should be on one side of the bed opposite the stretcher. Two more workers should be on the other side of the stretcher.
10. Each worker should roll up the sides of the draw sheet and prepare to move the resident (Fig. 10-26). Protect the resident's arms and legs during the transfer.
11. On the count of three, the workers lift and move the resident to the stretcher. All should move at once. Make sure the resident is centered on the stretcher (Fig. 10-27).

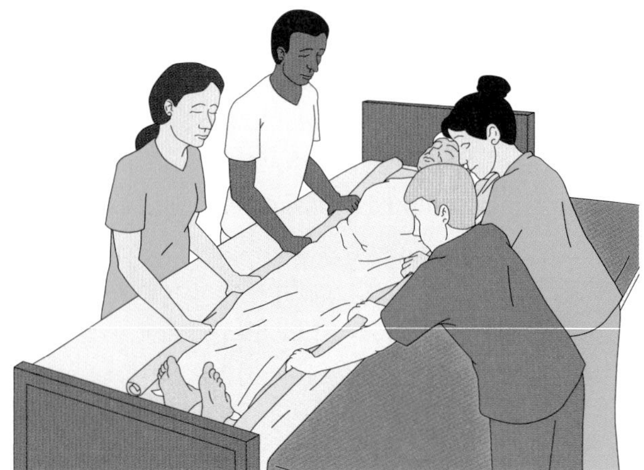

Fig. 10-26. *With two workers on each side, roll up the sides of the draw sheet and prepare to move the resident.*

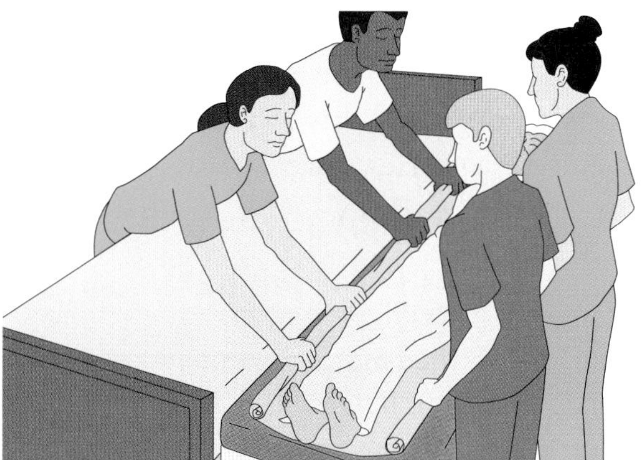

Fig. 10-27. *On the count of three, all workers should lift and move at once.*

12. Place a pillow under the resident's head. Make sure resident is still covered with the blanket.
13. Place the safety straps across the resident. Raise side rails on stretcher.
14. Unlock stretcher's wheels. Move resident to proper place, staying with him until another staff member takes over.
15. Wash your hands.
16. Report any changes in resident to the nurse. Document procedure using facility guidelines.

To return the resident to bed, the bed height should be equal to or slightly below the stretcher.

Mechanical Lifts

Facilities often have mechanical, or hydraulic, lifts available to transfer residents. This equipment helps prevent injury to staff and residents. Nursing assistants may assist residents with many types of transfers using a mechanical or hydraulic lift. Using these lifts requires special training. Nursing assistants should not use equipment they have not been trained to use, as doing this could cause injury.

There are many different types of mechanical lifts (Fig. 10-28). Using these devices helps prevent common workplace injuries and may be mandatory at facilities that have no-lift policies. Nursing assistants should always ask for help if there is anything that they do not understand about the provided lift equipment.

Guidelines: Mechanical or Hydraulic Lifts

- **G** Be careful when moving a resident using a mechanical lift. If possible, have another person assist you when transferring with these lifts. It is safer for at least two people to do these types of transfers.
- **G** Keep the chair or wheelchair to which the resident is to be moved close to the bed so that the resident is only moved a short distance in the lift.
- **G** Check that the valves are working on the lift before using it.
- **G** Check the sling and straps for any fraying or tears. Do not use the lift if there are tears or holes.
- **G** Open the legs of the stand to the widest position before helping the resident into the lift.
- **G** Once the resident is in the sling and the straps are connected, pump up the lift only to the point where the resident's body clears the bed or chair.

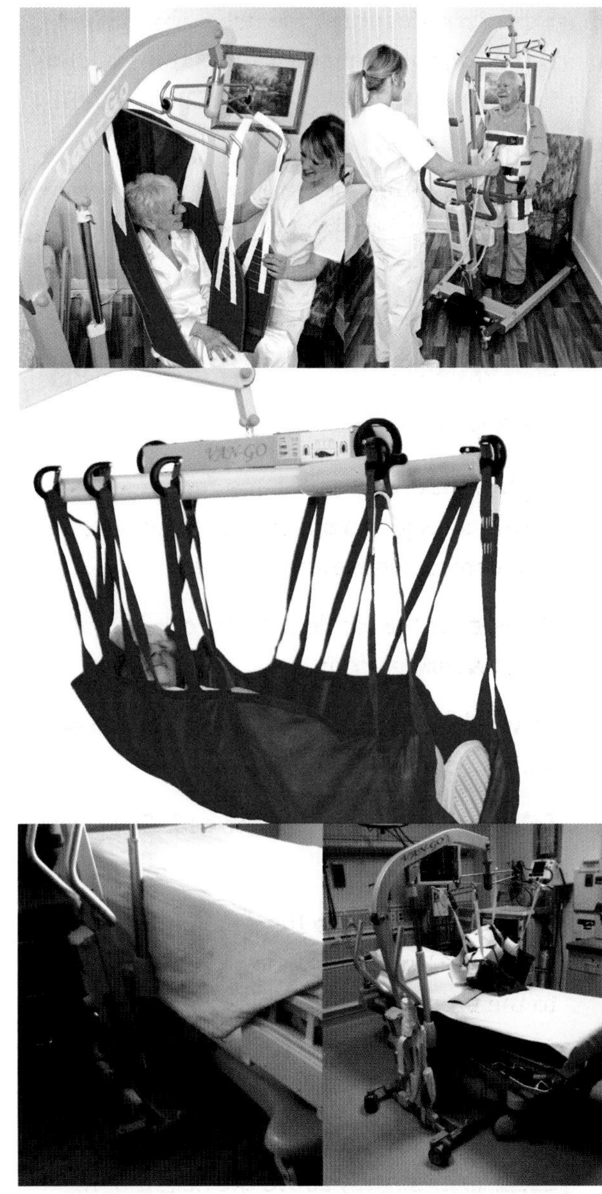

Fig. 10-28. *There are different types of lifts that transfer completely dependent residents and residents who can bear some weight.* (PHOTOS COURTESY OF VANCARE INC., 800-694-4525)

Transferring a resident using a mechanical lift

Equipment: wheelchair or chair, coworker (if available), mechanical or hydraulic lift

The following is a basic procedure for transferring using a mechanical lift. Ask someone to help you before starting.

1. Identify yourself by name. Identify the resident by name.
2. Wash your hands.

3. Explain procedure to the resident. Speak clearly, slowly, and directly. Maintain face-to-face contact whenever possible.
4. Provide for the resident's privacy with curtain, screen, or door.
5. Lock bed wheels.
6. Position wheelchair next to bed. Lock brakes.
7. Help the resident turn to one side of the bed. Position the sling under the resident, with the edge next to the resident's back, fanfolding if necessary. Adjust the bottom of the sling so that it is even with the resident's knees. Help the resident roll back to the middle of the bed, and then spread out the fanfolded edge of the sling.
8. Roll the mechanical lift to bedside. Make sure the base is opened to its widest point. Push the base of the lift under the bed.
9. Position the overhead bar directly over the resident (Fig. 10-29).

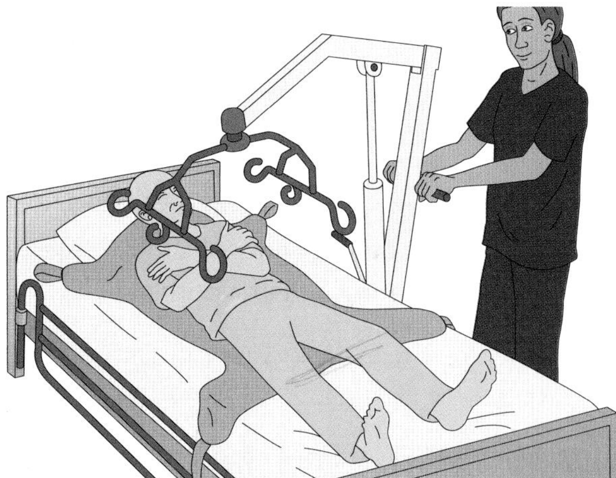

Fig. 10-29. *Position the overhead bar directly over the resident.*

10. With the resident lying on his back, attach one set of straps to each side of the sling. Attach one set of straps to the overhead bar. Have a coworker support the resident at the head, shoulders, and knees while being lifted. The resident's arms should be folded across his chest (Fig. 10-30). If the device has S hooks, they should face away from resident. Make sure all straps are connected properly and are smooth and straight.

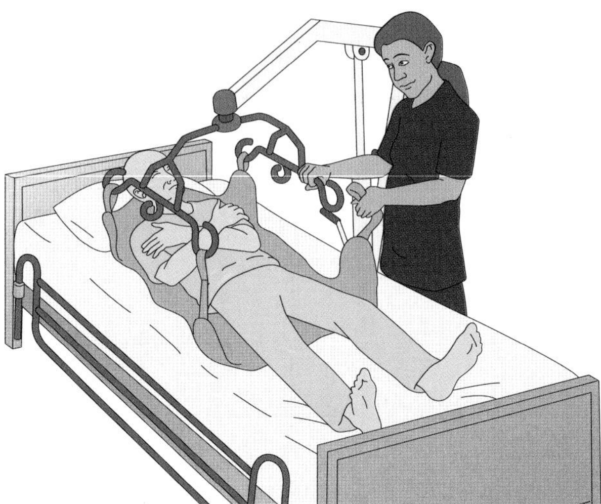

Fig. 10-30. *With the resident's arms folded across his chest, attach the straps to the sling.*

11. Following manufacturer's instructions, raise the resident two inches above the bed. Pause a moment for the resident to gain balance.
12. The coworker can help support and guide the resident's body while you roll the lift so that the resident is positioned over the chair or wheelchair (10-31).

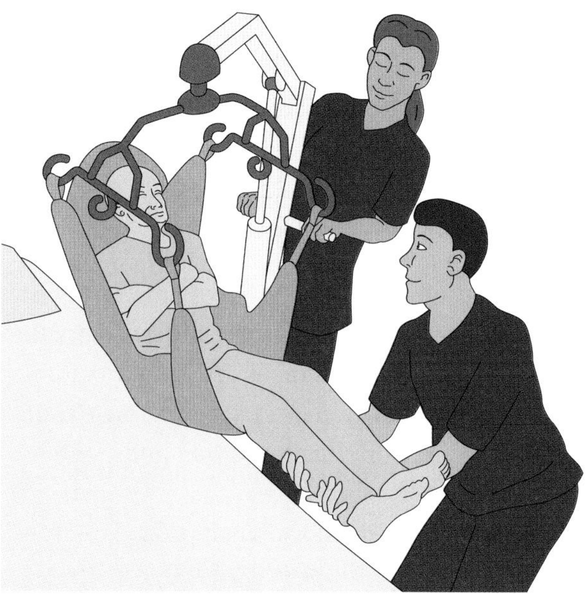

Fig. 10-31. *Having another person help to support and guide the resident promotes safety during the transfer and lessens the chance of injury.*

13. Slowly lower the resident into the chair or wheelchair. Push down gently on the resident's knees to help the resident into a sitting, rather than reclining, position.
14. Undo the straps from the overhead bar to the sling. Remove sling or leave in place for transfer back to bed.
15. Be sure the resident is seated comfortably and correctly in the chair or wheelchair. Remove privacy measures.
16. Place call light within resident's reach.
17. Wash your hands.
18. Report any changes in resident to the nurse. Document procedure using facility guidelines.

A stand-up, or standing lift, is used when a person can bear some weight on his legs, but has poor leg strength and/or balance (Fig. 10-28, image at top right). The resident must be able to stand and have some arm strength in order to use this lift. There are different types of stand-up lifts, including manual and battery-powered.

The stand-up lift consists of both user and operator support bars (the user support bars may consist of two vertical bars or one crossbar), padded swivel swing-out seats (and/or straps, vest, or belt for some models), knee pads, a platform base with foot plate, and four small wheels with locking brakes.

When using a stand-up lift, the nursing assistant must be sure that the brakes are locked before beginning a transfer. The NA should have the resident begin in a sitting position and place his feet firmly on the foot plate of the platform, with knees pressing against the knee pads. The resident should grasp the support bar(s) and gently pull himself to a standing position, using his own strength. Then the NA can lower both sides of the padded swing-out seat into position. The NA should adjust straps, vest, or belt if these are used. The resident should slowly lower himself onto the seat while holding the support bars and pressing knees against knee pads. The NA should unlock the wheel brakes and use the operator bars to transfer the resident to the location desired and then perform these steps in reverse order to release the resident from the lift.

Toilet Transfers

The bladder empties more efficiently when a person is able to use the toilet. In order to use the toilet, residents must be able to bear some weight on their legs.

Nursing assistants should offer trips to the bathroom often and respond to call lights quickly. Chapter 16 has more information on bedpan and urinal use.

Transferring a resident onto and off of a toilet

Equipment: 2 pairs of gloves, toilet paper or disposable wipes, transfer belt, wheelchair

1. Identify yourself by name. Identify the resident by name.
2. Wash your hands.
3. Explain procedure to the resident. Speak clearly, slowly, and directly. Maintain face-to-face contact whenever possible. Make sure resident is wearing non-skid shoes.
4. Provide for the resident's privacy with curtain, screen, or door.
5. Position wheelchair at a right angle to the toilet to face the hand bar/wall rail. Place wheelchair on the resident's stronger side.
6. Remove wheelchair footrests. Lock wheels.
7. Put on gloves.
8. Apply a transfer belt around the resident's waist over clothing (not on bare skin). Grasp belt securely on both sides.
9. Ask resident to push against the armrests of the wheelchair and stand, reaching for and

grasping the hand bar. Move wheelchair out of the way (Fig. 10-32).

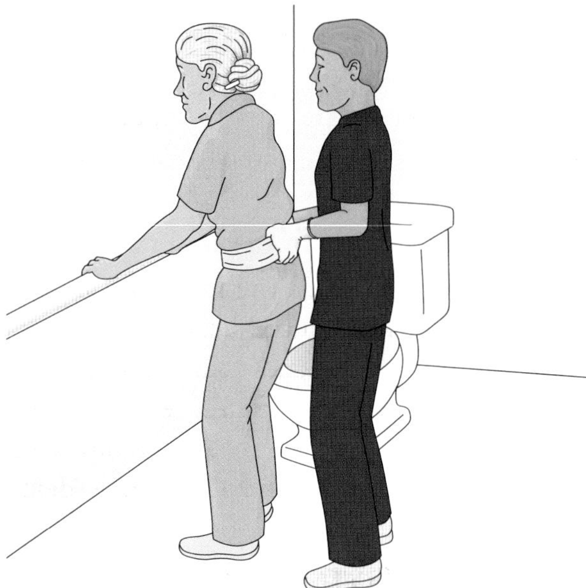

Fig. 10-32. The resident should be standing while grasping the hand bar for support.

10. Ask resident to pivot her foot and back up until she can feel the front of the toilet with the back of her legs (Fig. 10-33).

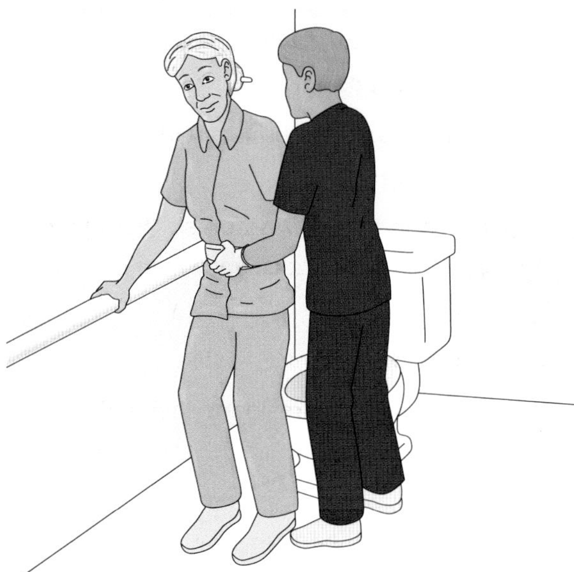

Fig. 10-33. Have the resident pivot and feel the toilet with the back of her legs. Assist as needed.

11. Help resident to pull down pants and underwear. You may need to keep one hand on the transfer belt while helping to remove clothing.
12. Help resident slowly sit down on the toilet. Ask resident to pull the emergency cord if she needs help. Remove and discard gloves. Wash your hands. Leave bathroom and close door.
13. When called, return and don clean gloves. Assist with perineal care as necessary (Chapter 13). Ask her to stand and reach for the hand bar.
14. Use toilet paper or disposable wipes to clean the resident. Make sure she is clean and dry before pulling up clothing. Remove and discard gloves.
15. Help resident to the sink to wash hands.
16. Wash your hands.
17. Help resident back into wheelchair. Be sure the resident is seated comfortably and correctly in the wheelchair. Remove transfer belt. Replace footrests.
18. Help resident to leave the bathroom. Make sure resident is comfortable. Remove privacy measures.
19. Place call light within resident's reach.
20. Wash your hands again.
21. Report any changes in resident to the nurse. Document procedure using facility guidelines.

Vehicle Transfers

When a resident is leaving a facility, he or she may need help getting into a vehicle. The front seat is wider and is usually easier to get into.

Transferring a resident into a vehicle

Equipment: wheelchair

1. Identify yourself by name. Identify the resident by name.
2. Wash your hands.

3. Explain procedure to the resident. Speak clearly, slowly, and directly. Maintain face-to-face contact whenever possible.
4. Place wheelchair close to the vehicle at a 45-degree angle. Open the door on the resident's stronger side.
5. Lock wheelchair.
6. Ask the resident to push against the armrests of the wheelchair and stand.
7. Ask the resident to stand, grasp the vehicle, and pivot his foot so the side of the seat touches the back of the legs.
8. The resident should then sit in the seat and lift one leg, and then the other, into the vehicle (Fig. 10-34).

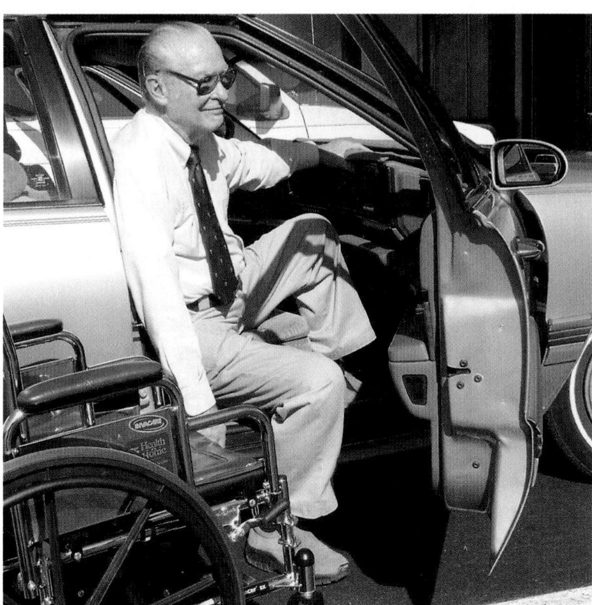

Fig. 10-34. *After resident sits in the vehicle seat, he should put his legs in one at a time.*

9. Carefully position the resident comfortably in the vehicle. Help fasten seat belt.
10. Safely shut the door.
11. Return the wheelchair to the appropriate place for cleaning.
12. Wash your hands.
13. Document procedure using facility guidelines.

4. Discuss how to safely ambulate residents

Ambulation is walking. A resident who is **ambulatory** is one who can get out of bed and walk. Many older residents are ambulatory, but need assistance to walk safely. Several tools, including gait belts, canes, walkers, and crutches, assist with ambulation.

Nursing assistants should check the care plan before helping a resident ambulate. The NA should discuss the resident's abilities, limitations, and disabilities with the nurse. Any time an NA helps a resident, she should communicate what she would like to do and allow the resident to do what he can.

Assisting a resident to ambulate

Equipment: gait belt, non-skid shoes

1. Identify yourself by name. Identify the resident by name.
2. Wash your hands.
3. Explain procedure to resident. Speak clearly, slowly, and directly. Maintain face-to-face contact whenever possible.
4. Provide for resident's privacy with curtain, screen, or door.
5. Adjust bed to lowest position so that the feet are flat on the floor. Lock bed wheels.
6. Before ambulating, put non-skid footwear on the resident and securely fasten.
7. Stand in front of the resident, facing the resident, with your feet about shoulder-width apart.
8. Place gait belt around resident's waist over clothing (not on bare skin). Grasp belt securely on both sides.
9. Always allow resident to do whatever he is able to do for himself. If the resident is unable to stand without help, brace (support) the resident's lower extremities. Bend your knees. If the resident has a weak knee, brace it against your knee (Fig. 10-35).

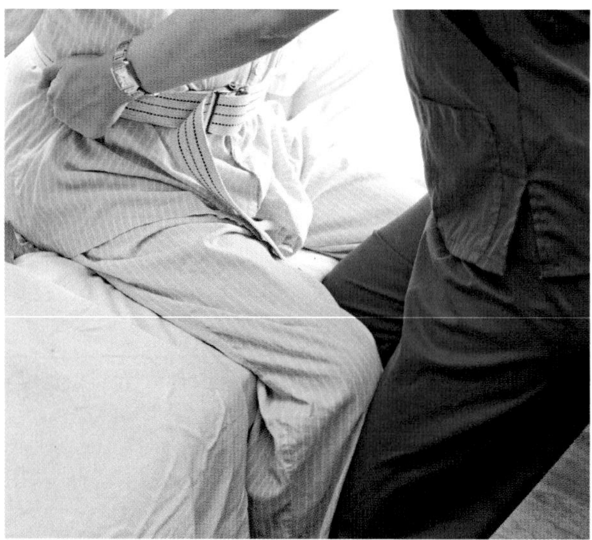

Fig. 10-35. If resident has a weak knee, brace it against your knee.

10. Hold the resident close to your center of gravity. Provide instructions to allow resident to help with standing. Tell the resident to lean forward, push down on the bed with his hands, and stand on the count of three. On three, with hands still grasping the gait belt on both sides and moving upward, slowly help resident to stand.
11. Walk slightly behind and to one side of resident for the full ordered distance, while holding onto the gait belt (10-36). If the resident has a weaker side, stand on the weaker side. Use the hand that is not holding the belt to offer support on the weak side. Ask resident to look forward, not down at the floor, during ambulation.

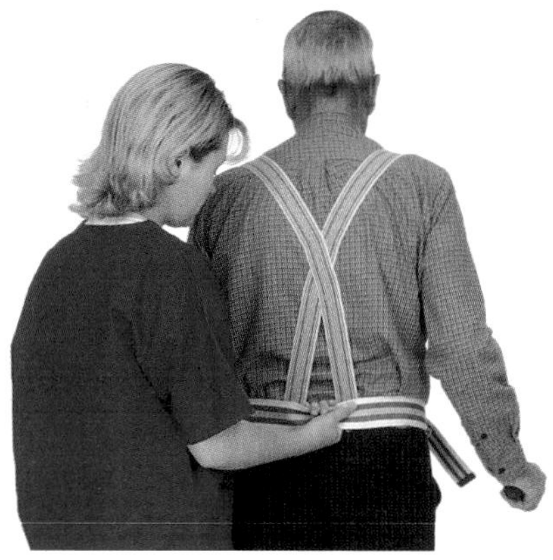

Fig. 10-36. Walk behind and to one side while holding onto the gait belt when assisting with ambulation.

12. Observe the resident's strength while you walk together. Provide a chair if the resident becomes dizzy or tired.
13. After ambulation, remove gait belt. Help resident to the bed or chair and check that the resident is in proper alignment. Make resident comfortable.
14. Leave bed in lowest position. Remove privacy measures.
15. Place call light within resident's reach.
16. Wash your hands.
17. Report any changes in resident to nurse. Document procedure using facility guidelines.

When helping a visually-impaired resident walk, the nursing assistant should let the person walk beside and slightly behind her, as he rests a hand on the NA's elbow. The NA should walk at a normal pace. She should let the resident know when they are about to turn a corner, or when a step is approaching, and whether they will be stepping up or down.

Residents who have difficulty walking may use adaptive or assistive devices, such as canes, walkers, or crutches to help themselves. The purpose of a cane is to help with balance. Residents using canes should be able to bear weight on both legs. If one leg is weaker, the cane should be held in the hand on the strong side.

Types of canes include the C cane, the functional grip cane, and the quad cane. The **C cane** is a straight cane with a curved handle at the top. It has a rubber-tipped bottom to prevent slipping. A C cane is used to improve balance. A **functional grip cane** is similar to the C cane, except that it has a straight grip handle, rather than a curved handle. The grip handle helps improve grip control and provides a little more support than the C cane. A **quad cane**, with four rubber-tipped feet and a rectangular base, is designed to bear more weight than the other canes (Fig. 10-37).

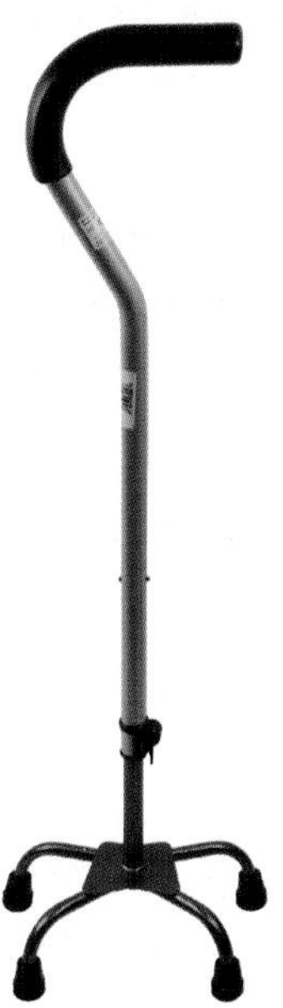

Fig. 10-37. A quad cane has four rubber-tipped feet and can bear more weight than other canes.

A **walker** is used when the resident can bear some weight on the legs. The walker provides stability for residents who are unsteady or lack balance. The metal frame of the walker may have rubber-tipped feet and/or wheels (Fig. 10-38). Other types of walkers are designed with a seat in the back to allow a person to rest during ambulation (Fig. 10-39).

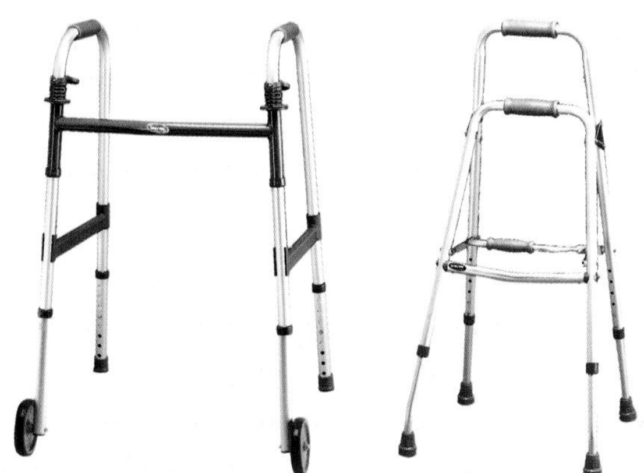

Fig. 10-38. The photo on the left shows a standard walker and the photo on the right shows a Hemi Walker, which is a walker that is designed for people who have difficulty using an arm or a hand. (© INVACARE CORPORATION. USED WITH PERMISSION. WWW.INVACARE.COM)

Crutches are used for residents who can bear no weight or limited weight on one leg. Some people use one crutch, and some use two.

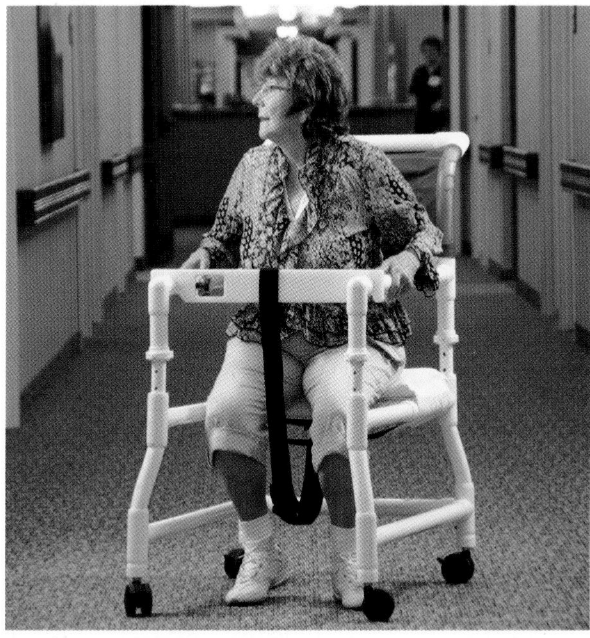

Fig. 10-39. There are different types of walkers. This type has a posterior seat to allow the person to sit and rest when necessary.

Whichever device is being used, the nursing assistant's role is to ensure safety. The NA should stay near the person, on the weak side. She should make sure the equipment is in proper condition. It must be sturdy, and it must have rubber tips or wheels on the bottom.

Guidelines: Cane or Walker Use

- **G** Be sure the walker or cane is in good condition. It must have rubber tips on bottom. The tips should not be cracked. Walkers may have wheels. If so, roll the walker to make sure the wheels are moving properly.
- **G** Be sure the resident is wearing securely fastened, non-skid shoes before ambulating.
- **G** When using a cane, the resident should place it on his stronger side.
- **G** When using a walker, have the resident place both hands on the walker. The walker should not be over-extended; it should be placed no more than six inches in front of the resident.
- **G** Stay near the resident on the weaker side.

G Do not hang purses or clothing on the walker.

G If the height of the cane or walker does not appear to be correct (too short, too tall, etc.), inform the nurse.

Assisting with ambulation for a resident using a cane, walker, or crutches

Equipment: gait belt, non-skid shoes, cane, walker, or crutches

1. Identify yourself by name. Identify resident by name.
2. Wash your hands.
3. Explain procedure to resident. Speak clearly, slowly, and directly. Maintain face-to-face contact whenever possible.
4. Provide for resident's privacy with curtain, screen, or door.
5. Adjust bed to lowest position so that the feet are flat on the floor. Lock bed wheels.
6. Before ambulating, put non-skid footwear on the resident and securely fasten.
7. Stand in front of the resident, facing the resident, with your feet about shoulder-width apart.
8. Place gait belt around resident's waist over clothing (not on bare skin). Grasp belt securely on both sides.
9. If the resident is unable to stand without help, brace (support) the resident's lower extremities. Bend your knees. If the resident has a weak knee, brace it against your knee. Help the resident to stand as described in the previous procedure.
10. Help as needed with ambulation.

a. ***Cane***: Resident places cane about six inches, or a comfortable distance, in front of his stronger leg. He brings weaker leg even with cane. He then brings stronger leg forward slightly ahead of cane (Fig. 10-40). Repeat.

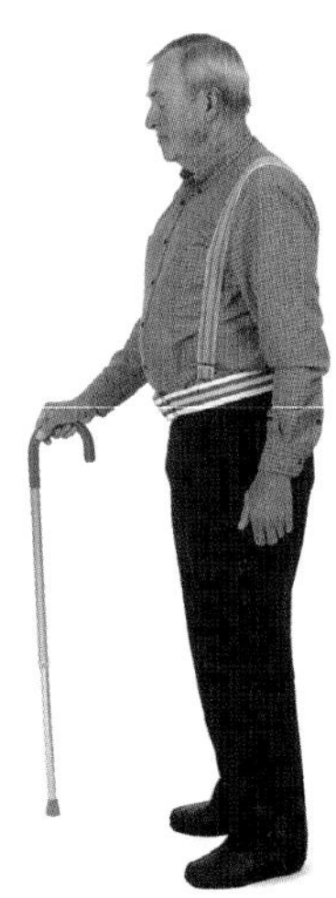

Fig. 10-40. *The cane moves in front of the stronger leg first.*

b. **Walker**: Resident picks up or rolls the walker and places it about six inches, or a comfortable distance, in front of him. All four feet or wheels of the walker should be on the ground before resident steps forward to the walker. The walker should not be moved again until the resident has moved both feet forward and is in a steady position (Fig. 10-41). The resident should never put his feet ahead of the walker.

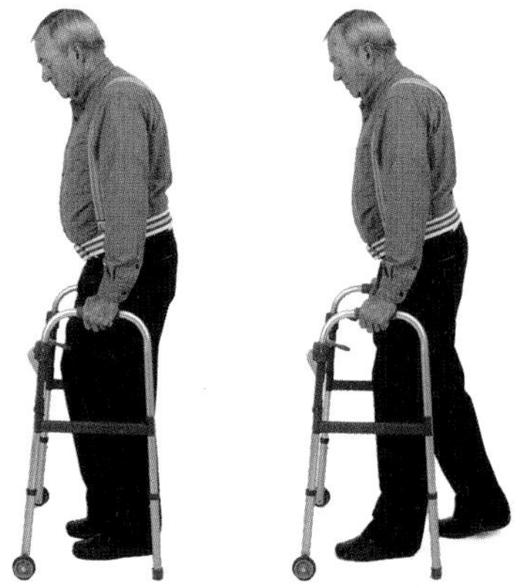

Fig. 10-41. *The walker can be moved after the resident is steady and both feet are forward.*

c. **Crutches**: Resident should be fitted for crutches and taught to use them correctly by a physical therapist or nurse. The resident may use the crutches several different ways, depending on what his weakness is. No matter how they are used, weight should be on the hands and arms. Weight should not be on the underarm area (Fig. 10-42).

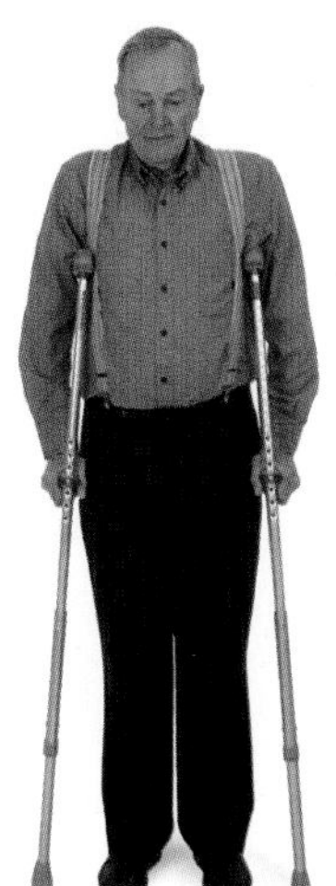

Fig. 10-42. *When using crutches, weight should be on the hands and arms, not on the underarms.*

11. Walk slightly behind and to one side of resident. Stay on the weaker side if resident has one. Hold the gait belt.
12. Watch for obstacles in the resident's path. Ask resident to look forward, not down at the floor, during ambulation.
13. Encourage the resident to rest if he is tired. When a person is tired, it increases the chance of a fall. Let the resident set the pace. Discuss how far he plans to go based on the care plan.
14. After ambulation, remove gait belt. Help resident to the bed or chair and check that the resident is in proper alignment. Make resident comfortable.
15. Leave bed in lowest position. Remove privacy measures.
16. Place call light within resident's reach.
17. Wash your hands.
18. Report any changes in resident to nurse. Document procedure using facility guidelines.

Chapter Review

1. List nine guidelines for using proper body mechanics.
2. What is positioning?
3. How often should bedbound residents be repositioned?
4. In which position is a resident lying on his side?
5. In which position is a resident lying on his stomach?
6. In which position is a resident lying flat on his back?
7. In which position is a resident lying on his left side with the lower arm behind the back and the upper knee bent and raised toward the chest?
8. In which position is a resident in a semi-sitting position (45 to 60 degrees) with the head and shoulders elevated?
9. What is a draw sheet?
10. What is shearing?
11. When is logrolling necessary?
12. How does dangling benefit a resident?
13. Describe how a transfer belt is applied.
14. Before helping a resident into or out of a wheelchair, what should a nursing assistant do?
15. If a resident has a weaker side, which side moves first in a transfer—the weaker or stronger side?
16. When may stretchers be used for residents?
17. List five guidelines for using a mechanical lift.
18. What is one benefit of using the toilet rather than a bedpan or urinal?
19. Define *ambulation*.
20. What is the purpose of canes?

21. How many feet does a quad cane have? 4
22. Which type of adaptive device for walking can be used when a resident can bear no weight on one leg—cane, walker, or crutches?
23. Which side should a nursing assistant stand near when a resident is using adaptive equipment—the weaker or stronger side?

1) Assess the weight load. What are the policies of your facility. Do not attempt to do it by yourself if you don't know if you can.
2) Plan the move & communicate the move to the resident. Check area for safety
3) Check your own body positioning & use a wide base support. Wear non-skid shoes (both)
4) Face what you are lifting. Face direction with your feet you are moving.
5) Keep back straight, shoulders back, head up.
6) Begin in squatting position & lift with legs. Bend at the hips & knees
7) Tighten stomach muscles when you begin to lift.
8) Keep the object close to your body. Lift objects only as high as your waist
9) If you can push, rather than lift, it's easier

Guidelines for using mechanical lifts:
1) Try to have another person help you.
2) Have wheelchair to which resident is to be moved close to bed so move is short as possible.
3) Check that the valves are working before using it.
4) Check for any fraying or tears on sling & straps
5) Open the legs on the lift to the widest position before lifting anyone.
6) Pump up the lift only to the position where the residents body clears the bed.

11 Admitting, Transferring, and Discharging

1. Describe how residents may feel when entering a facility

Chapter 8 described some of the many feelings residents may be having as they make the transition into a care facility. Losses, such as the loss of a familiar environment, or the loss of independence, can cause a person to feel scared, angry, sad, lonely, worried, helpless, or depressed. A new resident may yell at caregivers or may cry often. He may refuse to join in activities and want to be left alone. A new resident may want to talk to staff members as much as possible until he becomes more comfortable. These are just a few of the ways that new residents may show their emotions.

Moving always requires an adjustment, but as a person ages, it can be even harder (Fig. 11-1). This is especially true if illness, disability, and mobility problems are present. Perhaps at age 50 a new resident began to live alone as his children left the house. Then he lived alone, happily, for 20 years before having a stroke. He was no longer able to live alone safely, and his children did not live nearby to help him with his daily care. Living with his children was not an option, so he had to move into a care facility. He might feel worried and scared because he has never known any other home than the one he lived in for so many years. He might feel angry or depressed about moving into a new place filled with people he does not know. When independence is restricted and health declines, people are faced with difficult decisions about care. Moving into a facility is not an easy choice to make, and it is important for staff to remember this and empathize with residents.

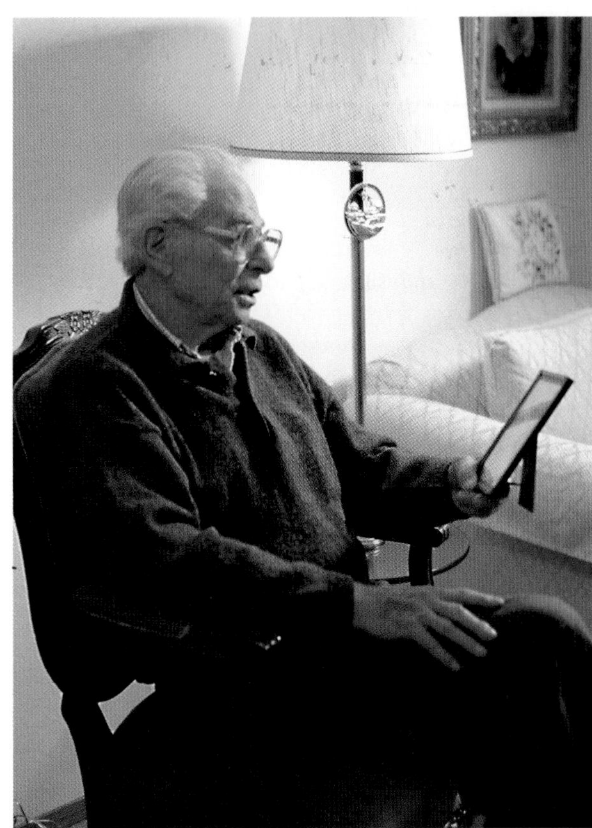

Fig. 11-1. *A new resident must leave familiar places and things. He may have just lost someone very close to him. He may be experiencing other losses as well. Nursing assistants should be supportive and welcoming.*

Nursing assistants play an important role in helping residents make a successful transition to long-term care facilities. By giving emotional support such as listening, as well as being kind, compassionate, and helpful, NAs can help residents feel better about their new homes. Guidelines for assisting new residents are found in the next learning objective.

Residents' Rights

New LGBT Residents

Entering a long-term care facility can be especially difficult for lesbian, gay, bisexual, or transgender (LGBT) residents. In addition to the challenges all residents face when giving up the independence of living in their own homes, LGBT residents may fear that they will not be accepted by staff or other residents. They may worry that their partners will not receive the same welcome the spouse or partner of a heterosexual resident would receive.

In addition, paperwork, such as the admission form, is usually written with the assumption that a resident is heterosexual. If a resident is not legally married but has a partner of the same gender, there may be no way for him to indicate this on the form. Staff can help residents by asking questions like, "Who is important in your life?"

More and more communities are recognizing the challenges of aging specific to LGBT elders. Organizations offering training to LTC workers may exist in the community. A nursing assistant might suggest to a supervisor that staff at her facility receive such training. It is essential that NAs not judge residents, even if they believe that homosexuality is wrong. Every resident deserves professional, caring service from facility staff. The facility is the resident's home, and NAs should make every effort to make all residents feel comfortable and welcome.

2. Explain the nursing assistant's role in the admission process

When a new resident is admitted, he is first directed to the admitting office. Paperwork is signed. The admission staff member makes copies of insurance information, Medicare cards, and other types of information. Both parties sign an agreement or contract, outlining the services provided and the costs for them. Emergency contact information and names of doctors are obtained. The Patient Self-Determination Act (PSDA), an amendment to OBRA, requires staff to explain information on advance directives and to find out if the resident has advance directives in place or wants to create them. A copy of the resident's rights is given to the new resident and his family. The rights are explained in a language the resident can understand. A facility handbook of policies and procedures may be given. The procedure on how to file grievances and complaints is explained. Pictures of new residents may be taken. These photos are used to identify residents and may be posted outside of their rooms.

Admission is often the first time a nursing assistant meets a new resident. This is a time of first impressions. The NA should try to make sure the resident has a good impression of her and her facility. Because change is difficult, staff must communicate with new residents. NAs can explain what to expect during the process and answer any questions that are within their scope of practice. If residents have questions that an NA cannot answer, she should find the nurse. It is a good idea for the NA to ask a new resident questions to find out her personal preferences and routines.

Each facility will have a procedure for admitting residents to their new home. However, these guidelines will help make the experience pleasant and successful:

Guidelines: Admission

G Prepare the room before the resident arrives. This helps him to feel expected and welcome. Make sure the bed is made and the room is tidy. Restock supplies that are low. Make sure there is an admission kit available if used. Admission kits often contain personal care items, such as a bath basin, an emesis basin, a water pitcher and drinking glass, toothpaste, soap, a comb, lotion, and tissues (Fig. 11-2). Admission kits may also contain a urine specimen cup, label, and transport bag.

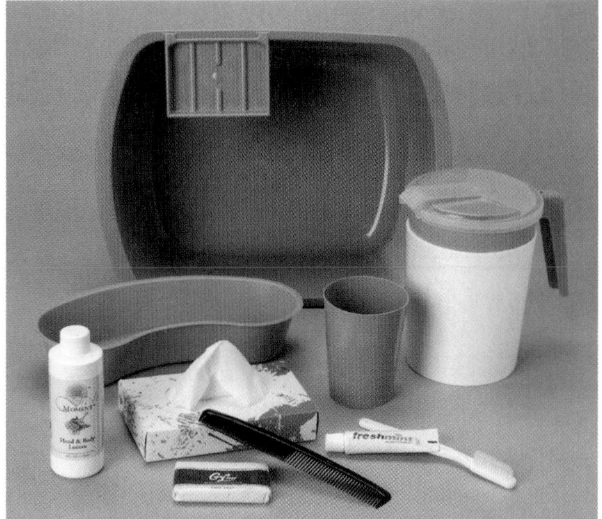

Fig. 11-2. An admission kit is usually placed in a resident's room before he or she is admitted. It may contain personal care items that the resident will need. (REPRINTED WITH PERMISSION OF BRIGGS CORPORATION, 800-247-2343, WWW.BRIGGSCORP.COM)

G When a new resident arrives at the facility, note the time and her condition. Is she using a wheelchair, is she on a stretcher, or is she walking? Who is with her? Observe the new resident for level of consciousness and if she seems confused. She will probably be feeling anxiety; look for signs of nervousness. Note any tubes she has, such as IVs or catheters.

G Introduce yourself and state your position. Smile and be friendly. Always call the person by her formal name until she tells you what she wants to be called.

G Never rush the process or the new resident. She should not feel like she is an inconvenience. Make sure that the new resident feels welcome and wanted.

G Explain day-to-day life in the facility. Offer to take the resident on a tour (Fig. 11-3). Show the resident the dining room, the activity room, the salon, the chapel, and any other important areas. During the tour, introduce the resident to other residents and staff members you see. Introduce the roommate if there is one.

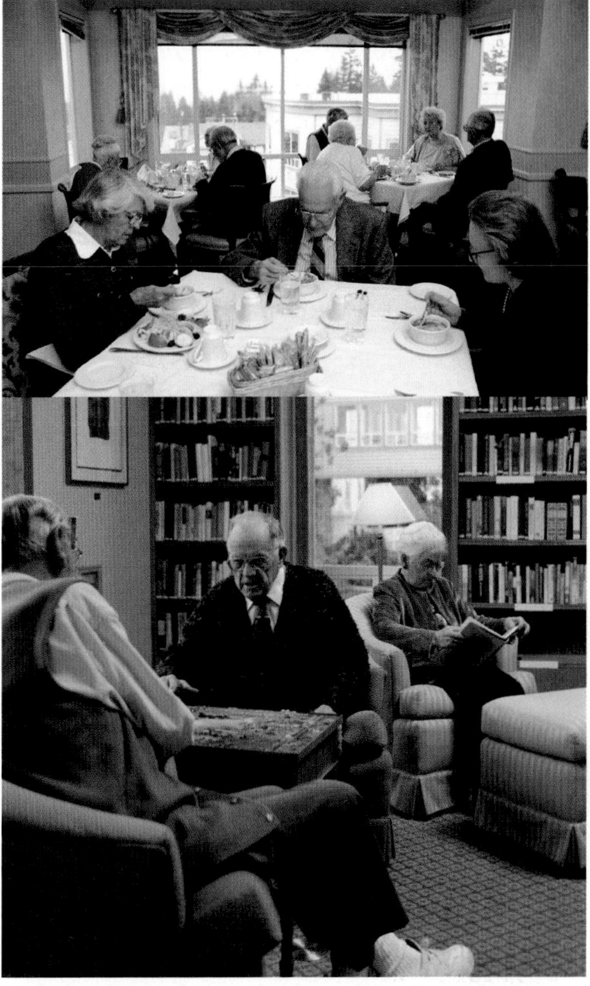

Fig. 11-3. Show the resident where the dining room is and review posted dining schedules. During the tour, be sure to introduce new residents to all other residents you see.

G Handle personal items with care and respect. A resident has a legal right to have her personal items treated carefully. These are the items she has chosen to bring with her. Some items may be stored in bags marked specifically for personal belongings. Ask the new resident if she brought any valuables with her. If so, offer to have them safely stored according to your facility's policy. If she refuses, follow the procedure to write an inventory and get the necessary signatures.

G When setting up the room, place personal items where the resident wants them (Fig. 11-4).

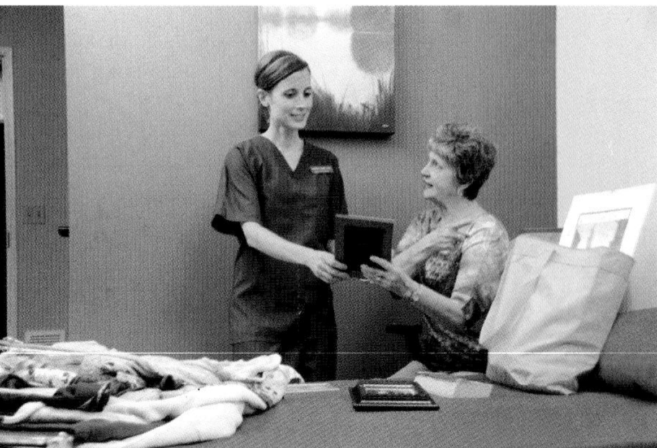

Fig. 11-4. *Handle personal items carefully, and set up the room as she prefers.*

G Admission is a stressful time. Be sure to observe the resident as she could have a problem or issue that is missed with the emphasis on transporting, paperwork, etc. It is important to observe the new resident's condition in order to recognize any changes that may take place later. Report to the nurse if you notice any of the following:

- Disconnected tubing
- Resident seems confused, combative, and/or unaware of surroundings
- Resident is having difficulty breathing or any other signs of distress
- Resident has missed a meal during admission process

G Follow facility policy on any other tasks that are required during the admission process.

G New residents may have good days followed by not-so-good days. Let residents adapt to their new homes at their own pace. Everyone is different. Getting used to a new home may take weeks or months.

Residents' Rights

Admission

OBRA requires that on admission, residents must be told of their legal rights. They must be provided with a written copy of these rights. This includes rights about their funds and the right to file a complaint with the state survey agency.

Admitting a resident

Equipment: may include admission paperwork (checklist and inventory form), gloves, and vital signs equipment

1. Identify yourself by name. Identify the resident by name.
2. Wash your hands.
3. Explain procedure to resident. Speak clearly, slowly, and directly. Maintain face-to-face contact whenever possible.
4. Provide for the resident's privacy with curtain, screen, or door (Fig. 11-5). If the family is present, ask them to step outside until the admission process is over. Show them where they can wait, and let them know approximately how long the process will take.

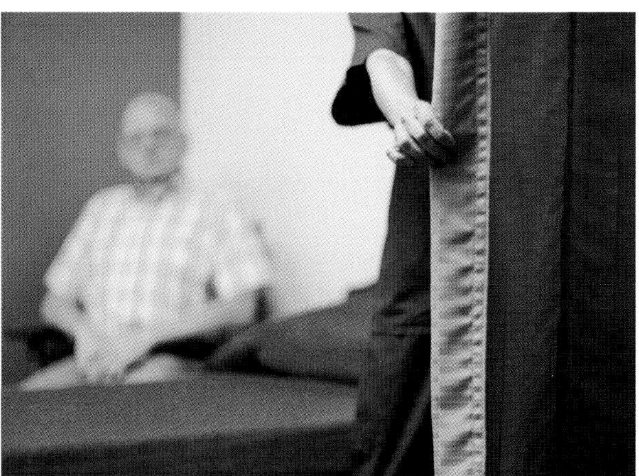

Fig. 11-5. *All residents have a legal right to privacy, and providing privacy is part of doing your job professionally. Your professional, respectful behavior can help put a new resident at ease.*

5. If part of facility policy, do these things:

- Measure the resident's height and weight (see procedures that follow).
- Measure the resident's baseline vital signs (Chapter 14). **Baseline** vital signs are initial values that can then be compared to future measurements.
- Obtain a urine specimen if required (Chapter 16).

- Complete the paperwork. Take an inventory of all the personal items.
- Help the resident put personal items away.
- Provide fresh water (Fig. 11-6).

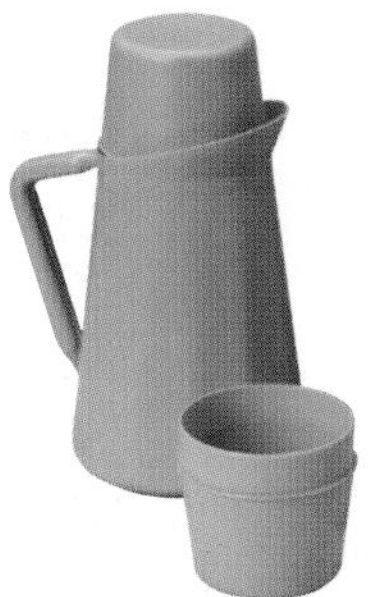

Fig. 11-6. *Providing fresh water is something you should do every time you leave a resident's room, unless he is on a fluid restriction. Doing this helps prevent dehydration. Make sure the pitcher and glass are light enough for the resident to lift. Provide ice if requested.* (REPRINTED WITH PERMISSION OF BRIGGS CORPORATION, 800-247-2343, WWW.BRIGGSCORP.COM)

6. Show the resident the room and bathroom. Explain how to work the bed controls and the call light. Show the resident the telephone, lights, and the television controls.
7. Introduce the resident to his roommate, if there is one. Introduce other residents and staff.
8. Make sure resident is comfortable. Remove privacy measures. Bring the family back inside if they were outside.
9. Place call light within resident's reach.
10. Wash your hands.
11. Document procedure using facility guidelines.

Residents' weight and height will be checked at admission. Nursing assistants also measure weight and height as part of regular care. Height is checked less frequently than weight. Weight changes can be signs of illness, so NAs must report any weight loss or gain, no matter how small.

Weight will be measured using pounds or kilograms. A pound is a unit of weight equal to 16 ounces. A kilogram is a unit of mass equal to 1000 grams; one kilogram equals 2.2 pounds.

Measuring and recording weight of an ambulatory resident

Equipment: standing/upright scale or bathroom scale, pen and paper

1. Identify yourself by name. Identify the resident by name.
2. Wash your hands.
3. Explain procedure to the resident. Speak clearly, slowly, and directly. Maintain face-to-face contact whenever possible.
4. Provide for resident's privacy with curtain, screen, or door.
5. If using a bathroom scale, set the scale on a hard surface in a place the resident can get to easily.
6. Make sure resident is wearing non-skid shoes that are securely fastened before walking to scale.
7. Start with scale balanced at zero before weighing the resident.
8. Help resident to step onto the center of the scale as needed. Be sure she is not holding, touching, or leaning against anything. This interferes with weight measurement. Do not force someone to let go. If you are unable to obtain a weight, notify the nurse.
9. Determine the resident's weight.

   Using a standing scale: Balance the scale by making the balance bar level. Move the small and large weight indicators until the bar balances. Read the two numbers shown (on the small and large weight indicators) when the bar is balanced. Add these two numbers together. This is the resident's weight (Fig. 11-7).

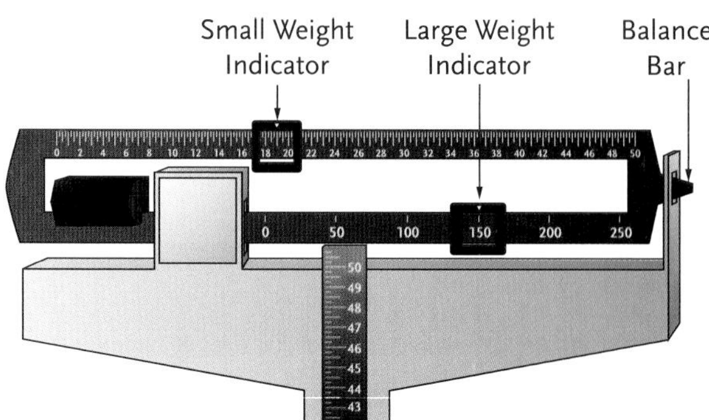

Fig. 11-7. Move the small and large weight indicators until the bar balances. The weight shown in the illustration is 169 pounds.

Using a bathroom scale: Read the weight when the dial has stopped moving.

10. Help resident to safely step off scale before recording weight.
11. Record the resident's weight.
12. Remove privacy measures.
13. Place call light within resident's reach.
14. Wash your hands.
15. Report any changes in resident's weight (when weighing resident after admission) to the nurse.
16. Document procedure using facility guidelines.

When residents are not able to get out of wheelchairs easily, they are weighed using a wheelchair scale. With this scale, wheelchairs are rolled directly onto the scale (Fig. 11-8). On some wheelchair scales, the nursing assistant will need to subtract the weight of the wheelchair from a resident's weight. If the weight of the wheelchair is not listed on the chair, the NA should weigh the empty wheelchair first and subtract the wheelchair's weight from the total.

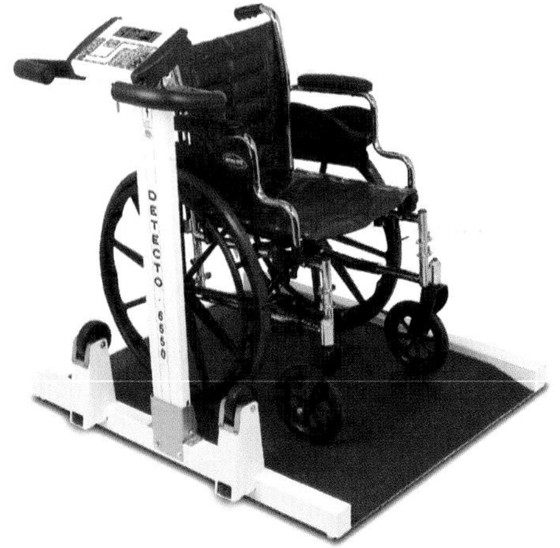

Fig. 11-8. Wheelchairs can be rolled directly onto wheelchair scales to determine weight. (PHOTO COURTESY OF DETECTO, WWW.DETECTO.COM, 800-641-2008)

When residents are not able to get out of bed, they are weighed on special bed scales (Fig. 11-9). Before using a bed scale, know how to use it properly and safely. Follow your facility's procedure and any manufacturer's instructions.

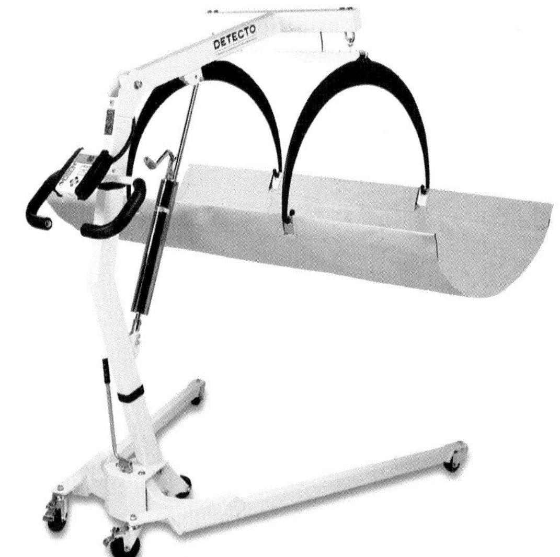

Fig. 11-9. A type of bed scale. (PHOTO COURTESY OF DETECTO, WWW.DETECTO.COM, 800-641-2008)

For measuring height, the rod measures in inches and fractions of inches. The nursing assistant should record the total number of inches. If the NA has to convert inches into feet, there are 12 inches in one foot.

Measuring and recording height of an ambulatory resident

For residents who can get out of bed, you will measure height using a standing scale.

Equipment: standing scale, pen, and paper

1. Identify yourself by name. Identify the resident by name.
2. Wash your hands.
3. Explain procedure to the resident. Speak clearly, slowly, and directly. Maintain face-to-face contact whenever possible.
4. Provide for resident's privacy with curtain, screen, or door.
5. Make sure resident is wearing non-skid shoes that are securely fastened before walking to scale.
6. Help resident to step onto scale, facing away from the scale.
7. Ask resident to stand straight if possible. Help as needed.
8. Pull up measuring rod from back of scale and gently lower the rod until it rests flat on the resident's head (Fig. 11-10).
9. Determine the resident's height.
10. Assist the resident in stepping off scale before recording height. Make sure that the measuring rod does not hit the resident in the head while trying to help the resident off of the scale.
11. Record height.
12. Remove privacy measures.
13. Place call light within resident's reach.
14. Wash your hands.
15. Document procedure using facility guidelines.

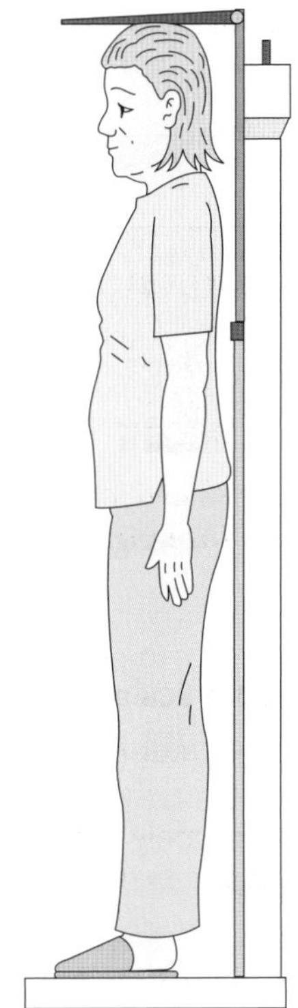

***Fig. 11-10.** To determine height on a standing scale, gently lower the measuring rod until it rests flat on the resident's head.*

Some residents will be unable to get out of bed. Height is sometimes measured by using a tape measure and making two pencil marks on the sheet that is underneath the resident. The NA makes a mark at the top of the resident's head and one at his feet and measures the distance between the marks (Figs. 11-11 and 11-12). Height of a bedridden resident can also be measured using other methods. Nursing assistants should follow the procedures used at their facilities.

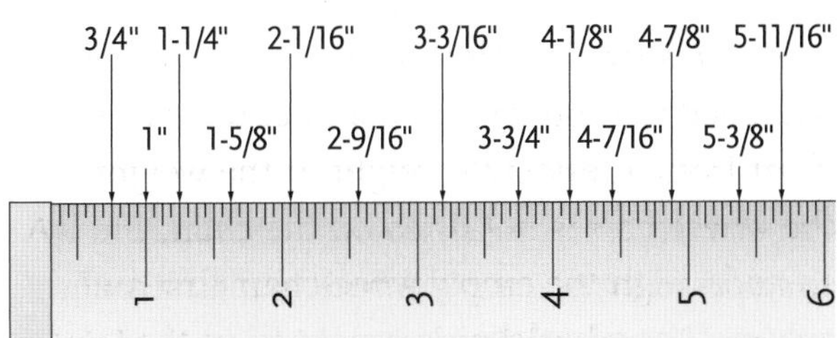

***Fig. 11-11.** Height can be measured in bed using a tape measure.*

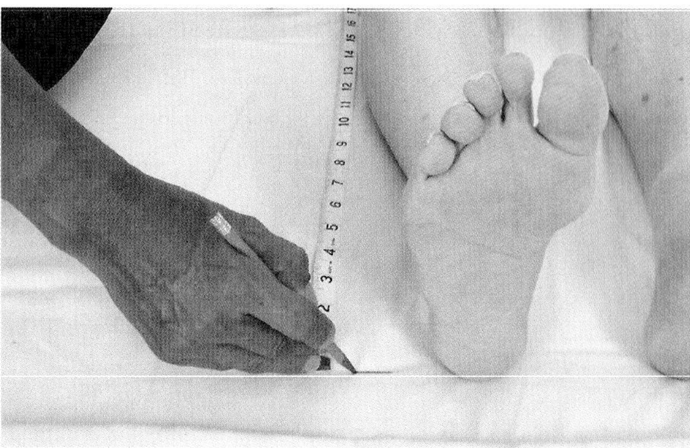

Fig. 11-12. *Make marks on the sheet at the resident's head and feet.*

3. Explain the nursing assistant's role during an in-house transfer of a resident

Residents may be transferred to a different area of the facility. In cases of acute illness, they may be transferred to a hospital. Change is difficult, and this is especially true when a person has an illness or her condition gets worse. Staff should work together to make transfers as smooth as possible for residents. A resident should be informed of the transfer as soon as possible so that she can begin to adjust to the idea. The nurse will inform the resident about the transfer and should explain how, where, when, and why the transfer will occur. Any questions the resident has should be answered.

Nursing assistants help residents pack their personal items before transferring. Because residents often worry about losing their belongings, NAs can involve them in the packing process. For example, the NA can let the resident see the empty closet, drawers, etc.

The resident may be transferred in a bed, stretcher, or wheelchair. To aid with planning, the NA should find out how the resident will be transferred beforehand. After the resident is in her new room or area, the NA should introduce her to all staff members she sees. The goal is to make the resident feel welcome, settled, and comfortable.

Transferring a resident

Equipment: may include a wheelchair, cart for belongings, the medical record, all of the resident's personal care items and packed personal items

1. Identify yourself by name. Identify the resident by name.
2. Wash your hands.
3. Explain procedure to the resident. Speak clearly, slowly, and directly. Maintain face-to-face contact whenever possible.
4. Collect the items to be moved onto the cart. Take them to the new location. If the resident is going into the hospital, they may be placed in temporary storage.
5. Help the resident into the wheelchair (stretcher may be used). Take him or her to proper area.
6. Introduce new residents and staff.
7. Help the resident to put personal items away.
8. Make sure that the resident is comfortable.
9. Place call light within resident's reach.
10. Wash your hands.
11. Report any changes in resident to the nurse.
12. Document procedure using facility guidelines.

When residents are being transferred out of the facility, nursing assistants should make sure residents' clothing is clean and appropriate for the weather. In addition, NAs should observe and report the following to the nurse:

- How the resident left the facility
- Who was with the resident
- Whether the resident left by stretcher or wheelchair

- If the resident understood where she was going
- The belongings the resident took with her
- The resident's vital signs before the transfer

If the resident will be returning soon, the nursing assistant should change the bed linens, tidy the room, and restock supplies.

4. Explain the nursing assistant's role in the discharge of a resident

To discharge a resident from a facility, a doctor must give the discharge order. The nurse then completes instructions for the resident to follow after discharge. The nurse will review these instructions and important information with the resident and her family and friends. Some of the following areas may be discussed:

- Future doctor or physical, speech, and occupational therapy appointments
- Home care, skilled nursing care
- Medications
- Ambulation instructions
- Medical equipment needed
- Medical transportation
- Any restrictions on activities
- Special exercises to keep the resident functioning at the highest level (Fig. 11-13)
- Special nutrition or dietary requirements
- Community resources

Nursing assistants help by collecting the resident's belongings and personal care items and packing them carefully. The NA should know what the resident's condition is at the time of discharge and find out if the resident will be using a wheelchair or stretcher.

The day of discharge is often a happy day for residents who are going home. However, some residents may experience uncertainty or fear about leaving the facility. They may be concerned that their health will suffer. Nursing assistants can help by being positive and reassuring. NAs can remind residents that their doctors believe they are ready to leave. However, if a resident has specific questions about care, the NA should inform the nurse.

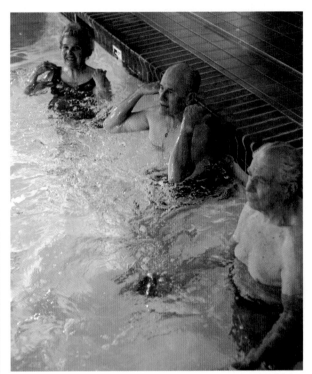

***Fig. 11-13.** After a resident is discharged, she may have instructions to exercise.*

Residents' Rights

Transfers or Discharges

OBRA requires that residents have the right to receive advance notice before being transferred out of or discharged from a facility. The written notice must contain the specifics of where and why they are being transferred or discharged, and it must be in a language they can understand. The staff must provide adequate preparation for the transfer or discharge.

Discharging a resident

Equipment: may include a wheelchair, cart for belongings, discharge paperwork, including the inventory list from admission, resident's care items

1. Identify yourself by name. Identify the resident by name.

2. Wash your hands.
3. Explain procedure to the resident. Speak clearly, slowly, and directly. Maintain face-to-face contact whenever possible.
4. Provide for resident's privacy with curtain, screen, or door.
5. Compare the inventory checklist to the items there. If all items are there, ask the resident to sign.
6. Put the personal items to be taken onto the cart and take them to pick-up area.
7. Help the resident dress and then into the wheelchair or onto stretcher if used.
8. Help the resident to say his goodbyes to the staff and residents.
9. Take resident to the pick-up area. Help him into vehicle. You are responsible for the resident until he is safely in the car and the door is closed.
10. Wash your hands.
11. Document procedure using facility guidelines. Include the following:
    - Time of discharge
    - Method of transport
    - Who was with the resident
    - The vital signs at discharge
    - What items the resident took with him (inventory checklist)

Residents' Rights

Privacy During Discharges

It is important for nursing assistants to always promote residents' privacy. The NA should close the door before talking about medical matters or other private things. He should pull the privacy curtain before the resident changes clothes or is bathed before transfer or discharge.

5. Describe the nursing assistant's role in physical exams

Some residents need a physical exam when arriving at a facility to help determine their needs and to provide important information for the care plan. Others need a physical exam periodically after they have been at the facility for a while. Doctors or nurses will perform the exam. Nursing assistants may help by bringing the resident to the proper area, gathering equipment, and providing emotional support.

Exams can make people fearful or anxious. They may fear what the examiner will do or what he or she will find. Exams can cause discomfort and embarrassment. Nursing assistants can provide support during this process by being comforting and by listening and answering questions within their scope of practice.

Nursing assistants are often responsible for gathering equipment for the nurse or doctor. Examples of equipment that may be needed include the following:

- Sphygmomanometer (for blood pressure)
- Stethoscope
- Alcohol wipes
- Flashlight
- Thermometer
- Tongue depressor
- Eye chart for vision screening
- Tuning fork (tests hearing with vibrations)
- Reflex hammer (taps body parts to test reflexes) (Fig. 11-14)
- Otoscope (lighted instrument that examines the outer ear and eardrum)
- Ophthalmoscope (lighted instrument that examines the eye)
- Specimen containers
- Lubricant
- Hemoccult card (tests for blood in stool)

- Vaginal speculum for females (opens the vagina so that it and the cervix can be examined)
- Gloves
- Drape

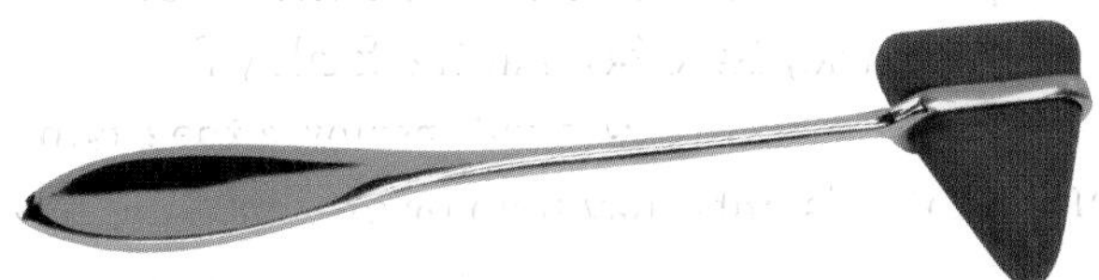

Fig. 11-14. *A reflex hammer is used to test reflexes.* (REPRINTED WITH PERMISSION OF BRIGGS CORPORATION, 800-247-2343, WWW.BRIGGSCORP.COM)

Nursing assistants may need to place residents in the correct position and drape them for the exam. Drapes cover the parts of the body that are not being examined. Some exam positions are embarrassing and uncomfortable. The nursing assistant can help by explaining why the position is needed and how long the resident can expect to stay in the position. In addition to draping the resident, the NA should close the door to the room and/or pull the privacy curtain to protect the resident's privacy. The NA should explain to the resident that he or she will not be exposed more than necessary during the exam. Common positions used during exams include the following:

The **dorsal recumbent** position is used to examine the breasts, chest, abdomen, and perineal area. A resident in the dorsal recumbent position is flat on her back with her knees flexed and feet flat on the bed. The drape is put over the resident, covering her body. Her head remains uncovered (Fig. 11-15).

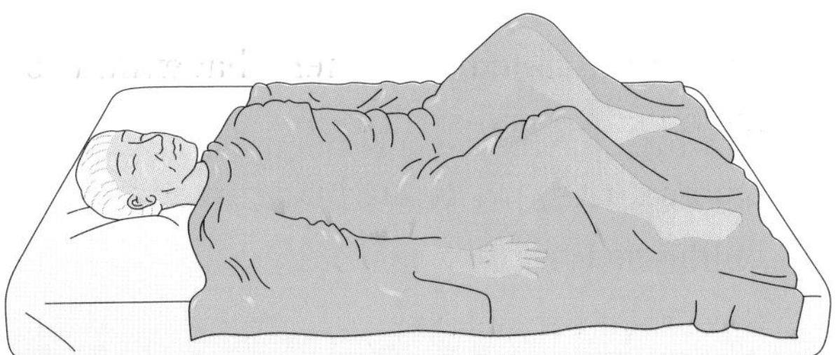

Fig. 11-15. *The dorsal recumbent position.*

The **lithotomy** position is used to examine the vagina. The resident lies on her back, and her hips are brought to the edge of the exam table. Her legs are flexed, and her feet are in padded stirrups. The drape is put over the resident, covering her body. Her head remains uncovered. The drape is also brought down to cover the perineal area and tops of the thighs (Fig. 11-16).

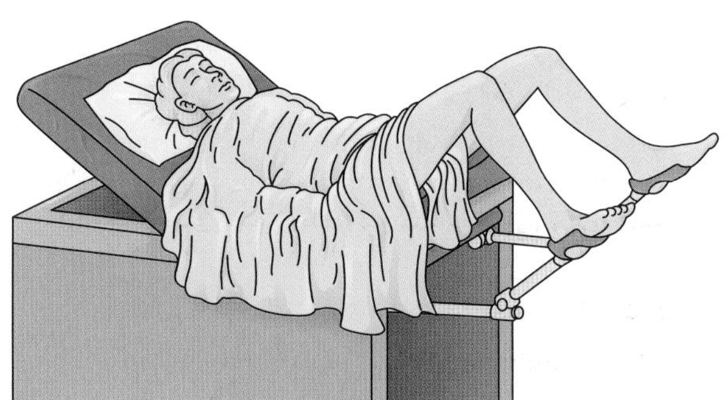

Fig. 11-16. *The lithotomy position.*

The **knee-chest** position may be used to examine the rectum or the vagina. A resident in the knee-chest position is lying on her abdomen. The knees are pulled toward the abdomen, and legs are separated. Arms are pulled up and flexed. The head is turned to one side. In the knee-chest position, the resident will be wearing a gown and possibly socks. The drape should be applied in a diamond shape to cover the back, buttocks, and thighs (Fig. 11-17).

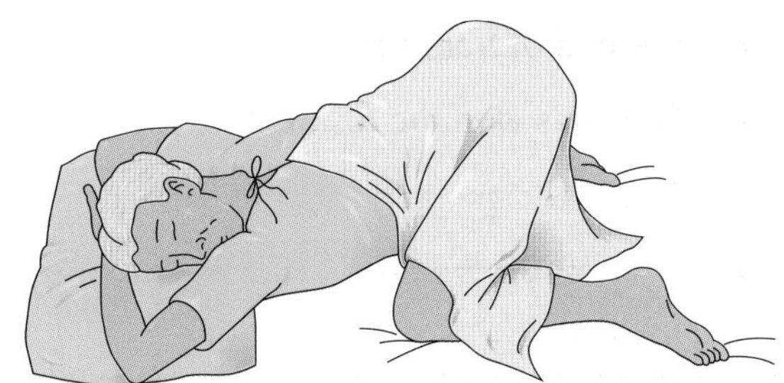

Fig. 11-17. *The knee-chest position.*

Guidelines: Physical Exams

G Wash your hands before and after the exam.

G Ask the resident to urinate before the exam. Collect any urine needed for a specimen at this time.

- Provide privacy throughout the exam. Use drapes and privacy screens. Expose only the body part being examined.
- Listen to and reassure the resident throughout the exam.
- Follow the directions of the examiner.
- Help the resident into the proper positions as needed.
- Protect the resident from falling.
- Provide enough light for the examiner.
- Put instruments in the proper place for the examiner. Hand instruments to the examiner as needed.
- Take and label specimens as needed.
- Follow Standard Precautions.
- For vision screenings, you may be asked to check that needed equipment is in place. Follow directions. Assist the screener to set up any equipment, such as the eye chart. If you transport residents to the site for screening, make sure to take their current eyeglasses or contact lenses with them. The screener will instruct you where to seat the residents or to have them stand. Operate the light switch as instructed. Make sure that the residents have their eyeglasses and other belongings when returning to their rooms.
- After the exam, the NA's responsibilities include the following:
  - Help the resident clean up and get dressed. Help the resident safely back to his or her room.
  - Dispose of any trash and disposable equipment in the exam area.
  - Bring all reusable equipment to the appropriate cleaning room. Clean and store reusable equipment according to facility policy.
  - Label and bring any specimens to the lab.

Residents' Rights

Exams

Residents have the right to know why exams are being performed and who is doing them. Residents have the right to choose examiners and to have family members present during the exam.

Chapter Review

1. What is one way that nursing assistants help residents make a successful transition to long-term care facilities?
2. List eight guidelines for nursing assistants to follow to help residents during the admission process.
3. Why is it important for nursing assistants to report any weight loss or gain that a resident has, no matter how small?
4. How many inches are in a foot?
5. What is one nursing assistant responsibility when assisting a resident with an in-house transfer?
6. List eight types of information that the nurse may cover with the resident and her family and friends during the discharge process.
7. What are two ways that nursing assistants can provide emotional support to residents who are having physical exams?
8. In which position is a resident lying on her abdomen with her knees pulled toward the abdomen, with her arms pulled up and flexed, and her head turned to one side?
9. Which position involves placing the woman's feet in padded stirrups and is generally used to examine the vagina?
10. In which position is a resident lying flat on her back with her knees flexed and feet flat on the bed?

12
The Resident's Unit

1. Explain why a comfortable environment is important for the resident's well-being

Illness and disability cause great stress. It helps residents feel better physically and psychologically if their environments are clean and comfortable. A comfortable and clean environment aids in relaxation and helps to reduce stress. A soothing environment may also help relieve pain and promote healing. Many things affect residents' comfort within their rooms. The more nursing assistants try to improve residents' environments, the more positive impact it may have on residents' health and well-being.

Many things can affect comfort level, such as noise, odors, temperature, lighting, diet, medications, illness, fear, and anxiety. Nursing assistants can use the following guidelines to avoid problems and promote comfort:

Guidelines: Promoting Comfort

G Common noises in facilities can upset and/or irritate residents. Help keep the noise level low by doing the following:

- Do not bang equipment or meal trays.
- Keep your voice low.
- Promptly answer ringing telephones and call lights.
- Close doors when residents ask you to.
- Turn off televisions when they are not in use.

G Odors may be caused by urine, feces, vomit, certain diseases, and wound drainage. Body and breath odors may be offensive, too. Help control odors by doing the following:

- Promptly clean up after episodes of incontinence.
- Change incontinence briefs as soon as they are soiled, and dispose of them properly.
- Empty and clean bedpans, urinals, commodes, and emesis basins promptly.
- Change soiled bed linens and clothing as soon as possible.
- Give regular oral care and personal care to help avoid body and breath odors.

G Temperature can affect comfort. OBRA requires that long-term care facilities have comfortable and safe environments by maintaining a temperature range of 71–81°F. As people age and lose protective fatty tissue, they may feel cold often. Illness can cause a person to feel cold, too. Help residents stay comfortable by doing the following:

- Layer clothing and bed covers for warmth.
- Keep residents away from drafty areas, such as near doors and windows.

- Offer blankets to residents in wheelchairs.
- Keep residents covered while giving personal care.

G Adequate lighting is important to promote safety and prevent falls. It also helps make a room pleasant. Residents may prefer darker rooms when they are ill, have a headache, or are sleeping. Keep lighting controls within the resident's reach.

G Foods ordered in special diets for residents may cause them discomfort. Heavy meals can also cause discomfort. Report resident complaints about food to the nurse. Chapter 15 contains information about nutrition and special diets.

G Foods and drinks that contain caffeine can prevent sleep or interfere with sleeping well. Caffeine may need to be decreased to promote better rest (Fig. 12-1).

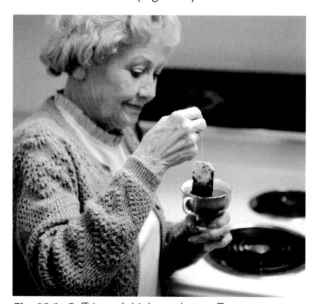

Fig. 12-1. *Caffeinated drinks, such as coffee or some teas, can prevent sleep and cause fatigue and irritability. They may need to be limited if they cause problems.*

G If residents seem sad, anxious, or fearful, help them by talking with them and listening to their concerns. Provide emotional support. If you think residents require more assistance than you can give, discuss this with the nurse.

2. Describe a standard resident unit

A resident's unit is the room or area where the resident lives. It contains the resident's furniture and personal possessions. The unit is the resident's home and must be treated with respect. Nursing assistants must always knock and wait to receive permission before entering.

Residents' units must be kept neat and clean. After providing care for a resident, the nursing assistant will clean the area and put equipment away. Providing a clean, safe, and orderly environment is an essential part of the NA's job.

Standard equipment that is generally found in each resident's unit includes the following:

Bed: Electric beds, also called hospital beds, are adjustable and can be raised and lowered (Fig. 12-2). Electric beds are operated by controls that hang on or near the side of the bed (Fig. 12-3). Buttons are used to raise and lower the head of the bed, the foot of the bed, sections of the bed, and the bed height. Most electric beds have a way to insert a crank so that they can be adjusted if there is a power failure. Manual beds have cranks to move them. The left crank usually raises and lowers the head of the bed. The right crank raises and lowers the foot of the bed. If the bed has a center crank, it will adjust the bed height. Normally beds are kept in their lowest horizontal position. Lowering the bed provides for residents' safety and helps reduce the risk of falls.

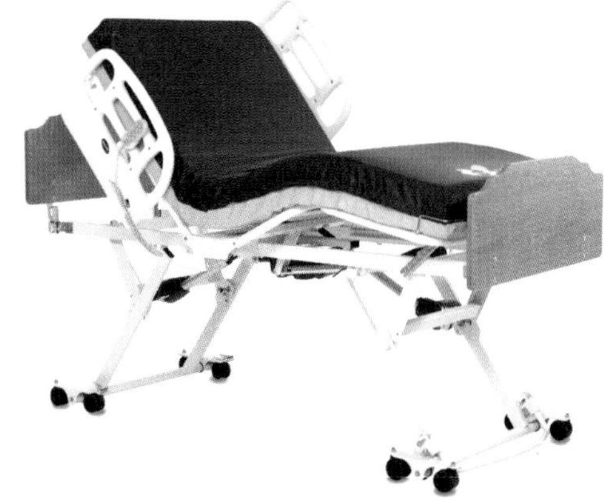

Fig. 12-2. *One type of electric bed.* (© INVACARE CORPORATION. USED WITH PERMISSION. WWW.INVACARE.COM)

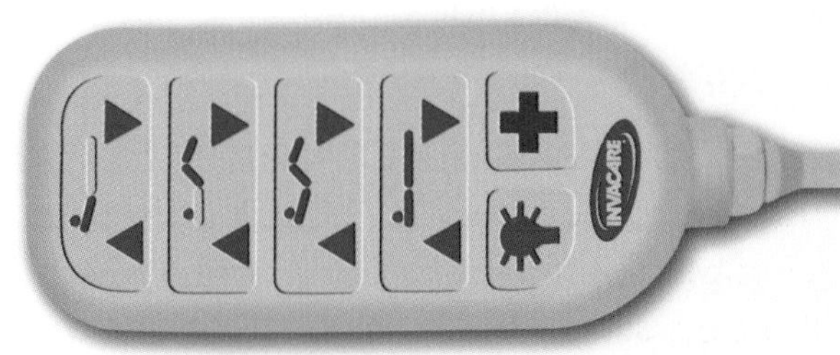

Fig. 12-3. Controls for an electric bed. (© INVACARE CORPORATION. USED WITH PERMISSION. WWW.INVACARE.COM)

Bedside stand: Small items are usually stored in bedside stands. The water pitcher and cup are often placed on top of the bedside stand. A telephone, radio, and other items, such as photos, may also be placed there (Fig. 12-4).

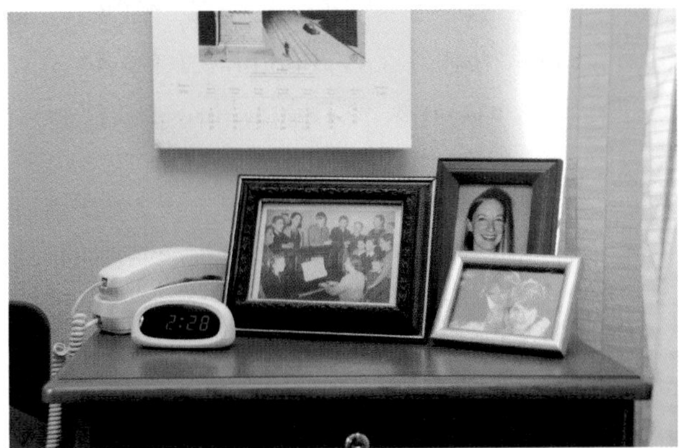

Fig. 12-4. Bedside stands often have personal items, such as photos, as well as things like telephones and remote controls placed on top of them.

These items may be stored inside the bedside stand:

- Urinal/bedpan and covers
- Wash basin
- Emesis basin (Fig. 12-5)
- Soap dish and soap
- Bath blanket
- Toilet paper
- Personal hygiene items

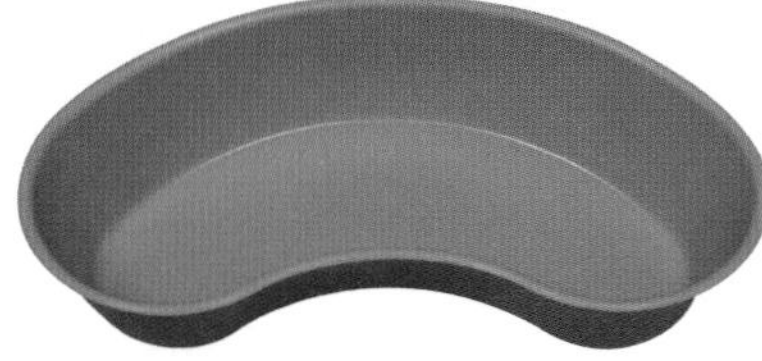

Fig. 12-5. An emesis basin is a kidney-shaped basin often used when giving mouth care. (REPRINTED WITH PERMISSION OF BRIGGS CORPORATION, 800-247-2343, WWW.BRIGGSCORP.COM)

Overbed table: The overbed table may be used for meals or personal care. It is a clean area and it must be kept clean and free of clutter (Fig. 12-6). Bedpans, urinals, soiled linen, and other contaminated items should not be placed on overbed tables.

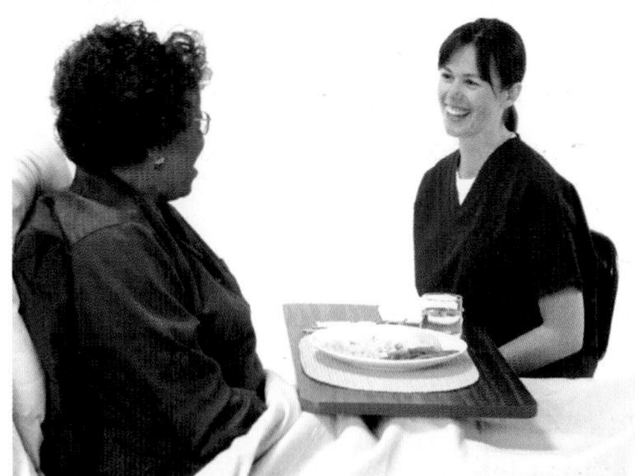

Fig. 12-6. Overbed tables are often used for residents' meals; they must be kept clean. Nursing assistants should never place bedpans, urinals, or soiled linens on overbed tables.

Call light: The intercom system is the most common call system used. When the resident presses the button, a light will be seen and/or a bell will be heard at the nurses' station. The call light allows the resident to communicate with staff whenever necessary. It is important for nursing assistants to always place the call light within the resident's reach and to answer all call lights immediately.

Privacy curtain: All residents in a facility have a legal right to personal privacy. This means that they must always be protected from public view when receiving care. Each bed usually has a privacy curtain that extends all the way around the bed (Fig. 12-7). Curtains keep others from seeing a resident undressed or while having care procedures done. To protect the resident's privacy, nursing assistants must keep this curtain closed when giving care. Although curtains and screens block vision, they do not block sound. NAs should keep their voices low and not discuss a resident's care near others. Closing the door when possible provides more complete privacy.

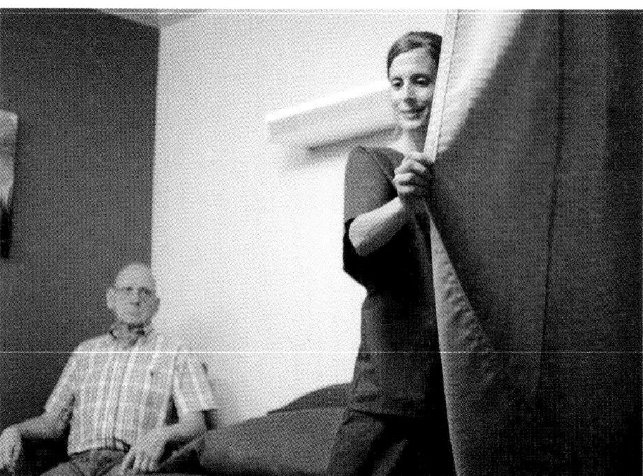

Fig. 12-7. Nursing assistants should pull the privacy curtain around the bed before giving care.

Bed Positions

Nursing assistants may be asked to position electric beds in specific positions. To position the bed in the Fowler's position, the head of the bed should be raised 45 to 60 degrees. To position the bed in the semi-Fowler's position, the head of the bed should be raised 30 to 45 degrees.

3. Discuss how to care for and clean unit equipment

There are many types of equipment in a care facility, and nursing assistants must know how to use and care for all equipment properly. This helps prevent infection and injury. If a nursing assistant does not know how to use a particular piece of equipment, she should ask for assistance. NAs should not try to use equipment that they do not know how to use.

Equipment that is discarded after one use is called disposable, or single-use, equipment. Disposable razors and latex gloves are examples of this type of equipment. Disposable equipment is used to prevent the spread of microorganisms. Nursing assistants should discard disposable equipment in the proper containers.

Some equipment, such as bedpans, urinals, and basins, need to be cleaned after each use. When handling this equipment, nursing assistants must wear gloves so that they do not come into contact with infectious wastes. NAs may need to clean and disinfect this equipment or place it in the proper area for cleaning.

Guidelines: Resident's Unit

- G Keep residents' units neat and clean. Clean the overbed table after use. Place the table within the resident's reach before leaving.
- G Keep the call light within the resident's reach. Check to see that it is within reach before you leave the room.
- G Keep equipment clean and in good condition. If any equipment appears broken or damaged, report it to the nurse and/or file the proper paperwork to get it repaired. Do not use broken or damaged equipment.
- G Remove meal trays right after meals. Check to make sure that there are no crumbs in the bed. Straighten bed linens as needed. Change linens if they become wet, soiled, or wrinkled.
- G Check to see if any personal supplies need to be restocked. Make sure the resident has fresh drinking water and a clean cup within reach and is able to lift the pitcher and the cup. Make sure that tissues, paper towels, toilet paper, soap, and other supplies that are used daily are stocked before you leave.
- G If trash needs to be emptied or the bathroom needs to be cleaned, notify the housekeeping department. Trash should be emptied at least daily.
- G Report signs of insects or pests immediately.
- G Do not move a resident's belongings or discard any personal items. Respect the resident's things. Ask residents where they want items stored. Offer to help residents arrange their space in a way that is pleasing to them. If residents control the heat and air conditioning in their rooms, do not change it for your comfort.
- G Clean equipment and return it to proper storage. Tidy the area. Providing a clean, safe, and orderly environment is part of your job.

4. Explain the importance of sleep and factors affecting sleep

Sleep is a natural period of rest for the mind and body. As a person sleeps, the mind and body's energy is restored. During sleep, vital functions are performed. These include repairing and renewing cells, processing information, and organizing memory. Sleep is essential to a person's health and well-being.

The circadian rhythm is an important factor in determining sleep patterns of humans. The **circadian rhythm** is the 24-hour day-night cycle. It also affects body temperature and hormone production, among other things.

When a person is sleep-deprived or suffers from **insomnia** (inability to fall asleep or remain asleep) or other sleep disorders, problems result. These include decreased mental function, reduced reaction time, and irritability. Sleep deprivation also decreases immune system function.

The elderly may take longer to go to sleep and can have more irregular sleep patterns. Some will take short naps during the day. Many elderly persons, especially those who are living away from their homes, have sleep problems. Many factors can affect sleep, such as fear, stress, noise, diet, medications, and illness. Sharing a room with another person can disturb sleep.

Observing and Reporting: Sleep Issues

When a resident complains that he or she is not sleeping well, observe and report the following:

- O/R Sleeping too much during the day
- O/R Eating or drinking items that contain too much caffeine late in the day
- O/R Wearing night clothes during the day
- O/R Eating heavy meals late at night
- O/R Refusing to take medication ordered for sleep
- O/R Taking new medications
- O/R Having TV, radio, computer, or light on late at night
- O/R Experiencing pain

5. Describe bedmaking guidelines and perform proper bedmaking

When residents spend much or all of their time in bed, careful bedmaking is essential to their comfort, cleanliness, and health (Fig. 12-8). Linens should always be changed after personal care procedures such as bed baths, or any time bedding or sheets are damp, soiled, or in need of straightening. Bed linens should be changed often for these reasons:

- Sheets that are damp, wrinkled, or bunched up under a resident are uncomfortable. They may prevent the resident from sleeping well.
- Microorganisms thrive in moist, warm places. Bedding that is damp or unclean encourages infection and disease.
- Residents who spend long hours in bed are at risk for pressure ulcers. Sheets that do not lie flat under the resident's body increase the risk of pressure ulcers because they cut off circulation.

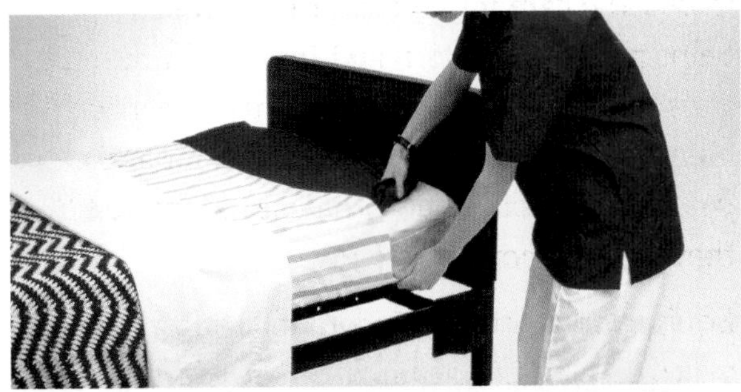

***Fig. 12-8.** Multiple layers of bedding, including a draw sheet, are used for residents who spend a lot of time in bed.*

Guidelines: Bedmaking

- G Keep linen wrinkle-free and tidy. Change linen whenever it is wet, damp, wrinkled, or dirty.
- G Wash your hands before handling clean linen (Fig. 12-9).

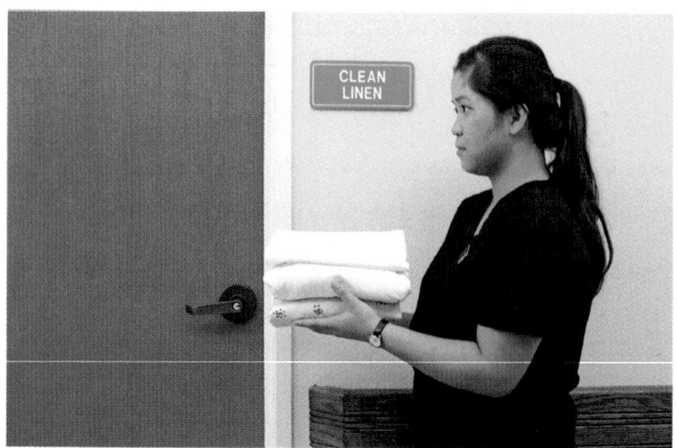

Fig. 12-9. *Make sure you have washed your hands before gathering clean linen.*

- Place clean linen on a clean surface, such as a chair or bedside stand. Do not place clean linen on the floor or on a contaminated area.
- Don (put on) gloves before removing bed linen from the bed.
- Look for personal items, such as dentures, hearing aids, jewelry, and glasses, before removing linen.
- When removing linen, fold or roll linen so that the dirtiest area is inside. Rolling puts the dirtiest surface of the linen inward. This lessens contamination.
- Do not shake linen or clothes. It may spread airborne contaminants.
- Bag soiled linen at the point of origin. Do not take it to other residents' rooms.
- Sort soiled linen away from resident care areas.
- Place wet linen in leakproof bags.
- Wear gloves when handling soiled linen. Hold soiled linen away from your body and place it in the proper container or area immediately. If dirty linen touches your uniform, your uniform becomes contaminated.
- Disposable bed protectors or pads are used for residents who are incontinent. Change bed protectors whenever they become soiled or wet, and dispose of them in the proper container. Put a clean bed protector on the bed when you change linen (Fig. 12-10).

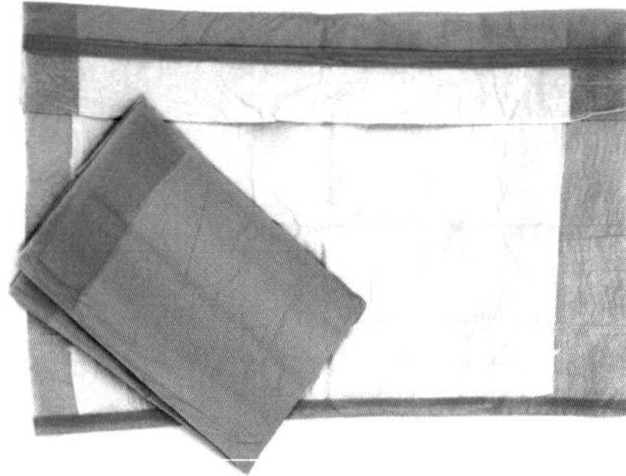

Fig. 12-10. *Disposable absorbent pads help protect sheets from sweat, urine, feces, and other fluids.*

If a resident cannot get out of bed, a nursing assistant must change the linens with the resident in bed. An **occupied bed** is a bed made while the resident is still in the bed. When making the bed, the NA should use a wide stance and bend her knees to avoid injury. Bending from the waist should also be avoided, especially when tucking sheets or blankets under the mattress. The height of the bed should be raised to make it easier and safer.

Mattresses can be heavy. It is easier to make an empty bed than one with a resident in it. An **unoccupied bed** is a bed made while no resident is in the bed. If the resident can be moved, the NA's job will be easier.

Making an occupied bed

Equipment: clean linen—mattress pad, fitted or flat bottom sheet, waterproof bed protector if needed, cotton draw sheet, flat top sheet, blanket(s), bath blanket, pillowcase(s), gloves

1. Identify yourself by name. Identify the resident by name.
2. Wash your hands.
3. Explain procedure to the resident. Speak clearly, slowly, and directly. Maintain face-to-face contact whenever possible.
4. Provide for resident's privacy with curtain, screen, or door.
5. Place clean linen on clean surface within reach (e.g., bedside stand, overbed table, or chair).

6. Adjust bed to a safe working level, usually waist high. Lower head of bed. Lock bed wheels.
7. Put on gloves.
8. Loosen top linen from the end of the bed on the working side.
9. Unfold bath blanket over the top sheet to cover the resident, and remove the top sheet. Keep the resident covered at all times with the bath blanket.
10. You will make the bed one side at a time. Raise side rail (if bed has them) on far side of bed. This protects the resident from falling out of the bed while you are making it. After raising side rail, go to the other side of the bed. Help resident to turn onto her side, moving away from you, toward the raised side rail (Fig. 12-11).

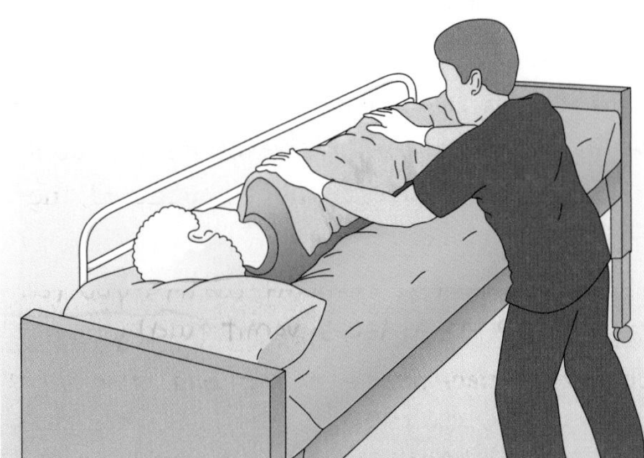

Fig. 12-11. *Turn resident onto her side, toward raised side rail.*

11. Loosen bottom soiled linen, mattress pad, and protector, if present, on the working side.
12. Roll bottom soiled linen toward resident, soiled side inside. Tuck it snugly against the resident's back.
13. Place the mattress pad (if used) on the bed, attaching elastic at corners on working side.
14. Place and tuck in clean bottom linen. Finish with bottom sheet free of wrinkles. If you are using a flat bottom sheet, leave enough overlap on each end to tuck under the mattress. If the sheet is only long enough to tuck in at one end, tuck it in securely at the top of the bed. Make hospital corners to keep bottom sheet wrinkle-free (Fig. 12-12).

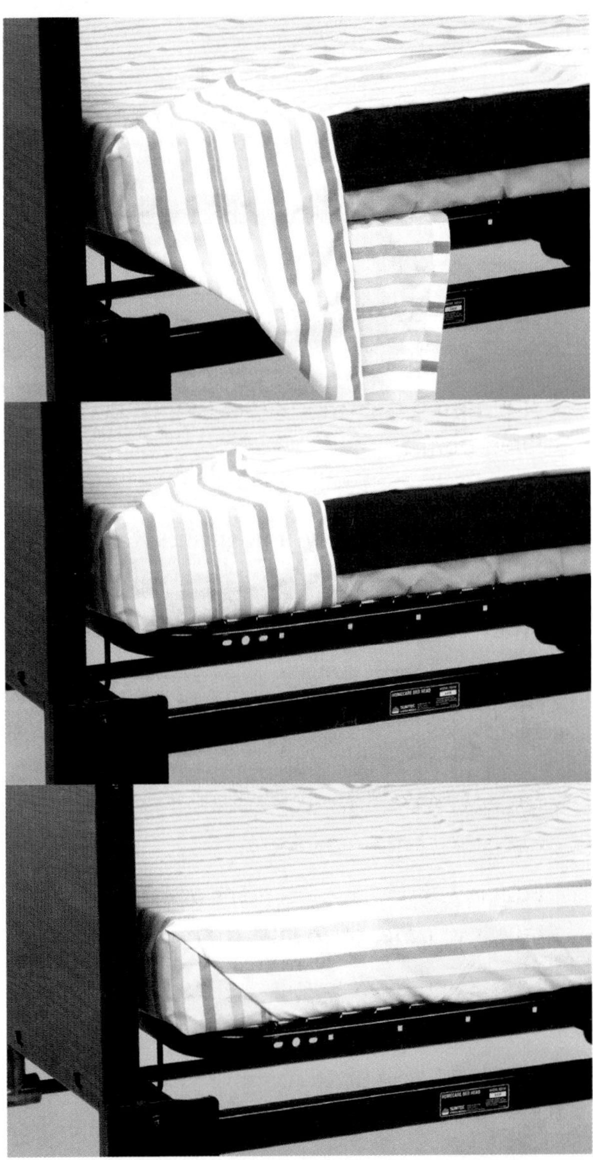

Fig. 12-12. *Hospital corners help keep the flat sheet smooth under the resident. They help prevent a resident's feet from being restricted by or tangled in linen when getting in and out of bed.*

15. Smooth the bottom sheet out toward the resident. Be sure there are no wrinkles in the mattress pad. Roll the extra material toward the resident. Tuck it under the resident's body (Fig. 12-13).

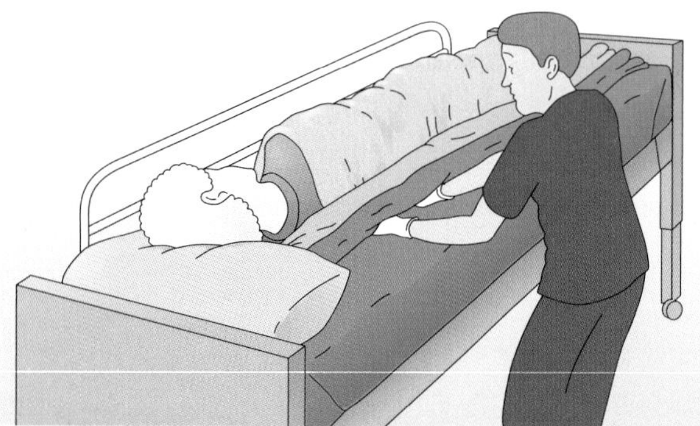

Fig. 12-13. Tuck extra material under the resident's body.

16. If using a waterproof bed protector, unfold it and center it on the bed. Tuck the side near you under the mattress. Smooth it out toward the resident. Tuck as you did with the sheet.

17. If using a draw sheet, place it on the bed. Tuck in on your side, smooth, and tuck as you did with the other bedding.

18. Raise side rail nearest you. Go to the other side of the bed, and lower the side rail on that side. Help resident turn onto clean bottom sheet (Fig. 12-14). Explain that she will be rolling over a pile of linen. Protect the resident from any soiled matter on the old linens.

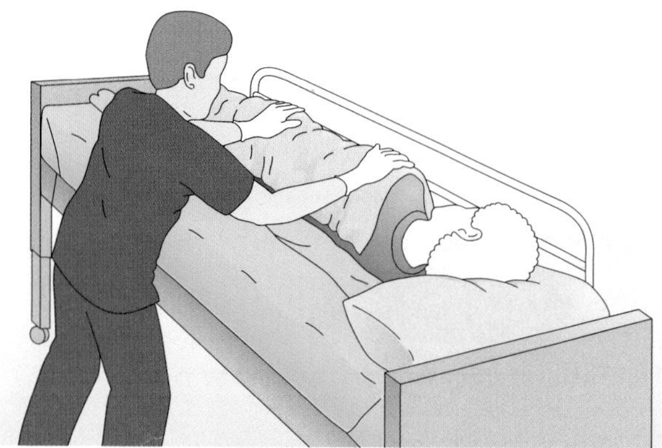

Fig. 12-14. While helping the resident turn onto the clean linen, try to avoid contact with soiled matter on dirty linen.

19. Loosen the soiled linen. Check for any personal items. Roll linen from head to foot of the bed. Avoid contact with your skin or clothes. Place it in a hamper or bag. Never put it on the floor or furniture. Never shake it. Soiled bed linens are full of microorganisms that should not be spread to other parts of the room.

20. Pull the clean linen through as quickly as possible. Start with the mattress pad and wrap around corners. Pull and tuck in clean bottom linen just like the other side. Pull and tuck in waterproof bed protector and draw sheet if used. Finish with bottom sheet free of wrinkles.

21. Ask resident to turn onto her back. Help as needed. Keep resident covered and comfortable, with a pillow under her head. Raise the side rail.

22. Unfold the top sheet. Place it over the resident and center it. Ask the resident to hold the top sheet. Slip the bath blanket or old sheet out from underneath (Fig. 12-15). Put it in the hamper or bag.

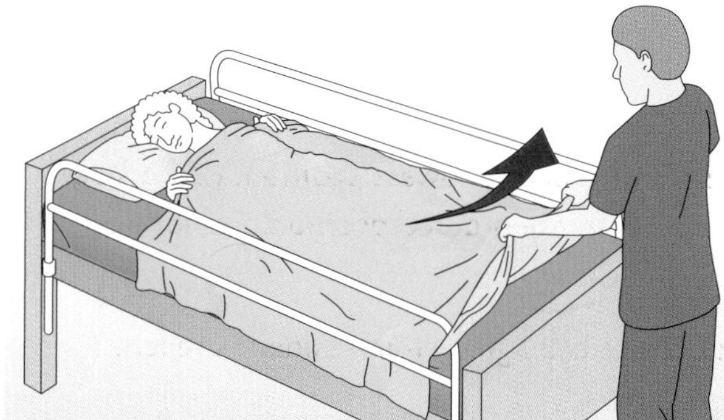

Fig. 12-15. With the resident holding on to the top sheet, pull the bath blanket out.

23. Place a blanket over the top sheet, matching the top edges. Tuck the bottom edges of top sheet and blanket under the bottom of the mattress. Make hospital corners on each side. Loosen the top linens over the resident's feet. This prevents pressure on the feet. At the top of the bed, fold the top sheet over the blanket about six inches.

24. Remove the pillow. Do not hold it near your face. Remove the soiled pillowcase by turning it inside out. Place it in the hamper or bag.

25. Remove and discard gloves. Wash your hands.

26. With one hand, grasp the clean pillowcase at the closed end. Turn it inside out over your arm. Next, using the same hand that has the pillowcase over it, grasp one narrow edge of the pillow. Pull the pillowcase over it with your free hand (Fig. 12-16). Do the same for any other pillows. Place them under resident's head with open end away from door.

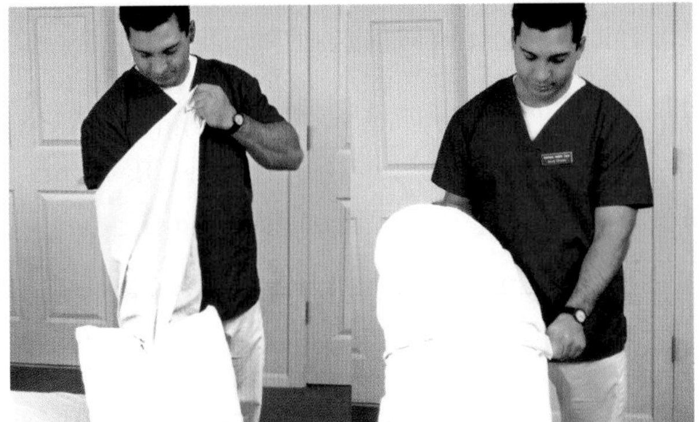

Fig. 12-16. *After the pillowcase is turned inside out over your arm, grasp one end of the pillow. Pull the pillowcase over the pillow.*

27. Make resident comfortable.

28. Return bed to lowest position. Leave side rails in the ordered position. Remove privacy measures.

29. Place call light within resident's reach.

30. Take laundry bag or hamper to proper area.

31. Wash your hands.

32. Report any changes in resident to the nurse.

33. Document procedure using facility guidelines.

Making an unoccupied bed

Equipment: clean linen—mattress pad, fitted or flat bottom sheet, waterproof bed protector if needed, blanket(s), cotton draw sheet, flat top sheet, pillowcase(s), gloves

1. Wash your hands.

2. Place clean linen on clean surface within reach (e.g., bedside stand, overbed table, or chair).

3. Adjust bed to a safe working level, usually waist high. Put bed in flattest position. Lock bed wheels.

4. Put on gloves.

5. Loosen soiled linen. Roll soiled linen (soiled side inside) from head to foot of bed. Avoid contact with your skin or clothes. Place it in a hamper or bag. Do not put it on the floor or furniture.

6. Remove and discard gloves. Wash your hands.

7. Remake the bed. Start with the mattress pad and wrap around corners. Place bottom sheet, tucking under mattress. Make hospital corners to keep the bottom sheet wrinkle-free. Put on waterproof bed protector and draw sheet, if used, smooth, and tuck under sides of bed.

8. Place top sheet and blanket over bed. Center these, tuck under end of bed and make hospital corners. Fold down the top sheet over the blanket about six inches. Fold both top sheet and blanket down so resident can easily get into bed. If resident will not be returning to bed immediately, leave bedding up.

9. Remove pillows and pillowcases. Put on clean pillowcases. Replace pillows.

10. Return bed to lowest position.

11. Take laundry bag or hamper to proper area.

12. Wash your hands.

13. Document procedure using facility guidelines.

A **closed bed** is a bed completely made with the bedspread and blankets in place. It is made for residents who will be out of bed most of the day.

It is also made when a resident is discharged. A closed bed is converted to an **open bed** by folding the linen down to the foot of the bed. An open bed is a bed that is ready to receive a resident who has been out of bed all day or who is being admitted to the facility.

A **surgical bed** is made to accept residents who are returning to bed on stretchers, or gurneys. These residents may be coming from a hospital or returning from a test or procedure. A surgical bed is opened to receive residents by loosening the linens on one side and folding them to the other side. This leaves one side open. Chapter 10 has information on transferring residents into bed from a stretcher.

Making a surgical bed

Equipment: clean linen, gloves

1. Wash your hands.
2. Place clean linen on clean surface within reach (e.g., bedside stand, overbed table, or chair).
3. Adjust bed to a safe working level, usually waist high. Lock bed wheels.
4. Put on gloves.
5. Remove all soiled linen, rolling it (soiled side inside) from head to foot of bed. Avoid contact with your skin or clothes. Place it in a hamper or bag.
6. Remove and discard gloves. Wash your hands.
7. Make an unoccupied, closed bed. See procedure *Making an unoccupied bed.*
8. Loosen linens on the side of bed that is away from the door (where the stretcher will be).
9. Fanfold linens lengthwise to the side away from door (Fig. 12-17). Fanfolded means folded several times into pleats.

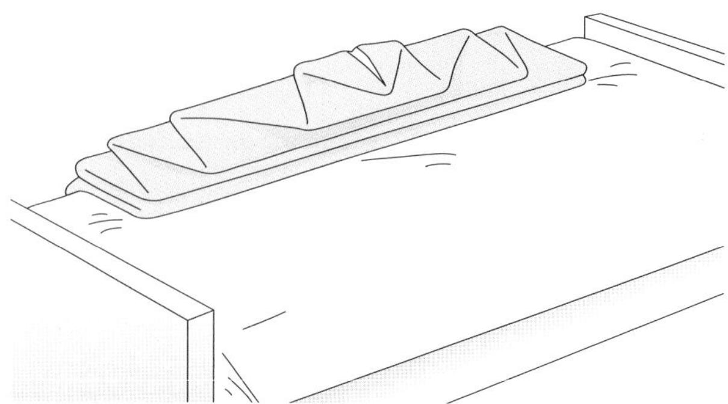

Fig. 12-17. *Fanfold the linen so that it is in pleated layers and position linen opposite the stretcher side of bed.*

10. Put on clean pillowcases. Replace pillows.
11. Leave bed in its locked position with both side rails down.
12. Make sure the pathway to the bed is clear.
13. Take laundry bag or hamper to proper area.
14. Wash your hands.
15. Document procedure using facility guidelines.

Chapter Review

1. What are three ways that nursing assistants can keep the noise level low in facilities?
2. What are three ways that nursing assistants can help control odors in facilities?
3. What is the temperature range for long-term care facilities that is required by OBRA?
4. Why are beds usually kept in their lowest positions?
5. What is the overbed table used for? Can bedpans and soiled linen be placed on an overbed table?
6. Where should call lights always be placed?
7. How do privacy curtains help protect residents' privacy?
8. What is disposable equipment? Why is it used?

9. List two functions that sleep performs for the body. Sleep helps the immune system function well. It helps hormones being produced & body temperature

10. What problems can result from not getting enough sleep? Mental function decreases. Reaction time decreases, People are irritable. Decreased immune system function.

11. When should bed linens be changed?
when a bath is given in bed. If sheets are damp or soiled or wrinkled.

12. List three reasons why it is important that bed linens be changed frequently.
To help with discouraging the growth of microorganisms. It makes the resident more comfortable and less stressful. It lessens the bed sores when sheets are clean & flat.

13. Which way should pillows face while under residents' heads? The open end of the pillow should be away from the door.

13 Personal Care Skills

1. Explain personal care of residents

Personal care is different from other tasks that nursing assistants may perform for residents, such as measuring vital signs or tidying a unit. The term *personal* refers to tasks that are concerned with the person's body, appearance, and hygiene, and suggests privacy may be important. **Hygiene** is the term used to describe practices to keep bodies clean and healthy. Bathing and brushing teeth are two examples. **Grooming** refers to practices like caring for fingernails and hair. Hygiene and grooming activities, as well as dressing, eating, transferring, and toileting are called **activities of daily living** (**ADLs**).

Some people who are recovering from an illness or an accident may not have the energy to care for themselves. Other reasons someone may need help with personal care include the following:

- A person has a long-term, chronic condition
- A person is frail because of advanced age
- A person is permanently disabled
- A person is dying

These residents may need assistance with their personal care, or they may need nursing assistants to provide it for them entirely. NAs may provide any or all of the personal care, including bathing, **perineal care** (care of genitals and anal area), toileting, mouth care, shampooing and combing the hair, nail care, shaving, dressing, eating, walking, and transferring. NAs will assist residents with these tasks every day. These activities are often referred to as *a.m. care* or *p.m. care*, which refers to the time of day that they are done.

Assisting with a.m. care includes the following:

- Offering a bedpan or urinal or helping the resident to the bathroom
- Helping the resident wash face and hands
- Assisting with mouth care before or after breakfast

Assisting with p.m. care includes the following:

- Offering a bedpan or urinal or helping the resident to the bathroom
- Helping the resident wash face and hands
- Giving a snack
- Assisting with mouth care
- Giving a back rub

Some residents will never be able to care for themselves, while other residents will regain strength and be able to perform their own personal care. An important part of a nursing assistant's job is to help residents be as independent as possible. This means showing residents with disabilities how to care for themselves and encouraging other residents to perform self-care as soon as they are able. Promoting independence is an important part of care.

All people have routines for personal care and activities of daily living. They also have preferences for how they are done. These routines remain important even when people are elderly, sick, or disabled. NAs should be aware of residents' individual preferences concerning their personal care. Residents may prefer certain soaps or skin care products. They may choose to bathe in the morning or at night. It is important for NAs to ask residents about their routines and preferences.

Many people have been doing personal care tasks for themselves their entire lives. They may feel uncomfortable with having others do or help them do these tasks. Some residents may not like to be touched by someone else. Nursing assistants must be sensitive to these issues and should remain professional when helping with these tasks.

Before beginning any task, the NA should explain to the resident exactly what she will be doing. Explaining care to a resident is not only his legal right, but it may also help lessen anxiety. The NA should ask the resident if he would like to use the bathroom or bedpan first. She should also provide privacy and let the resident make as many decisions as possible about when, where, and how a procedure will be done (Fig. 13-1). This promotes dignity and independence. In order to promote respect, dignity, and privacy, nursing assistants must do the following:

- Encourage residents to do as much as they are able to do and be patient.
- Knock and wait for permission to enter the resident's room.
- Not interrupt residents while they are in the bathroom.
- Leave the room when residents receive or make phone calls.
- Respect residents' private time and personal things.
- Not interrupt residents while they are dressing.
- Keep residents covered whenever possible when helping with dressing.

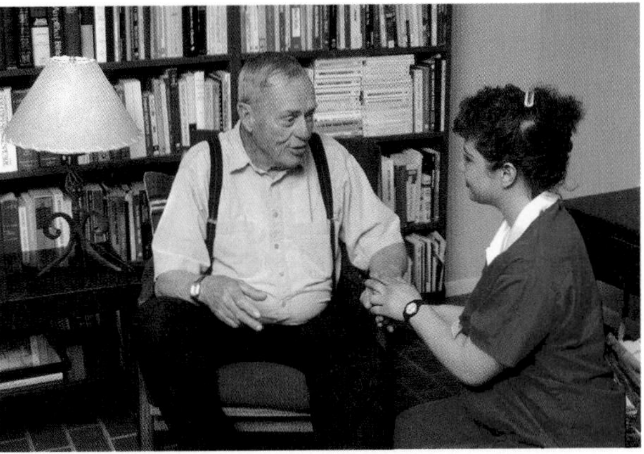

***Fig. 13-1.** Nursing assistants should let the resident make as many decisions as possible about the personal care they will perform.*

Personal care gives an NA the opportunity to observe a resident's skin, mental state, mobility, flexibility, comfort level, and ability to perform ADLs. While assisting with personal care, the NA should look for any problems or changes that have occurred. Communication is especially important during personal care. Some residents will talk about symptoms they are experiencing during personal care. They may say that they have been itching or that their skin feels dry. They may complain of numbness and tingling in a certain part of the body. The NA should keep a small notepad in a pocket to note exactly how the resident describes these symptoms. These comments should be reported to the nurse and documented immediately after the procedure.

Nursing assistants can also observe the resident's mental and emotional state during personal care. Is the resident depressed or confused? Can the resident concentrate on the activity or hold a conversation? Is the resident short of breath? Does the resident tremble or shake? The focus should be on changes from the resident's normal state. Is there a change in behavior, level of activity, skin color, movement, or anything else? NAs are in the best position to observe, report, and document any small change in residents. No matter what care task is assigned, performing it is only half the job.

During a personal care procedure, if the resident appears tired, the NA should stop so the resident can take a short rest. The resident should not be rushed. After care, the NA should always ask if the resident would like anything else. She should leave the resident's area clean and tidy and make sure that the call light is within reach. Before leaving, the NA must check to see that the room has proper lighting and is a comfortable temperature. There should not be any electrical cords or other objects in the walkways. The bed should be left in its lowest position unless the care plan indicates otherwise.

Observing and Reporting: Personal Care

- O/R Skin color, temperature, redness (more information listed in next Learning Objective)
- O/R Mobility
- O/R Flexibility
- O/R Comfort level, or pain or discomfort
- O/R Strength and the ability to perform ADLs
- O/R Mental and emotional state
- O/R Resident's complaints

2. Identify guidelines for providing skin care and preventing pressure ulcers

Immobility reduces the amount of blood that circulates to the skin. Residents who are bedbound are at an increased risk of skin deterioration at pressure points. **Pressure points** are areas of the body that bear much of its weight. Pressure points are mainly located at bony prominences. **Bony prominences** are areas of the body where the bone lies close to the skin. The skin here is at a much higher risk for skin breakdown. These areas include elbows, shoulder blades, sacrum (tailbone), hips and knees (inner and outer parts), ankles, heels, toes, and the backs of the neck and head. Other areas at risk are the ears, the area under the breasts or scrotum, the area between the folds of the buttocks or abdomen, and skin between the legs (Fig. 13-2).

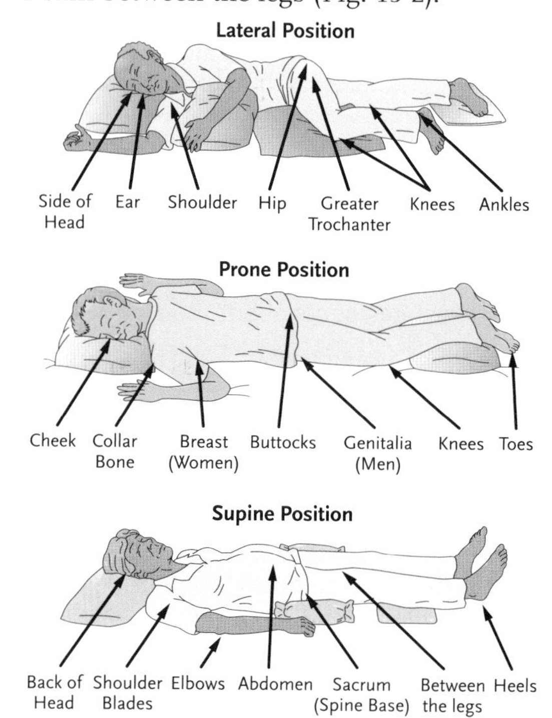

Fig. 13-2. *Pressure ulcer danger zones.*

The pressure on these areas reduces circulation, decreasing the amount of oxygen the cells receive. Warmth and moisture also contribute to skin breakdown. Once the surface of the skin is weakened, pathogens can invade and cause infection. When infection occurs, the healing process slows down.

When skin begins to break down, it becomes pale, white, or a reddened color. Darker skin may look purple. The resident may also complain of tingling or burning in the area. This discoloration does not go away, even when the resident's position is changed. If pressure is allowed to continue, the area will further break down. The resulting wound is called a **pressure ulcer**, pressure sore, bed sore, or decubitus ulcer. If caught early, a break or tear in the skin can heal fairly quickly without other complications. Once a pressure ulcer forms, it can get bigger, deeper, and infected. Pressure ulcers are painful and difficult to heal. They can lead to life-threatening infections. Prevention is very important and is the key to skin health.

There are four stages of pressure ulcers (Fig. 13-3):

- Stage 1: Skin is intact but there is redness that is not relieved within 15 to 30 minutes after removing pressure.
- Stage 2: There is partial skin loss involving the outer and/or inner layer of skin. The ulcer is superficial. It looks like a blister or a shallow crater.
- Stage 3: There is full skin loss involving damage or death of tissue that may extend down to the tissue that covers muscle. The ulcer looks like a deep crater.
- Stage 4: There is full skin loss with major destruction, tissue death, and damage to muscle, bone, or supporting structures.

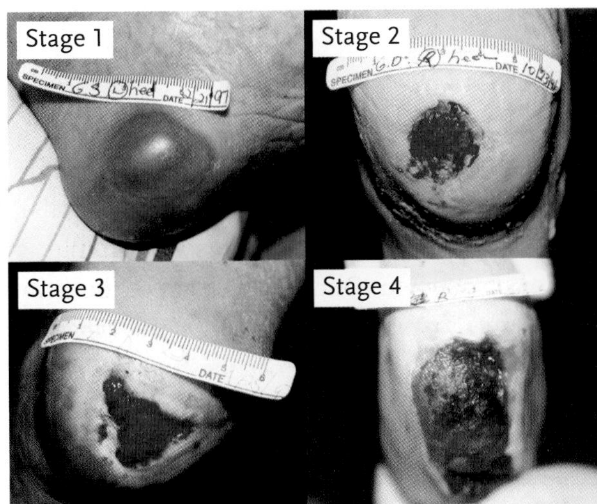

Fig. 13-3. *Pressure ulcers are categorized by four stages.* (PHOTOS COURTESY OF DR. TAMARA D. FISHMAN AND THE WOUND CARE INSTITUTE, INC.)

Observing and Reporting: Resident's Skin

Report any of these to the nurse:

- O/R Pale, white, reddened, or purple areas
- O/R Blisters or bruises
- O/R Complaints of tingling, warmth, or burning of the skin
- O/R Dry or flaking skin
- O/R Itching or scratching
- O/R Rash or any skin discoloration
- O/R Swelling
- O/R Fluid or blood draining from skin
- O/R Broken skin
- O/R Wounds or ulcers on the skin
- O/R Changes in wound or ulcer (size, depth, drainage, color, odor)
- O/R Redness or broken skin between toes or around toenails

In darker complexions, also look for

- O/R Any change in the feel of the tissue; any change in the appearance of the skin, such as the "orange-peel" look; a purplish hue; or extremely dry, crust-like areas that might be covering a tissue break

Breaks in the skin can cause serious, even life-threatening, complications. It is much easier to prevent skin problems and keep the skin healthy than it is to treat skin problems.

Guidelines: Basic Skin Care

- G Report any changes you observe in a resident's skin.
- G Provide regular, daily care for skin to keep it clean and dry. Check the skin daily, even when complete baths are not given or taken every day.
- G Reposition immobile residents often (at least every two hours).
- G Give frequent and thorough skin care as often as needed for incontinent residents. Change clothing and linens often as well. Check on them every two hours or as needed.
- G Avoid scratching or irritating the skin in any way. Keep rough, scratchy fabrics away from the resident's skin. Report to the nurse if a resident wears shoes that cause blisters.
- G Massage the skin often. Use light, circular strokes to increase circulation. Use little or

no pressure on bony areas. Do not massage a white, red, or purple area or put any pressure on it. Massage the healthy skin and tissue around the area.

- Elderly residents may have very fragile, thin skin. This makes the skin more susceptible to injury. Be gentle during transfers. Avoid pulling or tearing fragile skin.
- Residents who are overweight may have poor circulation and extra folds of skin. The skin under the folds may be difficult to clean and keep dry. Pay careful attention to these areas and give regular skin care. Report signs of skin irritation.
- Encourage residents to eat well-balanced meals. Proper nutrition is important for keeping skin healthy. Nutrition affects the color and texture of the skin. Very thin residents may be malnourished, which puts them at risk for skin injuries. Be gentle when moving and positioning them. More information about nutrition is in Chapter 15.
- Keep plastic or rubber materials from coming into contact with the resident's skin. These materials prevent air from circulating, which causes the skin to sweat.
- The care plan may include instructions on giving special skin care for dry, closed wounds or other conditions. The skin may have to be washed with a special soap or a brush may have to be used on the skin. Follow the care plan and nurse's instructions.

For residents who are confined to bed or who cannot change positions easily:

- Keep the bottom sheet tight and free from wrinkles. Keep the bed free from crumbs. Keep clothing or gowns free of wrinkles, too.
- Do not pull the resident across sheets during transfers or repositioning. This causes shearing, which can lead to skin breakdown.
- Place a sheepskin, chamois skin, or bed pad under the back and buttocks to absorb moisture or perspiration that may build up (Fig. 13-4). This also protects the skin from irritating bed linens. Sheepskin covers are also available for wheelchairs.

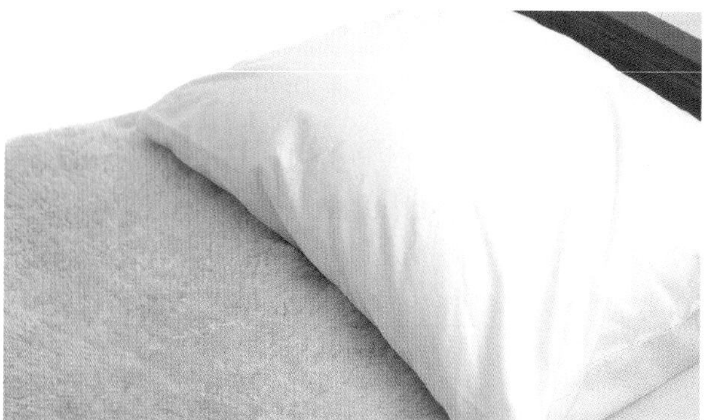

Fig. 13-4. *A sheepskin or chamois skin may be placed under the resident to absorb moisture.* (REPRINTED WITH PERMISSION OF BRIGGS CORPORATION, 800-247-2343, WWW.BRIGGSCORP.COM)

- Relieve pressure under bony prominences. Place foam rubber or sheepskin pads under them. Heel and elbow protectors made of foam and sheepskin are available (Fig. 13-5).

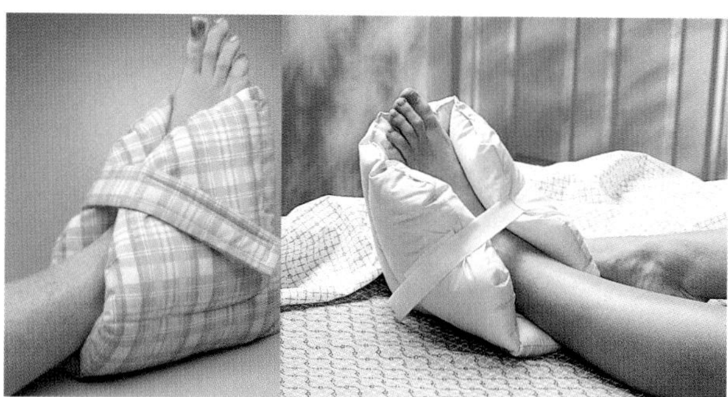

Fig. 13-5. *Padded heel protectors help keep feet properly aligned and prevent pressure ulcers.* (REPRINTED WITH PERMISSION OF BRIGGS CORPORATION, 800-247-2343, WWW.BRIGGSCORP.COM)

- A bed or chair can be made softer with flotation pads.
- Use a bed cradle to keep top sheets from rubbing the resident's skin.
- Residents seated in chairs or wheelchairs need to be repositioned often, too. Reposition residents every 15 minutes if they are in a wheelchair or chair and cannot change positions easily.

Applying Nonprescription Ointments, Lotions, or Powders

Nursing assistants may need to apply ointments, lotions, or powders to a resident's skin (Fig. 13-6). However, not all NAs are allowed to do this so they should make sure they understand the rules in their facility. If instructed to apply an ointment, lotion, or powder by the nurse, an NA should follow these rules and ask questions if anything is unclear:

- Read the directions.
- Know exactly where it is to be applied.
- Know if it should be rubbed in or left on the top of the skin.
- Wash her hands before and after application.
- Wear gloves.
- Avoid getting any on clothing, as it may stain.

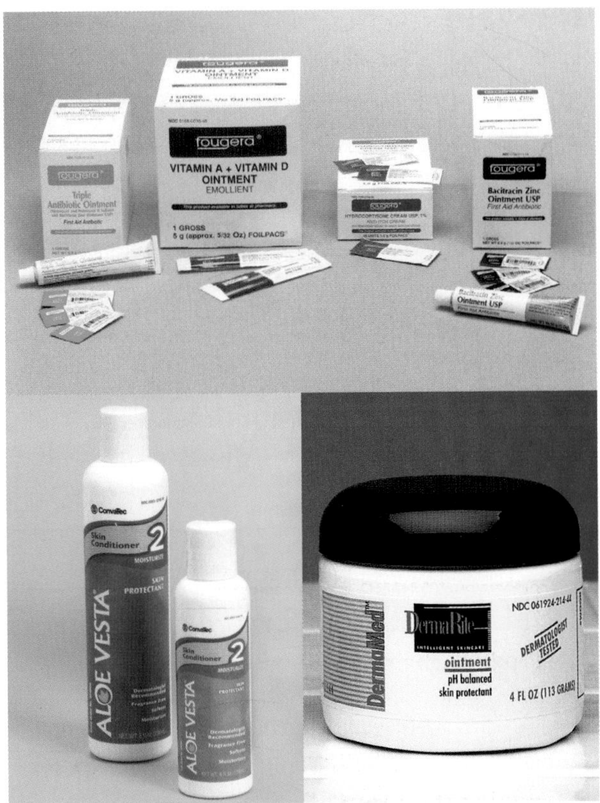

Fig. 13-6. There are many types of ointments, creams, and lotions that are used to treat, soften, and protect the skin. (REPRINTED WITH PERMISSION OF BRIGGS CORPORATION, 800-247-2343, WWW.BRIGGSCORP.COM)

Many positioning devices are available to help make residents safer and more comfortable.

Guidelines: Positioning Devices

- **G** Backrests provide support and comfort. They can be regular pillows or special wedge-shaped foam pillows.
- **G** Bed cradles or foot cradles are used to keep the bed covers from resting on residents' legs and feet (Fig. 13-7).

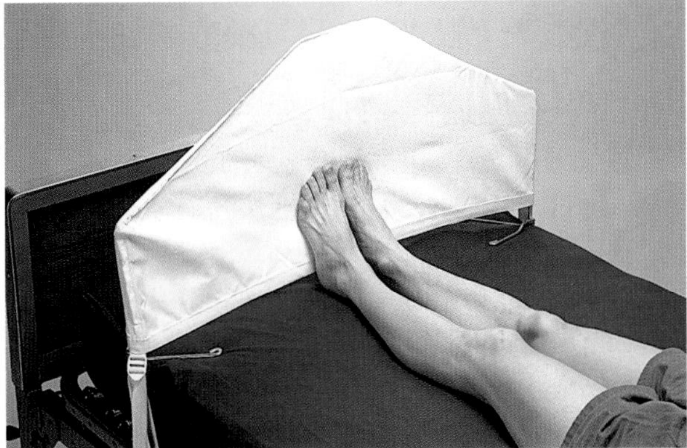

Fig. 13-7. Bed cradles help prevent bed covers from resting on the legs and feet. (REPRINTED WITH PERMISSION OF BRIGGS CORPORATION, 800-247-2343, WWW.BRIGGSCORP.COM)

- **G** Draw sheets may be placed under residents who cannot help with turning, lifting, or moving up in bed. Draw sheets help prevent skin damage that can be caused by shearing. A regular bed sheet folded in half can be used as a draw sheet.
- **G** Footboards are padded boards placed against the resident's feet to keep them properly aligned. They help prevent foot drop. **Foot drop** is a weakness of muscles in the feet and ankles that causes difficulty with the ability to flex the ankles and walk normally. Footboards are also used to keep bed covers off the feet. Rolled blankets or pillows can also be used as footboards.
- **G** Handrolls are cloth-covered or rubber items that keep the fingers from curling tightly (Fig. 13-8). A rolled washcloth, gauze bandage, or a rubber ball placed inside the palm may be used to keep the hand in a natural position. Handrolls can help prevent finger, hand, or wrist contractures.

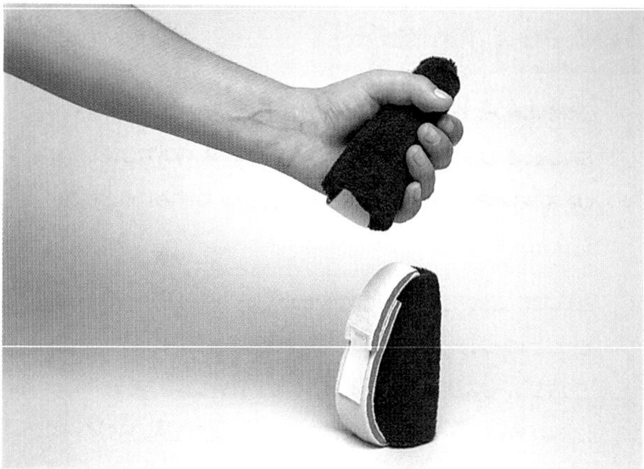

Fig. 13-8. Handrolls keep the fingers and hand in a natural position, helping to prevent contractures. (REPRINTED WITH PERMISSION OF BRIGGS CORPORATION, 800-247-2343, WWW.BRIGGSCORP.COM)

G An **orthotic device**, or **orthosis**—commonly referred to as a splint or brace—is a device that helps support and align a limb and improve its functioning (Fig. 13-9). It may be prescribed by a doctor to keep a resident's joints in the correct position. Orthoses also help prevent or correct deformities. Splints are a type of orthotic device. Splints and the skin area around them should be cleaned at least once daily and as needed.

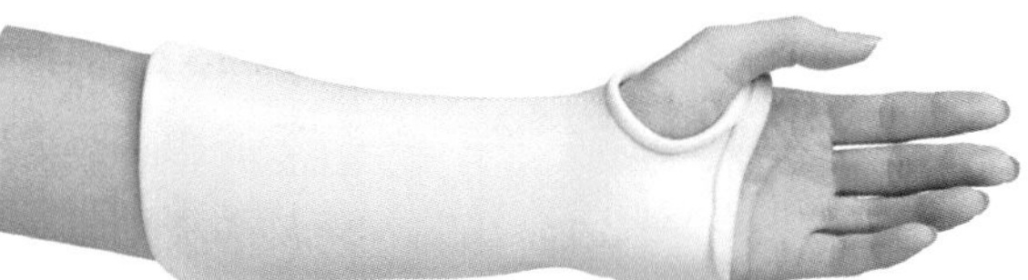

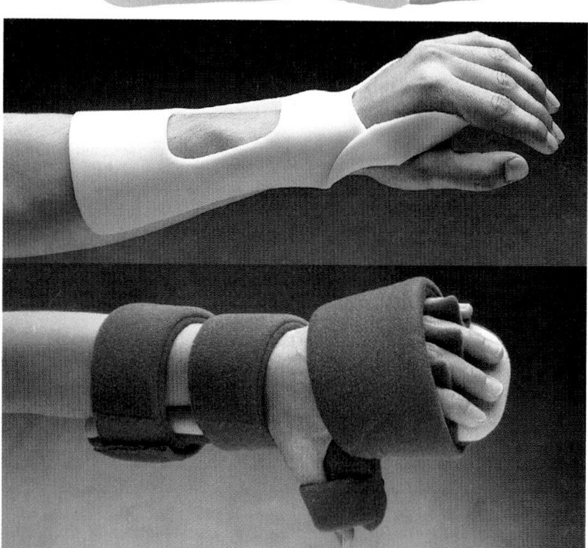

Fig. 13-9. Different types of orthotic splints. (PHOTOS COURTESY OF NORTH COAST MEDICAL, INC., WWW.NCMEDICAL.COM, 800-821-9319)

G Trochanter rolls are rolled towels or blankets used to keep a resident's hips from turning outward (Fig. 13-10).

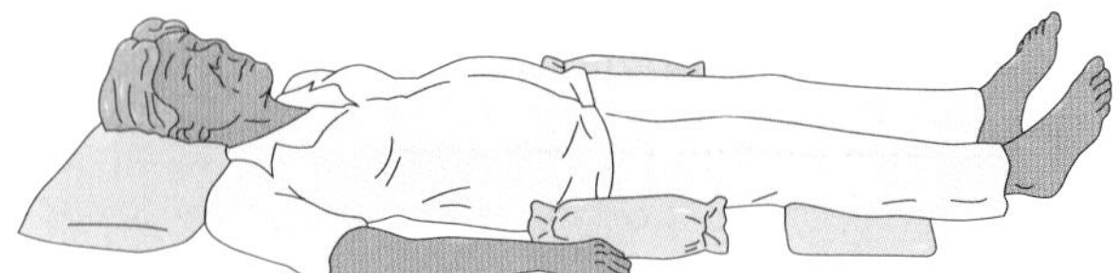

Fig. 13-10. Trochanter rolls help keep the hips in their proper position.

G Knee pillows are padded wedges that can help keep the spine, hips, and knees in the proper position and ease pain in the back, leg, hip, and knee areas (Fig. 13-11).

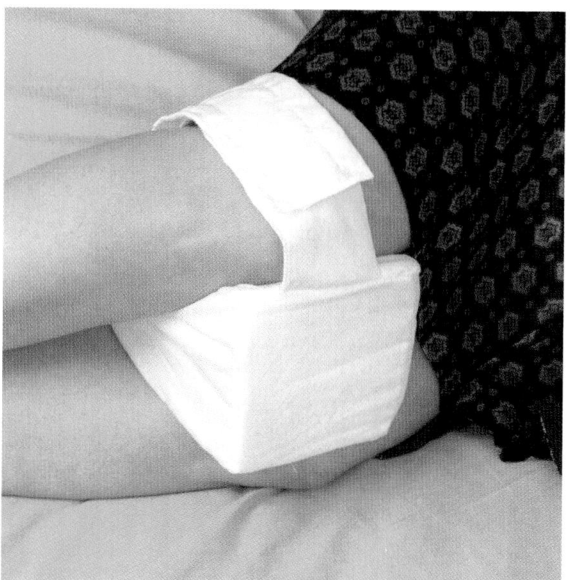

Fig. 13-11. Knee pillows help keep the knees, hip, and spine in the proper alignment. (REPRINTED WITH PERMISSION OF BRIGGS CORPORATION, 800-247-2343, WWW.BRIGGSCORP.COM)

3. Explain guidelines for assisting with bathing

Bathing promotes health and well-being. It removes perspiration, dirt, oil, and dead skin cells that collect on the skin. It helps to prevent skin irritation and body odor. Bathing can also be relaxing. The bed bath is an excellent time for moving arms and legs and increasing circulation. Bathing gives nursing assistants an opportunity to observe residents' skin carefully.

Residents may be given a complete bath in bed, or they may take a shower or have a tub bath. They may have a **partial bath**, which is a bath given on days when a complete bed bath, tub bath, or shower is not done. It includes washing the face, hands, **axillae** (underarms), and perineum. The **perineum** is the genital and anal area.

Most people have specific preferences for bathing. Some like to take long, hot baths, while others prefer a quick shower. Usually they have been bathing the same way most of their lives. Doctors have factors to consider about whether or not to honor residents' personal preferences regarding bathing. They include the resident's capabilities and his or her safety, as well as the safety of the caregiver. The doctor, along with the resident, will decide which type of bath is appropriate.

A doctor may order a special bath using an additive. An **additive** is a substance added to another substance, changing its effect. Examples of some common bath additives and their purpose include the following:

- Bran helps to relieve itching.
- Oatmeal baths are used for inflamed skin. Oatmeal helps to relieve itching and irritation and is soothing.
- Sodium bicarbonate (baking soda) is used to treat psoriasis (non-contagious skin disorder that causes red, scaly patches on the skin) and helps relieve itching.
- Epsom salts baths or soaks reduce pain and swelling and relax muscles.
- Pine products help refresh, calm, and cool.
- Tar coal baths are used to treat eczema and other skin conditions.
- Sulfur baths may be used for skin rashes, eczema, and to help relieve inflammation related to arthritis.

Guidelines: Bathing

- **G** The face, hands, underarms, and perineum should be washed every day. A complete bath or shower can be taken every other day or less often.
- **G** Older skin produces less perspiration and oil. Elderly people with dry and fragile skin should bathe only once or twice a week. This prevents further dryness. Be gentle with the skin when bathing residents.
- **G** Use only products approved by the facility or that the resident prefers.
- **G** Before bathing a resident, make sure the room is warm enough.
- **G** Be familiar with available safety and assistive devices.
- **G** Gather supplies before giving a bath so that the resident is not left alone.
- **G** Before bathing, make sure the water temperature is safe and comfortable. Test the water temperature to make sure it is not too hot. Then have the resident test the water temperature. The resident is best able to choose a comfortable water temperature.
- **G** Make sure all soap is removed from the skin before completing the bath.
- **G** Keep a record of the bathing schedule for each resident. Follow the care plan.

Giving a complete bed bath

Equipment: bath blanket, bath basin, soap, bath thermometer, 2-4 washcloths, 2-4 bath towels, clean gown or clothes, 2 pairs of gloves, orangewood stick or nail brush, lotion, deodorant

1. Identify yourself by name. Identify the resident by name.
2. Wash your hands.
3. Explain procedure to the resident. Speak clearly, slowly, and directly. Maintain face-to-face contact whenever possible.

4. Provide for the resident's privacy with curtain, screen, or door. Be sure the room is a comfortable temperature and there are no drafts.

5. Adjust bed to a safe level, usually waist high. Lock bed wheels.

6. Place a bath blanket or towel over resident (Fig. 13-12). Ask him to hold onto it as you remove or fold back top bedding. Remove gown, while keeping resident covered with bath blanket (or top sheet).

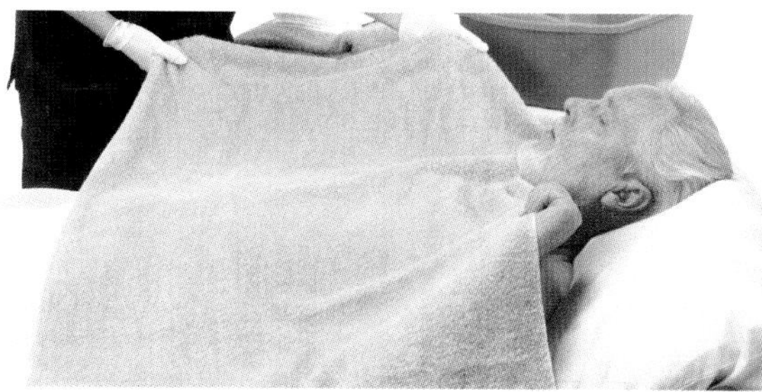

Fig. 13-12. *Cover the resident with a cotton blanket before removing top bedding.*

7. Fill the basin with warm water. Test water temperature with thermometer or against the inside of your wrist. Water temperature should not be over 105°F. Have resident check water temperature to see if it is comfortable. Adjust if necessary. The water will cool quickly. During the bath, change the water when it becomes too cool, soapy, or dirty.

8. Put on gloves.

9. Ask the resident to participate in washing. Help him do this whenever needed.

10. Uncover only one part of the body at a time. Place a towel under the part being washed.

11. Wash, rinse, and dry one part of the body at a time. Start at the head, work down, and complete the front first. When washing, use a clean area of the washcloth for each stroke.

    Eyes, Face, Ears, and Neck: Wash face with wet washcloth (no soap). Begin with the eye farther away from you. Wash inner area to outer area (Fig. 13-13). Use a different area of the washcloth for each stroke. Wash the face from the middle outward using firm but gentle strokes. Wash the ears and behind the ears and the neck. Rinse and pat dry.

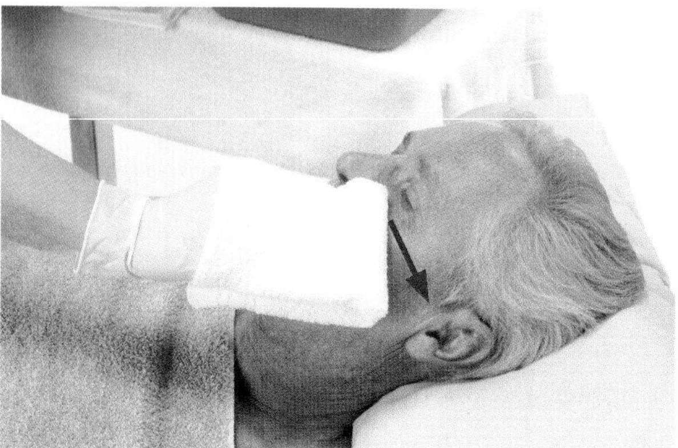

Fig. 13-13. *Wash the eye from the inner to outer area, using a different area of the washcloth for each stroke.*

    Arms and Axillae: Remove the resident's top clothing. Cover him with the bath blanket or towel. Remove one arm from under the towel. With a soapy washcloth, wash the upper arm and underarm. Use long strokes from the shoulder down to the wrist (Fig. 13-14). Rinse and pat dry. Repeat for the other arm.

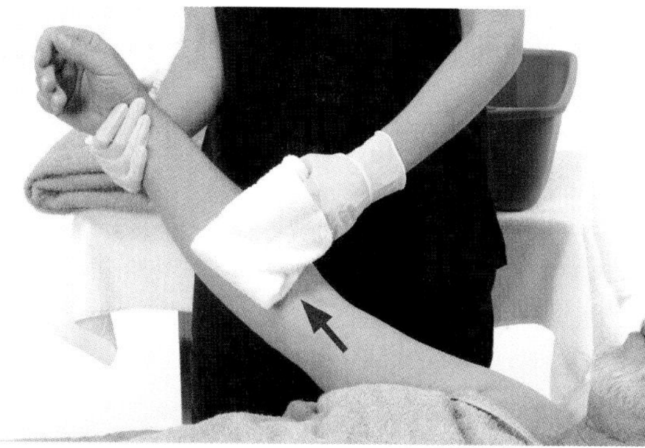

Fig. 13-14. *Support the wrist while washing the shoulder, arm, underarm, and elbow.*

    Hands: Wash one hand in a basin. Clean under the nails with an orangewood stick or nail brush if available (Fig. 13-15). Rinse and pat dry. Give nail care (see procedure later in this chapter) if it has been assigned. Repeat for the other hand. Put lotion on the resident's elbows and hands if ordered.

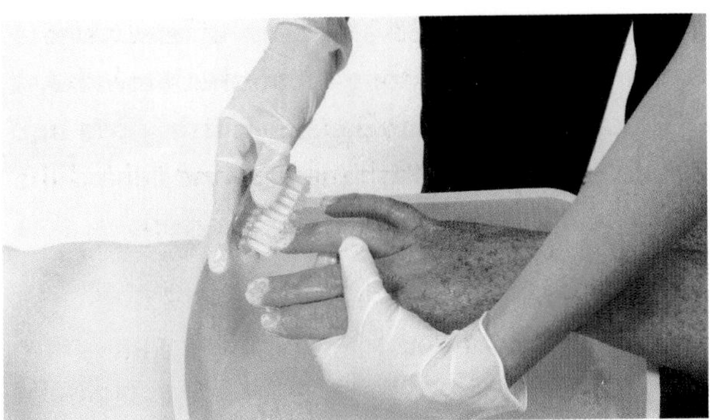

Fig. 13-15. Wash each hand in a basin. Thoroughly clean under the nails with a nail brush.

Chest: Place the towel again across the resident's chest. Pull the blanket down to the waist. Lift the towel only enough to wash the chest, rinse it, and pat dry. For a female resident, wash, rinse, and dry breasts and under breasts. Check the skin in this area for signs of irritation.

Abdomen: Keep the towel across chest. Fold the blanket down so that it still covers the pubic area. Wash the abdomen, rinse, and pat dry. If the resident has an ostomy, or opening in the abdomen for getting rid of body wastes, give skin care around the opening (Chapter 17 has information about ostomies). Cover with the towel. Pull the cotton blanket up to the resident's chin. Remove the towel.

Legs and Feet: Expose one leg and place a towel under it. Wash the thigh. Use long, downward strokes when washing. Rinse and pat dry. Do the same from the knee to the ankle (Fig. 13-16).

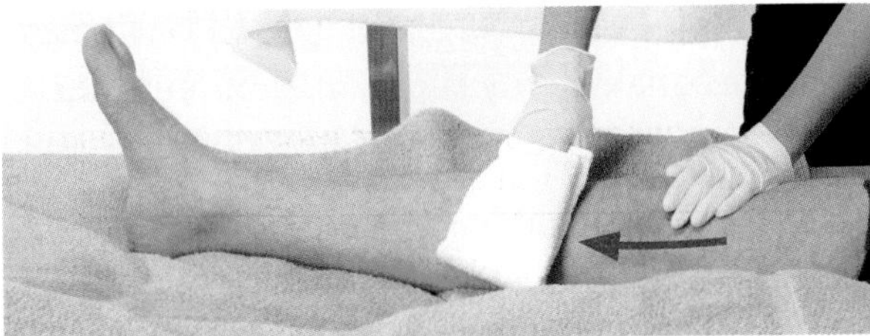

Fig. 13-16. Use long, downward strokes when washing the legs.

Place another towel under the foot. Move the basin to the towel. Place the foot into the basin. Wash the foot and between the toes (Fig. 13-17). Rinse foot and pat dry, making sure areas between toes are dry. Give nail care (see procedure later in this chapter) if it has been assigned. **Never clip a resident's toenails**. Apply lotion to the foot if ordered, especially at the heels. Do not apply lotion between the toes. Repeat steps for the other leg and foot.

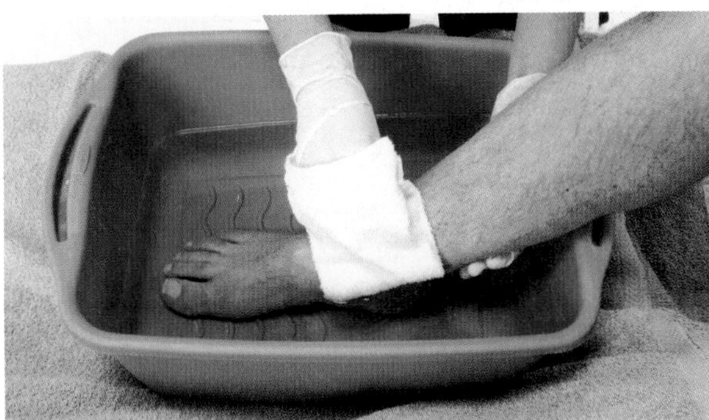

Fig. 13-17. Washing the feet includes cleaning between the toes.

Back: Help resident move to the center of the bed. Ask resident to turn onto his side so his back is facing you. If the bed has rails, raise the rail on the far side for safety. Fold the blanket away from the back. Place a towel lengthwise next to the back. Wash the back and neck with long, downward strokes (Fig. 13-18). Rinse and pat dry. Apply lotion if ordered.

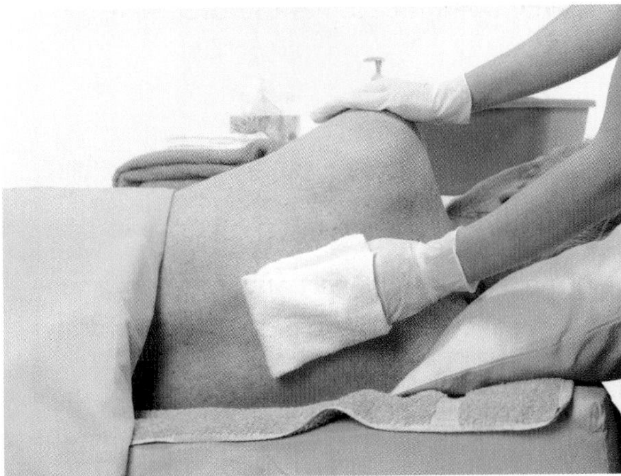

Fig. 13-18. Wash the back with long downward strokes.

12. Place the towel under the buttocks and upper thighs. Help the resident turn onto his back. Ask if he is able to wash the perineal area.

If so, place a basin of clean, warm water, a washcloth, and towel within reach. Hand items to the resident as needed. If the resident wants you to leave the room, remove and discard gloves. Wash your hands. Leave supplies and the call light within reach. If the resident has a urinary catheter in place, remind him not to pull it.

13. If the resident is unable to provide perineal care, you will do it. Remove and discard your gloves. Wash your hands and put on clean gloves. Provide privacy at all times.

14. **Perineal area and buttocks**: Change the bath water. Wash, rinse, and dry perineal area, working from front to back (clean to dirty).

    For a female resident: Using water and small amount of soap, wash the perineum from front to back, using single strokes (Fig. 13-19). Do not wash from the back to the front, as this may cause infection. Use a clean area of washcloth or a clean washcloth for each stroke.

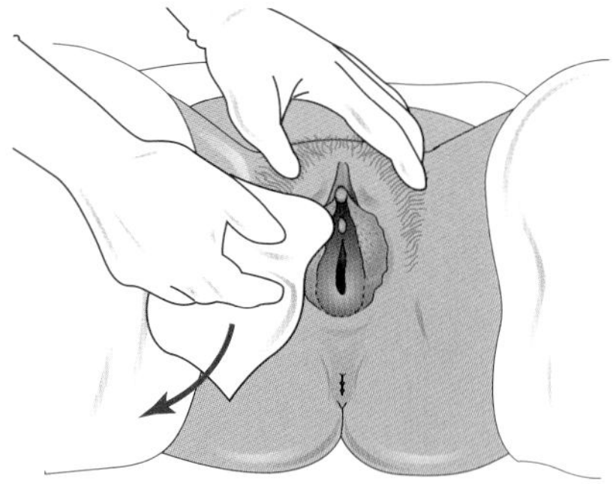

Fig. 13-19. Always work from front to back when performing perineal care. This helps prevent infection.

    First spread the labia majora, the outside folds of perineal skin that protect the urinary meatus and the vaginal opening. Wipe from front to back on one side with a clean washcloth. Then wipe the other side from front to back, using a clean part of the washcloth. Clean the perineum (area between the vagina and anus) last with a front to back motion. Rinse the area thoroughly in the same way. Make sure all soap is removed.

    Dry entire perineal area moving from front to back, using a blotting motion with towel. Ask resident to turn on her side. Wash, rinse, and dry buttocks and anal area. Clean the anal area without contaminating the perineal area.

    For a male resident: If the resident is uncircumcised, pull back the foreskin first. Gently push skin toward the base of penis. Hold the penis by the shaft. Wash in a circular motion from the tip down to the base. Use a clean area of washcloth or clean washcloth for each stroke (Fig. 13-20).

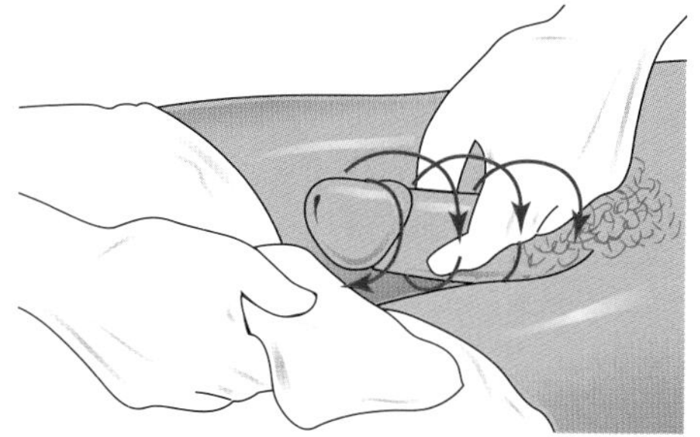

Fig. 13-20. Wash the penis in a circular motion from the tip down to the base.

    Thoroughly rinse the penis. If resident is uncircumcised, gently return foreskin to normal position. Then wash the scrotum and groin. The **groin** is the area from the pubis (area around the penis and scrotum) to the upper thighs. Rinse and pat dry. Ask the resident to turn on his side. Wash, rinse, and dry buttocks and anal area. Clean the anal area without contaminating the perineal area.

15. Cover the resident with the blanket.

16. Empty, rinse, and dry bath basin. Place basin in designated dirty supply area or return to storage, depending on facility policy.

17. Place soiled clothing and linens in proper containers.

18. Remove and discard gloves.

19. Wash your hands.

20. Provide resident with deodorant. Brush or comb the resident's hair (see procedure later in this chapter). Help resident put on clean

clothing and get into a comfortable position with proper body alignment.

21. Return bed to lowest position. Remove privacy measures.
22. Place call light within resident's reach.
23. Wash your hands.
24. Report any changes in resident to the nurse.
25. Document procedure using facility guidelines.

A back rub can help relax residents. It can make them more comfortable and increase circulation. Back rubs are often given after baths. After giving a back rub, the nursing assistant should note any changes in a resident's skin.

Giving a back rub

Equipment: cotton blanket or towel, lotion

1. Identify yourself by name. Identify the resident by name.
2. Wash your hands.
3. Explain procedure to the resident. Speak clearly, slowly, and directly. Maintain face-to-face contact whenever possible.
4. Provide for resident's privacy with curtain, screen, or door.
5. Adjust bed to a safe working level, usually waist high. Lower the head of the bed. Lock bed wheels.
6. Position the resident so he is lying on his side or his stomach. Many elderly people find that lying on their stomachs is uncomfortable. If so, have the resident lie on his side. Cover the resident with a cotton blanket, then fold back bed covers. Expose the resident's back to the top of the buttocks. Back rubs can also be given with the resident sitting up.
7. Warm lotion by putting bottle in warm water for five minutes. Run your hands under warm water. Pour lotion on your hands and rub them together to spread it. Always put lotion on your hands first, rather than directly on the resident's skin.
8. Place your hands on each side of upper part of the buttocks. Use the full palm of each hand. Make long, smooth upward strokes with both hands. Move along each side of the spine, up to the shoulders (Figs. 13-21 and 13-22). Circle your hands outward. Then move back along outer edges of the back. At the buttocks, make another circle. Move your hands back up to the shoulders. Without taking your hands from resident's skin, repeat this motion for three to five minutes.

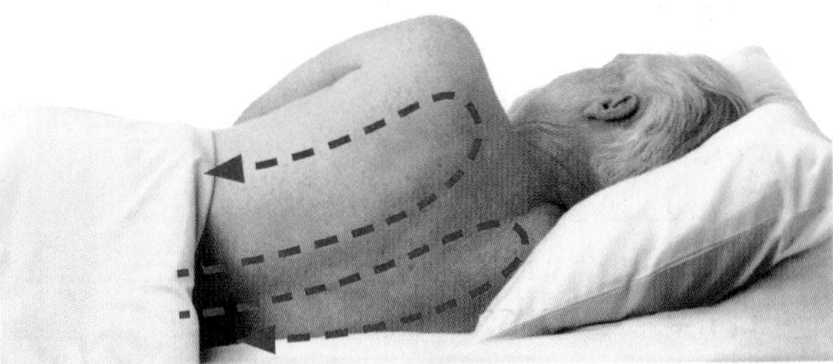

Fig. 13-21. *Move along each side of the spine, up to the shoulders.*

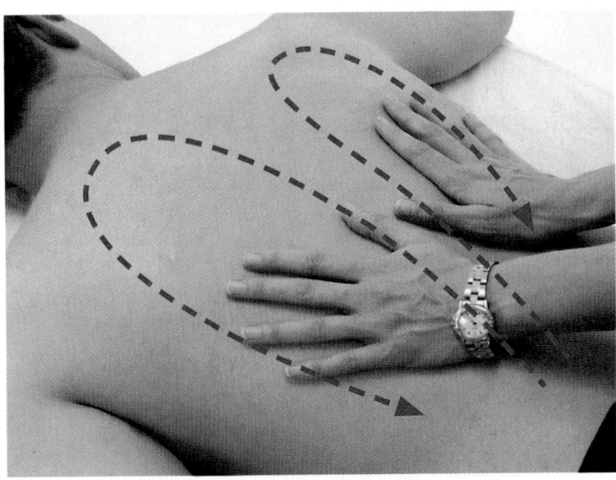

Fig. 13-22. *Long, upward strokes help release muscle tension.*

9. Knead with the first two fingers and thumb of each hand. Place them at base of the spine. Move upward together along each side of the spine. Apply gentle downward pressure with fingers and thumbs. Follow the same direction as with the long smooth strokes, circling at shoulders and buttocks.

10. Gently massage bony areas (spine, shoulder blades, hip bones). Use circular motions of your fingertips. Gentle massage stimulates circulation and helps prevent skin damage. However, if any of these areas are pale, white, or red, massage around them rather than on them. The redness indicates that the skin is already irritated and fragile. Include this information in your report to the nurse.
11. Let the resident know when you are almost through. Finish with some long smooth strokes, like the ones you used at the beginning of the massage.
12. Dry the back if extra lotion remains on it.
13. Remove blanket and towel.
14. Help the resident get dressed. Help the resident into a comfortable position.
15. Store supplies. Place soiled clothing and linens in proper containers.
16. Return bed to lowest position. Remove privacy measures.
17. Place call light within resident's reach.
18. Wash your hands.
19. Report any changes in resident to the nurse.
20. Document procedure using facility guidelines.

Hair care is an important part of cleanliness. Shampooing the hair removes dirt, bacteria, oils, and other materials from the hair. Residents who can get out of bed may have their hair shampooed in the sink, tub, or shower. For residents who cannot get out of bed, special troughs are available for shampooing hair in bed (Fig. 13-23). Troughs fit under the resident's head and neck and have a spout or hose that drains the water into a basin at the side of the bed. There are also special types of shampoos that do not require the use of water (Fig. 13-24). Nursing assistants should follow the care plan regarding the type of shampoo to use.

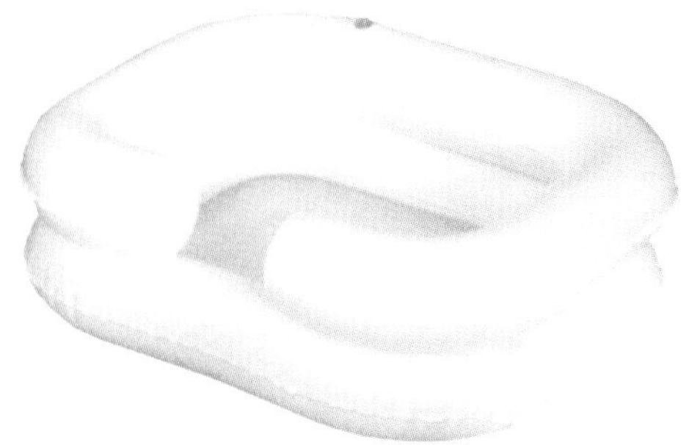

Fig. 13-23. *An inflatable bed shampoo trough can be used to shampoo hair while the person is in bed.* (REPRINTED WITH PERMISSION OF BRIGGS CORPORATION, 800-247-2343, WWW.BRIGGSCORP.COM)

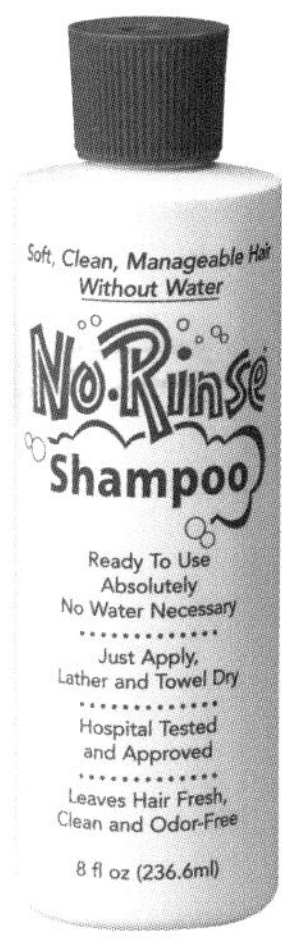

Fig. 13-24. *One type of shampoo that does not require water.* (REPRINTED WITH PERMISSION OF BRIGGS CORPORATION, 800-247-2343, WWW.BRIGGSCORP.COM)

Shampooing hair

Equipment: shampoo, hair conditioner (if requested), 2 bath towels, washcloth, bath thermometer, pitcher or handheld shower or sink attachment, waterproof pad (for washing hair in bed), bath blanket (for washing hair in bed), trough and catch basin (for washing hair in bed), chair (for washing hair in sink), protective plastic sheet or drape (for washing hair in sink), comb and brush, hair dryer

1. Identify yourself by name. Identify the resident by name.
2. Wash your hands.
3. Explain procedure to the resident. Speak clearly, slowly, and directly. Maintain face-to-face contact whenever possible.
4. Provide for the resident's privacy with curtain, screen, or door. Be sure the room is a

comfortable temperature and there are no drafts.

5. Test water temperature with thermometer or against the inside of your wrist. Water temperature should be no higher than 105°F. Have resident check water temperature. Adjust if necessary.

6. Position the resident and wet the resident's hair.

a. **For washing hair in the sink**, seat the resident in a chair covered with a protective plastic drape or sheet. Use a pillow under the plastic to support the head and neck. Have the resident lean her head back toward the sink. Give the resident a folded washcloth to hold over her forehead or eyes. Wet hair using a plastic cup or a hand-held sink attachment (Fig. 13-25).

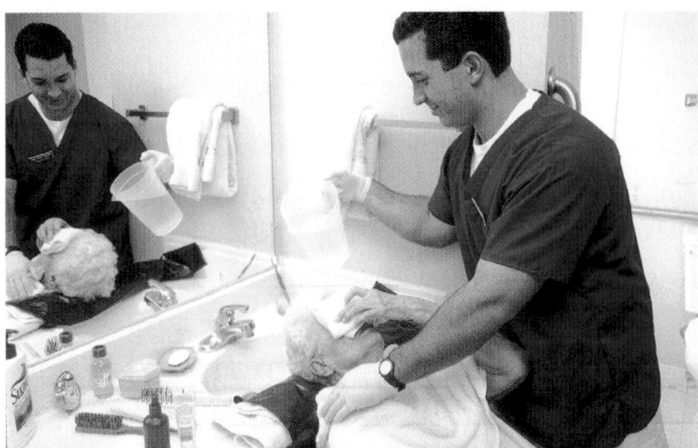

Fig. 13-25. *Make sure that the resident's head and neck are supported and her eyes are covered when washing hair in the sink.*

b. **For washing hair in bed**, arrange the supplies within reach on a nearby table. Remove all pillows, and place the resident in a flat position. Adjust bed to a safe level, usually waist high. Lock bed wheels. Place a waterproof pad beneath the resident's head and shoulders. Cover the resident with the blanket, and fold back the top sheet and regular blankets. Place the trough under the resident's head and connect trough to the catch basin. Place one towel across the resident's shoulders. Protect resident's eyes with a dry washcloth. Using the pitcher or attachment, pour enough water on the resident's hair to make it thoroughly wet.

7. Apply a small amount of shampoo to your hands and rub them together. Using both hands, massage the shampoo to a lather in the resident's hair. With your fingertips (not fingernails), massage the scalp in a circular motion, from front to back (Fig. 13-26). Do not scratch the scalp.

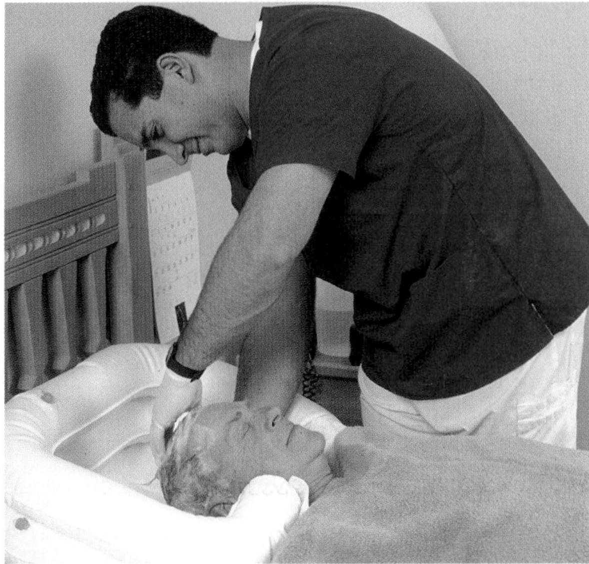

Fig. 13-26. *Use your fingertips, not your fingernails, to work shampoo into a lather. Be gentle so that you do not scratch the scalp.*

8. Rinse the hair in the same way you wet it. Rinse until water runs clear. Repeat the shampoo, rinse again, and use conditioner if the resident wants it. Be sure to rinse the hair thoroughly to prevent the scalp from getting dry and itchy.

9. Wrap the resident's hair in a clean towel. If shampooing at the sink, return the resident to an upright position. If shampooing in bed, remove the trough. Using the washcloth or towel, wipe water from the face, head, and neck.

10. Remove the hair towel and gently rub scalp and hair with the towel. Comb or brush hair (see procedure later in the chapter).

11. Dry hair with a hair dryer on the low setting. Style hair as the resident prefers.

12. Make resident comfortable.
13. Return bed to lowest position. Remove privacy measures.
14. Place call light within resident's reach.
15. Empty, rinse, and wipe bath basin/pitcher. Take to proper area.
16. Clean comb or brush. Return hair dryer and comb or brush to proper storage.
17. Place soiled linen in proper container.
18. Wash your hands.
19. Report any changes in resident to nurse.
20. Document procedure using facility guidelines.

Many people prefer showers or tub baths to bed baths (Fig. 13-27). It is important for a nursing assistant to check with the nurse first to make sure a shower or tub bath is allowed.

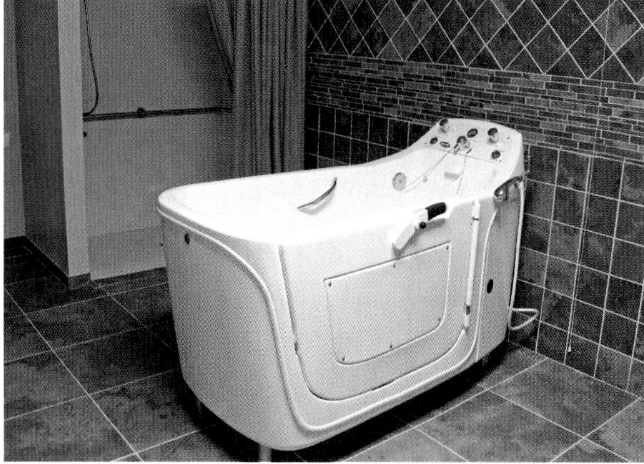

Fig. 13-27. *A common style of tub used in long-term care facilities.*

Guidelines: Safety for Showers and Tub Baths

- G Clean tub or shower before and after use.
- G Make sure bathroom or shower room floor is dry.
- G Be familiar with available safety and assistive devices. Check that handrails, grab bars, and lifts are in working order.
- G Have resident use safety bars to get into or out of the tub or shower.
- G Place all needed items within reach.
- G Do not leave the resident alone.
- G Do not use bath oils, lotions, or powders in showers or tubs. They make surfaces slippery and dangerous.
- G Test water temperature with thermometer or your wrist before resident gets into shower. Water temperature should be no higher than 105°F. Make sure temperature is comfortable for resident.

Residents' Rights

Privacy When Bathing

Privacy is very important when residents are having a shower or tub bath. Just as with a bed bath, NAs should keep residents covered when possible. Residents' bodies should not be unnecessarily exposed.

Some residents will have whirlpool baths. In a whirlpool bath, the water moves around the tub. The water movement helps clean, stimulates circulation, and promotes wound healing. To take a whirlpool bath, a resident is first covered, placed in a chairlift, and lowered into the whirlpool. The resident may feel faint or dizzy after the bath. The nursing assistant should remain with the resident while he or she is bathing.

Giving a shower or tub bath

Equipment: bath blanket, soap, shampoo, bath thermometer, 2-4 washcloths, 2-4 bath towels, clean gown and robe or clothes, non-skid footwear, 2 pairs of gloves, lotion, deodorant

1. Wash your hands.
2. Place equipment in shower or tub room. Put on gloves. Clean shower or tub area and shower chair. Place bucket under shower chair (in case resident has a bowel movement). Turn on heat lamp to warm the room, if available.
3. Remove and discard gloves. Wash your hands.

4. Go to resident's room. Identify yourself by name. Identify the resident by name.
5. Wash your hands.
6. Explain procedure to the resident. Speak clearly, slowly, and directly. Maintain face-to-face contact whenever possible.
7. Provide for resident's privacy with curtain, screen, or door.
8. Help resident put on non-skid footwear. Transport resident to shower or tub room.
9. Put on clean gloves.
10. Help resident remove clothing and shoes.

For a shower:

11. If using a shower chair, place it close to resident and lock its wheels (Fig. 13-28). Safely transfer resident into shower chair.

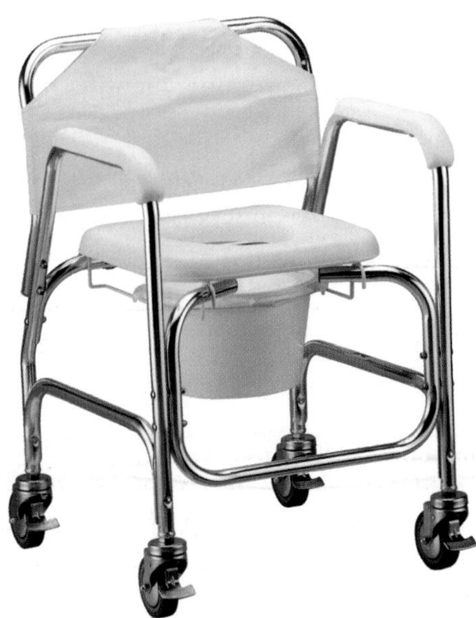

Fig. 13-28. *A* ***shower chair*** *is a sturdy chair designed to be placed in a bathtub or shower. It is water- and slip-resistant. The chair or bench enables a person who is unable to get into a tub or is too weak to stand in a shower to bathe in the tub or shower, rather than in bed. A shower chair must be locked before transferring a resident into it.* ((PHOTO COURTESY OF NOVA MEDICAL PRODUCTS, WWW.NOVAMEDICALPRODUCTS.COM)

12. Turn on water. Test water temperature with thermometer. Water temperature should be no higher than 105°F. Have resident check water temperature. Adjust if necessary. Check temperature throughout the shower.

For a tub bath:

11. Safely transfer resident onto chair or tub lift.
12. Fill the tub halfway with warm water. Test water temperature with thermometer. Water temperature should be no higher than 105°F. Have resident check water temperature. Adjust if necessary.

Remaining steps for either procedure:

13. Help the resident into shower or tub. Unlock shower chair, and move it into shower. Lock wheels.
14. Stay with resident during procedure.
15. Let resident wash as much as possible on his or her own. Help to wash his or her face.
16. Help resident shampoo and rinse hair thoroughly.
17. Using soap, help to wash and rinse the entire body. Move from head to toe (clean to dirty).
18. Turn off water or drain the tub. Cover resident with bath blanket while tub drains.
19. Unlock shower chair wheels if used. Roll resident out of shower, or help resident out of tub and onto a chair.
20. Give resident towel(s) and help to pat dry. Pat dry under the breasts, between skin folds, in the perineal area, and between toes.
21. Apply lotion and deodorant as needed.
22. Place soiled clothing and linens in proper containers.
23. Remove and discard gloves.
24. Wash your hands.
25. Help resident dress and comb hair before leaving shower room. Put on non-skid footwear. Return resident to room.

26. Make sure resident is comfortable.
27. Place call light within resident's reach.
28. Report any changes in resident to nurse.
29. Document procedure using facility guidelines.

After a resident showers or bathes, the nursing assistant may need to return to the shower room and clean the shower, shower chair, chair lift, or the tub. She should follow facility policy.

4. Explain guidelines for assisting with grooming

Grooming affects the way people feel about themselves and how they appear to others. A well-groomed person is more likely to feel better physically and emotionally (Fig. 13-29). When helping with grooming, nursing assistants should always let residents do all they can for themselves. Residents should make as many choices as possible. Some residents may be embarrassed, depressed, or anxious because they need help with grooming tasks that they have performed for themselves all their lives. Nursing assistants should be sensitive to this. Professional, respectful assistance with grooming can help residents maintain self-respect and feel good about themselves.

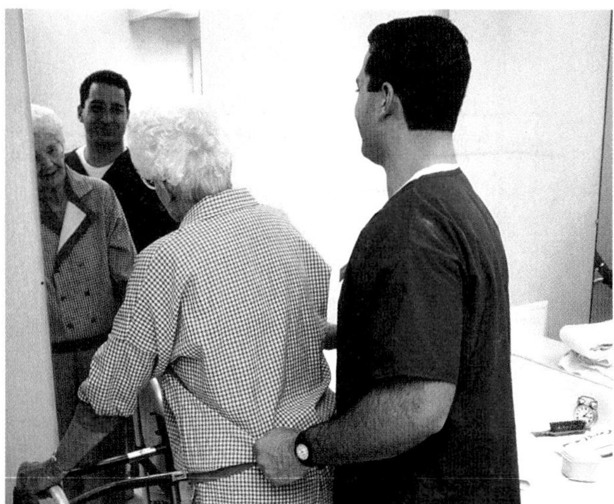

Fig. 13-29. *A well-groomed appearance helps a person feel good about herself.*

Fingernail Care

Fingernails can harbor bacteria. It is important to keep hands and nails clean to help prevent infection. Nail care should be given when assigned and when nails are dirty or have jagged edges. Nursing assistants should never cut a resident's fingernails or toenails. For some residents, poor circulation can lead to infection if skin is accidentally cut while caring for nails. For a diabetic resident, such an infection can lead to a severe wound or even amputation. Chapter 18 contains more information on diabetes. If assigned to provide nail care, the nursing assistant should know exactly what care to provide. She should never use the same nail equipment on more than one resident.

Providing fingernail care

Equipment: orangewood stick, emery board, lotion, basin, soap, washcloth, 2 towels, bath thermometer, gloves

1. Identify yourself by name. Identify the resident by name.
2. Wash your hands.
3. Explain procedure to the resident. Speak clearly, slowly, and directly. Maintain face-to-face contact whenever possible.
4. Provide for resident's privacy with curtain, screen, or door.
5. If resident is in bed, adjust bed to a safe level, usually waist high. Lock bed wheels.
6. Fill the basin halfway with warm water. Test water temperature with thermometer or against the inside of your wrist to ensure it is safe. Water temperature should be no higher than 105°F. Have resident check water temperature. Adjust if necessary. Place basin at a comfortable level for the resident.
7. Put on gloves.
8. Soak the resident's hands and nails in the water. Soak all 10 fingertips for at least five minutes.

9. Remove hands from water. Wash hands with soapy washcloth. Rinse. Pat hands dry with towel, including between fingers. Remove the hand basin.
10. Place the resident's hands on the towel. Gently clean under each fingernail with the orangewood stick (Fig. 13-30).

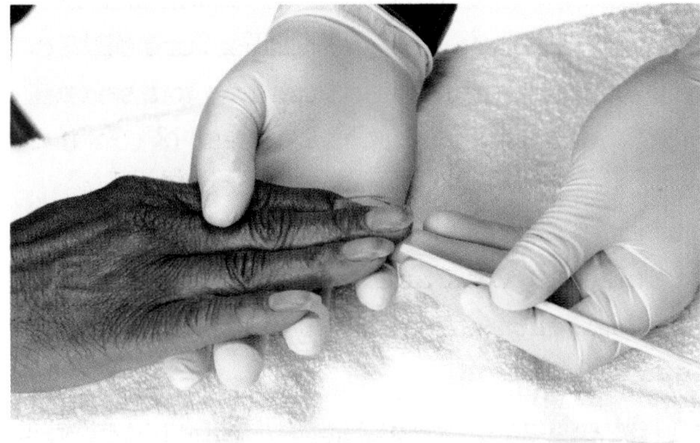

Fig. 13-30. *Be gentle when removing dirt from under the nails with an orangewood stick.*

11. Wipe orangewood stick on towel after cleaning under each nail. Wash resident's hands again. Dry them thoroughly, especially between the fingers.
12. Shape fingernails with an emery board or nail file. File in a curve. Finish with nails smooth and free of rough edges.
13. Apply lotion from fingertips to wrists.
14. Empty, rinse, and dry basin. Place basin in designated dirty supply area or return to storage, depending on facility policy.
15. Place soiled clothing and linens in proper containers.
16. Remove and discard gloves. Wash your hands.
17. Make resident comfortable.
18. Return bed to lowest position. Remove privacy measures.
19. Place call light within resident's reach.
20. Wash your hands.
21. Report any changes in resident to the nurse.
22. Document procedure using facility guidelines.

Foot Care

Careful foot care is extremely important; it should be a part of daily care of residents. Keeping the feet clean and dry helps prevent complications, especially for diabetic residents. When nursing assistants provide foot care, they should observe the feet for any of the following:

Observing and Reporting: Foot Care

Report any of these to the nurse:

- O/R Dry, flaking skin
- O/R Non-intact or broken skin
- O/R Discoloration of the feet, such as reddened, gray, white, or black areas
- O/R Blisters
- O/R Bruises
- O/R Blood or drainage
- O/R Long, ragged toenails
- O/R Ingrown toenails
- O/R Swelling
- O/R Soft, fragile heels
- O/R Differences in temperature of the feet

Providing foot care

Equipment: basin, bath mat, soap, lotion, washcloth, 2 towels, bath thermometer, clean socks, gloves

1. Identify yourself by name. Identify the resident by name.
2. Wash your hands.
3. Explain procedure to the resident. Speak clearly, slowly, and directly. Maintain face-to-face contact whenever possible.

4. Provide for resident's privacy with curtain, screen, or door.
5. If resident is in bed, adjust bed to a safe level, usually waist high. Lock bed wheels.
6. Fill the basin halfway with warm water. Test water temperature with thermometer or against the inside of your wrist to ensure it is safe. Water temperature should be no higher than 105°F. Have resident check water temperature. Adjust if necessary.
7. Place basin on a bath mat or bath towel on the floor (if the resident is sitting in a chair) or on a towel at the foot of the bed (if the resident is in bed). Make sure basin is in a comfortable position for the resident. Support the foot and ankle throughout the procedure.
8. Put on gloves.
9. Remove resident's socks. Completely submerge resident's feet in water. Soak the feet for 10 to 20 minutes. Add warm water to the basin as necessary.
10. Put soap on wet washcloth. Remove one foot from water. Wash entire foot, including between the toes and around nail beds (Fig. 13-31).

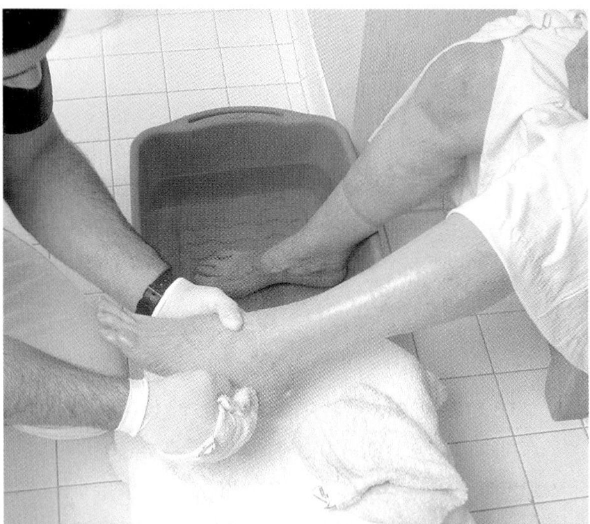

Fig. 13-31. *Soak the resident's feet before washing the entire foot, including the nail beds.*

11. Rinse entire foot, including between the toes.
12. Using towel, thoroughly dry entire foot, especially between the toes.
13. Repeat steps 10 through 12 for the other foot.
14. Put lotion in one hand and warm lotion by rubbing hands together. Massage lotion into entire foot (top and bottom), except between the toes. Remove excess, if any, with a towel.
15. Help resident put on clean socks.
16. Empty, rinse, and dry basin. Place basin in designated dirty supply area or return to storage, depending on facility policy.
17. Place soiled clothing and linens in proper containers.
18. Remove and discard gloves. Wash your hands.
19. Make resident comfortable.
20. Return bed to lowest position. Remove privacy measures.
21. Place call light within resident's reach.
22. Wash your hands.
23. Report any changes in resident to the nurse.
24. Document procedure using facility guidelines.

Shaving

Before assisting with shaving, the NA should make sure the resident wants her to shave him or help him shave. Personal preferences for shaving must be respected. NAs must wear gloves when shaving a resident due to the risk of being exposed to blood. This is a part of following Standard Precautions; it helps prevent infection.

If a resident has a beard or mustache, it will need daily care. Washing and combing a beard or mustache every day is usually enough. The

NA can ask the resident how he would like it done. She should not trim or shave a beard or mustache without a resident's permission.

There are different types of razors. NAs should check with the nurse to know which type of razor the resident uses:

- A **safety razor** has a sharp blade, which comes with a special safety casing to help prevent cuts. This type of razor requires shaving cream or soap.
- A **disposable razor** requires shaving cream or soap. It is discarded in a sharps container after use.
- An **electric razor** is the safest and easiest type of razor to use. It does not require soap or shaving cream.

Shaving a resident

Equipment: razor, basin filled halfway with warm water (if using safety or disposable razor), 2 towels, washcloth, mirror, shaving cream or soap (if using safety or disposable razor), after-shave lotion, gloves

1. Identify yourself by name. Identify the resident by name.
2. Wash your hands.
3. Explain procedure to the resident. Speak clearly, slowly, and directly. Maintain face-to-face contact whenever possible.
4. Provide for resident's privacy with curtain, screen, or door.
5. If resident is in bed, adjust bed to safe level, usually waist high. Lock bed wheels.
6. Raise the head of the bed so that the resident is sitting up. Place towel across the resident's chest, under his chin.
7. Put on gloves.

Shaving using a safety or disposable razor:

8. If using a safety or disposable razor, use a blade that is sharp. A dull blade can irritate the skin. Soften the beard with a warm, wet washcloth on the face for a few minutes before shaving. Lather the face with shaving cream or soap and warm water. Warm water and lather make shaving more comfortable.
9. Hold skin taut. Shave in the direction of hair growth. Shave beard in downward strokes on face and upward strokes on neck (Fig. 13-32). Rinse the blade often in the basin to keep it clean and wet.

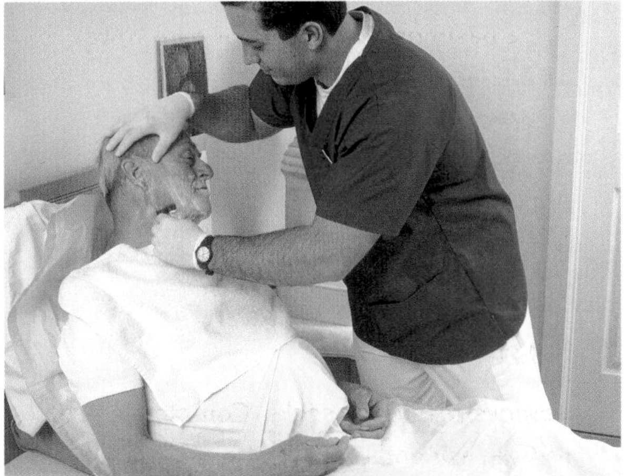

Fig. 13-32. Holding the skin taut, shave in downward strokes on face and upward strokes on neck.

10. When you have finished, wash and rinse the resident's face with a warm, wet washcloth. If he is able, let him use the washcloth himself. Use towel to dry the resident's face. Offer a mirror to the resident.

Shaving using an electric razor:

8. Use a small brush to clean the razor. Do not use an electric razor near any water source or when oxygen is in use. Electricity near water may cause electrocution. Electricity near oxygen may cause an explosion.
9. Turn on the razor and hold skin taut. Shave with smooth, even movements (Fig. 13-33). Shave beard with back and forth motion in direction of beard growth with foil shaver. Shave beard in circular motion with three-head shaver. Shave the chin and under the chin.

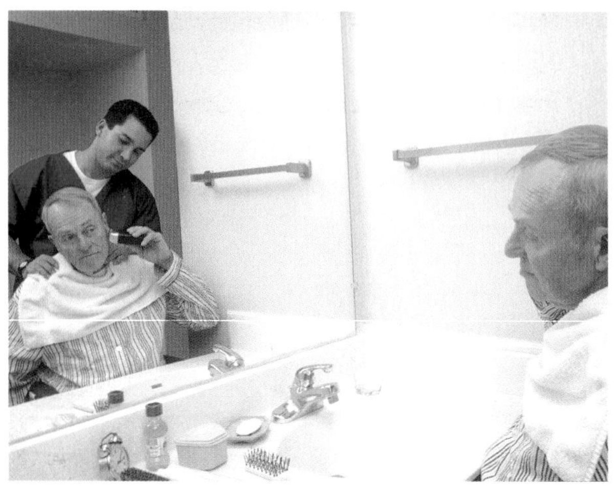

Fig. 13-33. Shave, or have the resident shave, with smooth, even movements.

10. When you have finished, offer a mirror to the resident.

Final steps:

11. If the resident wants after-shave lotion, moisten your palms with the lotion and pat it onto the resident's face.
12. Remove the towel. Place the towel and washcloth in proper container.
13. Clean the equipment and store it. For safety razor, rinse the razor. For disposable razor, dispose of it in a sharps container. For electric razor, clean head of razor. Remove whiskers from razor. Recap shaving head and return razor to case.
14. Remove and discard gloves. Wash your hands.
15. Make resident comfortable.
16. Return bed to lowest position. Remove privacy measures.
17. Place call light within resident's reach.
18. Wash your hands.
19. Report any changes in resident to the nurse.
20. Document procedure using facility guidelines.

Hair Care

Nursing assistants help keep residents' hair clean and styled. Hair ornaments should be used only as requested, and residents' hair should never be combed or brushed into childish styles. Because hair thins as people age, pieces of hair can be pulled out of the head while combing or brushing it. Nursing assistants must handle residents' hair very gently.

Pediculosis is the medical term for an infestation of lice. Lice are tiny insects that bite into the skin and suck blood to live and grow. Three types of lice are head lice, body lice, and crab or pubic lice. Head lice are usually found on the scalp. Lice are usually difficult to see. Symptoms include itching, bite marks on the scalp, skin sores, and matted, bad-smelling hair and scalp. Sometimes lice eggs can be seen on the hair, behind the ears, and on the neck. The eggs (nits) are small and round and may be brown or white. Lice droppings may be visible on sheets or pillows. They look like a fine black powder.

If nursing assistants notice any of these symptoms, they should report to the nurse immediately. Lice can spread very quickly. Special creams, shampoos, lotions, or sprays may be used to treat the lice. People who have lice spread it to others. To help prevent the spread of lice, residents' combs, brushes, clothes, wigs, and hats should not be shared with anyone else.

Dandruff is an excessive shedding of dead skin cells from the scalp. It is the result of the normal growing process of the skin cells of the scalp. The most common symptom is flaking of small, round, white patches from the head. Itching can also occur. Dandruff is a natural process. It cannot be stopped; it can only be controlled. Residents who have dandruff may use a special medicated dandruff shampoo to help control it.

Combing or brushing hair

Equipment: comb, brush, towel, mirror, hair care items requested by resident.

Use hair care products that the resident prefers for his or her type of hair.

1. Identify yourself by name. Identify the resident by name.
2. Wash your hands.
3. Explain procedure to the resident. Speak clearly, slowly, and directly. Maintain face-to-face contact whenever possible.
4. Provide for resident's privacy with curtain, screen, or door.
5. If resident is in bed, adjust bed to a safe level, usually waist high. Raise the head of the bed to have resident in an upright sitting position. Lock bed wheels. If resident is ambulatory, provide a chair.
6. Place a towel under the resident's head or around the shoulders.
7. Remove any hairpins, hair ties, or clips.
8. If the hair is tangled, work on the tangles first. Remove tangles by dividing hair into small sections. Hold lock of hair just above the tangle so you do not pull at the scalp. Gently comb or brush through the tangle. If resident agrees, you can use a small amount of detangler or leave-in conditioner.
9. After tangles are removed, brush two-inch sections of hair at a time. Brush from ends to roots (Fig. 13-34).

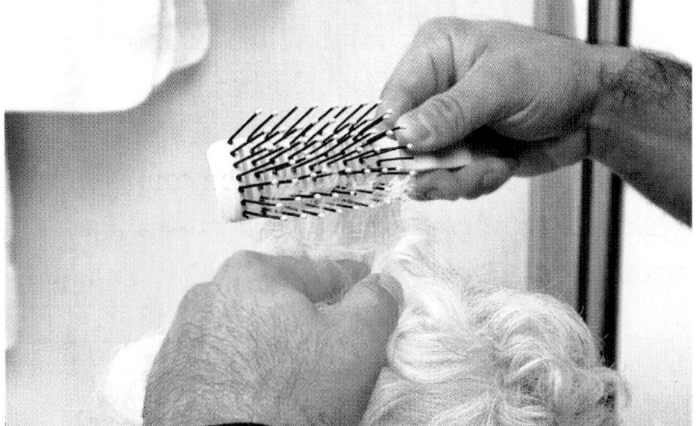

Fig. 13-34. *Gently brush hair after tangles are removed.*

10. Neatly style hair as resident prefers (Fig. 13-35). Avoid childish hairstyles. Each resident may prefer different styles. Offer mirror to the resident.

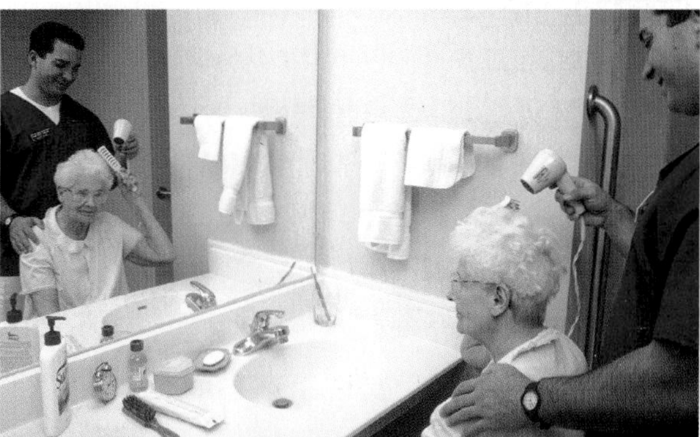

Fig. 13-35. *Assist the resident in styling her hair as she prefers it.*

11. Return supplies to proper storage. Clean hair from comb or brush. Clean comb or brush.
12. Dispose of soiled linen in the proper container.
13. Make resident comfortable.
14. Return bed to lowest position. Remove privacy measures.
15. Place call light within resident's reach.
16. Wash your hands.
17. Report any changes in resident to nurse.
18. Document procedure using facility guidelines.

5. List guidelines for assisting with dressing

Dressing and undressing residents is an important part of daily care. When helping with dressing, the NA should know what limitations the resident has. Residents may have one side of the body that is weaker than the other side due to stroke or injury. This side is called the **affected side**. It will be weaker. The NA should never refer to the weaker side as the "bad side" or talk about the "bad" leg or arm. The terms weaker or

involved should be used to refer to the affected side. When dressing residents, the NA should always begin with the weaker side of the body to reduce the risk of injury. The weaker arm is placed through a sleeve first (Fig. 13-36). When a leg is weak, it is easier if the resident sits down to pull the pants over both legs.

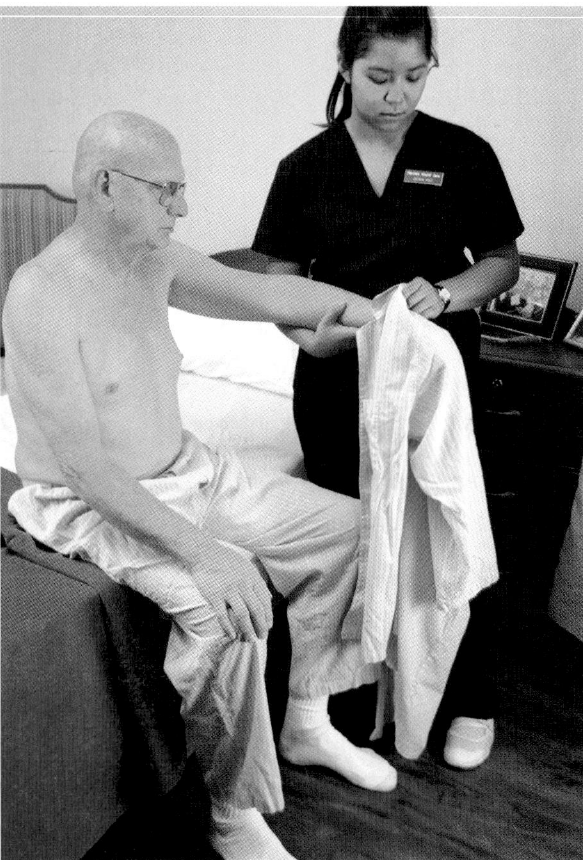

Fig. 13-36. *When dressing, the NA should start with the affected (weaker) side first.*

Guidelines: Dressing and Undressing

- G As with all care, ask about and follow the resident's preferences. Remember, resident-directed care is the resident's legal right and your responsibility.
- G Let the resident choose clothing for the day. However, check to see if it is clean, appropriate for the weather, and in good condition.
- G Encourage the resident to dress in regular clothes rather than nightclothes. Wearing regular daytime clothing encourages more activity and out-of-bed time. Elastic-waist pants or skirts are easy to pull on over legs and hips. Be sure the elastic waistband of underpants, slip, pantyhose, pants, or skirt fits comfortably at the waist. Clothing that is a size larger than the resident would normally wear is easier to put on.
- G The resident should do as much to dress or undress himself as possible. It may take longer, but it helps maintain independence and regain self-care skills. Ask where your help is needed.
- G Provide privacy. If the resident has just had a bath, cover him with the bath blanket. Put on undergarments first. Never expose more than you need to.
- G When putting on socks or stockings, roll or fold them down. They can then be slipped over the toes and foot, then unrolled up into place. Make sure toes, heels, and seams of socks or stockings are in the right place.
- G For a female resident, make sure bra cups fit over the breasts. Front-fastening bras are easier for residents to fasten by themselves. Bras that fasten in back can be put around the waist and fastened first, then rotated around and moved up. Arms can be put through the straps last. This can be done in reverse for undressing.
- G For residents who have weakness or paralysis on one side, place the weaker arm or leg through the garment first, then the strong arm or leg. When undressing, do the opposite—start with the stronger, or unaffected side.
- G Several types of adaptive aids for dressing are available to help residents maintain independence in dressing themselves (Fig. 13-37). An occupational therapist may teach residents to perform ADLs using adaptive equipment.

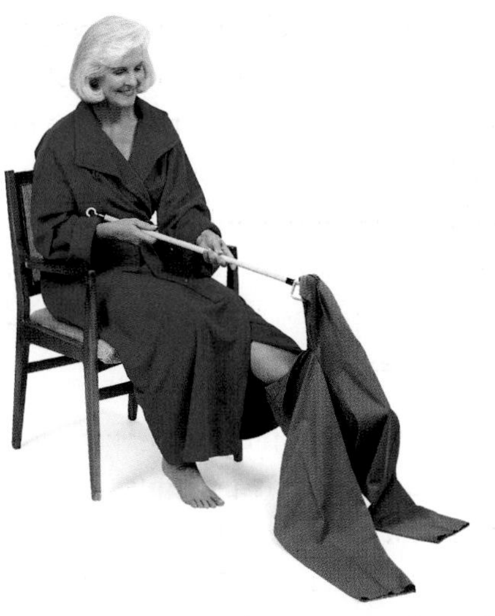

Fig. 13-37. Special dressing aids promote independence by helping residents dress themselves. (PHOTO COURTESY OF NORTH COAST MEDICAL, INC., WWW.NCMEDICAL.COM, 800-821-9319)

Dressing a resident

Equipment: clean clothes of resident's choice, non-skid footwear

When putting on all items, move resident's body gently and naturally. Avoid force and over-extension of limbs and joints.

1. Identify yourself by name. Identify the resident by name.
2. Wash your hands.
3. Explain procedure to the resident. Speak clearly, slowly, and directly. Maintain face-to-face contact whenever possible.
4. Provide for resident's privacy with curtain, screen, or door.
5. Ask resident what she would like to wear. Dress her in outfit of choice (Fig 13-38).
6. Remove resident's gown or top without completely exposing the resident. Take clothes off the unaffected, or stronger, side first when undressing. Then remove from weaker side.
7. Help resident put affected, or weaker, arm through the sleeve of the shirt, sweater, or slip before placing garment on the unaffected arm.

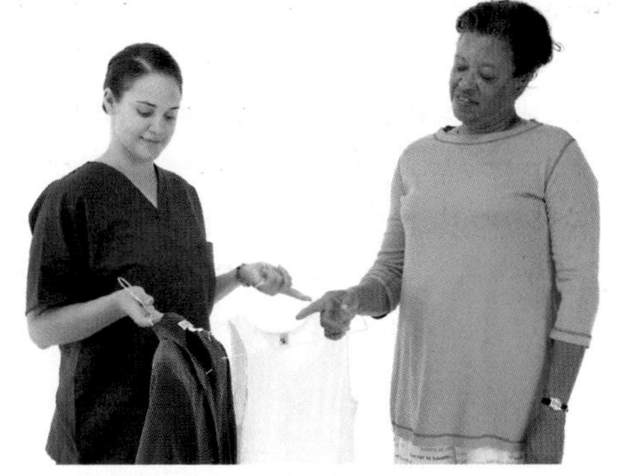

Fig. 13-38. Residents have a legal right to choose the clothing they want to wear for the day.

8. Help resident put on skirt, pants, or dress. Put the affected (weaker) leg through the skirt or pants first. Then place unaffected (stronger) leg through the skirt or pants.
9. Place bed at the lowest position. Lock bed wheels.
10. Have resident sit down and help put on socks and non-skid footwear. Tie laces.
11. Finish with resident dressed appropriately. Make sure clothing is right-side-out and zippers and buttons are fastened.
12. Place gown in soiled linen container.
13. Keep bed in lowest position. Remove privacy measures.
14. Place call light within resident's reach.
15. Wash your hands.
16. Report any changes in resident to the nurse.
17. Document procedure using facility guidelines.

6. Identify guidelines for proper oral care

Oral care, or care of the mouth, teeth, and gums, is performed at least twice each day to clean the mouth. Oral care should be done after breakfast and after the last meal or snack of the day. It may also be done before a resident eats. Oral care includes brushing teeth, tongue, and gums; flossing teeth with dental floss; caring for lips; and caring for dentures (Fig. 13-39). **Dental floss** is a special kind of string used to clean between teeth. When giving oral care, nursing assistants must wear gloves and follow Standard Precautions.

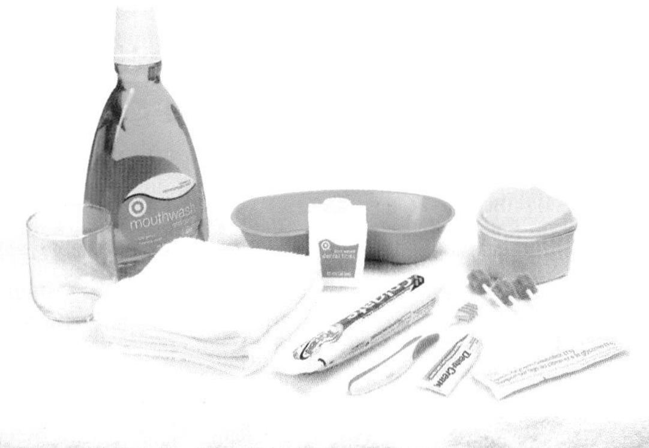

Fig. 13-39. *Some supplies needed for oral care.*

Proper, regular oral care can help prevent disease and bad breath (**halitosis**). Regular oral care also promotes a healthy appetite. Cleaning the mouth removes particles and leftover food, which makes eating more pleasant. Residents who are unconscious, are on oxygen, or have tubes in their noses or mouths need frequent oral care. Also, if they are not taking any fluids by mouth or are taking medications which dry their mouths, they will need oral care more often. When an NA performs oral care, he should observe the resident's mouth carefully.

Observing and Reporting: Oral Care

Report any of these to the nurse:

- O/R Irritation
- O/R Infection
- O/R Raised areas
- O/R Coated or swollen tongue
- O/R Ulcers, such as canker sores or small, painful, white sores
- O/R Flaky, white spots
- O/R Dry, cracked, bleeding, or chapped lips
- O/R Loose, chipped, broken, or decayed teeth
- O/R Swollen, irritated, bleeding, or whitish gums
- O/R Breath that smells bad or fruity
- O/R Resident reports of mouth pain

Providing oral care

Equipment: toothbrush, toothpaste, emesis basin, gloves, towel, glass of water, lip moisturizer

Maintain clean technique with placement of the toothbrush throughout procedure.

1. Identify yourself by name. Identify the resident by name.
2. Wash your hands.
3. Explain procedure to the resident. Speak clearly, slowly, and directly. Maintain face-to-face contact whenever possible.
4. Provide for resident's privacy with curtain, screen, or door.
5. If resident is in bed, adjust bed to a safe level, usually waist high. Raise the head of the bed to have resident in an upright sitting position. Lock bed wheels.
6. Put on gloves.
7. Place a towel across the resident's chest.
8. Wet toothbrush and put on small amount of toothpaste.
9. Clean entire mouth, including the tongue and all surfaces of teeth and the gumline, using gentle strokes. First brush inner, outer, and chewing surfaces of the upper teeth, then do the same with the lower teeth. Use short strokes. Brush back and forth. Brush tongue.
10. Give the resident the glass of water to rinse the mouth. Place the emesis basin under the resident's chin, with the inward curve under the chin. Have resident spit water into emesis basin (Fig. 13-40). Wipe resident's mouth and remove towel. Apply lip moisturizer.

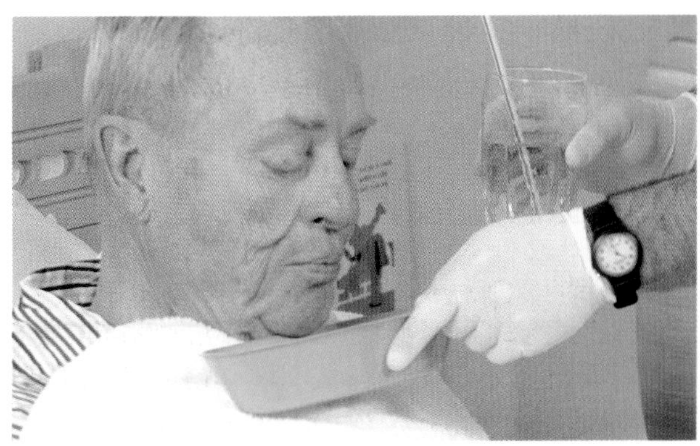

Fig. 13-40. Rinsing and spitting removes food particles and toothpaste.

11. Empty, rinse, and dry basin. Place basin in designated dirty supply area or return to storage, depending on facility policy.
12. Place soiled clothing and linens in proper containers.
13. Remove and discard gloves. Wash your hands.
14. Make resident comfortable.
15. Return bed to lowest position. Remove privacy measures.
16. Place call light within resident's reach.
17. Wash your hands.
18. Report any problems with teeth, mouth, tongue, and lips to nurse. This includes odor, cracking, sores, bleeding, and any discoloration.
19. Document procedure using facility guidelines.

Oral care does not just involve taking care of the teeth. Residents who do not have teeth will need oral care performed, too. **Edentulous** means having no teeth. For edentulous residents, NAs will clean the mouth, tongue, and gums using mouthwash or other solution on gauze or swabs. The gauze can be wrapped on a tongue blade and moistened with mouthwash or solution if swabs are not available.

Even though residents who are unconscious cannot eat, breathing through the mouth causes saliva to dry in the mouth. Oral care needs to be performed more frequently to keep the mouth clean and moist.

With unconscious residents, NAs must use as little liquid as possible when giving mouth care. Because the person's swallowing reflex is weak, he or she is at risk for aspiration. **Aspiration** is the inhalation of food, fluid, or foreign material into the lungs. Aspiration can cause pneumonia or death. Turning unconscious residents on their sides before giving oral care can also help prevent aspiration. For these residents, only swabs soaked in tiny amounts of fluid should be used to clean the mouth.

Providing oral care for the unconscious resident

Equipment: sponge swabs, tongue depressor, towel, emesis basin, gloves, glass of water, lip moisturizer, cleaning solution (check the care plan)

1. Identify yourself by name. Identify the resident by name. Even residents who are unconscious may be able to hear you. Always speak to them as you would to any resident.
2. Wash your hands.
3. Explain procedure to the resident. Speak clearly, slowly, and directly. Maintain face-to-face contact whenever possible.
4. Provide for resident's privacy with curtain, screen, or door.
5. Adjust bed to a safe level, usually waist high. Lock bed wheels.
6. Put on gloves.
7. Turn resident on his side or turn his head to the side. Place a towel under his cheek and chin. Place an emesis basin next to the cheek and chin so that excess fluid flows into the basin.
8. Hold mouth open with the tongue depressor.

9. Dip the sponge swab in the cleaning solution. Squeeze excess solution to prevent aspiration. Wipe teeth, gums, tongue, and inside surfaces of mouth. Remove debris with the swab. Change swab often. Repeat this step until the mouth is clean (Fig. 13-41).

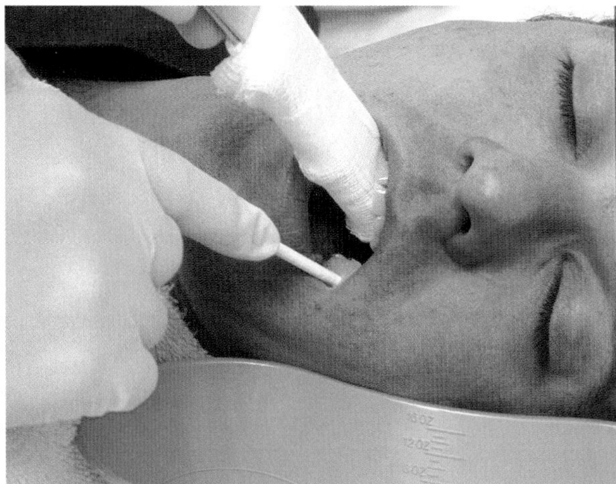

Fig. 13-41. *Wipe all inside surfaces of the mouth to clean the mouth, stimulate the gums, and remove mucus.*

10. Rinse with clean swab dipped in water. Squeeze swab first to remove excess water.
11. Remove the towel and basin. Pat lips or face dry if needed. Apply lip moisturizer.
12. Empty, rinse, and dry basin. Place basin in designated dirty supply area or return to storage, depending on facility policy.
13. Place soiled linens in the proper container.
14. Remove and discard gloves. Wash your hands.
15. Return bed to lowest position. Remove privacy measures.
16. Place call light within resident's reach.
17. Wash your hands.
18. Report any problems with teeth, mouth, tongue, and lips to nurse. This includes odor, cracking, sores, bleeding, and any discoloration.
19. Document procedure using facility guidelines.

Flossing the teeth removes plaque and tartar buildup around the gum line and between the teeth. Teeth may be flossed immediately after or before they are brushed, as the resident prefers. Nursing assistants should follow the care plan's instructions regarding flossing.

Flossing teeth

Equipment: dental floss, glass of water, emesis basin, gloves, towel

1. Identify yourself by name. Identify the resident by name.
2. Wash your hands.
3. Explain procedure to the resident. Speak clearly, slowly, and directly. Maintain face-to-face contact whenever possible.
4. Provide for resident's privacy with curtain, screen, or door.
5. If resident is in bed, adjust bed to a safe level, usually waist high. Raise the head of the bed to have resident in an upright sitting position. Lock bed wheels.
6. Put on gloves.
7. Wrap the ends of floss securely around each of your index fingers (Fig. 13-42).

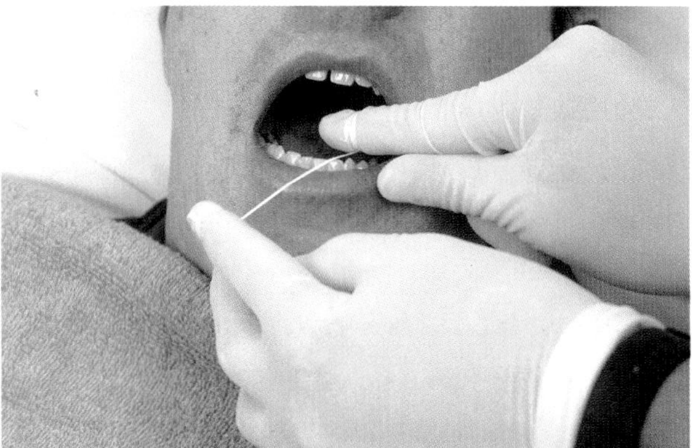

Fig. 13-42. *Before beginning, wrap floss securely around each index finger.*

8. Starting with the back teeth, place the floss between teeth. Move it down the surface of the tooth using a gentle sawing motion (Fig. 13-43).

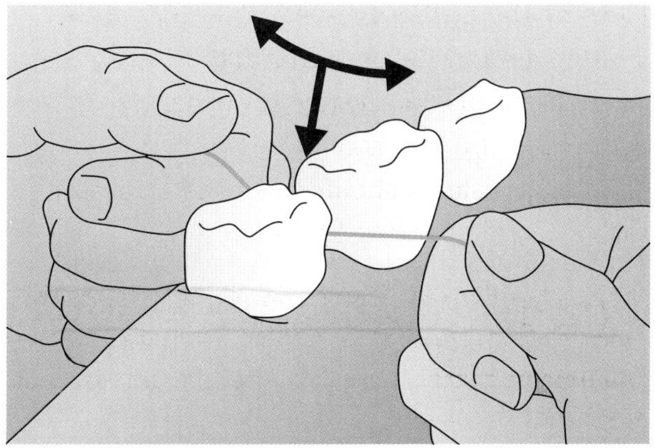

Fig. 13-43. Being gentle protects the gums.

Continue to the gum line. At the gum line, curve the floss. Slip it gently into the space between the gum and tooth, then go back up, scraping that side of the tooth (Fig. 13-44). Repeat this on the side of the other tooth.

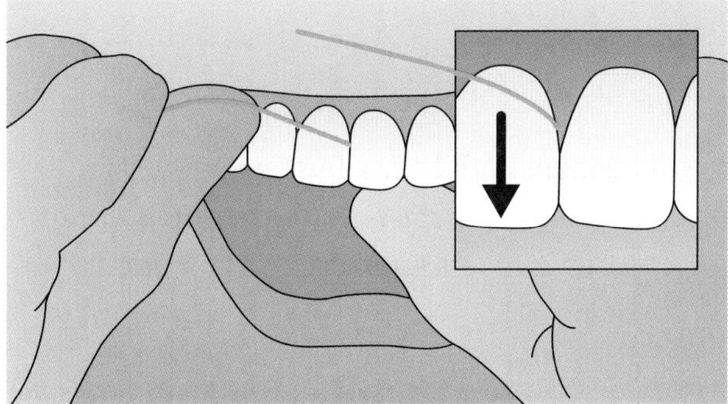

Fig. 13-44. Floss gently in the space between the gum and tooth. This removes food and prevents tooth decay.

9. After every two teeth, unwind floss from your fingers. Move it so you are using a clean area. Floss all teeth.
10. Occasionally offer water so that the resident can rinse debris from the mouth into the emesis basin.
11. Offer resident a face towel when done flossing all teeth.
12. Discard floss. Discard water and rinse and dry the basin. Place basin in designated dirty supply area or return to storage, depending on facility policy.
13. Place soiled linens in the proper container.
14. Remove and discard gloves. Wash your hands.
15. Make resident comfortable.
16. Return bed to lowest position. Remove privacy measures.
17. Place call light within resident's reach.
18. Wash your hands.
19. Report any problems with teeth, mouth, tongue, and lips to nurse. This includes odor, cracking, sores, bleeding, and any discoloration.
20. Document procedure using facility guidelines.

7. Define *dentures* and explain how to care for dentures

Dentures are artificial teeth. They are expensive, so it is important to take good care of them. Dentures must be handled carefully to avoid breaking or chipping them. If a resident's dentures break, he or she cannot eat. Nursing assistants must wear gloves when handling and cleaning dentures. The NA should notify the nurse if a resident's dentures do not fit properly, are chipped, or are missing.

Each person has his own preference about when and how denture care should be done. The NA should ask the resident how she can assist with denture care. Dentures should be stored in a denture cup labeled with the resident's name and room number. The dentures should be matched to the correct resident. Dentures should be stored in solution or in cool or moderate/tepid water. Hot water may damage dentures.

Residents' Rights

Denture Care

Denture care is very personal. The NA should always pull the privacy curtain and close the door before beginning. Many people who have dentures do not want to be seen without their teeth in place. When the NA removes the teeth, he should clean and return them immediately.

Cleaning and storing dentures

Equipment: denture brush or toothbrush, denture cleanser or tablet, labeled denture cup, 2 towels, gloves

1. Wash your hands.
2. Put on gloves.
3. Line the sink or a basin with one or two towels and partially fill sink with water. The towel and water will prevent the dentures from breaking if they slip from your hands and fall into the sink.
4. Rinse dentures in cool or tepid running water before brushing them. Do not use hot water, or dentures may warp.
5. Apply toothpaste or cleanser to denture brush or toothbrush.
6. Brush dentures on all surfaces (Fig. 13-45).

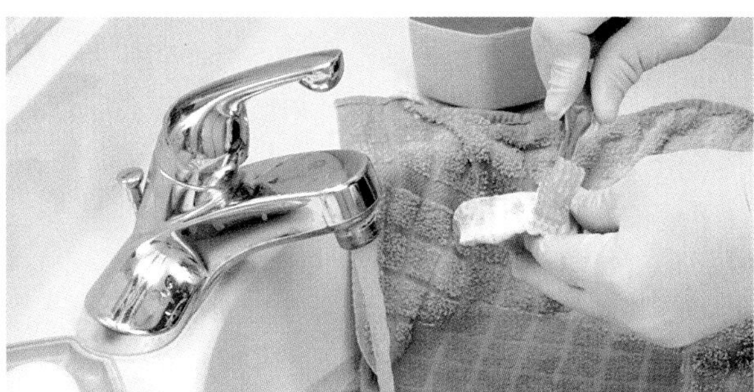

Fig. 13-45. *Brush dentures on all surfaces to properly clean them.*

7. Rinse all surfaces of dentures under cool or tepid running water. Do not use hot water.
8. Rinse denture cup before placing clean dentures in the cup.
9. Place dentures in clean denture cup with solution or cool or tepid water to prevent them from warping. Place lid on cup. Make sure cup is labeled with resident's name and room number. Put denture cup where it is normally stored. Some residents will want to wear dentures all of the time. They will only remove them for cleaning. If the resident wants to continue wearing dentures, return them to him or her. Do not place them in denture cup.
10. Clean, dry, and return the equipment to proper storage. Drain sink. Place soiled linens in the proper container.
11. Remove and discard gloves. Wash your hands.
12. Document procedure using facility guidelines. Report any changes in appearance of dentures to the nurse.

Removing and Reinserting Dentures

If a resident cannot remove her dentures, the NA must do it if trained and allowed to do so. The NA should make sure the resident is sitting upright, and she should don gloves before beginning. The lower denture should be removed first. The lower denture is easier to remove because it floats on the gum line of the lower jaw. The NA should grasp the lower denture with a gauze square (for a good grip) and remove it. She should place it in a denture cup filled with solution or moderate-temperature water.

The upper denture is sealed by suction. The NA should firmly grasp the upper denture with a gauze square and give a slight downward pull to break the suction. She should turn it at an angle to take it out of the mouth.

When inserting dentures, the NA should ask the resident to sit upright, and she should don gloves. If needed, she should apply denture cream or adhesive to the dentures. When the resident's mouth is open, the upper denture should be placed into the mouth by turning it at an angle. The NA should straighten it and press it onto the upper gum line firmly and evenly (Fig. 13-46). She should insert the lower denture onto the gum line of the lower jaw and press firmly.

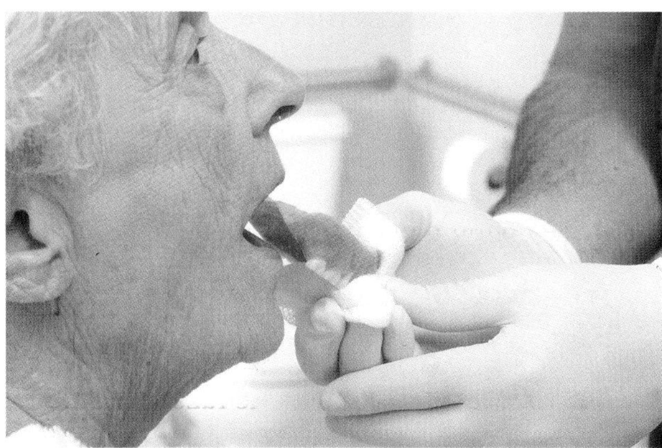

Fig. 13-46. *The NA should press the upper denture onto the upper gum line firmly and evenly.*

Chapter Review

1. List four examples of activities of daily living (ADLs). Eating, Getting dressed, Going to the toilet, Brushing teeth, Combing hair, transferring etc.
2. List five reasons that a resident may need help with personal care. 1) A person has a long-term, chronic condition 2) They may be weak & frail 3) They may be disabled 4) Ready to Die 5) Dizzy or ill
3. Give four examples of how to promote dignity and independence while giving personal care. 1) Let the resident make as many decisions as possible 2) Don't interrupt resident while they are in bathroom 3) Knock before you enter their room. 4) Leave the room if they make phone calls.
4. What are five things about a resident that a nursing assistant can observe during personal care? 1) any complaints about skin etc. or observations. 2) Do they have numbness or tingling anywhere? 3) How is their mental or emotional status? 4) Is resident short of breath? 5) Do they tremble or shake?
5. Why is preventing pressure ulcers extremely important? When a pressure ulcer forms, it can get bigger & deeper & infected quickly and becomes difficult, dangerous & life threatening
6. When skin begins to break down, what does it look like? pale or white or a reddened color. Darker skin may look purple.
7. List ten signs to observe and report about a resident's skin.
   Signs about a resident's skin
   1) Pale, white or reddened or purple
   2) Bruises or blisters
   3) c/o burning skin or tingling, warmth
   4) Dry or flaking skin
   5) Itching or scratching
   6) Rash or skin discoloration.
   7) Swelling
   8) Fluid or blood draining from skin
   9) Tears or rips in skin (broken)
   10) ulcers on skin
   11) change in wound or ulcer, foul odor, size depth etc.
   12) Broken skin, redness of skin around toes & fingernails.
   13) Feel of tissue is different (bumpy, rough)
8. At a minimum, how often should residents be repositioned? Every 2 hours if bed ridden and every hour if in a wheelchair. Every 15 minutes is preferable though in a wheelchair.
9. List four examples of positioning devices and explain how they can help. 1) Handrolls keep fingers and hand in a natural position, 2) Knee pillows help keep knees, hips & spine aligned, 3) Padded heel protectors keep feet aligned & pressure off... Footboards prevent foot drop. Bed cradles keep heavy covers off feet. Draw sheets prevent ...
10. Why is it unnecessary for many elderly people to have a complete bath or shower every day? Because their skin is dry & fragile & they don't perspire like we do when younger. Bathing often makes skin more dry.
11. Why should residents, as well as NAs, test the water temperature before bathing? It might be too hot for them or cold even at 105°F
12. Why should the nursing assistant wipe from front to back when giving perineal care? You always work from less dirty to more dirty to control the bacteria load.
13. List two benefits of back rubs. It is very comforting and it increases circulation
14. Why should bath oils, lotions, or powders NOT be used in showers or tubs? Because they could be very slippery & there would be a fall risk.
15. Explain why NAs must be especially careful while giving nail care to diabetic residents. Because a cut or tear could lead to infection, become serious and even a limb or arm might need amputation.
16. Why should an NA wear gloves while shaving residents? Transmission based precautions. Because of the Standard Precautions rules with blood involved if there was a cut. Blood-borne pathogen precautions
17. List the reasons why electric razors should not be used near water or when oxygen is in use. Electricity near water can cause electrocution & electricity near oxygen could cause an explosion.
18. What are the symptoms of head lice? Itching, bite marks on the scalp, matted bad smelling hair. Eggs white or brown on hair shaft. Lice droppings look like fine black powder.
19. If a resident has an affected side due to a stroke or an injury, how should the NA refer to that side? As the involved side or the affected or weaker side.
20. When dressing a resident with a weaker side, which arm is usually placed through the sleeve first—the weaker or stronger arm?
21. What does oral care consist of? Taking care to clean the mouth, teeth & gums, tongue & flossing teeth, care of dentures if they have them.
22. What is the minimum number of times per day that oral care is done? At least twice a day. AM & PM.
23. How can NAs help prevent aspiration during oral care of unconscious residents? Turn resident to the side or lay on his side. Put a basin next to cheek & chin so excess water flows into it. Squeeze out excess water from sponge to prevent aspiration. Use less water
24. Why should hot water not be used on dentures? Hot water can cause dentures to warp or become damaged.

14 Basic Nursing Skills

1. Explain the importance of monitoring vital signs

Nursing assistants monitor, document, and report residents' **vital signs**. Vital signs are important. They show how well the vital organs of the body, such as the heart and lungs, are working. They consist of the following:

- Measuring the body temperature
- Counting the pulse
- Counting the rate of respirations
- Measuring the blood pressure
- Observing and reporting the level of pain

Watching for changes in vital signs is very important. Changes can indicate that a resident's condition is worsening. Nursing assistants do not make diagnoses based on vital signs, but they do record accurate measurements and report changes and observations to the nurse. An NA should always notify the nurse if

- The resident has a fever (temperature is above average for the resident or outside the normal range)
- The resident has a respiratory or pulse rate that is too rapid or too slow
- The resident's blood pressure changes
- The resident's pain is worse or is not relieved by pain management

Ranges for Adult Vital Signs

Temp. Site	Fahrenheit	Celsius
Mouth (oral)	97.6°–99.6°	36.5°–37.5°
Rectum (rectal)	98.6°–100.6°	37.0°–38.1°
Armpit (axilla)	96.6°–98.6°	36.0°–37.0°
Ear (tympanic)	96.6°–99.7°	35.8°–37.6°
Temporal Artery	97.2°–100.1°	36.2°–37.8°

Normal Pulse Rate: 60–100 beats per minute
Normal Respiratory Rate: 12–20 respirations per minute

Blood Pressure

Normal	Systolic 100–119 Diastolic 60–79
Low	Below 100/60
Prehypertensive	Systolic 120–139 Diastolic 80–89
High	140/90 or above

Residents' Rights

Vital Signs

Nursing assistants should protect residents' privacy while taking vital signs by not exposing them. If an NA needs to measure blood pressure or move clothing out of the way, she should pull the privacy curtain around the bed and close the door. NAs should not discuss residents' vital sign measurements when near other people. They should report the information to the nurse.

2. List guidelines for measuring body temperature

Body temperature is normally very close to 98.6°F (Fahrenheit) or 37°C (Celsius). Body temperature reflects a balance between the heat created by the body and the heat lost to the environment. Many factors affect body temperature: age, illness, stress, environment, exercise, and the circadian rhythm can all cause changes in body temperature. The circadian rhythm is the 24-hour day-night cycle. Average temperature readings change throughout the day. People tend to have lower temperatures in the morning. Increases in body temperature may indicate an infection or disease.

There are different sites for measuring the body's temperature: the mouth (oral), the rectum (rectal), the armpit (axilla), the ear (tympanic), and the temporal artery (the artery under the skin of the forehead). The different sites require different thermometers. Temperatures are most often taken orally. A nursing assistant should not take an oral temperature on a person who

- Is unconscious
- Has recently had facial or oral surgery
- Is younger than 5 years old
- Is confused or disoriented
- Is heavily sedated
- Is likely to have a seizure
- Is coughing
- Is using oxygen
- Has facial paralysis
- Has a nasogastric tube (a feeding tube that is inserted through the nose and goes into the stomach)
- Has sores, redness, swelling, or pain in the mouth
- Has an injury to the face or neck

There are several types of thermometers, including the following:

- Mercury-free
- Digital
- Electronic
- Disposable
- Tympanic
- Temporal artery

Mercury-free thermometers can be used to take oral, rectal, or axillary temperatures. Thermometers are usually color-coded to show which is an oral and which is a rectal thermometer. Oral thermometers are usually green or blue; rectal thermometers are usually red (Fig. 14-1).

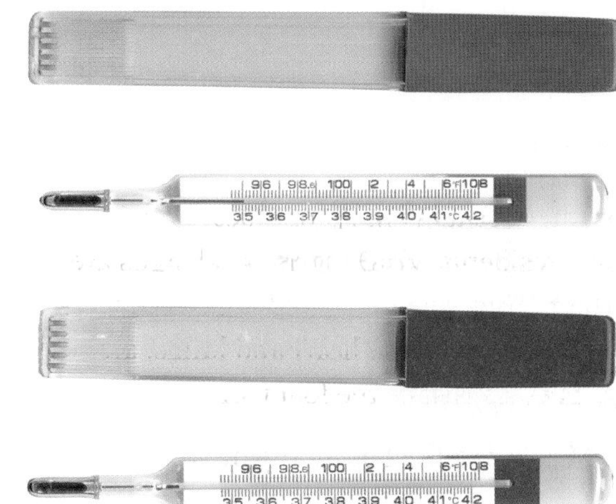

Fig. 14-1. *A mercury-free oral thermometer and a mercury-free rectal thermometer. Oral thermometers are usually green or blue; rectal thermometers are usually red.* (PHOTOS COURTESY OF RG MEDICAL DIAGNOSTICS OF WIXOM, MI, RGMD.COM)

Numbers on the thermometer allow the temperature to be read after it registers. Most thermometers show the temperature in degrees Fahrenheit (F). Each long line represents one degree, and each short line represents two-tenths of a degree. Some thermometers show the temperature in degrees Celsius (C), with the long lines representing one degree and the short lines representing one-tenth of a degree. Small arrows or highlighted numbers show the normal temperature: 98.6°F and 37°C (Fig. 14-2).

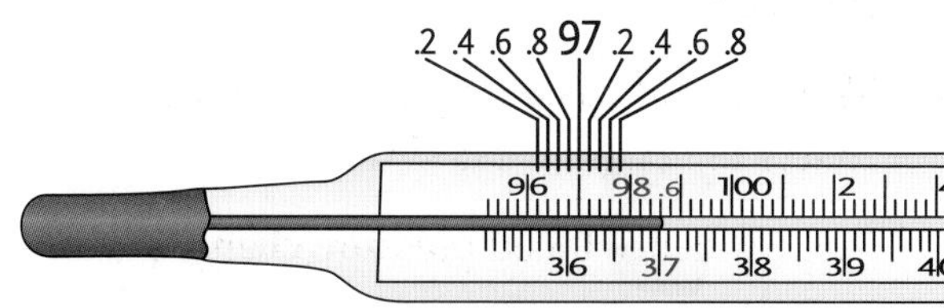

Fig. 14-2. *This shows a normal temperature reading: 98.6°F and 37°C.*

Digital or electronic thermometers can be used to take oral, rectal, or axillary temperatures (Figs. 14-3 and 14-4). These thermometers display the results digitally and register the temperature more quickly than mercury-free thermometers. These thermometers usually take two to sixty seconds to register the temperature. The thermometer will beep or flash when the temperature has registered. A digital thermometer may require a disposable plastic sheath to cover the probe to help prevent infection. The electronic thermometer must have a probe cover applied before use. The manufacturer's instructions explain the proper use of these thermometers.

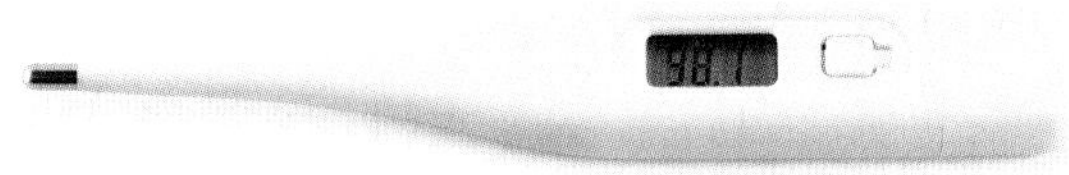

Fig. 14-3. A digital thermometer.

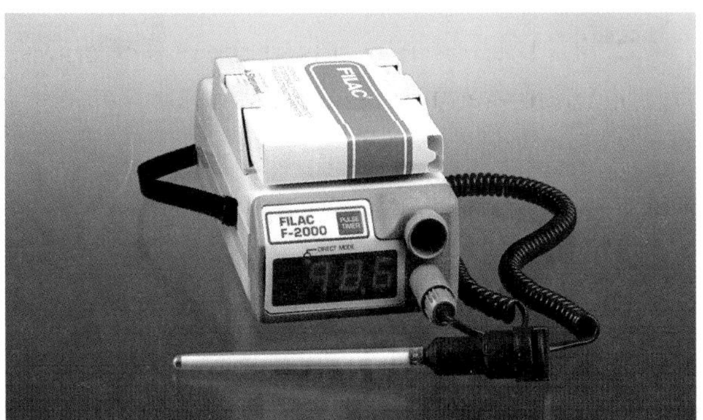

Fig. 14-4. An electronic thermometer.

Disposable thermometers register temperatures in 60 seconds. Usually a colored dot shows the temperature (Fig. 14-5). Disposable thermometers are often individually wrapped. They are only used once and then discarded in the proper container. Disposable, or single-use, equipment helps prevent infection.

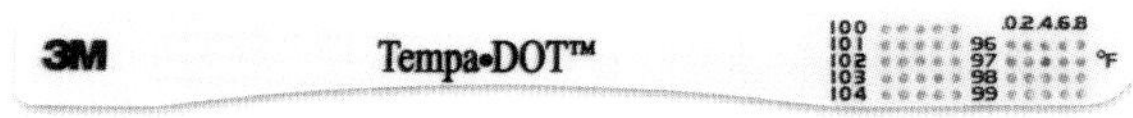

Fig. 14-5. One type of disposable thermometer.

The tympanic thermometer, or ear thermometer, registers a temperature quickly (Fig. 14-6). These thermometers require more practice to be able to take accurate temperatures.

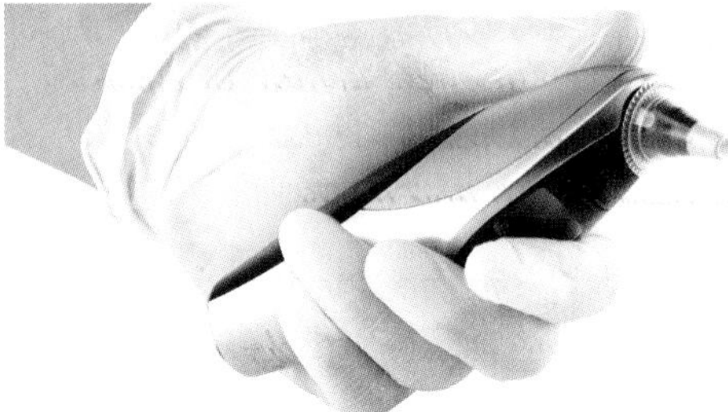

Fig. 14-6. A tympanic thermometer with a disposable sheath on the earpiece.

Temporal artery thermometers determine temperature readings by measuring the heat from the skin over the temporal artery. This is done by a gentle stroke or scan across the forehead (Fig. 14-7). Temporal artery thermometers are non-invasive, which means that they are not inserted into the body.

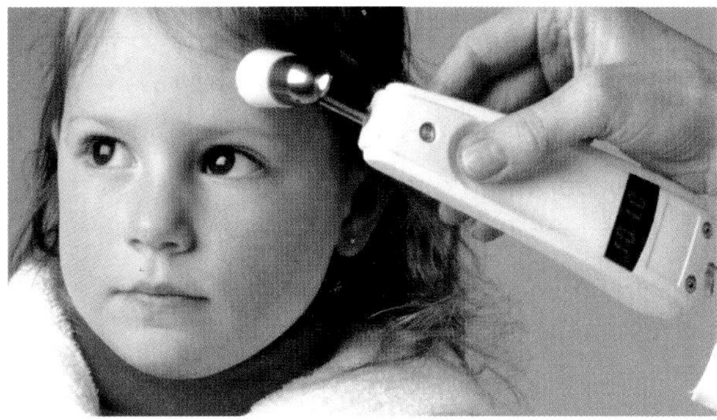

Fig. 14-7. A temporal artery thermometer. (PHOTO COURTESY OF EXERGEN CORPORATION, 800-422-3006, WWW.EXERGEN.COM)

There is a range of normal temperatures. Some people's temperatures normally run low. Others will run slightly higher temperatures, even in good health. Normal temperature readings also vary by the method used to take the temperature. A rectal temperature is considered to be the most accurate. However, taking a rectal temperature on an uncooperative person, such as a resident with dementia, can be dangerous. An axillary temperature is considered the least accurate.

Measuring and recording an oral temperature

Do not take an oral temperature on a resident who has smoked, eaten or drunk fluids, chewed gum, or exercised in the last 10-20 minutes.

Equipment: clean mercury-free, digital, or electronic thermometer, gloves, disposable sheath/cover for thermometer, tissues, pen and paper

1. Identify yourself by name. Identify the resident by name.
2. Wash your hands.
3. Explain procedure to the resident. Speak clearly, slowly, and directly. Maintain face-to-face contact whenever possible.
4. Provide for resident's privacy with curtain, screen, or door.
5. Put on gloves.
6. **Mercury-free thermometer**: Hold the thermometer by the stem. Before inserting it in the resident's mouth, shake thermometer down to below the lowest number (at least below 96°F or 35°C). To shake the thermometer down, hold it at the end opposite the bulb with the thumb and two fingers. With a snapping motion of the wrist, shake the thermometer (Fig. 14-8). Stand away from furniture and walls while doing so.

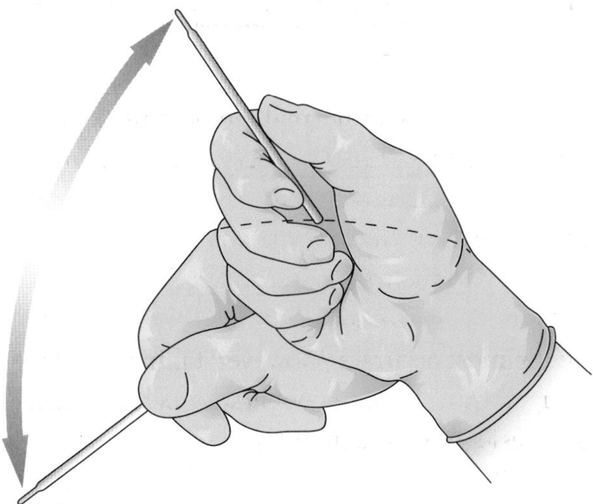

Fig. 14-8. *Shake thermometer down to below the lowest number before inserting in a resident's mouth.*

   Digital thermometer: Put on the disposable sheath. Turn on thermometer and wait until *ready* sign appears.

   Electronic thermometer: Remove the probe from base unit. Put on probe cover.

7. **Mercury-free thermometer**: Put on disposable sheath if available. Insert bulb end of the thermometer into resident's mouth, under tongue and to one side (Fig. 14-9).

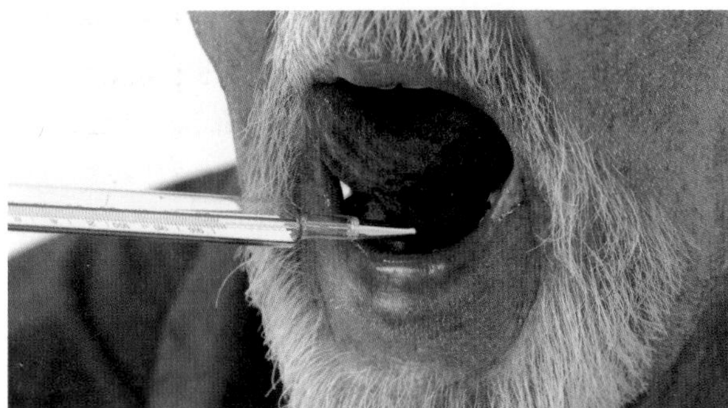

Fig. 14-9. *Insert thermometer under the resident's tongue and to one side.*

   Digital thermometer: Insert the end of digital thermometer into resident's mouth, under tongue and to one side.

   Electronic thermometer: Insert the end of electronic thermometer into resident's mouth, under tongue and to one side.

8. **Mercury-free thermometer**: Tell the resident to hold the thermometer in his mouth with lips closed. Assist as necessary. Resident should breathe through his nose. Ask resident not to bite down or to talk. Leave thermometer in place for at least three minutes.

   Digital thermometer: Leave in place until thermometer blinks or beeps.

   Electronic thermometer: Leave in place until you hear a tone or see a flashing or steady light.

9. **Mercury-free thermometer**: Remove the thermometer. Wipe with a tissue from stem to bulb or remove sheath. Dispose of the tissue or sheath. Hold the thermometer at eye level. Rotate until line appears, rolling the

thermometer between your thumb and forefinger. Read the temperature. Remember the temperature reading.

Digital thermometer: Remove the thermometer. Read temperature on display screen. Remember the temperature reading.

Electronic thermometer: Read the temperature on the display screen. Remember the temperature reading. Remove the probe.

10. **Mercury-free thermometer**: Clean thermometer with soap and water. Rinse with clean water and dry. Return it to case.

    Digital thermometer: Using a tissue, remove and dispose of sheath. Replace the thermometer in case.

    Electronic thermometer: Press the eject button to discard the cover (Fig. 14-10). Return the probe to the holder.

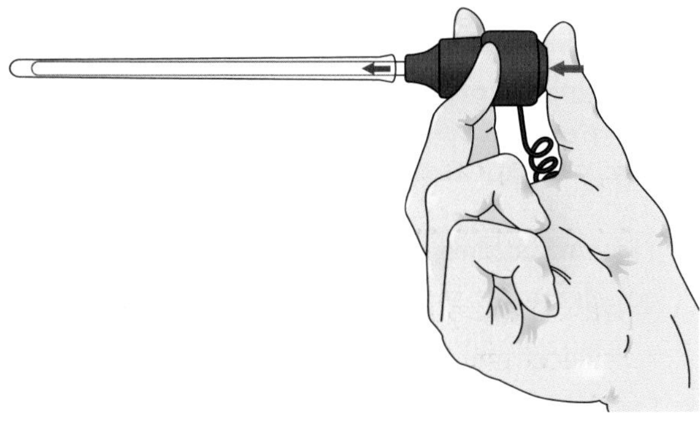

Fig. 14-10. *Eject and discard the probe cover after use.*

11. Remove and discard gloves.
12. Wash your hands.
13. Immediately record the temperature, date, time, and method used (oral).
14. Place call light within resident's reach.
15. Report any changes in resident to the nurse.

Rectal temperatures can be necessary when caring for unconscious residents, residents who have seizures, residents with poorly-fitting dentures or missing teeth, and anyone having trouble breathing through the nose. Rectal thermometers should be lubricated and inserted one-half to one inch for adults. Nursing assistants must always explain what they will do before starting this procedure. NAs need the resident's cooperation to take a rectal temperature. They should ask the resident to hold still and reassure him that the procedure will only take a few minutes. It is important to hold onto the thermometer at all times while taking a rectal temperature.

Measuring and recording a rectal temperature

Equipment: clean rectal mercury-free, digital, or electronic thermometer, lubricant, gloves, tissues, disposable sheath/cover, pen and paper

1. Identify yourself by name. Identify the resident by name.
2. Wash your hands.
3. Explain procedure to the resident. Speak clearly, slowly, and directly. Maintain face-to-face contact whenever possible.
4. Provide for resident's privacy with curtain, screen, or door.
5. Adjust bed to a safe level, usually waist high. Lock bed wheels.
6. Help the resident to the left side-lying (Sims') position (Fig. 14-11).

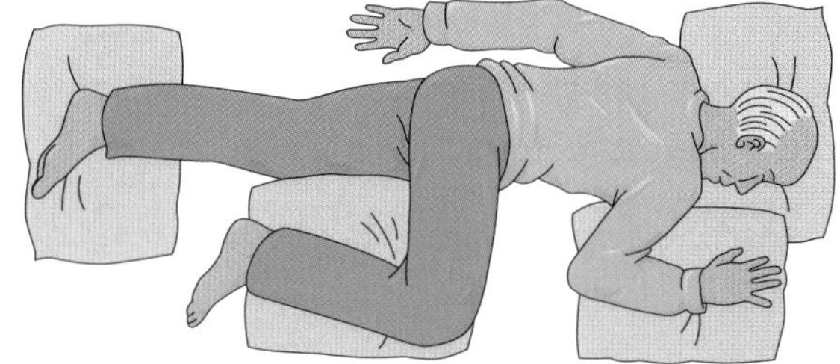

Fig. 14-11. *The resident must be in the left side-lying (Sims') position.*

7. Fold back the linens to expose only the rectal area.
8. Put on gloves.
9. **Mercury-free thermometer**: Hold thermometer by stem. Shake the thermometer down to below the lowest number.

Digital thermometer: Put on the disposable sheath. Turn on thermometer and wait until *ready* sign appears.

Electronic thermometer: Remove the probe from base unit. Put on probe cover.

10. Apply a small amount of lubricant to tip of bulb or probe cover (or apply pre-lubricated cover).
11. Separate the buttocks. Gently insert thermometer into rectum 1/2 to 1 inch. Stop if you meet resistance. Do not force the thermometer in (Fig. 14-12).

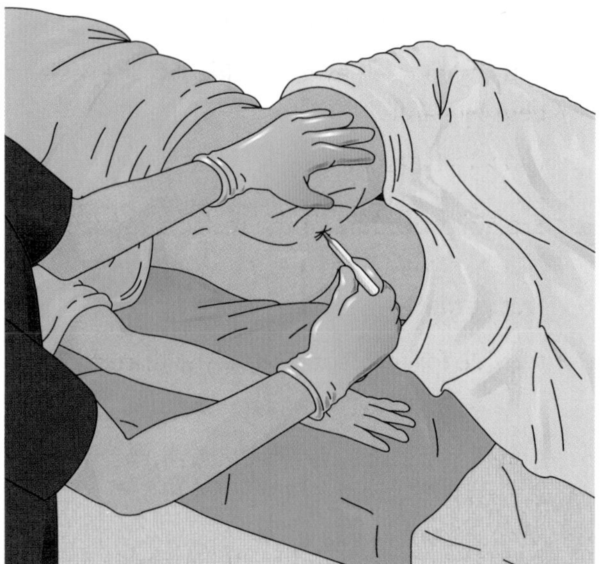

Fig. 14-12. *Gently insert a rectal thermometer one-half to one inch into the rectum.*

12. Replace the sheet over buttocks. Hold on to the thermometer at all times.
13. **Mercury-free thermometer**: Hold thermometer in place for at least three minutes.

    Digital thermometer: Hold thermometer in place until thermometer blinks or beeps.

    Electronic thermometer: Leave in place until you hear a tone or see a flashing or steady light.
14. Gently remove the thermometer. Wipe with tissue from stem to bulb or remove sheath. Discard tissue or sheath.
15. Read the thermometer at eye level as you would for an oral temperature. Remember the temperature reading.
16. **Mercury-free thermometer**: Clean thermometer with soap and water. Rinse with clean water and dry. Return it to case.

    Digital thermometer: Clean thermometer according to policy. Replace the thermometer in case.

    Electronic thermometer: Press the eject button to discard the cover. Return the probe to the holder.
17. Remove and discard gloves.
18. Wash your hands.
19. Assist the resident to a comfortable position.
20. Immediately record the temperature, date, time, and method used (rectal).
21. Place call light within resident's reach.
22. Report any changes in resident to the nurse.

Tympanic thermometers can be used to take a fast and accurate temperature reading. The nursing assistant should explain to the resident that she will be placing a thermometer in the ear canal. She should reassure the resident that this is painless. The short tip of the thermometer will only go into the ear one-quarter to one-half inch, depending upon the manufacturer's instructions.

Measuring and recording a tympanic temperature

Equipment: tympanic thermometer, gloves, disposable probe sheath/cover, pen and paper

1. Identify yourself by name. Identify the resident by name.
2. Wash your hands.

3. Explain procedure to the resident. Speak clearly, slowly, and directly. Maintain face-to-face contact whenever possible.
4. Provide for resident's privacy with curtain, screen, or door.
5. Put on gloves.
6. Put a disposable sheath over earpiece of the thermometer.
7. Position the resident's head so that the ear is in front of you. Straighten the ear canal by gently pulling up and back on the outside edge of the ear for an adult (Fig. 14-13). Insert the covered probe into the ear canal and press the button.

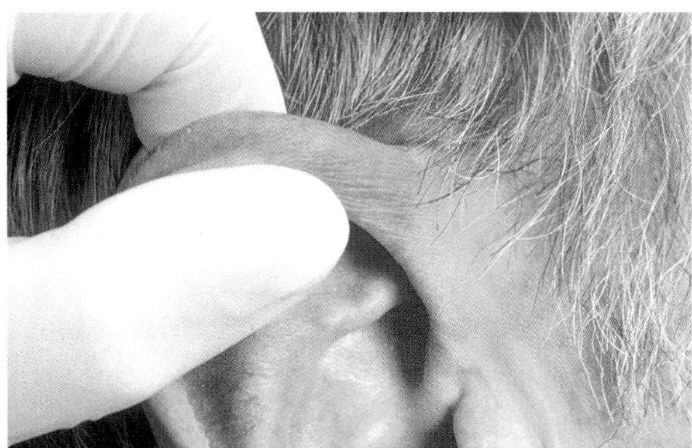

Fig. 14-13. *Straighten the ear canal by gently pulling up and back on the outside edge of the ear.*

8. Hold thermometer in place either for one second or until thermometer blinks or beeps (depends on model).
9. Read temperature. Remember the temperature reading.
10. Dispose of sheath. Return the thermometer to storage or to the battery charger if thermometer is rechargeable.
11. Remove and discard gloves.
12. Wash your hands.
13. Immediately record the temperature, date, time, and method used (tympanic).
14. Place call light within resident's reach.
15. Report any changes in resident to the nurse.

Axillary temperatures are much less reliable than temperatures taken at other sites. However, they can be safer if a resident is confused, disoriented, uncooperative, or has dementia.

Measuring and recording an axillary temperature

Equipment: clean mercury-free, digital, or electronic thermometer, gloves, tissues, disposable sheath/cover, pen and paper

1. Identify yourself by name. Identify the resident by name.
2. Wash your hands.
3. Explain procedure to the resident. Speak clearly, slowly, and directly. Maintain face-to-face contact whenever possible.
4. Provide for resident's privacy with curtain, screen, or door.
5. Put on gloves.
6. Remove resident's arm from sleeve of gown or shirt to allow skin contact with the end of the thermometer. Wipe axillary area with tissues before placing the thermometer.
7. **Mercury-free thermometer**: Hold the thermometer by the stem. Shake the thermometer down to below the lowest number.

   Digital thermometer: Put on the disposable sheath. Turn on thermometer and wait until *ready* sign appears.

   Electronic thermometer: Remove the probe from base unit. Put on probe cover.
8. Position thermometer (bulb end for mercury-free) in center of the armpit. Fold resident's arm over her chest.
9. **Mercury-free thermometer**: Hold the thermometer in place, with the arm close against the side, for eight to 10 minutes (Fig. 14-14).

   Digital thermometer: Leave in place until thermometer blinks or beeps.

Electronic thermometer: Leave in place until you hear a tone or see a flashing or steady light.

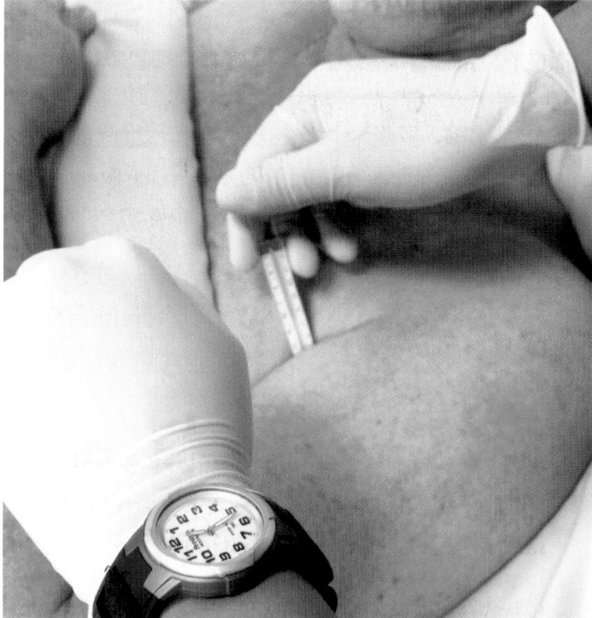

Fig. 14-14. After inserting the thermometer, fold the resident's arm over his chest and hold it in place for eight to 10 minutes.

10. **Mercury-free thermometer**: Remove the thermometer. Wipe with a tissue from stem to bulb or remove sheath. Dispose of the tissue or sheath. Read the thermometer at eye level as you would for an oral temperature. Remember the temperature reading.

    Digital thermometer: Remove the thermometer. Read temperature on display screen. Remember the temperature reading.

    Electronic thermometer: Read the temperature on the display screen. Remember the temperature reading. Remove the probe.

11. **Mercury-free thermometer**: Clean thermometer with soap and water. Rinse with clean water and dry. Return it to case.

    Digital thermometer: Using a tissue, remove and dispose of sheath. Replace the thermometer in case.

    Electronic thermometer: Press the eject button to discard the cover. Return the probe to the holder.

12. Remove and discard gloves.
13. Wash your hands.
14. Put resident's arm back into sleeve of gown.
15. Immediately record the temperature, date, time, and method used (axillary).
16. Place call light within resident's reach.
17. Report any changes in resident to the nurse.

3. List guidelines for measuring pulse and respirations

The pulse is the number of heartbeats per minute. The beat that is felt at certain pulse points in the body represents the wave of blood moving as a result of the heart pumping. The most common site for monitoring the pulse is on the inside of the wrist, where the radial artery runs just beneath the skin. This is called the **radial pulse**. The procedure for taking this pulse appears later in this chapter. The **brachial pulse** is the pulse inside the elbow, about one to one-and-a-half inches above the elbow. The radial and brachial pulses are involved in taking blood pressure, which is explained later in this chapter. Common pulse sites are shown in Fig. 14-15.

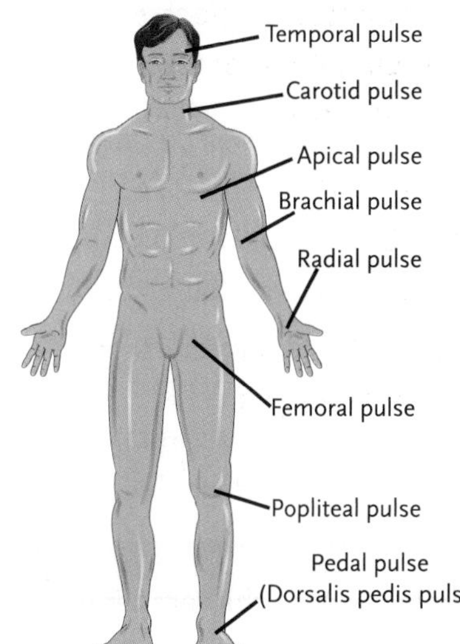

Fig. 14-15. Common pulse sites.

For adults, the normal pulse rate is 60 to 100 beats per minute. Small children have more rapid pulses, in the range of 100 to 120 beats per minute. A newborn baby's pulse may be as high as 120 to 140 beats per minute. Many things can affect the pulse rate, including exercise, fear, anger, anxiety, heat, infection, medications, and pain. A high or low rate does not necessarily indicate disease. However, sometimes the pulse rate can signal that illness exists. For example, a rapid pulse may result from fever, dehydration, or heart failure. A slow or weak pulse may indicate infection.

The **apical pulse** is heard by listening directly over the heart with a stethoscope. A **stethoscope** is an instrument designed to listen to sounds within the body, such as the heart beating or air moving through the lungs (Fig. 14-16). This is often the easiest method for measuring the pulse in infants and small children because their pulse points are harder to find.

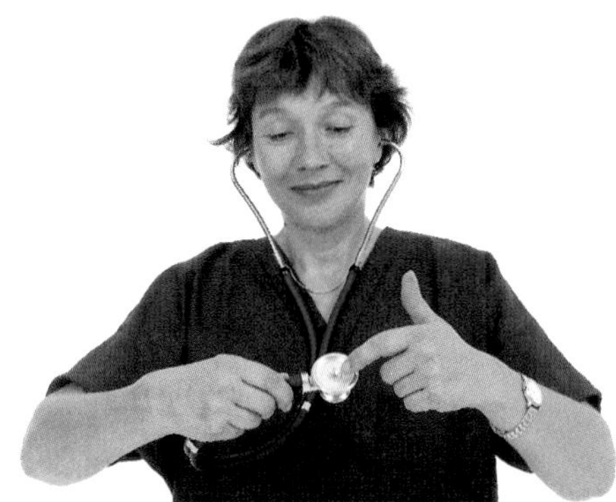

Fig. 14-16. *For adults, NAs should use the larger, round side of the stethoscope to hear a pulse and to take blood pressure. The smaller side is used for children or infants.*

The apical pulse is on the left side of the chest, just below the nipple. For adult residents, the apical pulse may be taken when the person has heart disease or takes medication that affects the heart. It may also be taken if residents have a weak radial pulse or an irregular pulse.

Measuring and recording apical pulse

Equipment: stethoscope, watch with second hand, alcohol wipes, pen and paper

1. Identify yourself by name. Identify the resident by name.
2. Wash your hands.
3. Explain procedure to the resident. Speak clearly, slowly, and directly. Maintain face-to-face contact whenever possible.
4. Provide for resident's privacy with curtain, screen, or door.
5. Before using stethoscope, wipe diaphragm and earpieces with alcohol wipes.
6. Fit the earpieces of the stethoscope snugly in your ears. Place the flat metal diaphragm on the left side of the chest, just below the nipple. Listen for the heartbeat.
7. Use the second hand of your watch. Count the heartbeats for one minute (Fig. 14-17). Each *lubdub* that you hear is counted as one beat. A normal heartbeat is rhythmical. Leave the stethoscope in place to count respirations (see procedure later in chapter).

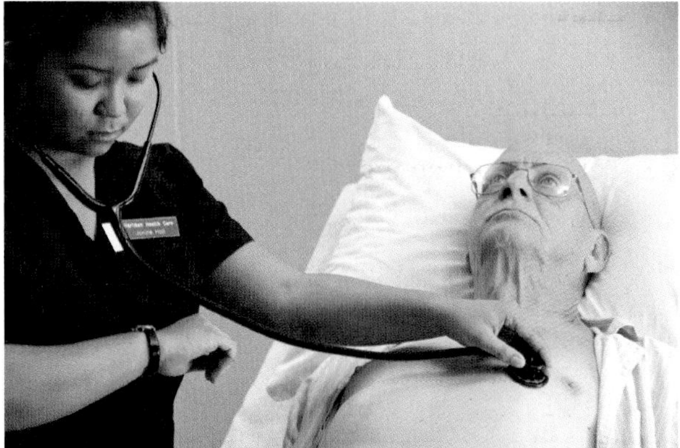

Fig. 14-17. *Count the heartbeats for one full minute to measure the apical pulse.*

8. Record pulse rate, date, time, and method used (apical). Note any irregularities in the rhythm.
9. Clean earpieces and diaphragm of stethoscope with alcohol wipes. Store stethoscope.
10. Wash your hands.
11. Place call light within resident's reach.
12. Report any changes in resident to the nurse.

Respiration is the process of breathing air into the lungs, or **inspiration**, and exhaling air out of the lungs, or **expiration**. Each respiration consists of an inspiration and an expiration. The chest rises during inspiration and falls during expiration.

The normal respiration rate for adults ranges from 12 to 20 breaths per minute. Infants and children have a faster respiratory rate. Infants normally breathe at a rate of 30 to 40 respirations per minute. The following are different types of respirations:

- **Apnea**: the absence of breathing
- **Dyspnea**: difficulty breathing
- **Eupnea**: normal breathing
- **Orthopnea**: shortness of breath when lying down that is relieved by sitting up
- **Tachypnea**: rapid breathing
- **Cheyne-Stokes**: alternating periods of slow, irregular breathing and rapid, shallow breathing

People may breathe more quickly if they know they are being observed. Because of this, respirations should be counted immediately after taking the pulse. The nursing assistant should keep her fingers on the resident's wrist or on the stethoscope over the heart. She should not make it obvious that she is watching the resident's breathing.

Measuring and recording radial pulse and counting and recording respirations

Equipment: watch with a second hand, pen and paper

1. Identify yourself by name. Identify the resident by name.
2. Wash your hands.
3. Explain procedure to the resident. Speak clearly, slowly, and directly. Maintain face-to-face contact whenever possible.
4. Provide for resident's privacy with curtain, screen, or door.
5. Place fingertips on the thumb side of resident's wrist. Locate pulse (Fig. 14-18).

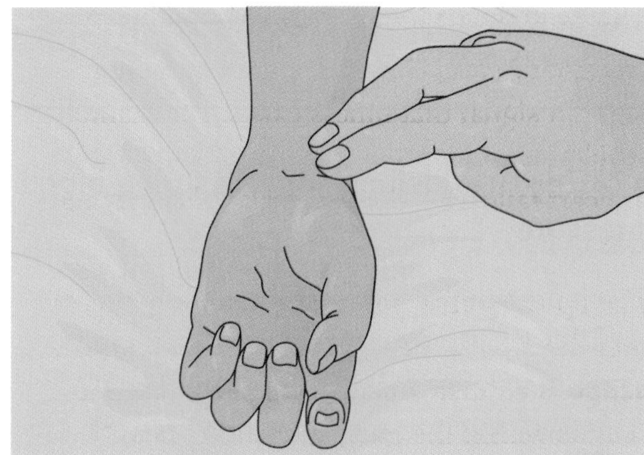

Fig. 14-18. *Measure the radial pulse by placing fingertips on the thumb side of the wrist.*

6. Using your watch, count the beats for one full minute.
7. Keeping your fingertips on the resident's wrist, count respirations for one full minute (Fig. 14-19). Observe the pattern and character of the resident's breathing. Normal breathing is smooth and quiet. If you see signs of troubled, shallow, or noisy breathing, such as wheezing, report it.

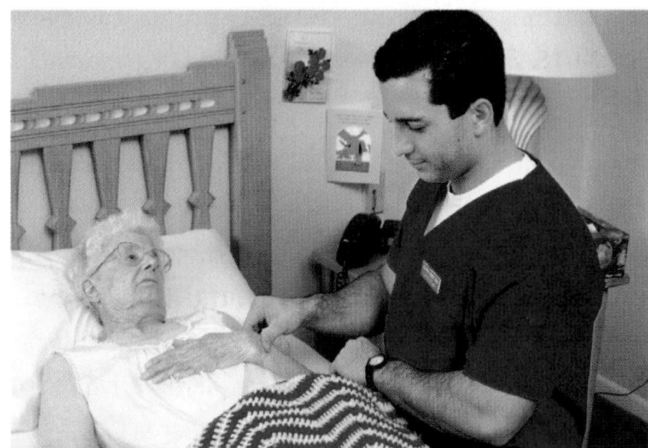

Fig. 14-19. *Count the respiratory rate directly after taking the radial pulse. Do not make it obvious that you are watching her breathing.*

8. Record pulse rate, date, time, and method used (radial). Record the respiratory rate and the pattern or character of breathing.

9. Place call light within resident's reach.
10. Wash your hands.
11. Report to the nurse if the pulse is less than 60 beats per minute, over 100 beats per minute, if the rhythm is irregular, or if breathing is irregular.

4. Explain guidelines for measuring blood pressure

Blood pressure is an important indicator of a person's health. Blood pressure is measured in millimeters of mercury (mmHg). The measurement shows how well the heart is working. There are two parts of blood pressure, the systolic measurement and the diastolic measurement.

In the **systolic** phase, the heart is at work, contracting and pushing the blood from the left ventricle of the heart. The reading shows the pressure on the walls of arteries as blood is pumped through the body. The normal range for systolic blood pressure is 100 to 119 mmHg.

The second measurement reflects the **diastolic** phase—when the heart relaxes. The diastolic measurement is always lower than the systolic measurement. It shows the pressure in the arteries when the heart is at rest. The normal range for adults is 60 to 79 mmHg.

People with high blood pressure, or **hypertension**, have elevated systolic and/or diastolic blood pressures. A blood pressure level of 140/90 mmHg or higher is considered high and should be reported to the nurse. However, if blood pressure is between 120/80 mmHg and 139/89 mmHg, it is called **prehypertension**. This means that the person does not have high blood pressure now but is likely to develop it in the future.

Many factors can increase blood pressure. These include aging, exercise, physical or emotional stress, pain, medications, and the volume of blood in circulation. For example, loss of blood will lead to abnormally low blood pressure (100/60 or lower), or **hypotension**. Hypotension can be life-threatening if not corrected.

Blood pressure is measured using a stethoscope and a blood pressure cuff, or **sphygmomanometer** (Fig. 14-20). Inside the cuff is an inflatable balloon that expands when air is pumped into the cuff. Two pieces of tubing are connected to the cuff. One leads to a rubber bulb that pumps air into the cuff. A pressure control valve lets a person control the release of air from the cuff after it is inflated. The other piece of tubing is connected to a pressure gauge with numbers. The gauge is either a mercury column or a round dial.

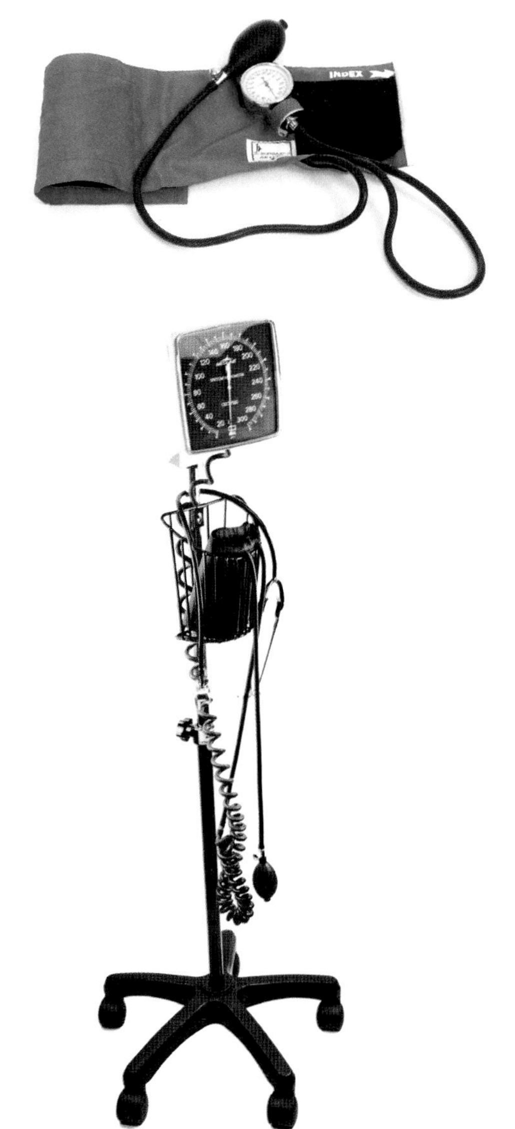

Fig. 14-20. Different types of sphygmomanometers.

There may be an electronic sphygmomanometer available. The systolic and diastolic pressure readings and pulse are displayed digitally (Fig. 4-21). Some units automatically inflate and deflate. The use of a stethoscope is not required with an electronic sphygmomanometer.

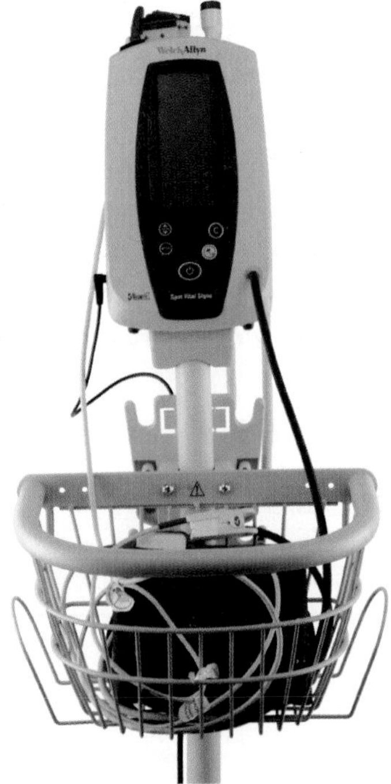

Fig. 14-21. *One type of electronic sphygmomanometer that measures other vital signs as well.*

When measuring blood pressure, the first sound heard is the systolic pressure (top number). When the sound changes to a soft muffled thump or disappears, this is the diastolic pressure (bottom number). Blood pressure is recorded as a fraction. The systolic reading is on top, and the diastolic reading is on the bottom (for example: 120/80).

Blood pressure should not be measured on an arm that has an IV, a dialysis shunt, or any medical equipment. A side that has a cast, recent trauma, paralysis from a stroke, burn(s), or has had breast surgery (mastectomy) should be avoided.

This textbook includes two methods for taking blood pressure: the one-step method and the two-step method. In the two-step method, the NA gets an estimate of the systolic blood pressure first. After obtaining an estimated systolic reading, she will deflate the cuff and begin again. If using the one-step method, she will not get an estimated systolic reading before obtaining the blood pressure reading. Requirements vary from state to state, and nursing assistants may need to know one or both methods to be certified. Some states do not allow NAs to measure blood pressure at all. Each nursing assistant must know her scope of practice and follow her facility's policies.

It is important to use a cuff that is the correct size when measuring blood pressure. Available sizes include standard, pediatric, and large.

Measuring and recording blood pressure (one-step method)

Equipment: sphygmomanometer (blood pressure cuff), stethoscope, alcohol wipes, pen and paper

1. Identify yourself by name. Identify the resident by name.
2. Wash your hands.
3. Explain procedure to the resident. Speak clearly, slowly, and directly. Maintain face-to-face contact whenever possible.
4. Provide for resident's privacy with curtain, screen, or door.
5. Ask the resident to roll up his sleeve so that the upper arm is exposed. Do not measure blood pressure over clothing.
6. Position resident's arm with palm up. The arm should be level with the heart.
7. With the valve open, squeeze the cuff. Make sure it is completely deflated.
8. Place blood pressure cuff snugly on resident's upper arm. The center of the cuff with sensor/arrow is placed over the brachial artery (1-1½ inches above the elbow, toward inside of elbow) (Fig. 14-22).
9. Before using stethoscope, wipe diaphragm and earpieces with alcohol wipes.

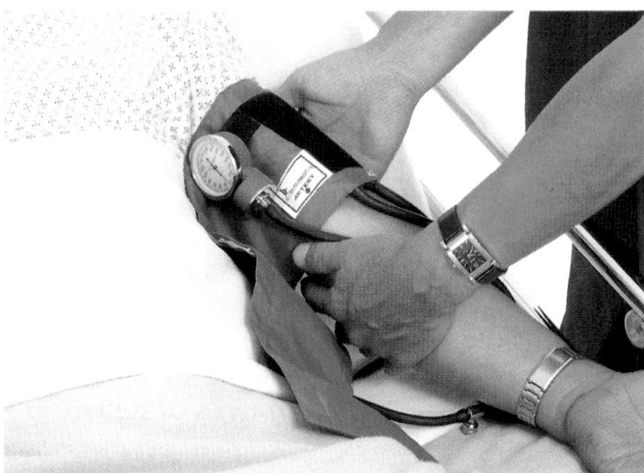

Fig. 14-22. *Place the center of the cuff over the brachial artery.*

10. Locate brachial pulse with fingertips.
11. Place diaphragm of stethoscope over brachial artery.
12. Place earpieces of stethoscope in your ears.
13. Close the valve (clockwise) until it stops. Do not over-tighten it (Fig. 14-23).

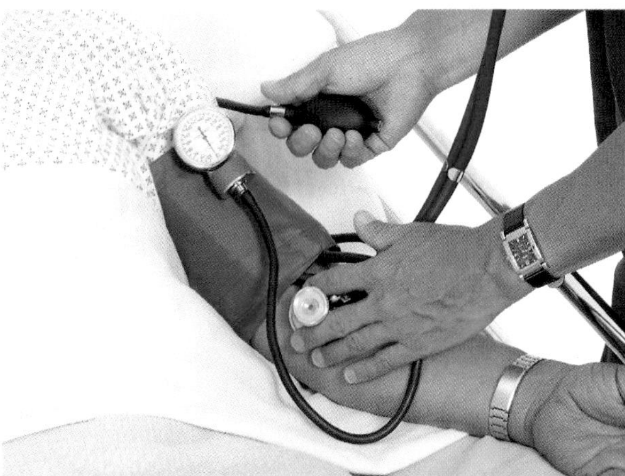

Fig. 14-23. *Close the valve, but do not over-tighten it; tight valves are difficult to release.*

14. Inflate cuff to 30 mmHg above the point at which the pulse is last heard or felt.
15. Open the valve slightly with thumb and index finger. Deflate cuff slowly. Releasing the valve slowly allows you to hear beats accurately.
16. Watch gauge. Listen for sound of the pulse.
17. Remember the reading at which the first pulse sound is heard. This is the systolic pressure.
18. Continue listening for a change or muffling of pulse sound. The point of change or the point the sound disappears is the diastolic pressure. Remember this reading.
19. Open the valve to deflate cuff completely. Remove cuff.
20. Record both the systolic and diastolic pressures. Write the numbers like a fraction, with the systolic reading on top and the diastolic reading on the bottom (for example: 120/80). Note which arm was used. Write *RA* for right arm and *LA* for left arm.
21. Wipe diaphragm and earpieces of stethoscope with alcohol wipes. Store equipment.
22. Place call light within resident's reach.
23. Wash your hands.
24. Report any changes in resident to the nurse.

Measuring and recording blood pressure (two-step method)

Equipment: sphygmomanometer (blood pressure cuff), stethoscope, alcohol wipes, pen and paper

1. Identify yourself by name. Identify the resident by name.
2. Wash your hands.
3. Explain procedure to the resident. Speak clearly, slowly, and directly. Maintain face-to-face contact whenever possible.
4. Provide for resident's privacy with curtain, screen, or door.
5. Ask the resident to roll up his sleeve so that the upper arm is exposed. Do not measure blood pressure over clothing.
6. Position resident's arm with palm up. The arm should be level with the heart.
7. With the valve open, squeeze the cuff. Make sure it is completely deflated.
8. Place blood pressure cuff snugly on resident's upper arm. The center of the cuff with

sensor/arrow is placed over the brachial artery (1-1½ inches above the elbow, toward inside of elbow).

9. Locate the radial (wrist) pulse with your fingertips.
10. Close the valve (clockwise) until it stops. Inflate cuff while watching gauge.
11. Stop inflating when you can no longer feel the radial pulse. Note the reading. The number is an estimate of the systolic pressure. This estimate helps you not to inflate the cuff too high later in this procedure. Inflating the cuff too high is painful and may damage small blood vessels.
12. Open the valve to deflate cuff completely.
13. Write down the estimated systolic reading.
14. Before using the stethoscope, wipe diaphragm and earpieces of stethoscope with alcohol wipes.
15. Locate brachial pulse with fingertips.
16. Place the earpieces of the stethoscope in your ears.
17. Place the diaphragm of the stethoscope over the brachial artery.
18. Close the valve (clockwise) until it stops. Do not over-tighten it.
19. Inflate the cuff to 30 mmHg above your estimated systolic pressure.
20. Open the valve slightly with thumb and index finger. Deflate cuff slowly. Releasing the valve slowly allows you to hear beats accurately.
21. Watch the gauge. Listen for sound of the pulse.
22. Remember the reading at which the first pulse sound is heard. This is the systolic pressure.
23. Continue listening for a change or muffling of pulse sound. The point of change or the point that the sound disappears is the diastolic pressure. Remember this reading.
24. Open the valve to deflate cuff completely. Remove cuff.
25. Record both the systolic and diastolic pressures. Write the numbers like a fraction, with the systolic reading on top and the diastolic reading on the bottom (for example: 120/80). Note which arm was used. Write *RA* for right arm and *LA* for left arm.
26. Wipe diaphragm and earpieces of stethoscope with alcohol wipes. Store equipment.
27. Place call light within resident's reach.
28. Wash your hands.
29. Report any changes in resident to the nurse.

Orthostatic Blood Pressures

Nursing assistants may be asked by the nurse to take an orthostatic blood pressure measurement. To do this, the resident must first lie down, and the nursing assistant should record the systolic and diastolic pressures. Next, the resident should sit up. The NA should wait two minutes and measure blood pressure again, recording the systolic and diastolic pressures. Finally, the resident should stand up. The NA should wait two minutes and measure blood pressure again, recording both pressures. Orthostatic blood pressures must be checked in this order: lying down, sitting, and standing up. All three blood pressure measurements should be reported to the nurse.

5. Describe guidelines for pain management

Pain is often referred to as the fifth vital sign because it is as important to monitor as the other vital signs. Nursing assistants must observe and report residents' pain carefully. Pain is uncomfortable. It can swiftly drain energy and hope. Pain is also a personal experience, which means it is different for each person. Because NAs spend the most time with residents, they play an important role in pain monitoring and prevention. Care plans are made based on NAs' reports.

Pain is not a normal part of aging. Sustained pain may lead to withdrawal, depression, and isolation. Nursing assistants must treat residents' complaints of pain seriously (Fig. 14-24). They should listen to what residents are saying about the way they feel and take action to help them. If a resident complains of pain, the following questions can be asked to get the most accurate information. NAs should then immediately report the information to the nurse.

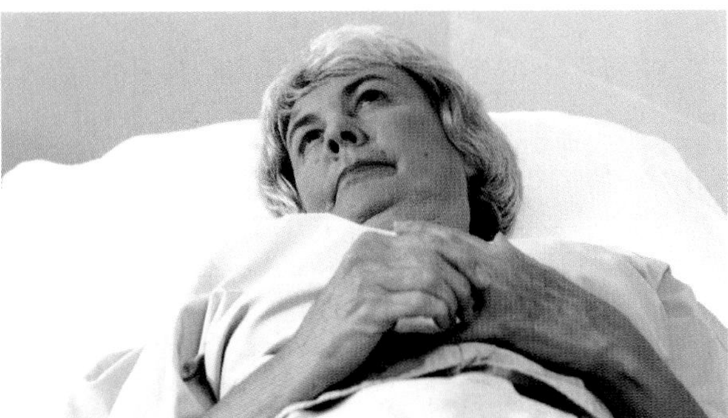

Fig. 14-24. *Nursing assistants should believe residents when they say they are in pain and take quick action to help them. Being in pain is unpleasant. NAs should be empathetic. They should ask questions and report their observations.*

- Where is the pain?
- When did the pain start?
- Is the pain mild, moderate, or severe? To help assess this, the NA can ask the resident to rate the pain on a scale of 0 to 10, with 0 being no pain and 10 being the worst pain the resident can imagine.
- Can you describe the pain? For example, is it a dull, aching, sharp, piercing, or stabbing pain? The NA should use the resident's words when reporting to the nurse.
- What were you doing before the pain started?
- How long does the pain last, and how often does it occur?
- What makes the pain better? What makes the pain worse?

Residents may have concerns about managing their pain. These concerns may make them hesitant to report their pain. Barriers to managing pain include the following:

- Fear of addiction to pain medication
- Feeling that pain is a normal part of aging
- Worrying about constipation and fatigue from pain medication
- Feeling that caregivers are too busy to deal with their pain
- Feeling that too much pain medication will cause death

NAs should be patient and caring when helping residents who are in pain. If residents are worried about the effects of pain medication or if they have questions about it, the NA should report to the nurse. Some people do not feel comfortable saying that they are in pain. A person's culture affects how he or she responds to pain. Some cultures believe that it is best not to react to pain. Other cultures believe in expressing pain freely. The NA should watch for body language or other messages that indicate that residents may be in pain. Signs and symptoms of pain are important to observe and report.

Observing and Reporting: Pain

Report any of these to the nurse:

- O/R Increased pulse, respirations, blood pressure
- O/R Sweating
- O/R Nausea
- O/R Vomiting
- O/R Tightening the jaw
- O/R Squeezing eyes shut
- O/R Holding or guarding a body part
- O/R Frowning
- O/R Grinding teeth
- O/R Increased restlessness
- O/R Agitation or tension
- O/R Change in behavior
- O/R Crying

- Sighing
- Groaning
- Breathing heavily
- Rocking
- Pacing
- Repetitive movements
- Difficulty moving or walking

Guidelines: Measures to Reduce Pain

- Report complaints of pain or unrelieved pain immediately.
- Gently position the body in proper alignment. Use pillows for support. Assist in frequent changes of position if the resident desires it.
- Give back rubs.
- Ask if the resident would like to take a warm bath or shower.
- Assist the resident to the bathroom or commode or offer the bedpan or urinal.
- Encourage slow, deep breathing.
- Provide a calm and quiet environment. Use soft music to distract the resident.
- Be patient, caring, gentle, and responsive to residents who are in pain.

6. Explain the benefits of warm and cold applications

Applying heat or cold to injured areas can have several positive effects. Heat relieves pain and muscular tension. It reduces swelling, elevates the temperature in the tissues, and increases blood flow. Increased blood flow brings more oxygen and nutrients to the tissues for healing.

Cold applications can help stop bleeding. They help prevent swelling, reduce pain, and bring down high fevers. Applying ice bags or cold compresses immediately after an injury can stop bleeding and prevent swelling.

Warm and cold applications may be dry or moist. Moisture strengthens the effect of heat and cold. This means that moist applications are more likely to cause injury. Paralysis, numbness, disorientation, confusion, dementia, and other conditions may cause a person to be unable to feel, notice, or understand damage that is occurring from a warm or cold application. For example, a resident recovering from a stroke who has paralysis on one side may not be able to feel if a warm pack is burning his skin. A resident with Alzheimer's disease may not understand that he is being burned and/or be able to communicate pain clearly.

Nursing assistants must be very careful when using these applications. They should know how long the application should be performed and should use the correct temperature as given in the care plan. When warm and cold applications are applied for too long, the opposite effect of what is intended results. Residents receiving warm or cold applications should be checked often, especially those who have conditions that may make them unaware of possible injury.

Moist applications include the following:

- Compresses (warm or cold)
- Soaks (warm or cold)
- Tub baths (warm)
- Sponge baths (warm or cold)
- Sitz baths (warm)
- Ice packs (cold)

Dry applications include the following:

- Aquamatic K-pad (warm or cold)
- Electric heating pads (warm)
- Disposable warm packs (warm)
- Ice bags (cold)
- Disposable cold packs (cold)

Nursing assistants may be allowed to prepare and apply warm and cold applications. NAs should only perform procedures that are assigned to them. They should never perform a procedure they are not trained or allowed to do.

Observing and Reporting: Warm and Cold Applications

Report the following to the nurse:

- O/R Excessive redness
- O/R Pain
- O/R Blisters
- O/R Numbness

These signs indicate that the application may be causing tissue damage.

Residents' Rights

Warm and Cold Applications

When applying warm or cold applications, NAs should keep residents' bodies covered and only expose the area that needs treatment. Doing this promotes dignity and honors a resident's legal right to privacy.

Warm Applications

A washcloth or a commercial warm compress may be used as a warm compress. There are different types of commercial compresses available (Fig. 14-25). If these are provided, the NA should follow the package directions and the nurse's instructions.

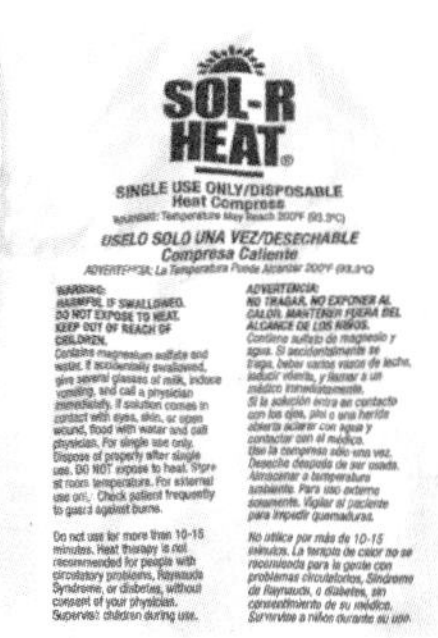

Fig. 14-25. Disposable heat compresses are used only once and then discarded. The compress shown here must be squeezed to activate and then applied. It maintains heat for a certain amount of time, usually up to 20 minutes. (REPRINTED WITH PERMISSION OF BRIGGS CORPORATION, 800-247-2343, WWW.BRIGGSCORP.COM)

Applying warm compresses

Equipment: washcloth or compress, plastic wrap, towel, basin, bath thermometer

1. Identify yourself by name. Identify the resident by name.
2. Wash your hands.
3. Explain procedure to the resident. Speak clearly, slowly, and directly. Maintain face-to-face contact whenever possible.
4. Provide for the resident's privacy with curtain, screen, or door.
5. Fill basin one-half to two-thirds full with warm water. Test water temperature with thermometer or against the inside of your wrist to ensure it is safe. Water temperature should be no higher than 105°F. Have resident check water temperature. Adjust if necessary.
6. Soak the washcloth in the water and wring it out. Immediately apply it to the area needing a warm compress. Note the time. Quickly cover the washcloth with plastic wrap and the towel to keep it warm (Fig. 14-26).

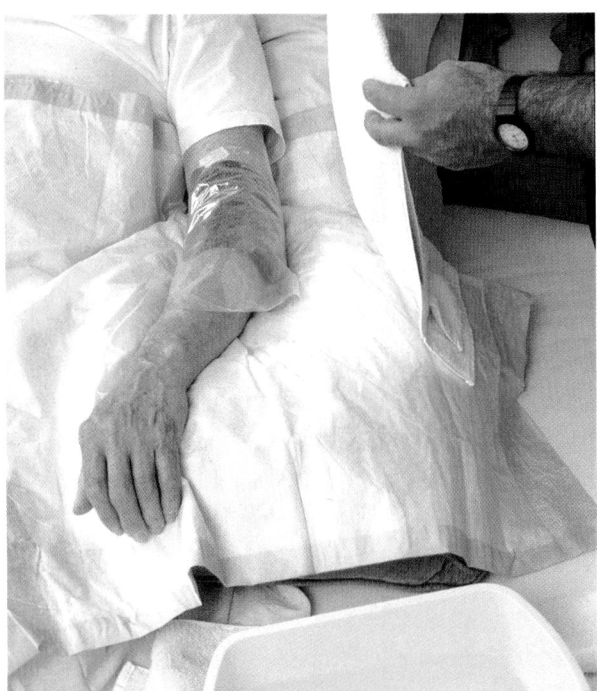

Fig. 14-26. Cover compresses to keep them warm.

7. Check the area every five minutes. Remove the compress if the area is red or numb or if the resident complains of pain or discomfort. Change the compress if cooling occurs. Remove the compress after 20 minutes.
8. Make resident comfortable.
9. Place soiled towels in proper container.
10. Empty, rinse, and wipe basin. Return to proper storage. Discard plastic wrap.
11. Place call light within resident's reach.
12. Wash your hands.
13. Report any changes in resident to the nurse.
14. Document procedure using facility guidelines.

Administering warm soaks

Equipment: towel, basin, bath thermometer, bath blanket

1. Identify yourself by name. Identify the resident by name.
2. Wash your hands.
3. Explain procedure to the resident. Speak clearly, slowly, and directly. Maintain face-to-face contact whenever possible.
4. Provide for the resident's privacy with curtain, screen, or door.
5. Fill the basin half full of warm water. Test water temperature with thermometer or against the inside of your wrist to ensure it is safe. Water temperature should be no higher than 105°F. Have resident check water temperature. Adjust if necessary.
6. Immerse the body part in the basin. Pad the edge of the basin with a towel (Fig. 14-27). Use a bath blanket to cover the resident if needed for extra warmth.

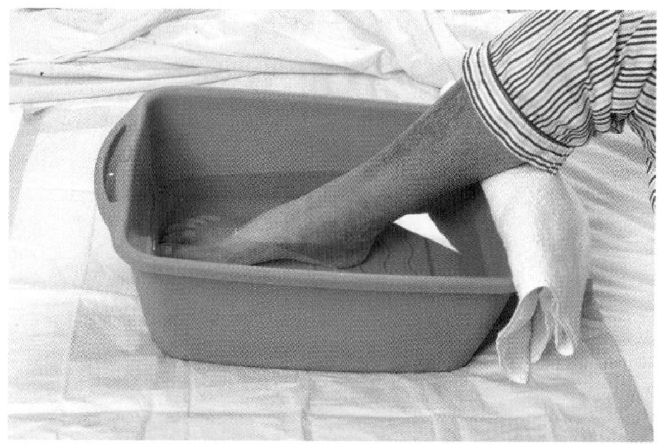

***Fig. 14-27.** Pad the edge of the basin to make the resident more comfortable.*

7. Check water temperature every five minutes. Add hot water as needed to maintain the temperature. Never add water hotter than 105°F to avoid burns. To prevent burns, ask the resident not to add hot water. Observe the area for redness. Discontinue the soak if the resident experiences pain or discomfort.
8. Soak for 15 to 20 minutes or as ordered.
9. Remove basin. Use the towel to dry resident.
10. Make resident comfortable.
11. Place soiled towel in proper container.
12. Empty, rinse, and wipe basin. Return to proper storage.
13. Place call light within resident's reach.
14. Wash your hands.
15. Report any changes in resident to the nurse.
16. Document procedure using facility guidelines.

Applying an Aquamatic K-Pad

Equipment: Aquamatic K-Pad and control unit (Fig. 14-28), covering for pad, distilled water

1. Identify yourself by name. Identify the resident by name.
2. Wash your hands.

3. Explain procedure to the resident. Speak clearly, slowly, and directly. Maintain face-to-face contact whenever possible.

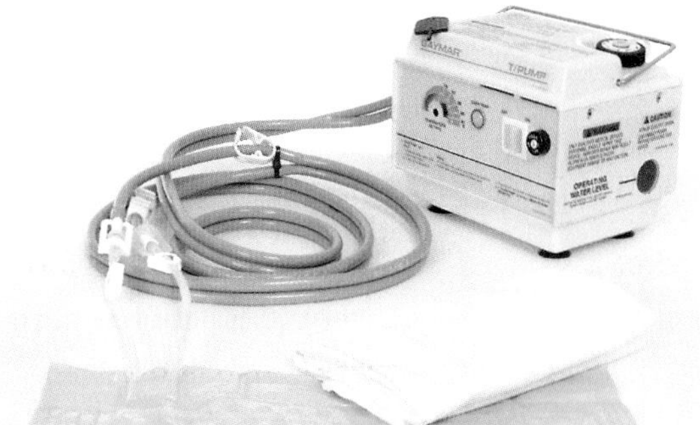

Fig. 14-28. An Aquamatic K-Pad.

4. Provide for the resident's privacy during procedure with curtain, screen, or door.
5. Place the control unit on the bedside table. Make sure cords are not frayed or damaged. Check that tubing between pad and unit is intact.
6. Remove cover of control unit to check level of water. If it is low, fill it with distilled water to the fill line.
7. Put the cover of control unit back in place.
8. Plug unit in and turn pad on. Temperature should have been pre-set. If it was not, check with the nurse for proper temperature.
9. Place the pad in the cover. Do not pin the pad to the cover.
10. Uncover area to be treated. Place the covered pad on the area. Note the time. Make sure the tubing is not hanging below the bed. It should be coiled on the bed.
11. Return and check area every five minutes. Remove the pad if the area is red or numb or if the resident reports pain or discomfort.
12. Check water level and refill when necessary.
13. Remove pad after 20 minutes.
14. Make resident comfortable.
15. Clean and store supplies.
16. Place call light within resident's reach.
17. Wash your hands.
18. Report any changes in resident to the nurse.
19. Document procedure using facility guidelines.

Another type of heat application is a **sitz bath**, or a warm soak of the perineal area. Sitz baths clean perineal wounds and reduce inflammation and pain. Circulation in the perineal area is increased. Voiding may be stimulated by a sitz bath. Residents with perineal swelling (such as hemorrhoids) or perineal wounds (such as those that occur during childbirth) may be ordered to take sitz baths. Because the sitz bath causes increased blood flow to the pelvic area, blood flow to other parts of the body is decreased. Residents may feel weak, faint, or dizzy after a sitz bath. Nursing assistants must always wear gloves when helping with a sitz bath.

A disposable sitz bath fits on the toilet seat and is attached to a rubber bag containing warm water (Fig. 14-29).

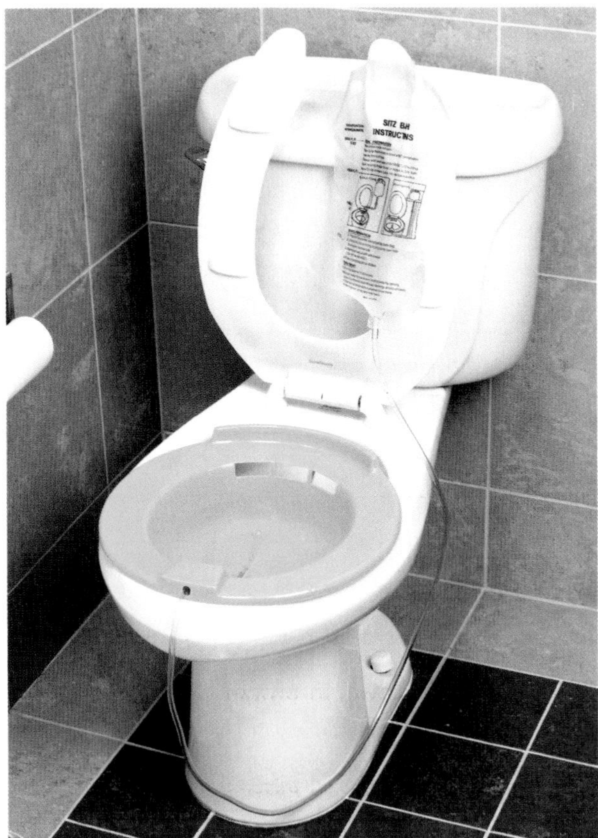

Fig. 14-29. A disposable sitz bath. (REPRINTED WITH PERMISSION OF BRIGGS CORPORATION, 800-247-2343, WWW.BRIGGSCORP.COM)

Assisting with a sitz bath

Equipment: disposable sitz bath, bath thermometer, towels, gloves

1. Identify yourself by name. Identify the resident by name.
2. Wash your hands.
3. Explain procedure to the resident. Speak clearly, slowly, and directly. Maintain face-to-face contact whenever possible.
4. Provide for the resident's privacy with curtain, screen, or door.
5. Put on gloves.
6. Fill the sitz bath two-thirds full with warm water. Place the disposable sitz bath on the toilet seat. Check the water temperature using the bath thermometer. Water temperature should be no higher than 105°F. If the sitz bath is being used to help relieve pain and to stimulate circulation, the water temperature may need to be higher. Follow instructions in the care plan.
7. Help the resident undress and sit on the sitz bath. A valve on the tubing connected to the bag allows the resident or you to refill the water in the sitz bath again with warm water.
8. You may be required to stay with the resident for safety reasons. If you leave the room, check on the resident every five minutes to make sure he is not dizzy or weak. Stay with a resident who seems unsteady.
9. Help the resident off of the sitz bath in 20 minutes. Provide towels and help with dressing if needed.
10. Make sure resident is comfortable.
11. Place soiled towel in proper container. Clean and store supplies.
12. Remove and discard gloves.
13. Wash your hands.
14. Place call light within resident's reach.
15. Report any changes in resident to the nurse.
16. Document procedure using facility guidelines.

Cold Applications

There are different types of commercial cold packs available (Fig. 14-30), which may be used instead of traditional ice packs. If these are provided, nursing assistants should follow the package directions and the nurse's instructions.

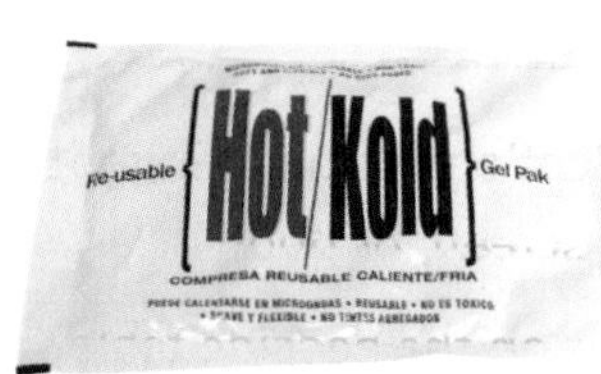

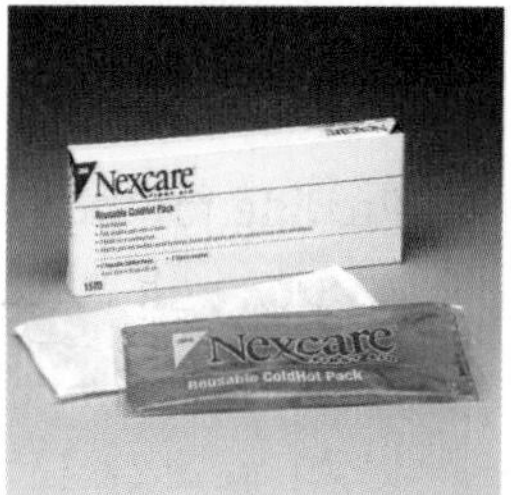

Fig. 14-30. *Some types of reusable packs may be used for heat or cold. They can be microwaved for heat or stored in the freezer for cold.* (REPRINTED WITH PERMISSION OF BRIGGS CORPORATION, 800-247-2343, WWW.BRIGGSCORP.COM)

Applying ice packs

Equipment: cold pack or sealable plastic bag and crushed ice, towel to cover pack or bag

1. Identify yourself by name. Identify the resident by name.
2. Wash your hands.
3. Explain procedure to the resident. Speak clearly, slowly, and directly. Maintain face-to-face contact whenever possible.
4. Provide for the resident's privacy with curtain, screen, or door.
5. Fill plastic bag one-half to two-thirds full with crushed ice. Seal bag. Remove excess air. Cover bag with towel (Fig. 14-31).
6. Apply bag to the area as ordered. Note the time. Use another towel to cover bag if it is too cold.
7. Check the area after ten minutes for blisters or pale, white, or gray skin. Stop treatment if resident reports numbness or pain.

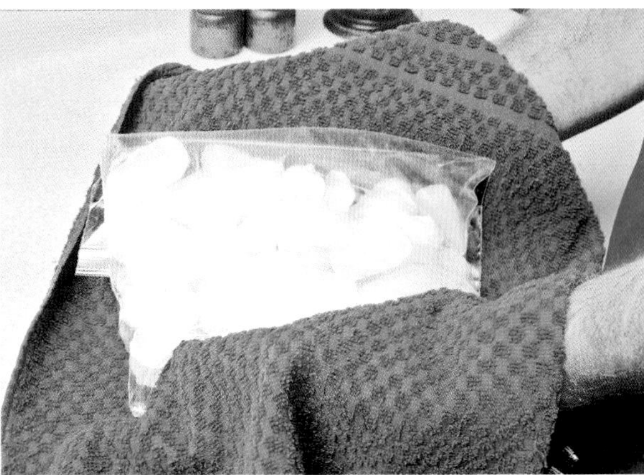

Fig. 14-31. *Seal the bag filled with ice and cover it with a towel.*

8. Remove ice after 20 minutes or as ordered.
9. Make resident comfortable.
10. Place soiled towel in proper container. Discard supplies or store in freezer if ordered.
11. Place call light within resident's reach.
12. Wash your hands.
13. Report any changes in resident to the nurse.
14. Document procedure using facility guidelines.

A washcloth dipped in cold water may be used as a cold compress; disposable or reusable compresses are also available (Fig. 14-32). Nursing assistants should follow instructions on the package.

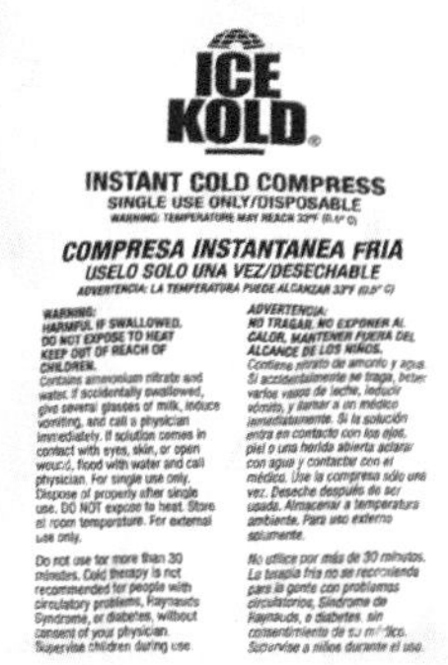

Fig. 14-32. *This type of cold compress is disposable. It must be squeezed to activate it, and it will last up to 30 minutes. It remains flexible when activated.* (REPRINTED WITH PERMISSION OF BRIGGS CORPORATION, 800-247-2343, WWW.BRIGGSCORP.COM)

Applying cold compresses

Equipment: basin filled with water and ice, two washcloths, disposable bed protector, towels

1. Identify yourself by name. Identify the resident by name.
2. Wash your hands.
3. Explain procedure to the resident. Speak clearly, slowly, and directly. Maintain face-to-face contact whenever possible.
4. Provide for the resident's privacy with curtain, screen, or door.
5. Place bed protector under area to be treated. Rinse washcloth in basin and wring out (Fig. 14-33). Cover the area to be treated with a towel. Apply cold washcloth to the area as directed. Change washcloths often to keep area cold.

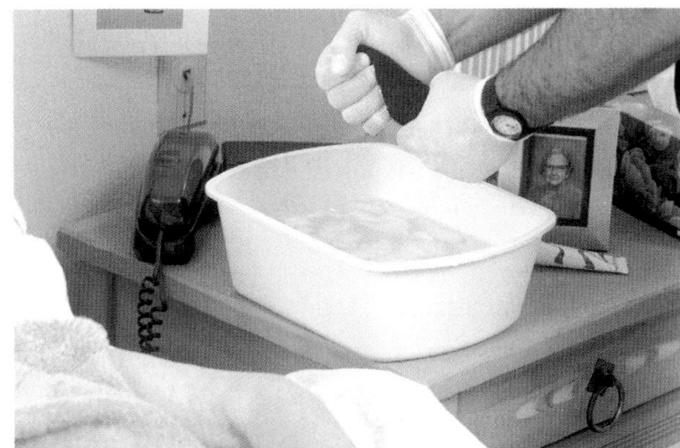

Fig. 14-33. *Wring out the washcloth before applying it to the area to be treated.*

6. Check the area after five minutes for blisters or pale, white, or gray skin. Stop treatment if resident complains of numbness or pain.
7. Remove compresses after 20 minutes or as ordered in the care plan. Give resident towels as needed to dry the area.
8. Make resident comfortable.
9. Place towels in proper container. Empty, clean, and store basin.
10. Place call light within resident's reach.
11. Wash your hands.

12. Report any changes in resident to the nurse.
13. Document procedure using facility guidelines.

7. Discuss non-sterile and sterile dressings

Sterile dressings cover new, open, or draining wounds. A nurse changes these dressings. Non-sterile dressings are applied to dry, closed wounds that have less chance of infection. Nursing assistants may change non-sterile dressings.

Changing a dry dressing using non-sterile technique

Equipment: package of square gauze dressings, adhesive tape, scissors, 2 pairs of gloves

1. Identify yourself by name. Identify the resident by name.
2. Wash your hands.
3. Explain procedure to the resident. Speak clearly, slowly, and directly. Maintain face-to-face contact whenever possible.
4. Provide for resident's privacy with curtain, screen, or door.
5. With scissors, cut pieces of tape long enough to secure the dressing. Hang tape on the edge of a table within reach. Open the four-inch gauze square package without touching the gauze. Place the opened package on a flat surface.
6. Put on gloves.
7. Remove soiled dressing by gently peeling tape toward the wound. Lift dressing off the wound. Do not drag it over the wound. Observe the dressing for any odor or drainage. Notice the color and size of the wound. Dispose of used dressing in proper container.
8. Remove and discard gloves. Wash your hands.
9. Put on new gloves. Touching only outer edges of new four-inch gauze, remove it from the package. Apply it to the wound. Tape gauze in place. Secure it firmly (Fig. 14-34).

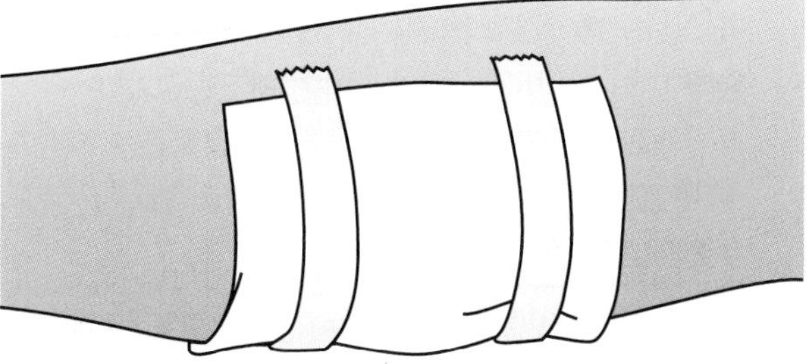

Fig. 14-34. *Tape gauze in place to secure the dressing. Do not completely cover all areas of the dressing with tape.*

10. Discard supplies.
11. Remove and discard gloves.
12. Wash your hands.
13. Make resident comfortable.
14. Place call light within resident's reach.
15. Report any changes in resident to the nurse.
16. Document procedure using facility guidelines.

Even though nursing assistants do not change sterile dressings, they can gather and store equipment and supplies, observe and report about the dressing site, and they may be allowed to clean the equipment. Duties may also include properly positioning the resident, cutting the tape, and disposing of the soiled dressing. Supplies that may be needed for changing a sterile dressing include the following:

- Special gauze has one side that has a shiny, non-stick surface, which will not stick to wounds when removed.
- Abdominal pads (ABDs) are large, heavy gauze dressings that cover smaller gauze dressings and help keep them in place and provide absorbency.

- Cotton bandages (sometimes called *Kerlix* or *Kling* bandages) can stretch and mold to a body part and help hold it in place; these are often used on bony areas, such as the knees and elbows.
- Binders are stretchable pieces of fabric that can be fastened. They hold dressings in place and give support to surgical wounds. Binders can also reduce swelling and ease discomfort.
- Medical-grade adhesive tape panels (sometimes called *Montgomery Straps*) help keep frequently-changed dressings in place. The adhesive is not removed with each dressing change so that skin is less likely to become irritated.

Guidelines: Sterile Dressings

G If the wrapper on the supply is torn, it is no longer considered sterile and cannot be used.

G The wrapper on the supply cannot be opened and closed again. Once a wrapper is opened, the supplies inside are no longer sterile.

G If a wrapper is wet or has wrinkles or marks that indicate it was once wet, it is no longer considered sterile.

G If the date on the supply shows it has expired, it is no longer considered sterile. All commercially-prepared supplies are dated. A sterile supply that has expired should not be used.

G If you are unsure whether a supply is sterile or not, do not use it.

G Because of the way the wound and the skin around it may look, the resident may feel embarrassed about having others see the area. Promote the resident's comfort and dignity when assisting the nurse with a sterile dressing change by being professional. Do not show any discomfort, even if you are bothered by the appearance of the resident's wound or skin.

G Observing and documenting your observations are very important parts of your job. While you are assisting with changing a sterile dressing, observe for any changes in the wound, especially the following:

- Skin that has changed color
- Scab that has come off
- Bleeding
- Swelling
- Odor
- Drainage

8. Discuss guidelines for elastic bandages

Elastic, or non-sterile, bandages (sometimes called *ACE bandages*) are used to hold dressings in place, secure splints, and support and protect body parts. In addition, these bandages may decrease swelling that occurs from an injury (Fig. 14-35).

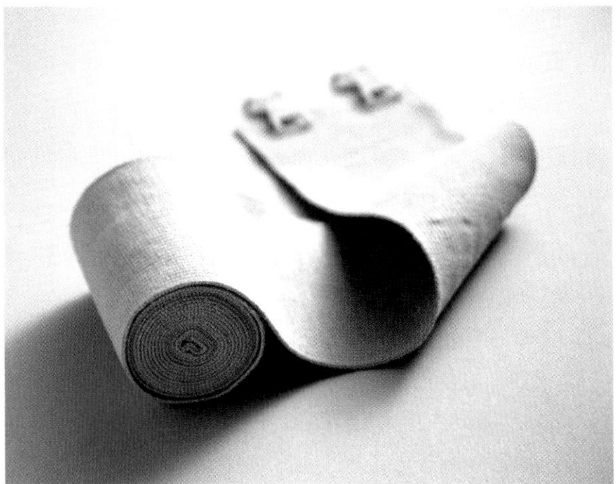

Fig. 14-35. *One type of elastic bandage.*

Nursing assistants may be required to assist with the use of an elast vic bandage. Duties may include bringing the bandage to the resident, positioning the resident to apply the bandage, washing and storing the bandage, and documenting observations. Some states allow NAs to apply and remove elastic bandages. They should follow their facility's policies and the care plan regarding elastic bandages.

Guidelines: Elastic Bandages

- G Keep the area to be wrapped clean and dry.
- G Apply elastic bandages snugly enough to control bleeding and prevent movement of dressings. However, make sure that the body part is not wrapped too tightly, which can decrease circulation.
- G Wrap the bandage upwards and evenly, in a figure-eight pattern, so that no part of the wrapped area is pinched.
- G Do not tie the bandage because this cuts off circulation to the body part; the end is held in place with special clips, tape, or fasteners.
- G Remove the bandage as often as indicated in the care plan.
- G Check the bandage often because it can become wrinkled or loose, which causes it to lose effectiveness, or it can become bunched up, which causes pressure and possible discomfort.
- G Check on the resident 15 minutes after the bandage is applied to check for signs of poor circulation. Signs and symptoms of poor circulation include the following:
  - Swelling
  - Bluish, or cyanotic, skin
  - Shiny, tight skin
  - Skin that is cold to the touch
  - Sores
  - Numbness
  - Tingling
  - Pain or discomfort

  Loosen the bandage if you note any signs of poor circulation, and notify the nurse immediately.

9. List care guidelines for a resident who has an IV

IV is the abbreviation for **intravenous**, or into a vein. A resident with an IV is receiving medication, nutrition, or fluids through a vein. When a doctor prescribes an IV, a nurse inserts a needle or tube into a vein. This allows direct access to the bloodstream. Medication, nutrition, or fluids either drip from a bag suspended on a pole or are pumped by a portable pump through a tube and into the vein (Fig. 14-36). Some residents with chronic conditions may have a permanent opening for IVs, called a *port*. This opening has been surgically created to allow easy access for IV fluids.

Nursing assistants never insert or remove IV lines. They are not responsible for care of the IV site. Their only responsibility for IV care is to report and document any observations of changes or problems with the IV.

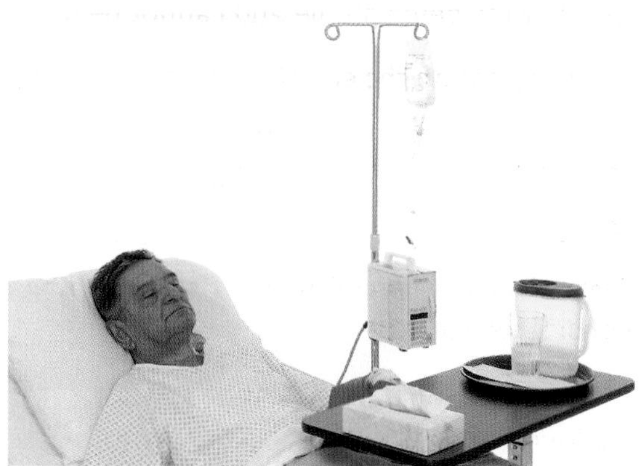

Fig. 14-36. *A resident receiving intravenous medication.*

Observing and Reporting: IVs

Report any of the following to the nurse:

- O/R The tube/needle falls out or is removed
- O/R The tubing disconnects
- O/R The dressing around the IV site is loose or not intact
- O/R Blood is in the tubing or around the IV site

- O/R The site is swollen or discolored
- O/R The resident complains of pain
- O/R The bag is broken, or the level of fluid does not seem to decrease
- O/R The IV fluid is not dripping or is leaking
- O/R The IV fluid is nearly gone
- O/R The pump beeps, indicating a problem
- O/R The pump is dropped

Nursing assistants should document their observations and the care provided. They should not do any of the following when caring for a resident who has an IV:

- Measure blood pressure on an arm with an IV
- Get the IV site wet
- Lower the IV bag below the IV site.
- Leave the tubing kinked
- Touch the clamp
- Pull or catch the tubing on anything, such as clothing
- Disconnect the IV from the pump or turn off the alarm

Assisting in changing clothes for a resident who has an IV

Equipment: clean clothes

1. Identify yourself by name. Identify the resident by name.
2. Wash your hands.
3. Explain procedure to the resident. Speak clearly, slowly, and directly. Maintain face-to-face contact whenever possible.
4. Provide for resident's privacy with curtain, screen, or door.
5. Adjust bed to lowest position. Lock bed wheels.
6. Assist resident to sitting position with feet flat on the floor.
7. Ask the resident to remove the arm without the IV from clothing. Assist as necessary.
8. Help the resident gather the clothing on the arm with the IV. Carefully lift the clothing over the IV site and move it up the tubing toward the IV bag (Fig. 14-37).

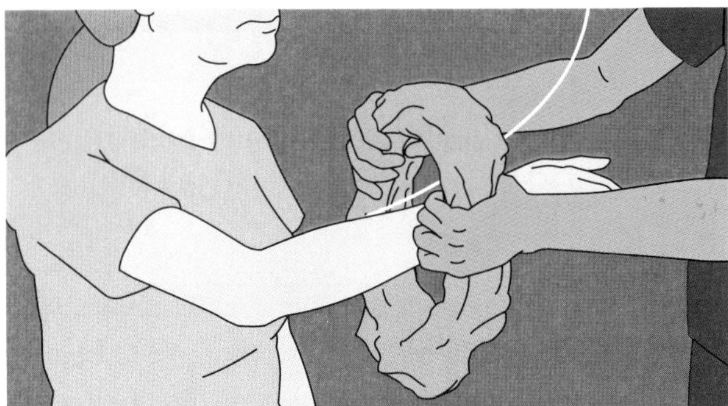

Fig. 14-37. *Make sure clothing does not catch on tubing.*

9. Lift the IV bag off of its pole, keeping it higher than the IV site. Carefully slide clothing over the bag. Place bag back on the pole.
10. Set the used clothing aside to be placed with soiled laundry.
11. Gather the sleeve of the clean clothing.
12. Lift the IV bag off its pole and, keeping it higher than the IV site, carefully slide the clothing over the bag (Fig. 14-38). Place the IV bag back on the pole.

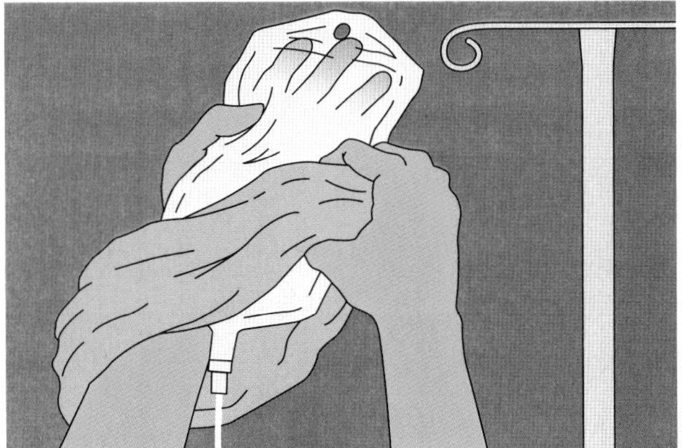

Fig. 14-38. *Always keep the IV bag higher than the IV site.*

13. Carefully move the clean clothing down the IV tubing, over the IV site, and onto the resident's arm.

14. Have the resident put her other arm in the clothing. Assist as necessary.
15. Check that the IV is dripping properly. Make sure none of the tubing is dislodged and that the IV site dressing is in place. Make sure tubing is not kinked after you are finished.
16. Assist the resident with changing the rest of her clothing as necessary.
17. Place soiled clothes in proper container.
18. Make resident comfortable.
19. Place call light within resident's reach.
20. Wash your hands.
21. Report any changes in resident to the nurse.
22. Document procedure using facility guidelines.

Special gowns with sleeves that snap and unsnap are available to lessen the risk of pulling out IVs.

Residents' Rights

IVs

Nursing assistants can protect the rights of residents with IVs by helping them be as independent as possible. The NA should set up the area so the resident may still feed herself, help with bathing and hair care if able, etc. NAs can ask the nurse how to transport residents to activities they want to attend.

10. Discuss oxygen therapy and explain related care guidelines

Oxygen therapy is the administration of oxygen to increase the supply of oxygen to the lungs. This increases the availability of oxygen to the body tissues. Oxygen therapy is used to treat breathing difficulties and is prescribed by a doctor. Nursing assistants should never stop, adjust, or administer oxygen for a resident.

Oxygen may be piped into a resident's room through a central system. It may be in tanks or produced by an oxygen concentrator. Compressed oxygen and liquid oxygen are stored in tanks of varying sizes (Fig. 14-39). An oxygen concentrator produces and distributes oxygen, but does not store oxygen.

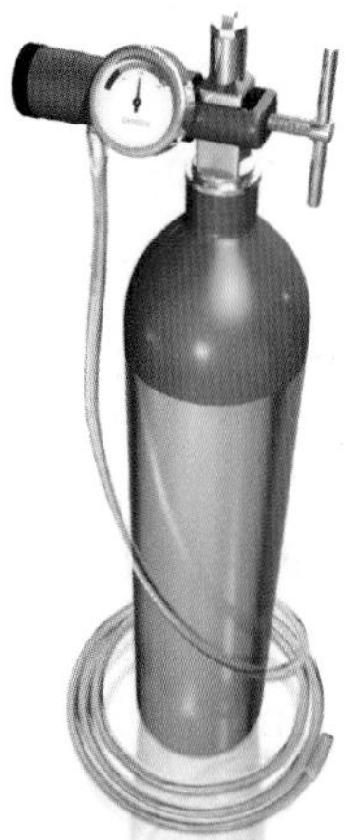

Fig. 14-39. *This is one type of oxygen tank.*

An **oxygen concentrator** is a box-like device that changes air in the room into air with more oxygen. Oxygen concentrators are quiet machines. They can be larger units or portable ones that can move or travel with the resident (Fig. 14-40). They have at least one filter that typically needs to be cleaned once per week. Oxygen concentrators run on electricity. They are plugged into wall outlets and are turned on and off by a switch. It may take a while for the oxygen concentrator to reach full power after it is turned on.

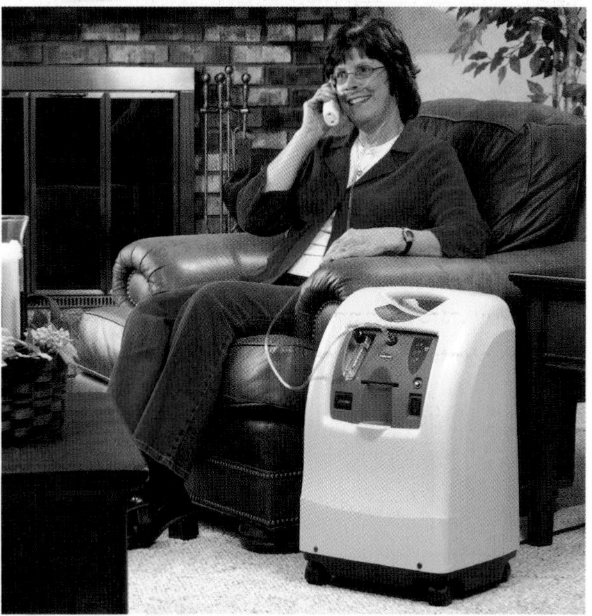

Fig. 14-40. *One type of oxygen concentrator.* (© INVACARE CORPORATION. USED WITH PERMISSION. WWW.INVACARE.COM)

Some residents receive oxygen through a nasal cannula. A **nasal cannula** is a piece of plastic tubing that fits around the face and is secured by a strap that goes over the ears and around the back of the head. The face piece has two short prongs made of tubing. These prongs fit inside the nose, pointing downward, and oxygen is delivered through them. A nurse or respiratory therapist fits the cannula. The length of the prongs (usually no more than half an inch) is adjusted for the resident's comfort. The resident can talk and eat while wearing the cannula (Fig. 14-41).

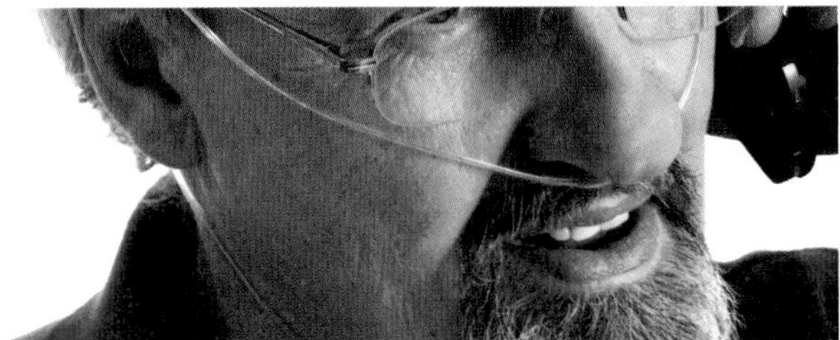

***Fig. 14-41.** Residents can still talk and eat while wearing a nasal cannula.*

Residents who do not need concentrated oxygen all the time may use a face mask when they need oxygen (Fig. 14-42). The face mask fits over the nose and mouth. It is secured by a strap that goes over the ears and around the back of the head. The mask should be checked to see that it fits snugly on the resident's face, but it should not pinch the face. It is difficult for a resident to talk when wearing an oxygen face mask. The mask must be removed for the resident to eat or drink anything.

Oxygen can be irritating to the nose and mouth. The strap of a nasal cannula or face mask can also cause irritation around the ears. NAs should wash and dry skin carefully and provide frequent mouth care. They should offer the resident plenty of fluids and report any irritation observed.

Oxygen is a very dangerous fire hazard because it makes other things burn (supports combustion). Safety guidelines for oxygen use are located in Chapter 6.

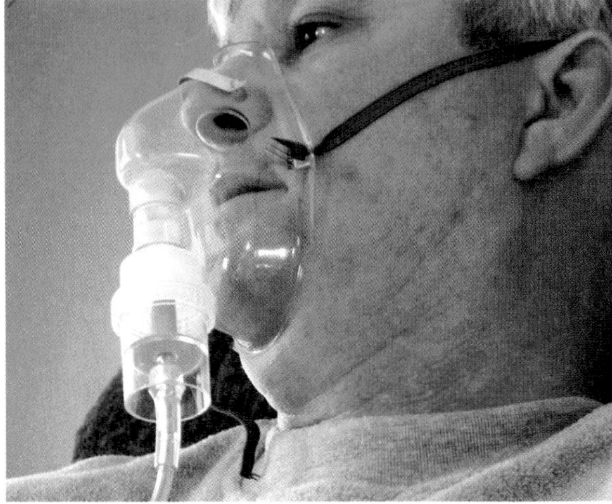

***Fig. 14-42.** Residents who need oxygen occasionally may use a face mask.*

Guidelines: Oxygen Delivery Devices

For residents using oxygen tanks:

- G Measure and record pulse and respirations before and after resident uses the oxygen tank to see if there are any changes.
- G The flow meter shows how much oxygen is flowing out to the resident at any time. It should be set at the amount stated on the care plan. If it is not, report this to the nurse. Do not adjust oxygen level.
- G Make sure the humidifying bottle has sterile water in it and is attached correctly. Wash the humidifying bottle according to the care plan or equipment supplier's instructions.
- G Change the nasal cannula when ordered. It will need to be changed when it is hard or cracked, at least once per week.
- G Make sure the oxygen tank is secured and will not tip over.

For residents using liquid oxygen:

- G Turn off supply valves when the reservoir is not in use.
- G Do not tip the reservoir on its side.
- G Make sure the reservoir is not in a closet, cupboard, or other closed-in space.

- Do not cover the reservoir with bed linens or clothing.
- When lifting the reservoir, lift with two hands. Do not roll the reservoir or walk it on edge.
- Do not touch frosted parts of the equipment, because the cold can cause frostbite. Do not touch liquid oxygen; it can cause frostbite. Report if the reservoir is leaking.

For residents using oxygen concentrators:

- Measure and record pulse and respirations before and after resident uses the oxygen concentrator to see if there are any changes.
- The oxygen concentrator dial must be set at the same rate as indicated in the care plan. If it is not, report this to the nurse. Do not adjust oxygen level.
- Check the humidifying bottle each time the device is used to see that it has sterile water in it and that it is screwed on tightly. Sterile water, not tap water, must be used because minerals in tap water may clog the tubing.
- Make sure the concentrator is in a well-ventilated area, at least six inches from a wall.
- Because the air filter cleans the air going into the machine, brush it off daily to remove dust.

Humidifiers

A humidifier is a device that puts moisture into the air. Residents who use oxygen equipment or who have breathing problems may use humidifiers. Making the air moist or humid can make residents more comfortable.

There are different types of humidifiers; some humidifiers put warm moisture into the air and some put cool moisture into the air.

Nursing assistants should follow the care plan's instructions for cleaning and care of a humidifier. Because pathogens grow in moist areas, the water tank of the humidifier should be washed often. Other responsibilities NAs may have include adding water to the humidifier when needed and possibly adding special tablets to prevent mineral build-up.

Chapter Review

1. List five vital signs that must be monitored.
2. What are the main sites for taking the body's temperature?
3. Which temperature site is considered to be the most accurate?
4. What is the most common site for monitoring the pulse? Where is it located?
5. Why should respirations be counted immediately after measuring the pulse rate?
6. List the two parts of measuring blood pressure and briefly define both phases.
7. List the two pieces of equipment normally used to monitor blood pressure.
8. How are blood pressure numbers written and recorded?
9. List 15 signs that may show that a resident is in pain.
10. List seven measures that can reduce pain.
11. What are the benefits of warm applications? What are the benefits of cold applications?
12. What four signs should an NA watch for at the site of a warm or cold application?
13. What is the purpose of a sitz bath?
14. When are non-sterile dressings usually used?
15. What duties may a nursing assistant have regarding sterile dressings?
16. List six signs of poor circulation that an NA should observe for when an elastic bandage is applied.
17. What is a nursing assistant's responsibility regarding care of an IV?
18. What is an oxygen concentrator?
19. What is a nasal cannula?
20. Why is oxygen a dangerous fire hazard?

15 Nutrition and Hydration

1. Describe the importance of proper nutrition and list the six basic nutrients

Proper nutrition is very important. **Nutrition** is how the body uses food to maintain health. Bodies need a well-balanced diet containing essential nutrients and plenty of fluids. This helps the body grow new cells, maintain normal body function, and have energy for activities. Proper nutrition in childhood and early adulthood helps ensure good health later in life. For the ill or elderly, a well-balanced diet helps maintain muscle and skin tissues and prevent pressure ulcers. A healthy diet promotes the healing of wounds. It also helps a person cope with physical and emotional stress.

A **nutrient** is something found in food that provides energy, promotes growth and health, and helps regulate metabolism. Metabolism is the process by which nutrients are broken down to be used by the body for energy and other needs. The body needs the following six nutrients for growth and development:

1. **Water**: Water is the most essential nutrient for life. Because one-half to two-thirds of the body's weight is water, a person needs about 64 ounces, or eight glasses, of water or other fluids per day. Without it, a person can only live a few days. Water assists in the digestion and absorption of food. It helps with the elimination of waste. Through perspiration, water also helps maintain normal body temperature. Maintaining enough fluid in the body is necessary for good health (Fig. 15-1).

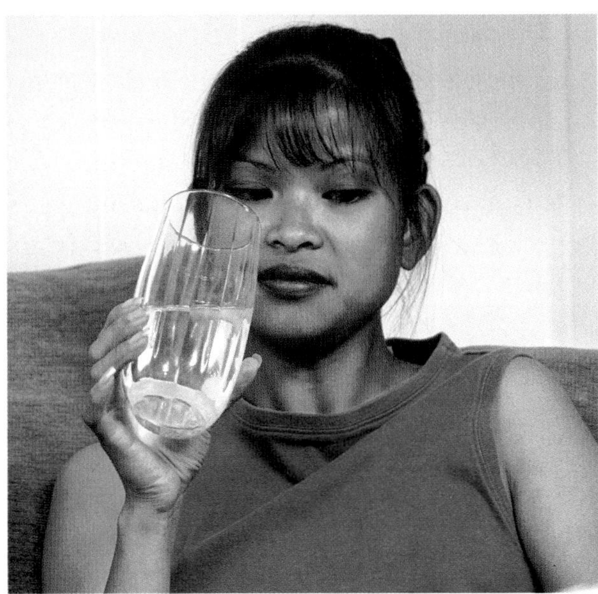

Fig. 15-1. *Water is the most essential nutrient for life. Drinking plenty of water promotes good health.*

The fluids a person drinks—water, juice, soda, coffee, tea, and milk—provide most of the water the body uses. Some foods are also sources of water, including soup, celery, lettuce, apples, and peaches.

2. **Carbohydrates**: Carbohydrates supply the body with energy and extra protein and help the body use fat efficiently. Carbohydrates also provide fiber, which is necessary for bowel elimination.

Carbohydrates can be divided into two basic types: complex and simple carbohydrates (Fig. 15-2). **Complex carbohydrates** are found in bread, cereal, potatoes, rice, pasta, vegetables, and fruits. **Simple carbohydrates** are found in foods such as sugars, sweets, syrups, and jellies. Simple carbohydrates do not have the same nutritional value that complex carbohydrates do.

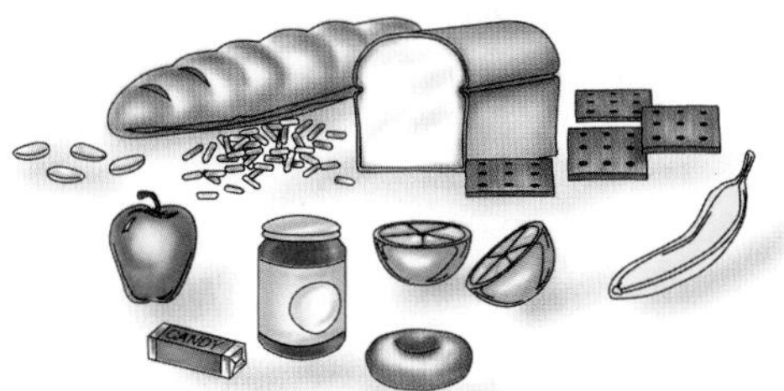

Fig. 15-2. *Sources of carbohydrates.*

3. **Protein**: Proteins are part of every body cell. They are needed for tissue growth and repair. Proteins also supply energy for the body. Excess proteins are excreted by the kidneys or stored as body fat. Sources of protein include seafood, poultry, meat, eggs, milk, cheese, nuts, nut butters, peas, dried beans or legumes, and soy products (tofu, tempeh, some veggie burgers) (Fig. 15-3). Whole grain cereals, pastas, rice, and breads contain some proteins, too.

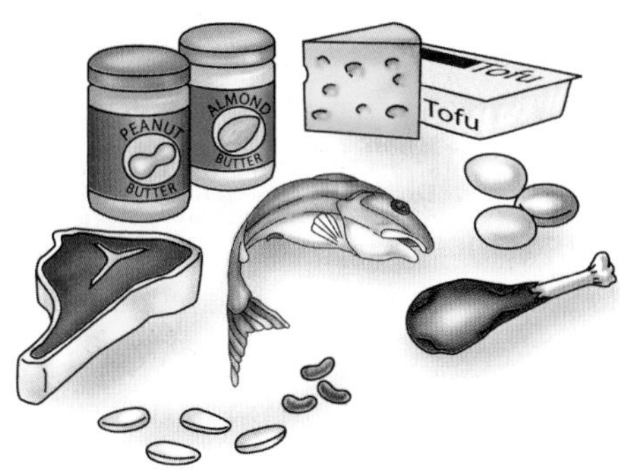

Fig. 15-3. *Sources of protein.*

4. **Fats**: Fat helps the body store energy. In addition, fats add flavor to food and are important for the absorption of certain vitamins. Excess fat in the diet is stored as fat in the body.

Examples of fats are butter, margarine, salad dressings, oils, and animal fats in meats, dairy products, fowl, and fish (Fig. 15-4). Monounsaturated vegetable fats (including olive oil and canola oil) and polyunsaturated vegetable fats (including corn and safflower oils) are healthier kinds of fats. Saturated fats, including animal fats like butter, lard, bacon, and other fatty meats, are not as healthy. They should be limited in most diets.

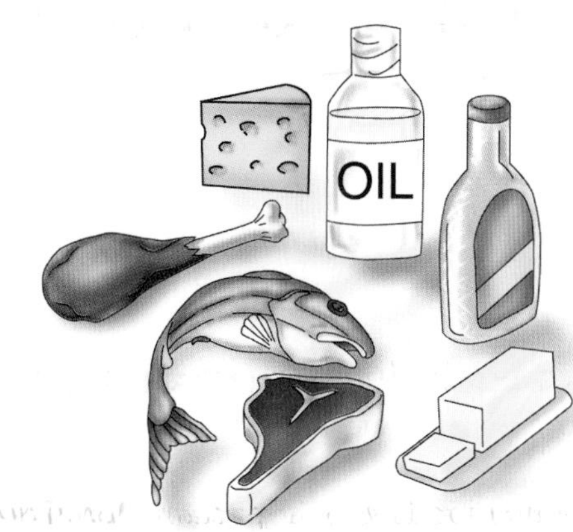

Fig. 15-4. *Sources of fat.*

5. **Vitamins**: Vitamins are substances that are needed by the body to function. The body cannot produce most vitamins; they can only be obtained by eating certain foods. Vitamins A, D, E, and K are fat-soluble vitamins. This means they are carried and stored in body fat. Vitamins B and C are water-soluble vitamins that are broken down by water in the body and used by the body, but cannot be stored. They are eliminated in urine and feces.

6. **Minerals**: Minerals maintain body functions. They provide energy and regulate body processes. Zinc, iron, calcium, and magnesium are examples of minerals. Minerals are found in many foods.

2. Describe the USDA's MyPlate

Most foods contain several nutrients, but no one food contains all the nutrients that are necessary to maintain a healthy body. That is why it is important to eat a daily diet that is well-balanced. There is not one single dietary plan that is right for everyone. People have different nutritional needs depending upon their age, gender, and activity levels.

In 2011, in response to increasing rates of people who are overweight or obese, the United States Department of Agriculture (USDA) developed MyPlate to help people build a healthy plate at meal times (Fig. 15-5). The MyPlate icon emphasizes vegetables, fruits, grains, protein, and low-fat dairy. It replaces the USDA's MyPyramid icon, which was introduced in 2005.

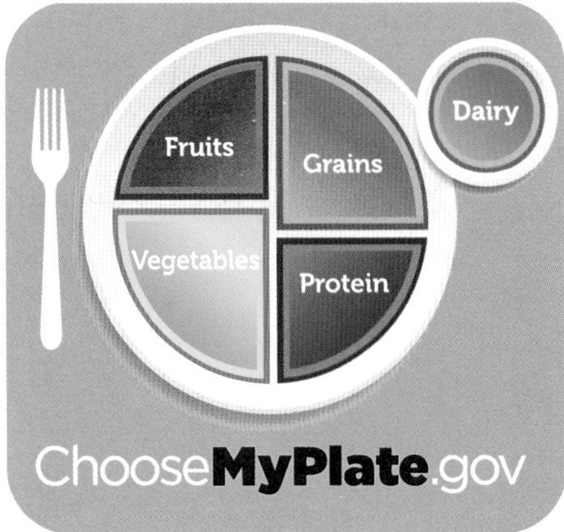

Fig. 15-5. *The MyPlate icon and web address was developed by the U.S. Department of Agriculture in 2011 to help promote healthy eating practices.*

MyPlate's message of adopting healthy eating habits supports the *2010 Dietary Guidelines for Americans*. The *Dietary Guidelines for Americans* issues recommendations for improving health by promoting healthy eating and physical activity. It is reviewed, revised (if necessary), and published every five years.

MyPlate gives suggestions and tools for making healthy choices; however, it does not provide specific messages about what a person should eat. The MyPlate icon includes the following food groups:

Vegetables and fruits: A person should make half his plate fruits and vegetables. Vegetables include all fresh, frozen, canned, and dried vegetables, and vegetable juices. There are five subgroups within the vegetable group, organized by their nutritional content. These are dark green vegetables, red and orange vegetables, dry beans and peas, starchy vegetables, and other vegetables. A variety of vegetables from these subgroups should be eaten every day. Dark green, red, and orange vegetables have the best nutritional content (Fig. 15-6).

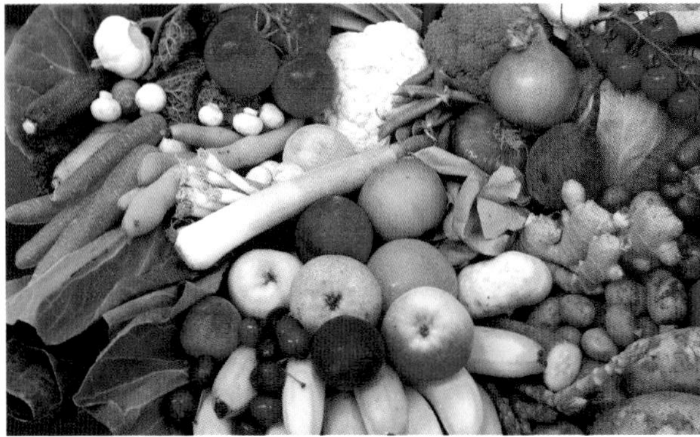

Fig. 15-6. *Eating a variety of vegetables every day, especially dark green, red, and orange vegetables, helps promote good health.*

Vegetables are low in fat and calories and have no cholesterol (although sauces and seasonings may add fat, calories, and cholesterol). They are good sources of dietary fiber, potassium, vitamin A, vitamin E, and vitamin C.

Fruits include all fresh, frozen, canned, and dried fruits, and 100% fruit juices. Most choices should be whole, cut-up, or pureed fruit, rather than juice, for the additional dietary fiber provided. Fruit can be added as a main dish, side dish, or as a dessert.

Fruits, like vegetables, are naturally low in fat, sodium, and calories and have no cholesterol. They are important sources of dietary fiber and many nutrients, including folic acid, potassium, and vitamin C. Foods containing dietary fiber help provide a feeling of fullness with fewer calories. Folic acid helps the body form red blood cells. Vitamin C is important for growth and repair of body tissues.

Grains: A person should make half his grain intake whole grains. Grains include all foods made from wheat, rice, oats, cornmeal, or barley, such as bread, pasta, oatmeal, breakfast cereals, tortillas, and grits. Grains can be divided into two groups: whole grains and refined grains. Whole grains contain bran and germ, as well as the endosperm. Refined grains retain only the endosperm. Examples of whole grains include brown rice, wild rice, bulgur, oatmeal, whole-grain corn, whole oats, whole wheat, and whole rye. Consuming foods rich in fiber reduces the risk of heart disease and other diseases and may reduce constipation.

Protein: MyPlate guidelines emphasize the importance of eating a variety of protein foods every week. Meat, poultry, seafood, and eggs are animal sources of proteins. Beans, peas, soy products, nuts, and seeds are plant sources of proteins.

Seafood should be eaten twice a week in place of meat or poultry. Seafood that is higher in oils and low in mercury, such as salmon or trout, is a better choice (Fig. 15-7). Lean meats and poultry, as well as eggs and egg whites, can be eaten on a regular basis. A person should eat plant-based protein foods more often. Beans and peas, soy products (tofu, tempeh, some veggie burgers), nuts, and seeds are low in saturated fat and high in fiber. Some nuts and seeds (flax, walnuts) are excellent sources of essential fatty acids. These acids may reduce the risk of cardiovascular disease. Sunflower seeds and almonds are good sources of vitamin E.

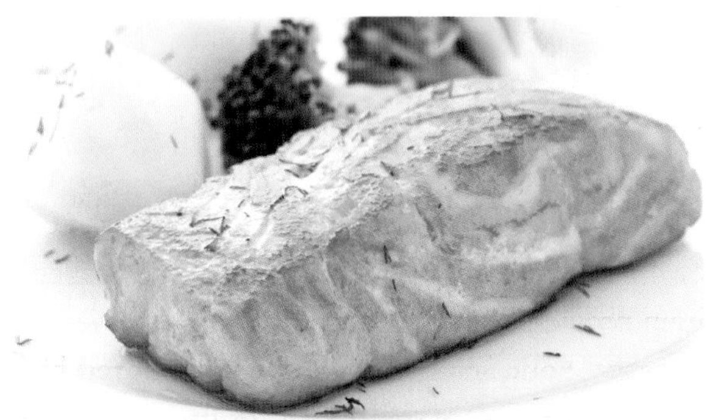

Fig. 15-7. *Fish, like this salmon, contains healthy oils and is a good source of protein.*

Dairy: All milk products and foods made from milk that retain their calcium content, such as yogurt and cheese, are part of the dairy category. Most dairy group choices should be fat-free or low-fat (1%). Fat-free or low-fat milk or yogurt should be chosen more often than cheese. Milk and yogurt contain less sodium than most cheeses.

Milk provides nutrients that are vital for the health and maintenance of the body. These nutrients include calcium, potassium, vitamin D, and protein. Fat-free or low-fat milk provides these nutrients without the extra calories and saturated fat (Fig. 15-8). Soy products enriched with calcium are an alternative to dairy foods.

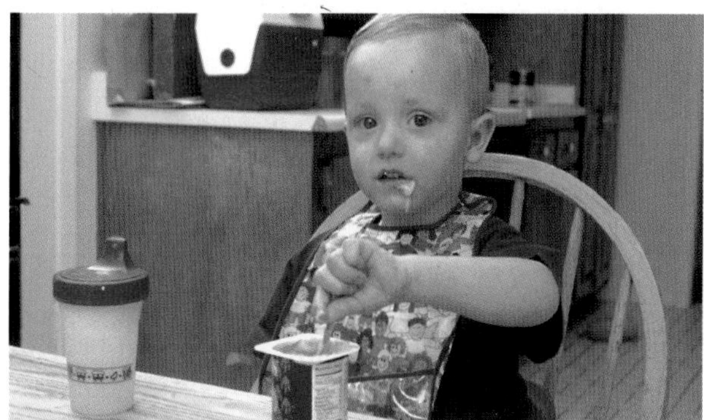

Fig. 15-8. *Low-fat milk or yogurt is a good source of calcium without the added saturated fat.*

ChooseMyPlate.gov has more information about the USDA's MyPlate. The following guidelines provide additional tips for making healthy food choices:

Guidelines: Healthy Food Choices

- G Balance calories. Calorie balance is the relationship between the calories obtained from food and fluids consumed and the calories used during normal body functions and physical activity. Proper calorie intake varies from person to person. To find the proper calorie intake, the USDA suggests visiting ChooseMyPlate.gov.
- G Enjoy your food, but eat less. Eating too fast or eating without paying attention to your food can lead to overeating. Recognize when you feel hungry and when you are full. Notice what you are eating. Stop eating when you feel satisfied.
- G Avoid oversized portions. Choose smaller-sized portions when eating. Portion out food before you eat it, and use smaller bowls and plates for meals. When eating out, split food with others or take part of your meal home.

- **G** Eat these foods more often: vegetables, fruits, whole grains, and fat-free or 1% milk and low-fat dairy products. These foods have better nutrients for health.
- **G** Eat these foods less often: foods high in solid fats, added sugars, and salt. These foods include fatty meats, like bacon and hot dogs, cheese, fried foods, ice cream, and cookies.
- **G** Compare sodium in foods. Read product labels to determine if they contain salt or sodium. Foods high in sodium include the following:
    - Cured meats, including ham, bacon, lunch meat, sausage, salt pork, and hot dogs
    - Salty or smoked fish, including herring, salted cod, sardines, anchovies, caviar, smoked salmon, or lox
    - Processed cheese and some other cheeses
    - Salted foods, including nuts, pretzels, potato chips, dips, and spreads, such as salted butter and margarine
    - Vegetables preserved in brine, such as pickles, sauerkraut, pickled vegetables, olives, and relishes
    - Sauces with high concentrations of salt, including Worcestershire, chili, steak, and soy sauces; ketchup; and mayonnaise
    - Commercially-prepared foods such as breads, canned soups and vegetables, and certain breakfast cereals

  Select canned foods that are labeled *sodium-free, very low sodium, low-sodium*, or *reduced sodium*.
- **G** Drink water instead of sugary drinks. Drinking water or unsweetened beverages reduces sugar and calorie intake. Sweetened beverages, such as soda, fruit punch, and sports drinks, are a major source of sugar and calories in diets.

3. Identify nutritional problems of the elderly or ill

Aging and illness can lead to emotional and physical problems that affect the intake of food. For example, people who are lonely or who suffer from illnesses that affect their ability to chew and swallow may have little interest in food. Weaker hands and arms due to paralysis and tremors make it hard to eat. People with illnesses that affect their ability to chew and swallow may not want to eat. In addition, people who are ill are often fatigued, nauseated, or in pain, which contributes to poor fluid and food intake. Other problems that affect nutritional intake include the following:

- Metabolism slows. Muscles weaken and lose tone, and body movement slows. Reduced activity or exercise affects appetite.
- A loss of vision may affect the way food looks, which can decrease appetite.
- Weakened senses of smell and taste affect appetite. Medication may impair these senses (Fig. 15-9).
- Less saliva production affects chewing and swallowing.
- Dentures, tooth loss, and poor dental health can make chewing difficult.
- Digestion takes longer and is less efficient.
- Certain medication or limited activity causes constipation. Constipation often interferes with appetite. Fiber, fluids, and exercise can improve this common problem.

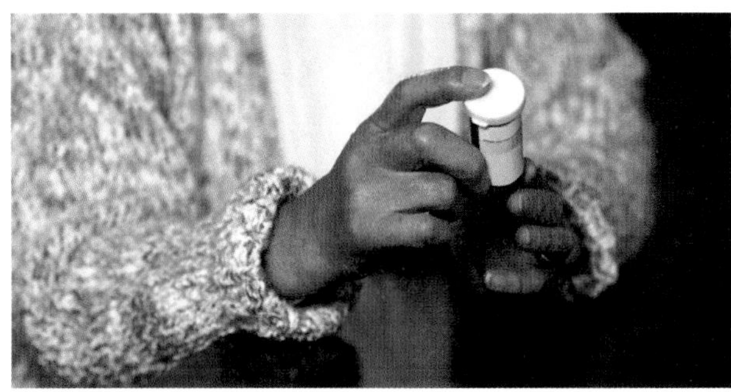

Fig. 15-9. *Many elderly people take a variety of medications, which can affect the way food smells and tastes.*

Unintended weight loss is a serious problem for the elderly. Weight loss can mean that the resident has a serious medical condition. It can lead to skin breakdown, which leads to pressure ulcers. It is very important for nursing assistants to report any weight loss, no matter how small. If a resident has diabetes, chronic obstructive pulmonary disease, cancer, HIV, or other diseases, he is at a greater risk for malnutrition. (Chapter 18 contains more information on these diseases.)

Guidelines: Preventing Unintended Weight Loss

- G Report observations and warning signs to the nurse.
- G Food should look, taste, and smell good, particularly since the resident may have a poor sense of taste and smell.
- G Encourage residents to eat. Talk about food that is being served in a positive tone of voice, using positive words (Fig. 15-10).

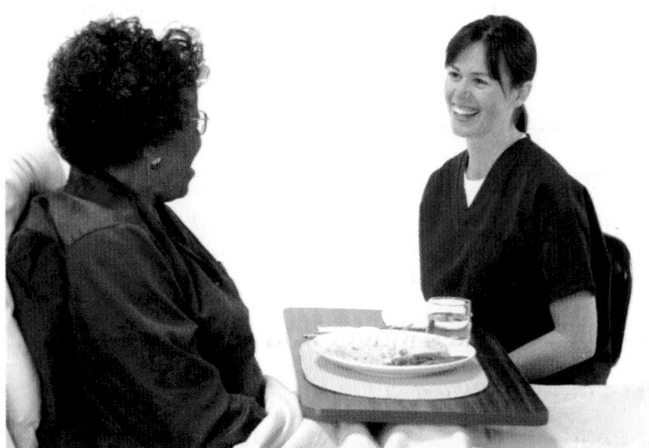

***Fig. 15-10.** Being friendly and positive while helping residents with eating helps promote appetite and prevent weight loss.*

- G Honor residents' food likes and dislikes.
- G Offer different kinds of foods and beverages.
- G Help residents who have trouble feeding themselves.
- G Season foods to residents' preferences.
- G Allow enough time for residents to finish eating.
- G Tell the nurse if residents have trouble using utensils.
- G Record the meal/snack intake.
- G Provide oral care before and after meals.
- G Position residents sitting upright for eating.
- G If a resident has had a loss of appetite and/or seems sad, ask about it.

Observing and Reporting: Unintended Weight Loss

Report any of these to the nurse:

- O/R Resident needs help eating or drinking
- O/R Resident eats less than 70% of meals served
- O/R Resident has mouth pain
- O/R Resident has dentures that do not fit properly
- O/R Resident has difficulty chewing or swallowing
- O/R Resident coughs or chokes while eating
- O/R Resident is sad, has crying spells, or withdraws from others
- O/R Resident is confused, wanders, or paces

Care must be taken in meal planning to ensure good nutrition for the elderly and ill. Many illnesses require restrictions of fluids, proteins, certain minerals, or calories. Conditions that make eating or swallowing difficult include the following:

- Stroke, or CVA, which can cause facial weakness and paralysis
- Nerve and muscle damage from head and neck cancer
- Multiple sclerosis
- Parkinson's disease
- Alzheimer's disease

If a resident has trouble swallowing, soft foods and liquids that have been thickened may be easier to swallow. Thickening improves the ability to control fluid in the mouth and throat.

Thickened liquids include milk shakes, pureed foods, sherbet, gelatin, thin hot cereal, cream soups, and fruit juices that have been frozen to a slushy consistency. There is more information about swallowing problems and thickened liquids later in the chapter.

When the digestive system does not function properly, hyperalimentation, or **total parenteral nutrition (TPN)**, may be necessary. With TPN, a solution of nutrients is administered directly into the bloodstream. It bypasses the digestive system.

When a person is unable to swallow, he or she may be fed through a tube. A **nasogastric tube** is inserted into the nose and goes to the stomach. A tube can also be placed into the stomach through the abdominal wall. This is called a **percutaneous endoscopic gastrostomy (PEG) tube**. The surgically-created opening into the stomach that allows insertion of a tube is called a **gastrostomy** (Fig. 15-11). Tube feedings are used when residents cannot swallow but can digest food. Conditions that may prevent residents from swallowing include coma, cancer, stroke, refusal to eat, or extreme weakness. It is important to remember that residents have the legal right to refuse treatment, which includes the insertion of tubes.

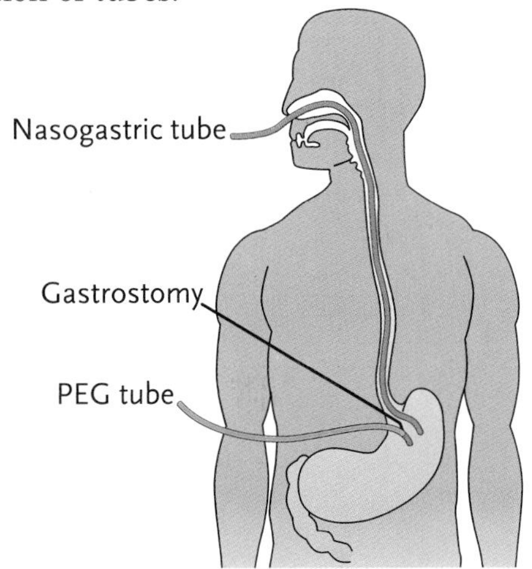

Fig. 15-11. *Nasogastric tubes are inserted through the nose, and PEG tubes are inserted through the abdominal wall into the stomach.*

Nursing assistants never insert tubes, do the feeding, or irrigate (clean) the tubes. However, they may assemble equipment and supplies and hand them to the nurse. NAs may need to position the resident in a sitting position for feeding. They may also discard or clean and store used equipment and supplies. In addition, NAs should observe, report, and document any observation of changes in the resident or problems with the feeding.

Guidelines: Tube Feedings

- Wash your hands before assisting with any aspect of tube feedings.
- Make sure the tubing is not coiled or kinked or resting underneath the resident.
- Be aware if the resident has an order for *nothing by mouth* or *NPO*.
- The tube is only inserted and removed by a doctor or nurse. If it comes out, report it immediately.
- A doctor will prescribe the type and amount of feeding. The feedings should be at room temperature and will be in liquid form.
- A resident with a feeding tube should always have the head of the bed elevated 30 degrees. However, during a feeding, the resident should remain in a sitting position with the head of the bed elevated at least 45 degrees. This helps prevent serious problems, such as aspiration. The elderly can develop pneumonia or even die from improper positioning during tube feedings. After the feeding, keep the resident upright for as long as ordered, at least 30 minutes.
- If the resident must remain in bed for long periods during feedings, give careful skin care. This helps to prevent pressure ulcers on the hips and sacral area.

Observing and Reporting: Tube Feedings

Report any of these to the nurse immediately:

- O/R Redness or drainage around the opening
- O/R Skin sores or bruises
- O/R Cyanotic skin
- O/R Resident complains of pain or nausea
- O/R Choking or coughing
- O/R Vomiting
- O/R Diarrhea
- O/R Swollen abdomen
- O/R Fever
- O/R Tube falling out
- O/R Problems with equipment
- O/R Sound of feeding pump alarm
- O/R Change of resident's inclined position

4. Describe factors that influence food preferences

Culture, ethnicity, income, education, religion, and geography all affect ideas about nutrition. Food preferences may be formed by what a person ate as a child, by what tastes good, or by personal beliefs about what should be eaten (Fig. 15-12). For example, some people choose not to eat any animals or animal products, such as steak, chicken, butter, or eggs. These people are called vegetarians or vegans, depending on what they eat.

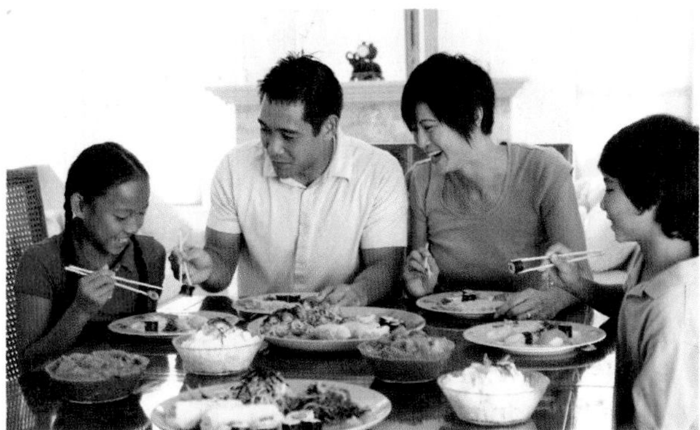

Fig. 15-12. Food likes and dislikes are influenced by what a person ate as a child.

The region or culture a person grows up in often influences his food preference. For example, people from the southwestern United States may like spicy foods. Southern cooking may include fried foods, such as fried chicken or fried okra. Ethnic groups often share common foods. These may be eaten at certain times of the year or all the time. Religious beliefs affect diet, too. For example, some Muslims and Jewish people do not eat any pork. Mormons may not drink alcohol, tea, or coffee.

Food preferences may change while a resident is living at a facility. Just as anyone may decide that he likes some foods for a time and then change his mind, so may residents. Whatever residents' food preferences may be, nursing assistants should respect them. It is never appropriate to make fun of personal preferences. If an NA notices that certain food is not being eaten—no matter how small the amount—she should report it to the nurse.

Residents' Rights

Food Choices

Residents have the legal right to make choices about their food. They can choose what kind of food they want to eat, and they can refuse the food and drink being offered. Nursing assistants must honor a resident's personal beliefs and preferences about selecting and avoiding specific foods. Although residents have the right to refuse, it is best to ask questions when they do. Communication is the key to understanding why a resident refuses something. For example, if a resident refuses his dinner, the NA can ask if there is something wrong with the food. The resident may tell the NA that he is Jewish and cannot eat a pork chop because it is not kosher. NAs should respond to requests for different food in a pleasant way. The NA can explain that she will report to the nurse and will get him another meal as quickly as possible. She should remove the tray and take it to the dietitian or dietary department so that an alternative may be offered.

5. Explain the role of the dietary department

The dietary department staff are responsible for planning meals for all residents. Residents have different nutritional needs. When planning meals, the dietary staff consider these needs, along with individual likes and dislikes. Meals must be balanced to provide proper nutrition.

In addition to planning meals, the dietary staff prepare food in such a way that each resident can manage it. The food must also look appealing. Staff create **diet cards** (Fig. 15-13), which list the resident's name and information about special diets, allergies, likes and dislikes, and other dietary instructions. A diet card is included with each meal that is served to residents who do not eat in the dining room. Nursing assistants are responsible for checking that the diet card matches the correct resident.

NAME ______ ROOM ______ DIETARY LABEL HERE
DIET ______ DIETARY LABEL HERE

BREAKFAST (LIKES)	LUNCH (LIKES)	DINNER (LIKES)
(DISLIKES)	(DISLIKES)	(DISLIKES)
☐ COF. ☐ DECAF. COF. ☐ TEA ☐ MILK	☐ COF. ☐ DECAF. COF. ☐ TEA ☐ MILK	☐ COF. ☐ DECAF. COF. ☐ TEA ☐ MILK

Form 20R BRIGGS, Des Moines, IA 50306 (800) 247-2343

Fig. 15-13. A sample diet card. (REPRINTED WITH PERMISSION OF BRIGGS CORPORATION, 800-247-2343, WWW.BRIGGSCORP.COM)

The dietary department staff must follow strict procedures when preparing food in order to prevent the spread of infection. Regular surveys are performed to check for cleanliness and to ensure that the staff is following proper guidelines.

6. Explain special diets

A doctor sometimes places residents who have certain illnesses on special diets. These diets are known as **therapeutic**, **modified**, or **special diets**. Certain nutrients or fluids may be restricted or eliminated. Some medications may also interact with certain foods, which then must be restricted. Residents who do not eat enough may be placed on special supplementary diets. Diets are also prescribed for weight control and food allergies.

Several types of modified diets are available for different illnesses. Some residents may be on a combination of restricted diets. The care plan should specify any special diets the resident is on. It should also explain any eating problems that a resident may have and how the resident's eating habits can be improved (Fig. 15-14). Nursing assistants must never modify a resident's diet. Special diets can only be prescribed by doctors and planned by dietitians, along with residents. NAs should follow each resident's diet plan without making judgments. Observations should be reported to the nurse.

	Diet Order: Low fat
✓	Meal Preparation
	Assist with Feeding
✓	Limit/Encourage Fluids
	Grocery Shopping

Fig. 15-14. The care plan specifies special diets or dietary restrictions.

Low-Sodium Diet: Residents with high blood pressure, heart disease, kidney disease, or fluid retention may be placed on a low-sodium diet. Many foods contain sodium, but people are most familiar with it as one of two ingredients in salt. Salt is the first food to be restricted in a low-sodium diet because it is high in sodium. For residents on a low-sodium diet, salt will not be used. Salt shakers or packets will not be on the diet tray. Common abbreviations for this diet are *Low Na*, which means low sodium or *NAS*, which stands for *No Added Salt*.

Fluid-Restricted Diet: The amount of fluid consumed through food and fluids must equal the amount of fluid that leaves the body through perspiration, stool, urine, and expiration. This is fluid balance. When fluid intake is greater than fluid output, body tissues become swollen with excess fluid. In addition, people with severe heart disease and kidney disease may have trouble processing fluid. To prevent further damage, doctors may restrict a resident's fluid intake. For residents on fluid restriction, the NA will need to measure and document exact amounts of fluid intake and report excesses to the nurse.

Additional fluids or foods that count as fluids, such as ice cream, puddings, gelatin, etc., should not be offered. If the resident complains of thirst or requests fluids, the NA should tell the nurse. A common abbreviation for this diet is *RF*, which stands for *Restrict Fluids*.

High-Potassium Diets (K+): Some residents are taking blood pressure medications or **diuretics**, which are medications that reduce fluid volume. These residents may be excreting so much fluid that their bodies are depleted of potassium. Other residents may be placed on a high-potassium diet for different reasons.

Foods high in potassium include bananas, grapefruits, oranges, orange juice, prune juice, prunes, dried apricots, figs, raisins, dates, cantaloupes, tomatoes, potatoes with skins, sweet potatoes and yams, winter squash, legumes, avocados, and unsalted nuts. *K+* is the common abbreviation for this diet.

Low-Protein Diet: People who have kidney disease may also be on low-protein diets. Protein is restricted because it breaks down into compounds that may lead to further kidney damage. The extent of the restrictions depends on the stage of the disease and whether the resident is on dialysis. Vegetables and starches, such as breads and pasta, are encouraged.

Low-Fat/Low-Cholesterol Diet: People who have high levels of cholesterol in their blood are at risk for heart attacks and heart disease. People with gallbladder disease, diseases that interfere with fat digestion, and liver disease are also placed on low-fat/low-cholesterol diets.

Low-fat/low-cholesterol diets permit skim milk, low-fat cottage cheese, fish, white meat of turkey and chicken, and vegetable fats (especially monounsaturated fats such as olive, canola, and peanut oils). Residents on this diet may need to follow these guidelines:

- Eat lean cuts of meat, including lamb, beef, and pork, and eat these only three times a week.
- Limit egg yolks to three or four per week (including eggs used in baking).
- Avoid organ meats, shellfish, fatty meats, cream, butter, lard, meat drippings, coconut and palm oils, and desserts and soups made with whole milk.
- Avoid fried foods and sweets.

People who have gallbladder disease or other digestive problems may be placed on a diet that restricts all fats. A common abbreviation for this diet is *Low-Fat/Low-Chol.*

Modified Calorie Diet: Some residents may need to reduce calories to lose weight or prevent additional weight gain. Other residents may need to gain weight and increase calories because of malnutrition, surgery, illness, or fever. Residents with certain conditions need more protein to promote growth and repair of tissue and regulation of body functions. Common abbreviations for this diet are *Low-Cal* or *High-Cal.*

Nutritional Supplements

Illness often causes residents to need extra nutrients, as well as additional calories. Sometimes a resident will be advised by his doctor or dietitian to add a high-nutrition supplement to the regular or modified diet. Usually this is done to encourage weight gain or the intake of proteins, vitamins, or minerals.

Nutritional supplements may come in a powdered or liquid form. Supplements may be pre-mixed and ready to consume. Powdered supplements need to be mixed with a liquid before being taken; the care plan will include instructions on how much liquid to add. When preparing supplements, the nursing assistant should make sure the supplement is mixed thoroughly.

The NA should make sure the resident takes the supplement at the ordered time. A resident who is ill, tired, or in pain may not have much of an appetite. It may take a long time for him to drink a large glass of a thick liquid. The NA should be patient and encouraging. If a resident does not want to drink the supplement, the NA should not insist that he do so, but should report this to the nurse.

Bland Diet: Gastric and duodenal ulcers can be irritated by foods that produce or increase levels of acid in the stomach, so these foods are eliminated. The bland diet is also used for people who have intestinal disorders, such as Crohn's disease or irritable bowel syndrome (IBS). The following foods and drinks should be avoided: alcohol; beverages containing caffeine, such as coffee, tea, and soft drinks; citrus juices; spicy foods; and spicy seasonings such as black pepper, cayenne, and chili pepper. Three meals or more per day are usually advised. If alcohol is allowed, it should be drunk with meals.

Diabetic Diet: People with diabetes must be very careful about what they eat (Fig. 15-15). Calories and carbohydrates are carefully regulated in the diets of residents who have diabetes. Protein and fats are also regulated. The types of foods and the amounts are determined by nutritional and energy needs. A dietitian and the resident will make up a meal plan, taking into account the person's health status, activity levels, and lifestyle. The meal plan will include all the right types and amounts of food for each day.

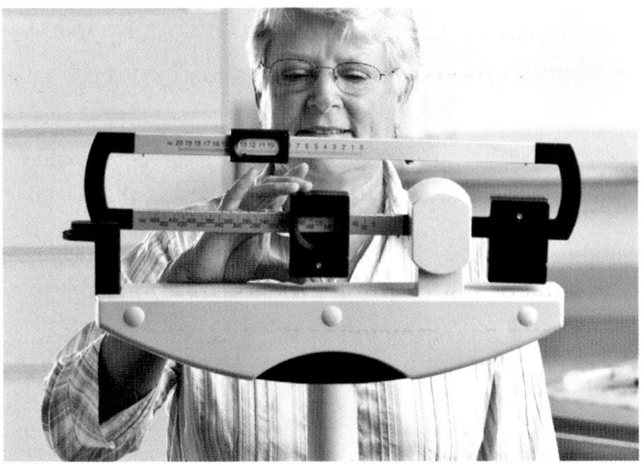

Fig. 15-15. *People who have diabetes must be very careful about what they eat and must keep their weight in a healthy range.*

The meal plan may use a carbohydrate-counting approach (often called *carb counting*). After the proper amount of carbohydrates is determined by the dietitian, they need to be counted in each meal or snack. Nutrition labels need to be read, paying attention to serving size and carbohydrate content. Food portions may need to be measured.

Meal planning can also be done by using the exchange system. Using this system, similar foods can be substituted for one another to make up a menu. Looking at the exchange list, the resident can choose food he wants to eat, while controlling his diet.

To keep their blood glucose levels near normal, diabetic residents must eat the right amount of the right type of food at the right time. They must eat all that is served. Nursing assistants should encourage them to do so and should not offer other foods without the nurse's approval. If a resident will not eat what is directed, or if the NA thinks that he or she is not following the diet, she should tell the nurse.

Diabetics should avoid foods that are high in sugar, such as candy, because sugary foods can cause problems with insulin balance. Foods and drinks high in sugar include candy, ice cream, cakes, cookies, jellies, jams, fruits canned in heavy syrup, soft drinks, and alcoholic beverages. Many foods are high in sugar that do not appear to be so, such as canned vegetables, many breakfast cereals, and ketchup.

A meal tray for a resident with diabetes may have artificial sweetener, low-calorie jelly, and/or low-calorie maple syrup. Residents with diabetes should use artificial sweetener, rather than sugar, in their coffee or tea. Common abbreviations for this diet are *NCS*, which stands for *No Concentrated Sweets* or *LCS*, which stands for *Low Concentrated Sweets*. The American Diabetic Association's (ADA) website, diabetes.org, has more information on diabetic diets.

Low-Residue (Low-Fiber) Diet: This diet decreases the amount of fiber, whole grains, raw fruits and vegetables, seeds, and other foods, such as dairy and coffee. The low-residue diet is used for people with bowel disturbances.

High-Residue (High-Fiber) Diet: High-residue diets increase the intake of fiber and whole grains, such as whole grain cereals, bread, and raw fruits and vegetables. This diet helps with problems such as constipation and bowel disorders.

Gluten-Free Diet: This diet is free of gluten, which is a protein found in wheat, rye, and barley. It is used for people with celiac disease, which is a disorder that can damage the intestines if gluten is consumed. Foods containing wheat flour, such as tortillas, crackers, breads, cakes, pastas, and cereals, are eliminated from the diet. Some sauces and dressings also have wheat in them. Other items that may contain gluten include beer, hot dogs, candy, broths, and medications.

Unlike celiac disease, gluten intolerance is a condition that does not cause damage to the intestines. It does, however, cause unpleasant symptoms such as abdominal pain, gas, and diarrhea when products containing gluten are consumed. If a person has a gluten intolerance, eliminating gluten from the diet is usually enough to manage symptoms.

Vegetarian Diet: Health issues may cause a person to require a vegetarian diet. A person may also choose to eat a vegetarian diet for religious reasons or due to a dislike of meat, a compassion for animals, a belief in non-violence, or financial issues. There are different types of vegetarian diets, including the following:

- A lacto-ovo vegetarian diet excludes all meats, fish, and poultry, but allows eggs and dairy products.
- A lacto-vegetarian diet eliminates poultry, meats, fish, and eggs, but allows dairy products.
- An ovo-vegetarian diet omits all meats, fish, poultry, and dairy products, but allows eggs.
- A vegan diet eliminates poultry, meats, fish, eggs, and dairy products, along with all foods that are derived from animals.

Liquid Diet: A liquid diet is usually ordered for a short time due to a medical condition or before or after a test or surgery. It is ordered when a resident needs to keep the intestinal tract free of food. A liquid diet consists of foods that are in a liquid state at body temperature. Liquid diets are usually ordered as *clear* or *full*. A clear liquid diet includes clear juices, broth, gelatin, and popsicles. A full liquid diet includes all the liquids served on a clear liquid diet, with the addition of cream soups, milk, and ice cream.

Soft Diet and Mechanical Soft Diet: The soft diet is soft in texture and consists of soft or chopped foods that are easier to chew and swallow. Foods that are hard to chew and swallow, such as raw fruits and vegetables and some meats, will be restricted. High-fiber foods, fried foods, and spicy foods may also be limited to help with digestion. Doctors order this diet for residents who have trouble chewing and swallowing due to dental problems or other medical conditions. It is also ordered for people who are making the transition from a liquid diet to a regular diet.

The mechanical soft diet consists of chopped or blended foods that are easier to chew and swallow. Foods are prepared with blenders, food processors, or cutting utensils. Unlike the soft diet, the mechanical soft diet does not limit spices, fat, and fiber. Only the texture of foods is changed. For example, meats and poultry can be ground and moistened with sauces or water to ease swallowing. This diet is used for people who are recovering from surgery or who have difficulty chewing and swallowing.

Pureed Diet: To **puree** a food means to chop, blend, or grind it into a thick paste of baby food consistency. The food should be thick enough to hold its form in the mouth. This diet does not require a person to chew his food. A pureed diet is often used for people who have trouble chewing and/or swallowing more textured foods.

Menus

Residents may receive daily menus for their meals, and nursing assistants may need to help residents complete them. If asked to help a resident with a menu, the NA should make sure the menu offered matches the resident. When reading the menu to the resident, the NA should make the food choices sound appetizing. He should mark the selection that the resident wants if the resident is unable to do this. After completing each category on the menu, he should submit the menu to the dietary department.

7. Explain thickened liquids and identify three basic thickened consistencies

Residents with swallowing problems may be restricted to consuming only thickened liquids. Thickened liquids have a thickening powder or agent added to them, which improves the ability to control fluid in the mouth and throat. A doctor orders the necessary thickness after the resident has been evaluated by a speech-language pathologist.

Some beverages arrive already thickened and ready to consume. Other beverages must have the thickening agent added before serving. If thickening is ordered, it must be used with all liquids. This means that nursing assistants should not offer regular liquids, such as water or other beverages, to residents who must have thickened liquids. There are three basic thickened consistencies:

1. **Nectar Thick**: This consistency is thicker than water. It is the thickness of a thick juice, such as a pear nectar or tomato juice. A resident can drink this from a cup.
2. **Honey Thick**: This consistency has the thickness of honey. It will pour very slowly. A resident will usually use a spoon to consume it.
3. **Pudding Thick**: With this consistency, the liquids have become semi-solid, much like pudding. A spoon should stand up straight in the glass when put into the middle of the drink. A resident must consume these liquids with a spoon.

8. Describe how to make dining enjoyable for residents

Mealtimes are often the most anticipated times of a resident's day. Not only are meals important for getting proper nourishment, but they are also times for socializing, which has a positive effect on eating. Socializing can help prevent weight loss, dehydration, and malnutrition. It can also prevent loneliness and boredom.

Promoting healthy eating is an important part of a nursing assistant's job. Mealtime should be pleasant and enjoyable.

Guidelines: Promoting Appetites

- G Assist residents with grooming and hygiene tasks before dining as needed.
- G Give oral care before eating if requested.
- G Offer a trip to the bathroom or help with toileting before eating.
- G Help residents wash their hands before eating.
- G Encourage the use of dentures, eyeglasses, and hearing aids. If these are damaged, notify the nurse.
- G Check the environment. The temperature should be comfortable. Address any odors. Keep noise level low. Television sets should be off. Do not shout or raise your voice. Do not bang plates or cups. Some facilities play quiet music while residents are dining.
- G Seat residents next to their friends or people with like interests. Encourage conversation.
- G Properly position residents for eating. Usually, the proper position is upright, at a 90-degree angle. This helps prevent swallowing problems. If residents use a wheelchair, make sure they are sitting at a table that is the right height. Most facilities have adjust-

able tables for wheelchairs. Residents who use geri-chairs—reclining chairs on wheels—should be upright, not reclined, while eating.

- Serve food promptly to maintain the correct temperature.
- Plates and trays should look appetizing. If they do not, inform your supervisor.
- Give the resident the proper eating tools. Use assistive or adaptive utensils if needed (Fig. 15-16).

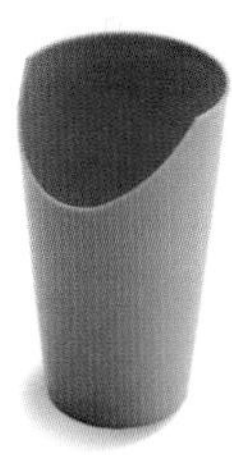

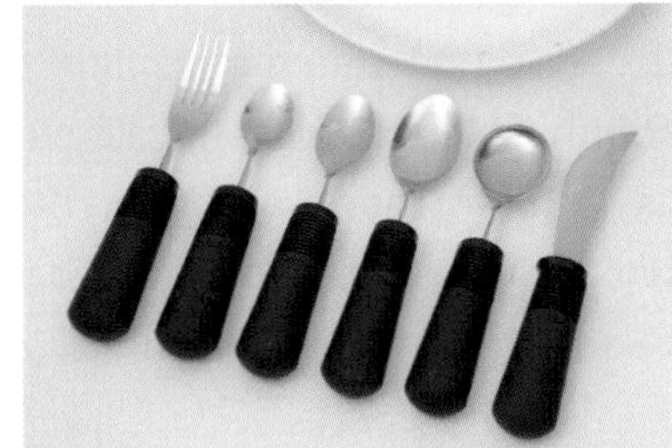

Fig. 15-16. *Types of assistive devices that can help with eating.* (PHOTOS COURTESY OF NORTH COAST MEDICAL, INC., 800-821-9319, WWW.NCMEDICAL.COM)

- Be cheerful, positive, and helpful. Make conversation if the resident wishes to talk.
- Honor requests regarding food. Residents have the legal right to ask for and receive different food. They can also ask for additional food.

9. Explain how to serve meal trays and assist with eating

Food may be served on trays or carried to residents from the kitchen. Nursing assistants must work quickly to make sure that food is served at the proper temperature and that residents do not have to wait too long for their food.

Guidelines: Serving Meal Trays

- Before you begin serving or helping residents, wash your hands.
- As you learned earlier in this textbook, it is very important to identify residents before serving a meal tray. Feeding a resident the wrong food can cause serious problems, even death. Identify each resident before placing food in front of him or her.
- Before you deliver trays or plates, check them closely. Make sure that you have the correct resident and the correct food and beverages for that person. Trays and plates should also be closely checked for added sugar and salt packets (Fig. 15-17). Be aware of residents who eat special diets. Watch for foods in residents' rooms or in the dining room that are not permitted by their doctors. Report any problems to the nurse.

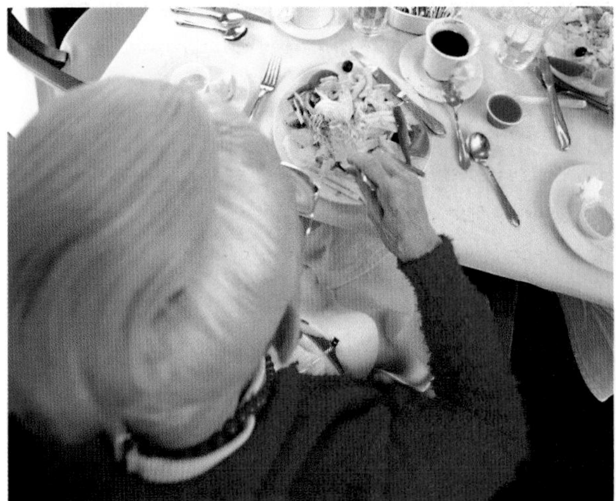

Fig. 15-17. *Observe residents' plates carefully to make sure they are receiving the correct food.*

- Serve all residents who are sitting together at one table before serving another table. Residents will then be able to eat together and not have to watch others eat.
- Prepare the food by following these steps, only doing what the resident cannot do for himself:
  - Remove the food and drink if it is on a tray and set it out on the table.
  - If you know residents need their food cut up, cut it before bringing it to the table. This promotes dignity. Cut food into small, bite-sized portions. Only cut meat and vegetables when necessary.

- Open milk or juice cartons. Open and insert a straw if the resident uses one. Place straws in the containers using the paper wrappers; do not touch them directly with your fingers. Some residents may not be able to use straws due to swallowing problems. This should be noted on their diet cards, and no straws should be on the tray. Residents may want you to pour the beverage into a cup. Do so if the resident wishes.
- Butter roll, bread, and vegetables as the resident prefers.
- Open any condiment packets. Offer to season food as resident prefers, including pureed food.

Residents will need different levels of assistance with eating. Some residents will not need any help. Other residents will only need help setting up; they may only need help opening cartons and cutting and seasoning their food. Once that is done, they can feed themselves. If this is the case, the NA should check in with these residents from time to time to see if they need anything else.

Other residents will be completely unable to feed themselves, and it will be the NA's job to feed them. Residents who must be fed are often embarrassed and depressed about their dependence on another person. Nursing assistants should be sensitive to this and give privacy while residents are eating. Residents should not be rushed through their meals.

NAs should only give assistance as specified, when necessary, or when residents request it. They should encourage residents to do whatever they can for themselves. For example, if a resident can hold and use a napkin, she should. If she can hold and eat finger foods, the NA should offer them. There are devices that help residents eat more independently (see Fig. 15-16 on previous page). More adaptive devices are shown in Chapter 21.

Mealtime involves more than eating. It is a chance for social interaction. Residents look forward to their interaction with nursing assistants and with others. It may be the highlight of their day. To avoid weight loss and dehydration, NAs must do all that they can to increase food and drink intake. Cheerful company and conversation can greatly increase how much a resident eats and drinks. Fewer digestive problems may occur. They also have a positive effect on residents' attitudes. The reverse is also true. Negative attitudes and poor communication can decrease how much a resident consumes. NAs should avoid making negative comments such as, "I don't know how you can eat this" or, "This looks awful." They should not judge residents' food preferences.

Guidelines: Assisting a Resident with Eating

G Verify that you have the right resident by checking the diet card against the name listed outside the door (or however the facility identifies its residents). Ask the resident to state his name. Check that the diet on the tray is correct and matches the diet card.

G Sit at a resident's eye level. Resident should be sitting upright, at a 90-degree angle. Make eye contact with the resident.

G If the resident wishes, allow time for prayer.

G Never treat the resident like a child. This is embarrassing and disrespectful. It is hard for many people to accept help with feeding. Be supportive and encouraging.

G Test the temperature of the food by putting your hand over the dish to sense the heat. Do not touch food to test its temperature. If you think the food is too hot, do not blow on it to cool it. Offer other food to give it time to cool.

G Cut foods and pour liquids as needed. Season foods to the resident's preference.

- Identify the foods and fluids that are in front of the resident. Call pureed foods by the correct name. For example, ask, "Would you like green beans?" rather than referring to it as "some green stuff."
- Ask the resident which food he prefers to eat first. Allow him to make the choice, even if he wants to eat dessert first.
- Do not mix foods unless the resident requests it.
- Do not rush the meal. Allow time for the resident to chew and swallow each bite. Be relaxed.
- Be social and friendly. Make simple conversation if the resident wishes to do so (Fig. 15-18). Try not to ask questions that require long answers. Use appropriate topics, such as the news, weather, the resident's life, things the resident enjoys, and food preferences. Say positive things about the food being served, such as "This smells really good," and "This looks really fresh."

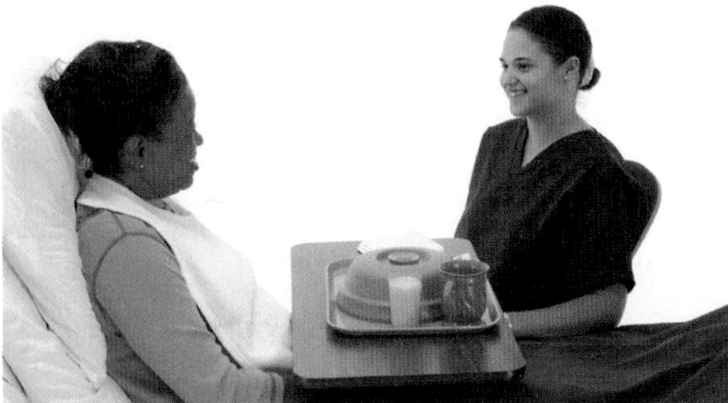

Fig. 15-18. Being friendly and social while helping residents with eating is important. Encourage residents to do whatever they can for themselves.

- Give the resident your full attention while he or she is eating. Do not talk to other staff members while helping residents eat.
- Alternate offering food and drink. Alternating cold and hot foods or bland foods and sweets can help increase appetite.
- If the resident wants a different food from what is being served, inform the dietitian so that an alternative may be offered.

Residents' Rights

Clothing Protectors

Residents have the right to refuse to wear a clothing protector (Fig. 15-19). The nursing assistant can offer a clothing protector, but should not insist that a resident wear one. She should respect the resident's wishes. In addition, NAs should not refer to a clothing protector as a *bib*. This promotes residents' dignity and avoids treating them like children.

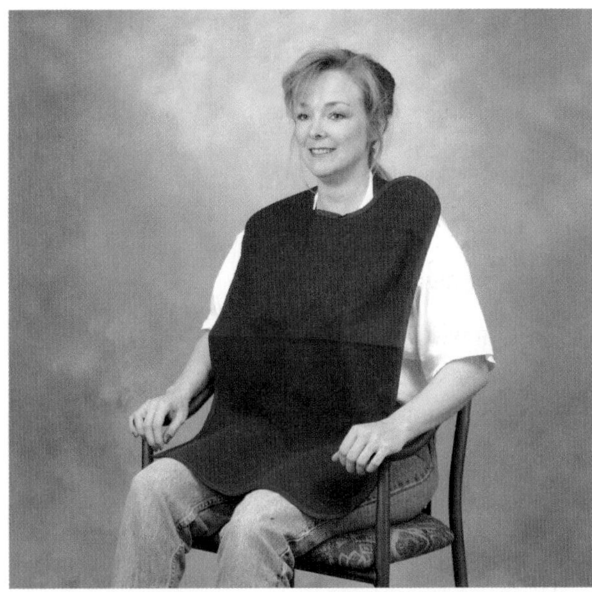

Fig. 15-19. *Residents have the right to choose whether or not to use a clothing protector. Nursing assistants must respect each resident's decision.* (REPRINTED WITH PERMISSION OF BRIGGS CORPORATION, 800-247-2343, WWW.BRIGGSCORP.COM)

Feeding a resident

Equipment: meal, eating utensils, clothing protector, washcloths or wipes

1. Identify yourself by name. Identify the resident by name.
2. Wash your hands.
3. Explain procedure to the resident. Speak clearly, slowly, and directly. Maintain face-to-face contact whenever possible.
4. Provide for resident's privacy with curtain, screen, or door.
5. Pick up diet card and ask resident to state her name. Verify that resident has received the right tray.

6. Raise the head of the bed. Make sure resident is in an upright sitting position (at a 90-degree angle).
7. Adjust bed height to where you will be able to sit at resident's eye level. Lock bed wheels.
8. Place meal tray where it can be easily seen by the resident, such as on the overbed table.
9. Help resident clean her hands with hand wipes if resident cannot do it herself.
10. Help resident put on clothing protector if desired.
11. Sit facing resident at the resident's eye level (Fig. 15-20). Sit on the stronger side if the resident has one-sided weakness.

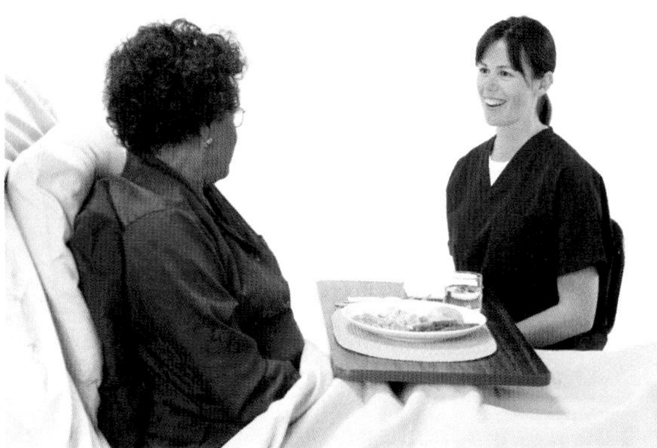

Fig. 15-20. *The resident should be sitting upright, and the nursing assistant should be sitting at her eye level.*

12. Tell the resident what foods are on the plate. Ask resident what she would like to eat first.
13. Check the temperature of the food. Using utensils, offer the food in bite-sized pieces. Tell the resident the content of each bite of food offered (Fig. 15-21). Alternate types of food offered, allowing for resident's preferences. Do not feed all of one type before offering another type. Make sure resident's mouth is empty before next bite or sip. Report any swallowing problems to the nurse immediately.
14. Offer drinks of beverage throughout the meal. If you are holding the cup, touch it to the resident's lips before you tip it. Give small, frequent sips.

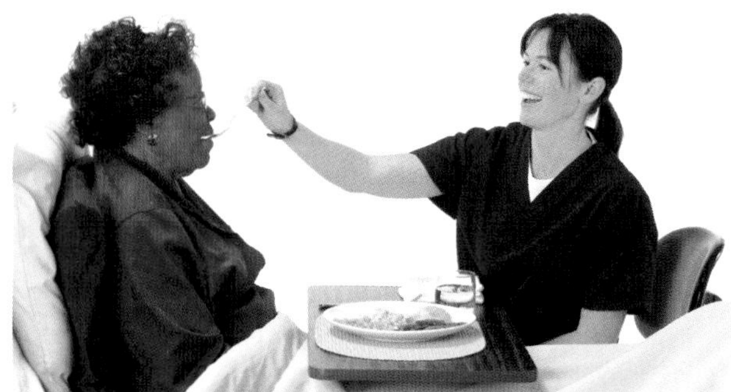

Fig. 15-21. *Offer the food in bite-sized pieces. Tell resident the content of each bite of food.*

15. Talk with resident during meal. It makes mealtime more enjoyable (Fig. 15-22). Do not rush the resident.

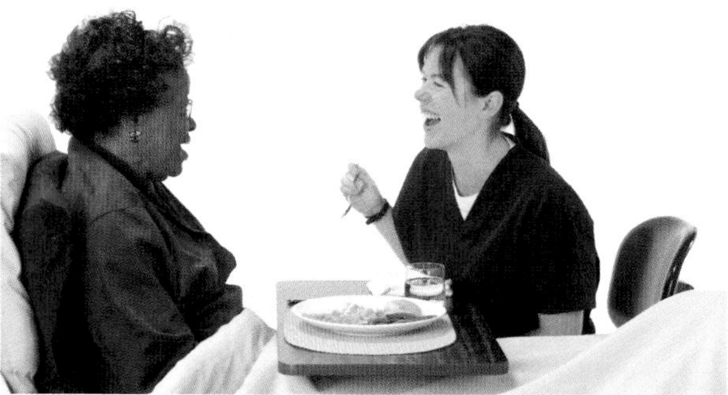

Fig. 15-22. *Socializing during mealtime makes eating more enjoyable for residents and may help promote a healthy appetite.*

16. Use washcloths or wipes to wipe food from resident's mouth and hands as needed during the meal. Wipe again at the end of the meal (Fig. 15-23).

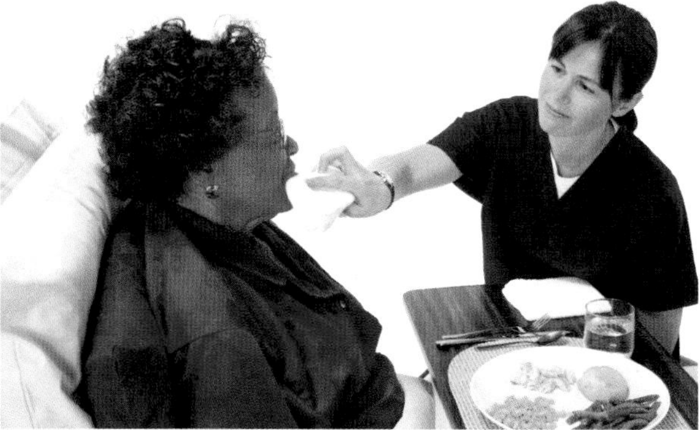

Fig. 15-23. *Wiping food from the mouth during the meal helps to maintain the resident's dignity.*

17. When the resident is finished eating, remove clothing protector if used. Dispose of protector in proper container.

18. Remove the food tray. Check for eyeglasses, dentures, or any personal items before removing tray. Place tray in proper area.
19. Make resident comfortable. Make sure the bed is free from crumbs.
20. Return bed to lowest position. Remove privacy measures.
21. Place call light within resident's reach.
22. Wash your hands.
23. Report any changes in resident to the nurse.
24. Document procedure using facility guidelines.

Food trays and plates should also be observed after the meal. This helps to identify residents with poor appetites. It may also signal illness, a problem such as dentures that do not fit properly, or a change in food preferences.

10. Describe how to assist residents with special needs

Residents with specific diseases or conditions, such as stroke, Parkinson's disease, Alzheimer's disease or other dementias, head trauma, blindness, or confusion may need special assistance when eating. These techniques can be helpful for residents who have special needs:

Guidelines: Dining Techniques

- G Use assistive devices such as utensils with built-up handle grips, plate guards, and drinking cups. Assistive or adaptive devices for eating help people feed themselves. These devices are ordered for specific residents and should be included on the meal tray.
- G To help maintain independence with eating, residents may benefit from physical and verbal cues. The hand-over-hand approach is an example of a physical cue. The resident lifts a utensil if he is able, and you put your hand over his to help with eating (Fig. 15-24). With your hand placed over the resident's hand, help in getting food on the utensil. Steer the utensil from the plate to the mouth and back. Repeat this until the resident is finished with his meal.

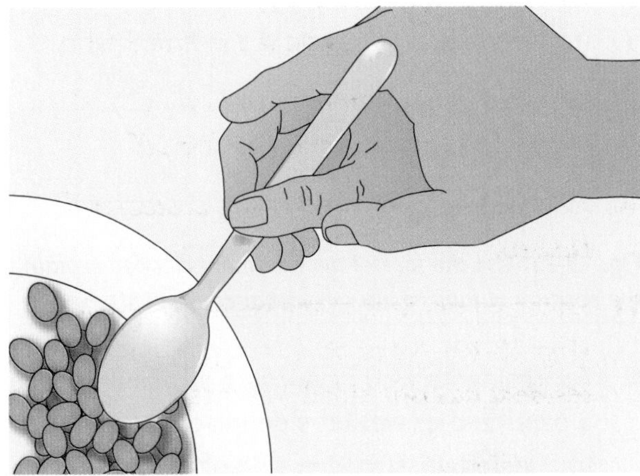

Fig. 15-24. *The hand-over-hand approach is used when a resident can help by lifting utensils. It helps promote independence.*

- G Verbal cues must be short and clear so that they are easily understood. The cues should prompt the resident to do something. Give verbal cues one at a time. Wait until the resident has finished one task before asking him to do another. The cues are repeated until the resident has finished eating. Examples of appropriate verbal cues include the following:
    - "Pick up your spoon."
    - "Put some carrots on your spoon."
    - "Raise the spoon to your lips."
    - "Open your mouth."
    - "Place the spoon in your mouth."
    - "Close your mouth."
    - "Take the spoon out of your mouth."
    - "Chew."
    - "Swallow."
    - "Drink some water."
- G For visually-impaired residents, use the face of an imaginary clock to explain the position of what is in front of them (Fig. 15-25).

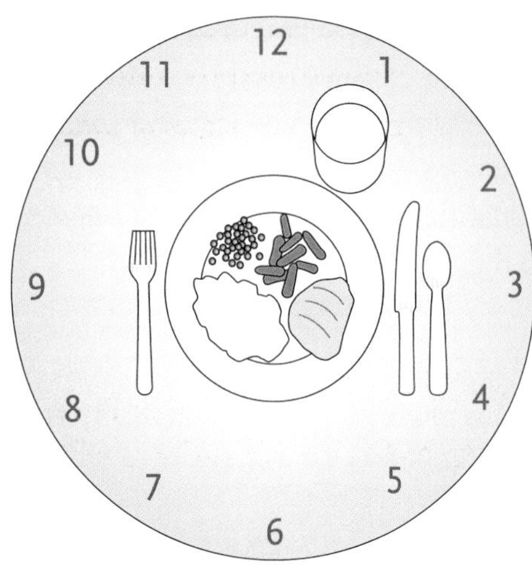

Fig. 15-25. *Use the face of an imaginary clock to explain the position of food to visually-impaired residents.*

- For residents who have had a stroke and have a paralyzed or weaker side, place food in the unaffected, or stronger, side of the mouth. Make sure food is swallowed before offering another bite.
- Place food in the resident's field of vision (Fig. 15-26). The nurse will determine a resident's field of vision.

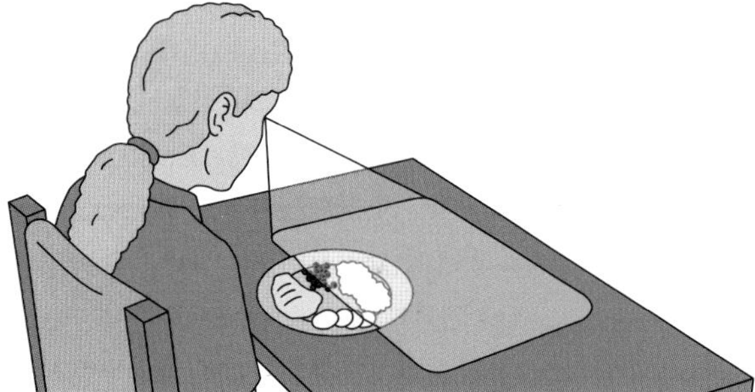

Fig. 15-26. *A resident who has had a stroke may have a limited field of vision. The nurse will determine the resident's field of vision. Make sure the resident can see what you place in front of him.*

- For residents who have Parkinson's disease, tremors or shaking can make it very difficult to eat. Help by using physical cues. Place food and drinks close so that the resident can easily reach them. Use assistive devices as needed.
- If a resident has poor sitting balance, seat him in a regular dining room chair with armrests, rather than in a wheelchair. Proper position in chair means hips are at a 90-degree angle, knees are flexed, and feet and arms are fully supported. Push the chair under the table. Place forearms on the table. If a resident tends to lean to one side, ask him to keep his elbows on the table.
- If a resident has poor neck control, a neck brace may be used to stabilize the head. Use assistive devices as needed. If resident is in a geri-chair, a wedge cushion behind the head and shoulders may be used.
- If the resident bites down on utensils, ask him to open his mouth. Do not pull the utensil out of the mouth. Wait until the jaw relaxes.
- If the resident pockets food in his cheeks, ask him to chew and swallow the food. Touch the side of his cheek. Ask him to use his tongue to get the food. Using your fingers on the cheek (near the lower jaw), gently push food toward teeth.
- If the resident holds food in his mouth, ask him to chew and swallow the food. You may need to trigger swallowing. To do this, gently press down on the tongue when taking the spoon out of the mouth. You can also try to gently press down on the top of his head with your hand (chin tuck, or a head position that positions the chin slightly downward toward the person's chest). Make sure the resident has swallowed the food before offering more.

Residents' Rights

Residents with Special Needs

Residents have the right to be treated with dignity and as adults. They have the right to self-determination. This means, in part, that they should be given the opportunity to choose and state their preferences for care and services. For example, a blind resident may want to feed herself without using utensils. This may not look dignified to others, but it is the resident's choice.

11. Define *dysphagia* and identify signs and symptoms of swallowing problems

Residents may have conditions that make eating or swallowing difficult. **Dysphagia** means difficulty in swallowing. A stroke, or CVA, can cause weakness and paralysis on one side of the body. Nerve and muscle damage from head and neck cancer, multiple sclerosis, Parkinson's disease, or Alzheimer's disease may also be present. If residents have difficulty swallowing, they will probably eat soft foods and drink thickened liquids. A special cup will help make swallowing easier.

Nursing assistants need to be able to recognize and report signs that a resident has a swallowing problem. Signs and symptoms of swallowing problems include the following:

- Coughing during or after meals
- Choking during meals
- Dribbling saliva, food, or fluid from the mouth
- Having food residue inside the mouth or cheeks during and after meals
- Gurgling during or after meals or losing voice
- Eating slowly
- Avoiding eating
- Spitting out pieces of food
- Swallowing several times per mouthful
- Clearing the throat frequently during and after meals
- Watering of the eyes when eating or drinking
- Food or fluid coming up into the nose
- Making a visible effort to swallow
- Breathing rapidly or with shorter breaths while eating or drinking
- Difficulty chewing food
- Difficulty swallowing medications

Swallowing problems put residents at high risk for choking on food or drink. Inhaling food, fluid, or foreign material into the lungs is called **aspiration**. Aspiration can cause pneumonia or death. An NA should alert the nurse immediately if he notices any signs of swallowing problems.

Guidelines: Preventing Aspiration

- G Position residents properly in a straight, upright position when eating or drinking. Do not try to feed residents in a reclining position.
- G Offer small pieces of food or small spoonfuls of pureed food.
- G Feed residents slowly; do not rush them.
- G Place food in the unaffected, or stronger, side of the mouth.
- G Make sure the mouth is empty before offering another bite of food or sip of drink.
- G If possible, keep residents in the upright position for about 30 minutes after eating and drinking.

12. Explain intake and output (I&O)

To maintain health, the body must take in a certain amount of fluid each day. Fluid comes in the form of liquids that a person drinks and is also found in semi-liquid foods like gelatin, soup, ice cream, pudding, and yogurt. Generally, a healthy person needs to take in from 64 to 96 ounces (oz.) of fluid each day. The fluid a person consumes is called **intake**, or **input**. When a person's intake is not in a healthy range, she can become dehydrated. Dehydration is a serious medical condition that requires immediate attention. More information on dehydration is in the next learning objective.

All fluid taken in each day cannot remain in the body. It must be eliminated as **output**. Output includes urine, feces (including diarrhea), vomitus, perspiration and moisture in the air that a person exhales, and wound drainage. If a person's intake exceeds her output, fluid builds up in body tissues. This fluid retention can cause medical problems and discomfort.

Fluid balance is maintaining equal input and output, or taking in and eliminating equal amounts of fluid. Most people maintain fluid balance naturally. But some residents must have their intake and output, or I&O, monitored and recorded. To monitor this, the nursing assistant will need to measure and document all fluids that the resident takes by mouth, as well as all urine and vomitus the resident produces. This is recorded on an Intake/Output (I&O) sheet (Fig. 15-27).

INTAKE AND OUTPUT RECORD

DATE	SHIFT	INTAKE (IN CC'S) ORAL	OUTPUT (IN CC'S) VOIDED	OUTPUT (IN CC'S) CATHETER	NUMBER OF INCONTINENT EPISODES (IF APPLICABLE)	DATE	SHIFT	INTAKE (IN CC'S) ORAL	OUTPUT (IN CC'S) VOIDED	OUTPUT (IN CC'S) CATHETER	NUMBER OF INCONTINENT EPISODES (IF APPLICABLE)
	7-3						7-3				
	3-11						3-11				
	11-7						11-7				
	24 HR. TOTAL						24 HR. TOTAL				
	7-3						7-3				
	3-11						3-11				
	11-7						11-7				
	24 HR. TOTAL						24 HR. TOTAL				
	7-3						7-3				
	3-11						3-11				
	11-7						11-7				
	24 HR. TOTAL						24 HR. TOTAL				
	7-3						7-3				
	3-11						3-11				
	11-7						11-7				
	24 HR. TOTAL						24 HR. TOTAL				
	7-3						7-3				
	3-11						3-11				
	11-7						11-7				
	24 HR. TOTAL						24 HR. TOTAL				
	7-3						7-3				
	3-11						3-11				
	11-7						11-7				
	24 HR. TOTAL						24 HR. TOTAL				
	7-3						7-3				
	3-11						3-11				
	11-7						11-7				
	24 HR. TOTAL						24 HR. TOTAL				

NAME-Last	First	Middle	Attending Physician	Record No.	Room/Bed

INTAKE AND OUTPUT RECORD

Fig. 15-27. *This is a sample intake and output record.*

Fluids are usually measured in milliliters (mL). Milliliters are units of measurement in the metric system. One milliliter is 1/1000 of a liter and is equal to one cubic centimeter (cc). Ounces (oz) are converted to milliliters. One ounce equals 30 milliliters, so to convert ounces to milliliters, the number of ounces must be multiplied by 30.

For example, an NA serves a resident a six-ounce glass of milk. The resident finishes most but not all of the milk, and the NA estimates the resident drank four ounces of milk. To convert ounces to milliliters, the number of ounces must be multiplied by 30. Four ounces multiplied by 30 equals 120 milliliters (mL). The NA would document 120 mL milk on her input sheet.

Conversions

One milliliter (mL) is a unit of measure equal to one cubic centimeter (cc). Follow your facility's policies on whether to document using mL or cc.

1 oz = 30 mL or 30 cc

2 oz = 60 mL

3 oz = 90 mL

4 oz = 120 mL

5 oz = 150 mL

6 oz = 180 mL

7 oz = 210 mL

8 oz = 240 mL

¼ cup = 2 oz = 60 mL

½ cup = 4 oz = 120 mL

1 cup = 8 oz = 240 mL

Before beginning, the NA should explain to the resident that she needs to keep track of his intake. She should ask the resident to let her know when he drinks something (if it is not something the NA served to him) and how much it was.

Measuring and recording intake and output

Equipment: I&O sheet, graduate (measuring container) (Fig. 15-28), pen and paper to record your findings

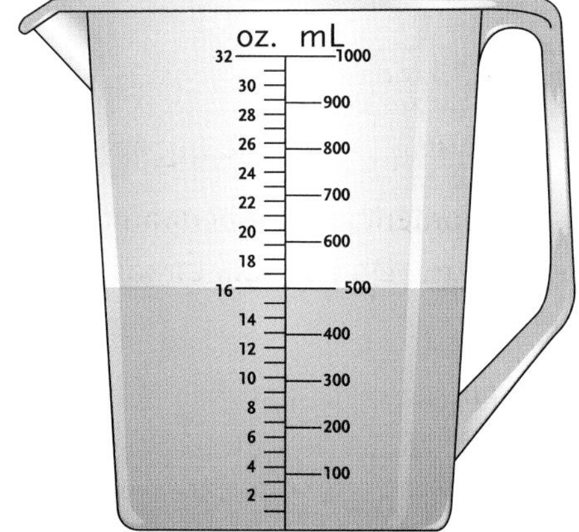

Fig. 15-28. *A graduate is a measuring container.*

Measure intake first.

1. Identify yourself by name. Identify the resident by name.
2. Wash your hands.
3. Explain procedure to the resident. Speak clearly, slowly, and directly. Maintain face-to-face contact whenever possible.
4. Provide for resident's privacy with curtain, screen, or door.
5. Using the graduate, measure how much fluid a resident is served. Note the amount on paper.
6. When resident has finished a meal or snack, measure any leftover fluids. Note this amount on paper.
7. Subtract the leftover amount from the amount served. If you have measured in ounces, convert to milliliters (mL) by multiplying by 30.
8. Document amount of fluid consumed (in mL) in input column on I&O sheet. Record the time and what fluid was taken. Report anything unusual that was observed, such as the resident refusing to drink, drinking very little, feeling nauseated, etc.
9. Wash your hands.

Measuring output is the other half of monitoring fluid balance.

Equipment: I&O sheet, graduate, gloves, pen and paper

1. Wash your hands.
2. Put on gloves before handling bedpan/urinal.
3. Pour the contents of the bedpan or urinal into graduate. Do not spill or splash any of the urine.
4. Place graduate on flat surface. Measure the amount of urine at eye level. Keep the container level (Fig. 15-29). Note the amount on paper, converting to mL if necessary.

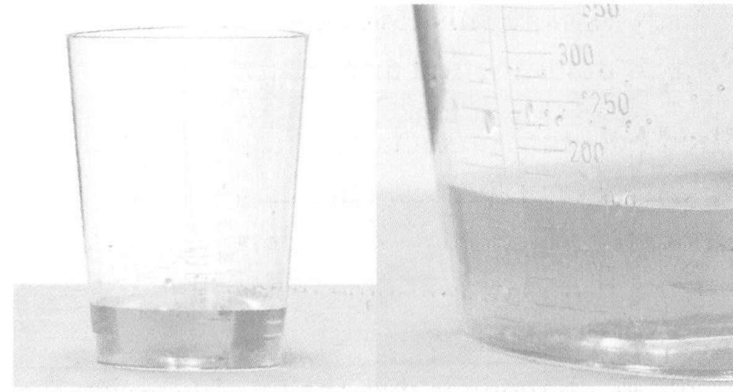

***Fig. 15-29.** Keep container on a flat surface while measuring output.*

5. After measuring urine, empty graduate into toilet without splashing.
6. Rinse graduate and pour rinse water into toilet.
7. Rinse bedpan/urinal and pour rinse water into toilet. Flush the toilet.
8. Place graduate and bedpan in area for cleaning or clean and store according to policy.
9. Remove and discard gloves.
10. Wash hands before recording output.
11. Document the time and amount of urine in output column on sheet. For example: 1545 hours, 200 mL urine. To measure vomitus, pour from basin into measuring container, then discard in the toilet. If resident vomits on the bed or floor, estimate the amount. Document emesis and amount on the I&O sheet.
12. Report any changes in resident to the nurse.

All facilities have methods to keep track of how much food and fluid a resident consumes. Percentages are often used to document food intake, but the specific method can vary (Fig. 15-30). The dietician calculates the percentages for meals. The NA may be asked to document how much of the entire meal a resident ate. For example, if the resident ate the entire meal served, the NA would document that 100% was eaten. If the resident ate about half of the meal, the NA would document 50% eaten, and so on.

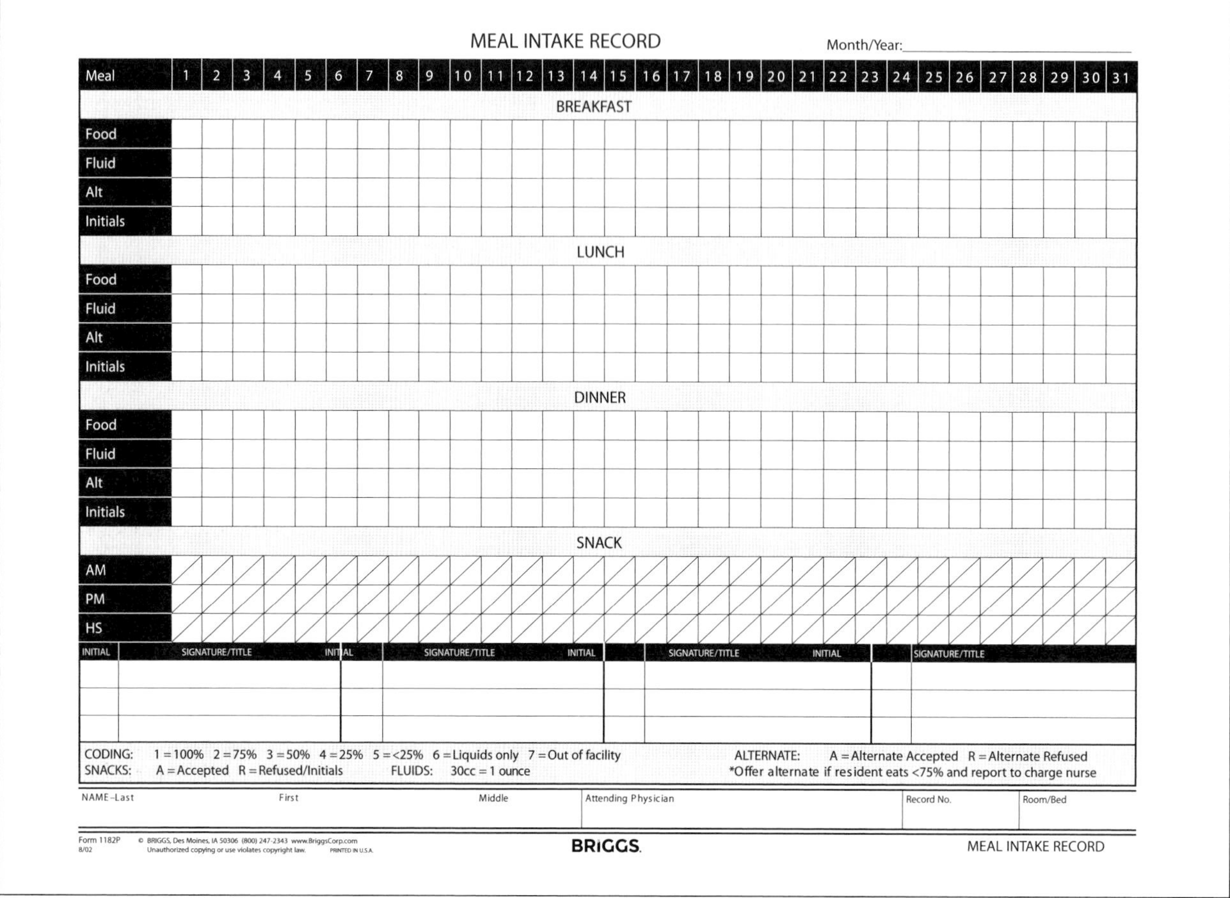

MEAL INTAKE RECORD

Month/Year:

Meal	1	2	3	4	5	6	7	8	9	10	11	12	13	14	15	16	17	18	19	20	21	22	23	24	25	26	27	28	29	30	31
BREAKFAST																															
Food																															
Fluid																															
Alt																															
Initials																															
LUNCH																															
Food																															
Fluid																															
Alt																															
Initials																															
DINNER																															
Food																															
Fluid																															
Alt																															
Initials																															
SNACK																															
AM																															
PM																															
HS																															

INITIAL	SIGNATURE/TITLE	INITIAL	SIGNATURE/TITLE	INITIAL	SIGNATURE/TITLE	INITIAL	SIGNATURE/TITLE

CODING: 1 = 100% 2 = 75% 3 = 50% 4 = 25% 5 = <25% 6 = Liquids only 7 = Out of facility
SNACKS: A = Accepted R = Refused/Initials FLUIDS: 30cc = 1 ounce

ALTERNATE: A = Alternate Accepted R = Alternate Refused
*Offer alternate if resident eats <75% and report to charge nurse

NAME–Last	First	Middle	Attending Physician	Record No.	Room/Bed

Form 1182P 8/02 © BRIGGS, Des Moines, IA 50306 (800) 247-2343 www.BriggsCorp.com Unauthorized copying or use violates copyright law. PRINTED IN U.S.A. BRIGGS. MEAL INTAKE RECORD

Fig. 15-30. *One type of form for documenting meal intake.* (REPRINTED WITH PERMISSION OF BRIGGS CORPORATION, 800-247-2343, WWW.BRIGGSCORP.COM)

Another percentage method requires that the NA calculate how much of each item served was consumed. For example, soup, salad, a roll, and fruit are on a lunch tray. The soup is worth 30% of her calories needed for lunch. If she finishes half of the soup, the NA would document that she ate 15% of that food, and so on.

It is very important for nursing assistants to follow their facility's policies and to document food intake accurately. If a resident eats less than 70% of his or her meal, the NA should report it to the nurse.

13. Identify ways to assist residents in maintaining fluid balance

Most residents should be encouraged to drink at least 64 ounces of water or other fluids a day. Water is an essential nutrient for life. Proper fluid intake is important. It helps prevent constipation and urinary incontinence. Without enough fluid, urine becomes concentrated. More concentrated urine creates a higher risk for infection. Proper fluid intake also helps to dilute wastes and flush out the urinary system. It may even help prevent confusion.

The sense of thirst can lessen as people age. Infection, fever, diarrhea, and some medications will also increase the need for fluid intake. Nursing assistants should remind elderly residents to drink fluids often (Fig. 15-31). Some residents will drink more fluids if they are offered in smaller amounts, rather than in one large glassful.

Some residents may have an order to force fluids or restrict fluids because of medical conditions. **Force fluids (FF)** means that the resident should be encouraged to drink as much fluid as possible. **Restrict fluids (RF)** means that the resident is allowed to drink, but must limit the daily amount to a level set by the doctor. When a resident has a restrict fluids order, the NA should not give the resident any extra fluids or a water pitcher unless the nurse approves it.

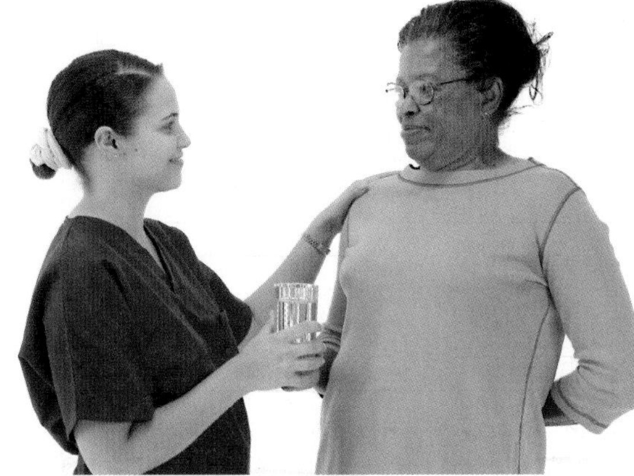

Fig. 15-31. Drinking enough water and other fluids promotes good health. NAs should encourage residents to drink fluids often.

The abbreviation **NPO** stands for *nothing by mouth*. This means that a resident is not allowed to have anything to eat or drink. Some residents have such a severe problem with swallowing that it is unsafe to give them anything by mouth. These types of residents will receive nutrition through a feeding tube or intravenously. Some residents may not be able to eat or drink for a short time before a medical test or surgery. Nursing assistants need to know this abbreviation and should never offer any food or drink, even water, to a resident with this order.

Dehydration occurs when a person does not have enough fluid in the body. Dehydration is a serious condition and is a major problem among the elderly. People can become dehydrated if they do not drink enough or if they have diarrhea or are vomiting. Preventing dehydration is very important.

Guidelines: Preventing Dehydration

- G Report observations and warning signs to the nurse immediately.
- G Encourage residents to drink every time you see them.
- G Offer fresh water or other fluids often. Offer drinks that the resident enjoys. Some residents may not like water and prefer other types of beverages, such as juice, soda, tea, or milk. Some residents do not want ice in their drinks. Honor personal preferences. Report to the nurse if the resident tells you he does not like the fluids being served.
- G Ice chips, frozen flavored ice sticks, and gelatin are also forms of liquids. Offer them often. Do not offer ice chips or sticks if a resident has a swallowing problem.
- G If appropriate, offer sips of liquid between bites of food at meals and snacks.
- G Make sure pitcher and cup are near enough and light enough for the resident to lift.
- G Offer assistance if resident cannot drink without help. Use adaptive cups as needed.
- G Record fluid intake and output.

Observing and Reporting: Dehydration

Report any of the following immediately:

- O/R Resident drinks less than six 8-ounce glasses of liquid per day
- O/R Resident drinks little or no fluids at meals
- O/R Resident needs help drinking from a cup or glass
- O/R Resident has trouble swallowing liquids
- O/R Resident has frequent vomiting, diarrhea, or fever
- O/R Resident is easily confused or tired

Report if resident has any of the following:

- O/R Dry mouth
- O/R Cracked lips
- O/R Sunken eyes

- Dark urine
- Strong-smelling urine
- Weight loss
- Complaints of abdominal pain

Serving fresh water

Equipment: water pitcher, ice scoop, glass, straw, gloves

1. Identify yourself by name. Identify the resident by name.
2. Wash your hands.
3. Put on gloves.
4. Scoop ice into water pitcher. Add fresh water.
5. Use and store ice scoop properly. Do not allow ice to touch your hand and fall back into container. Place scoop in proper receptacle after each use.
6. Take pitcher to resident.
7. Pour glass of water for resident. Leave pitcher and glass at the bedside.
8. Make sure that pitcher and glass are light enough for resident to lift. Leave a straw if the resident desires.
9. Place call light within resident's reach.
10. Remove and discard gloves.
11. Wash your hands.

Residents' Rights

Fluid Intake

Offering fresh fluids often helps prevent dehydration and helps keep residents healthy. Nursing assistants should encourage, but not force, fluids. NAs can ask residents which beverages they prefer and arrange for those to be available. They should respond to drink requests promptly unless there is a doctor's order restricting fluid intake. If this is the case, the NA should inform the resident about the order, and report the request to the nurse. If fluid intake is increased, the NA should offer additional trips to the bathroom and promote privacy. If urine is being measured, it should be done with the door closed.

Fluid overload occurs when the body cannot handle the amount of fluid consumed. This condition often affects people with heart or kidney disease.

Observing and Reporting: Fluid Overload

Report any of the following to the nurse:

- Swelling/edema of extremities (ankles, feet, fingers, hands); **edema** is swelling caused by excess fluid in body tissues
- Weight gain (daily weight gain of one to two pounds)
- Decreased urine output
- Shortness of breath
- Increased heart rate
- Skin that appears tight, smooth, and shiny

Chapter Review

1. How does a well-balanced diet help the ill and the elderly?
2. List the six basic nutrients and identify which nutrient is the most essential for life.
3. According to MyPlate's suggestions, what should half of a person's plate be mad e up of?
4. List some examples of plant sources of protein foods.
5. According to MyPlate, what should most dairy group choices be?
6. List four problems that may affect an elderly person's nutritional intake.
7. Why is it important for an NA to report any weight loss, no matter how small?
8. Describe ten ways that an NA can help prevent unintended weight loss.
9. What are two ways a resident may be fed if he has a digestive system that does not function properly or he cannot swallow?

1) Report to the nurse immediately any signs or symptoms
2) Encourage residents to drink everytime u see them.
3) offer drinks that the resident enjoys
4) offer popcycles, ice chips etc.
5) Make sure a pitcher of water is near & light enough to handle.
6) Record fluid intake & output.

10. List two factors that influence food preferences. Religion, Income, Your ethnic background, where you live in the world. How you are educated.

11. What information do diet cards contain? Name, special diets, allergies, likes & dislikes & other instructions.

12. What is the first food to be restricted in a low-sodium diet? Salt.

13. Why might a resident be placed on a low-fat/low-cholesterol diet? People that have high levels of cholesterol in their blood. Gallbladder disease, Liver disease.

14. What is the difference between a clear liquid diet and a full liquid diet? Clear diet has clear juices. — all food on a clear diet as well as cream soups, milk & ice cream

15. How is the mechanical soft diet different from the soft diet? The mechanical soft diet is more blenderized food. The soft diet is cut small & soft to swallow.

16. List five reasons that a person may choose to be a vegetarian. 1) Heath reasons 2) religious reasons 3) a compassion for animals. 4) for financial reasons. 5) Dislike meat.

17. How can thickened liquids help a person with swallowing problems? It helps the ability of the liquid to be controlled in the mouth & throat

18. What is the proper position to place a resident in for eating? 90% angle. Sitting upright.

19. How can being cheerful and positive while a resident eats affect the amount of food consumed? Socializing has a positive effect on mood & wanting to eat.

20. How can a nursing assistant verify that she has the correct resident for the meal tray that she is serving? Ask resident their name, check them closly. Check diet card & name on outside door.

21. How should a nursing assistant test the temperature of food? By feeling heat from food without touching it. Put hand over dish to sense heat.

22. What should the nursing assistant do if a resident wants a different food from what is being served? Inform the dietition so that an alternative may be given.

23. Should a nursing assistant insist that a resident wear a clothing protector if he does not want to wear one? Why or why not? No. You must respect each residents decision

24. When feeding a resident, how should the bed height be adjusted? So you are able to be on the same eye level.

25. How do verbal cues assist a resident with eating? It helps the resident maintain independence & self dignity.

26. When assisting a visually-impaired resident, how should the nursing assistant explain the position of food and objects in front of the resident? Like the face of a clock.

27. To which side of the mouth should food be directed if a resident has a weaker side—the weaker (affected) or stronger (unaffected) side?

28. What is the medical term for difficulty swallowing? Dysphagia = Difficulty swallowing.

29. List 12 signs that a resident may have a swallowing problem.

1) Coughing during or after meals
2) Choking during meals
3) Dribbling saliva, food or fluid from mouth
4) Having food or residue in mouth or cheeks during & after meals.
5) Gurgling during or after meals or losing voice
6) Eating slowly
7) Avoid eating
8) spitting out pieces of food
9) Swallowing several times per mouthful
10) Watering of eyes when eating or drinking
11) Food or fluid coming out the nose
12) Making a visible effort to swallow
13) Breathing rapidly or with shorter breaths while eating or drinking.
14) Difficulty swallowing med's.

30. Describe five guidelines to help prevent aspiration. 1) Have residents sit straight up 2) offer small pieces of food or small spoonfuls, 3) Feed residents slower 4) Put food in stronger side of mouth 5) Make sure mouth is empty 6) Keep resident in the upright position about 30 minutes after eating.

31. How many ounces of fluid does a healthy person need each day? 64 to 96

32. What is fluid balance? equal What gets taken in should come out in urine, feces, saliva etc.

33. How many milliliters (mL) equal one ounce (oz)? 30.

34. What counts as output? Urine, vomit, perspiration, moisture exhaled, wound drainage

35. What does the abbreviation *NPO* stand for? Nothing by mouth.

36. Describe six ways that a nursing assistant can help prevent dehydration.

37. List five signs about dehydration that a nursing assistant should report immediately. 1) Resident drinks less than 6 (8 oz) glasses of water a day. 2) He doesn't drink water at meals. 3) Needs help drinking from a cup or glass. 4) resident has trouble swallowing liquids 5) resident has diarrhea & vomiting Signs of fever Signs of Difficulty swallowing

38. List four signs about fluid overload that a nursing assistant should report. 1) swelling or edema in extremities 2) weight gain daily 3) ↓ urine output 4) short of breath 5) ↑ heart rate 6) skin is tight & shiny.

16 Urinary Elimination

1. List qualities of urine and identify signs and symptoms about urine to report

Urination, also known as *micturition* or *voiding*, is the act of passing urine from the bladder through the urethra to the outside of the body. Urine is made up of water and waste products filtered from the blood by the kidneys. Normal urine output varies with age and the amount and type of liquids consumed. Adults should produce about 1200 to 1500 mL of urine per day, although elderly adults may produce less.

Urine is normally pale yellow to amber in color (Fig. 16-1). However, there are many factors that can cause urine to be an abnormal color, such as medications, certain foods or food dyes, and vitamins and supplements. For example, beets can make urine appear pink or red, and B vitamins can make urine very bright yellow. Unusual urine color can also be a sign of illness.

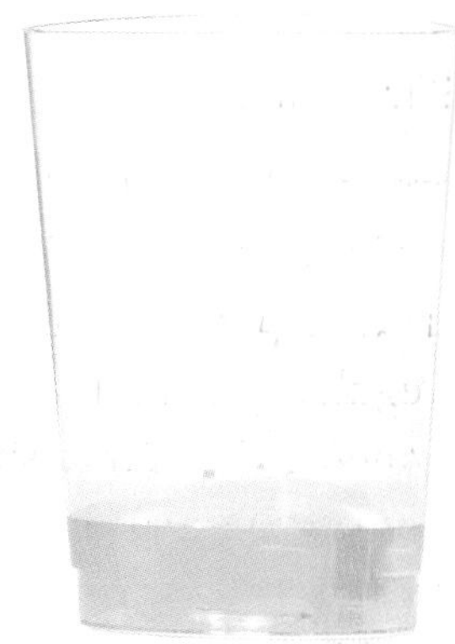

Fig. 16-1. *Urine is normally light or pale yellow in color. It should be clear, not cloudy.*

Normal urine should be clear or transparent when freshly voided and should have a faint smell. Urine that is cloudy or murky or that smells bad or fruity can be a sign of infection or illness.

Observing and Reporting: Urine

Report any of the following to the nurse:

- O/R Cloudy urine
- O/R Dark or rust-colored urine
- O/R Strong-, offensive-, or fruity-smelling urine
- O/R Resident complaints of pain, burning, or pressure when urinating
- O/R Blood, pus, mucus, or discharge in urine
- O/R Protein or glucose in urine (there is more information about this later in the chapter)
- O/R Urinary incontinence (the inability to control the bladder, which leads to an involuntary loss of urine)

2. List factors affecting urination and demonstrate how to assist with elimination

There are many factors that can affect normal urination, including the following:

Normal changes of aging: The ability of the kidneys to filter blood decreases. The bladder muscle tone weakens. The bladder is not able to hold the same amount of urine as it did when people were younger. Elderly people may need to urinate more frequently. Many awaken several times during the night to urinate. The bladder may not empty completely, causing susceptibility to infection.

To help promote normal urination, nursing assistants should offer frequent trips to the bathroom or bedpans and urinals. The best position for women to have normal urination is sitting. For men, it is standing. The supine (lying on the back) position should be avoided if possible because in this position a person cannot put pressure on the bladder and must work against gravity. NAs should follow a toileting schedule for residents if there is one.

When assisting with perineal care, NAs should wipe from front to back to prevent infection. They should help residents wash their hands after urinating.

Psychological factors: A lack of privacy, new environments, stress, anxiety, and depression can all affect urination. To promote normal urination, it is very important for an NA to provide plenty of privacy for elimination. She should close the bathroom door if a resident is in the bathroom. If the resident needs to use a bedpan or urinal, the NA should pull the privacy curtain and close the door. Residents should not be rushed or interrupted when they are in the bathroom. It is important for an NA to report signs of depression and anxiety (found in Chapter 20), as well as any changes in output.

Fluid intake: The sense of thirst lessens as a person ages. When a person drinks fewer fluids, urinary output decreases, and dehydration may result. Some beverages, such as those containing alcohol and caffeine, increase urine output.

To promote normal urination, NAs should encourage residents to drink fluids often. Because a healthy person needs to take in at least 64 ounces of fluid each day, the NA should provide fresh water and juices often (Fig. 16-2). Beverages that are high in vitamin C are especially good for preventing urinary tract infections. The NA must follow any fluid restrictions that a resident has.

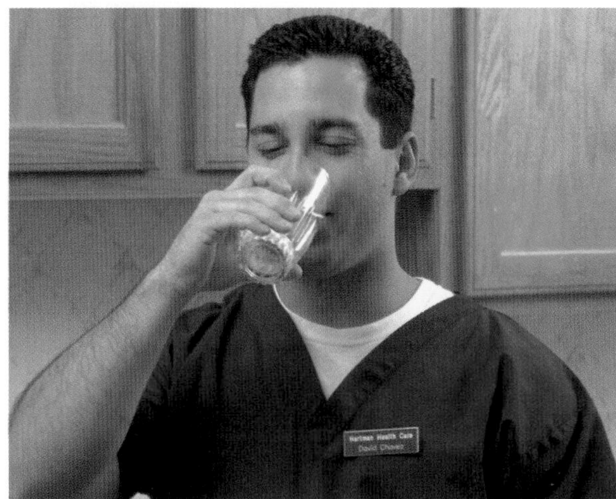

Fig. 16-2. *Drinking plenty of fluids is important to promoting a healthy urinary system.*

Medications: Medications can affect urinary output. For example, a resident who is taking diuretics (medications that reduce fluid in the body) will need to urinate frequently. To promote normal urination, NAs should regularly offer a trip to the bathroom or offer a bedpan or urinal. They should encourage fluid intake and report any changes in output or discoloration of urine.

Disorders: Many disorders and illnesses, such as bladder disease, infections, arthritis, congestive heart disease, neurological diseases, and diabetes, affect urination. Chapter 18 contains more information about these diseases.

Assisting with Elimination

Residents who are unable to get out of bed to use the toilet may be given a bedpan, a fracture pan, or a urinal. A **fracture pan** is a bedpan that is flatter than the regular bedpan. It is used for residents who cannot assist with raising their hips onto a regular bedpan (Fig. 16-3). Women will generally use a bedpan for urination and bowel movements. Men will generally use a urinal for urination and a bedpan for bowel movements (Fig. 16-4).

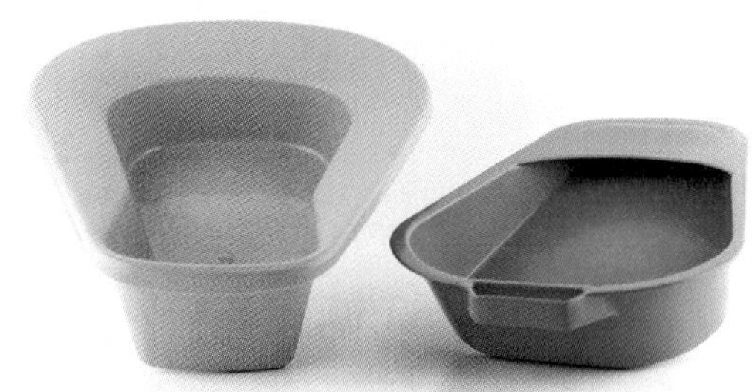

Fig. 16-3. *On the left is a standard pan and on the right is a fracture pan.*

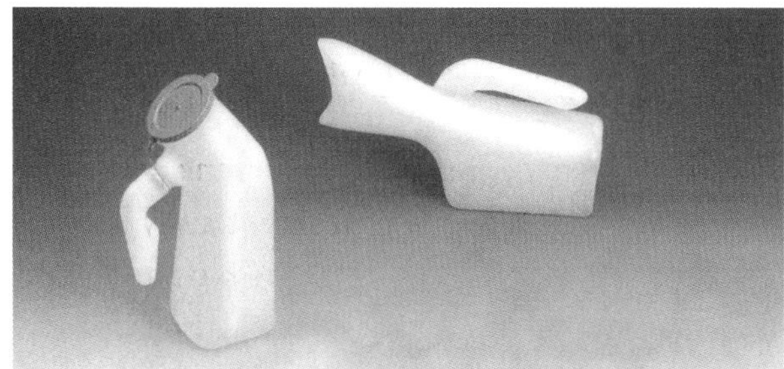

Fig. 16-4. *Two types of urinals.*

Elimination equipment is usually kept in the bathroom between uses. Residents who share bathrooms may need to have urinals and bedpans labeled. Nursing assistants should never place this equipment on overbed tables or on top of side tables.

Urine and feces are considered infectious wastes. Nursing assistants must always wear gloves when handling bedpans, urinals, or basins that contain wastes, including dirty bath water. NAs should be careful not to spill or splash wastes, and wastes should be discarded in the toilet. Immediately after use, containers used for elimination should be placed in the proper area for cleaning, or they should be cleaned and stored according to facility policy.

Residents' Rights

Rights with Elimination

Residents may be embarrassed about needing help with elimination. Nursing assistants should be professional when giving assistance and provide as much privacy as possible. To help promote dignity, NAs should treat residents as adults. NAs should be aware of the language they use when assisting with toileting needs. Proper terms for bodily functions should be used; childish words should be avoided.

Assisting a resident with the use of a bedpan

Equipment: bedpan, bedpan cover, protective pad, bath blanket, toilet paper, disposable wipes, towel, 2 pairs of gloves

1. Identify yourself by name. Identify the resident by name.
2. Wash your hands.
3. Explain procedure to the resident. Speak clearly, slowly, and directly. Maintain face-to-face contact whenever possible.
4. Provide for resident's privacy with curtain, screen, or door.
5. Adjust bed to a safe working level, usually waist high. Before placing bedpan, lower the head of the bed. Lock bed wheels.
6. Put on gloves.
7. Cover the resident with the bath blanket and ask him to hold it while you pull down the top covers underneath. Do not expose more of the resident than you need to.
8. Place a protective pad under the resident's buttocks and hips. To do this, have the resident roll toward you. If the resident cannot do this, you must turn the resident toward you (see Chapter 10). Be sure resident cannot roll off the bed. Move to the empty side of bed and place the protective pad on the area where the resident will lie on his back. The side of protective pad nearest the resident should be fanfolded (folded several times into pleats) and tucked under the resident (Fig. 16-5).

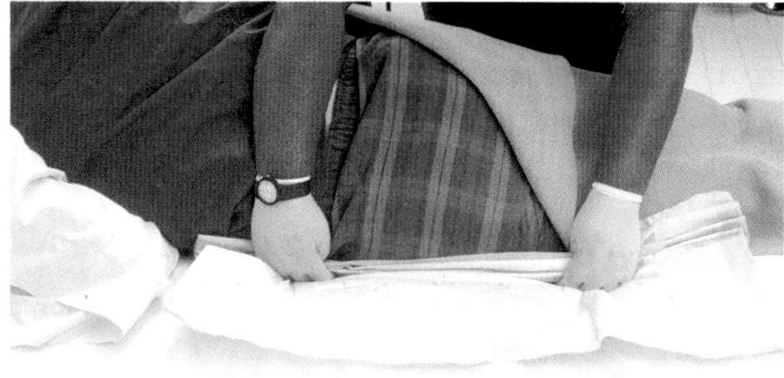

Fig. 16-5. *Fanfold the protective pad near the resident's back.*

Ask the resident to roll onto his back, or roll him as you did before. Unfold the rest of protective pad so it completely covers the area under and around the resident's hips (Fig. 16-6).

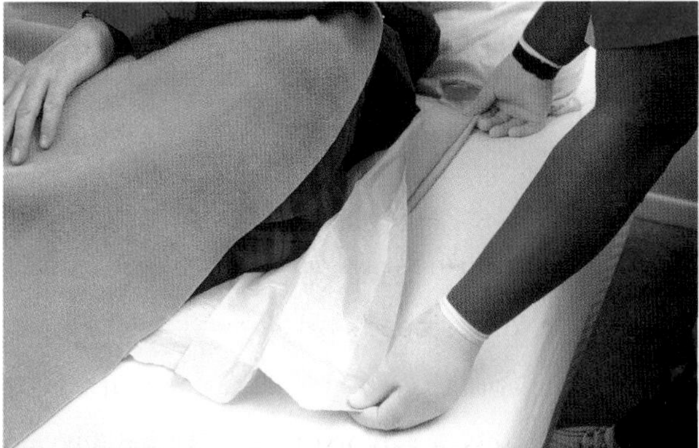

Fig. 16-6. *Unfold the rest of the protective pad so it completely covers area under and around the resident's hips.*

9. Ask the resident to remove undergarments, or help him do so.
10. Place the bedpan near his hips in the correct position. A **standard bedpan** should be positioned with the wider end aligned with the resident's buttocks. A **fracture pan** should be positioned with the handle toward the foot of bed.
11. If resident is able, ask him to raise his hips by pushing with feet and hands at the count of three (Fig. 16-7). Slide the bedpan under his hips.

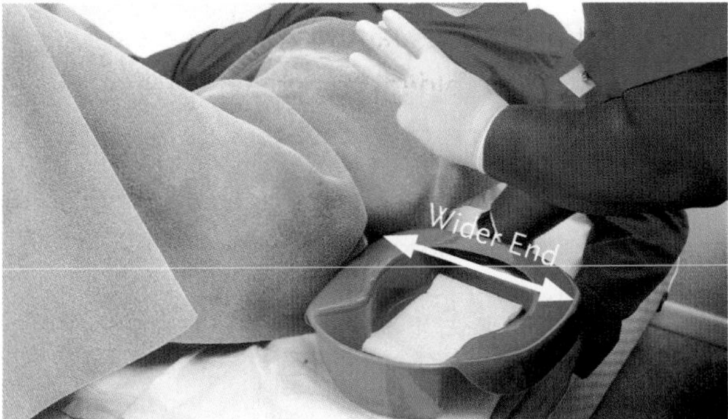

Fig. 16-7. *On the count of three, slide the bedpan under the resident's hips. The wider end of bedpan should be aligned with the resident's buttocks.*

If the resident cannot do this himself, place your arm under the small of his back and tell him to push with his heels and hands on your signal as you raise his hips (Fig. 16-8).

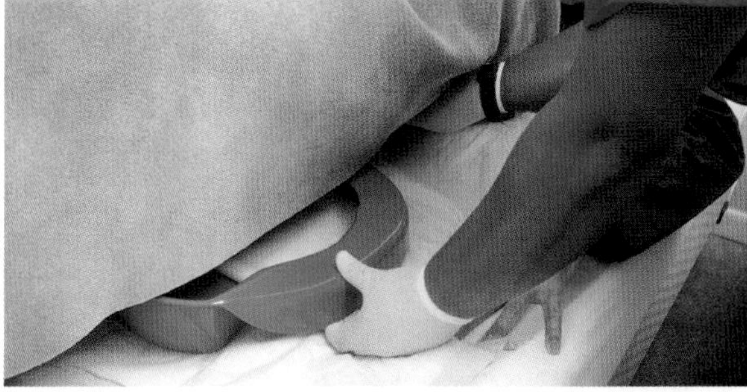

Fig. 16-8. *If a resident cannot raise his hips, you can raise his hips while he pushes with his heels and hands.*

If a resident cannot help you in any way, keep the bed flat and roll the resident away from you. Slip the bedpan under the hips and gently roll the resident back onto the bedpan. Keep the bedpan centered underneath.

12. Remove and discard gloves. Wash your hands.
13. Raise the head of the bed. Prop the resident into a semi-sitting position using pillows.
14. Make sure the bath blanket is still covering the resident. Place toilet paper and disposable wipes within resident's reach. Ask resident to clean his hands with a wipe when finished if he is able.
15. Place the call light within resident's reach. Ask resident to signal when done. Leave the room and close the door.
16. When called by the resident, return and put on clean gloves.
17. Lower the head of the bed. Make sure resident is still covered.
18. Remove bedpan carefully and cover bedpan.
19. Provide perineal care if help is needed. Wipe female residents from front to back. Dry the perineal area with a towel. Help the resident put on undergarment. Cover the resident and remove the bath blanket.
20. Place the towel and bath blanket in a hamper or bag, and discard disposable supplies.

21. Take bedpan to the bathroom. Empty the bedpan carefully into the toilet unless a specimen is needed or urine is being measured for intake/output monitoring. Note color, odor, and consistency of contents before flushing. If you notice anything unusual about the stool or urine (for example, the presence of blood), do not discard it. You will need to inform the nurse.
22. Turn the faucet on with a paper towel. Rinse the bedpan with cold water and empty it into the toilet. Flush the toilet. Place bedpan in proper area for cleaning or clean it according to facility policy.
23. Remove and discard gloves.
24. Wash your hands.
25. Make resident comfortable.
26. Return bed to lowest position. Remove privacy measures.
27. Place call light within resident's reach.
28. Report any changes in resident to the nurse.
29. Document procedure using facility guidelines.

Assisting a male resident with a urinal

Equipment: urinal, protective pad, disposable wipes, 2 pairs of gloves

1. Identify yourself by name. Identify the resident by name.
2. Wash your hands.
3. Explain procedure to the resident. Speak clearly, slowly, and directly. Maintain face-to-face contact whenever possible.
4. Provide for resident's privacy with curtain, screen, or door.
5. Adjust bed to a safe working level, usually waist high. Lock bed wheels.
6. Put on gloves.
7. Place a protective pad under the resident's buttocks and hips, as in earlier procedure.
8. Hand the urinal to the resident. If the resident is not able to help himself, place urinal between his legs and position the penis inside the urinal (Fig. 16-9). Replace covers.

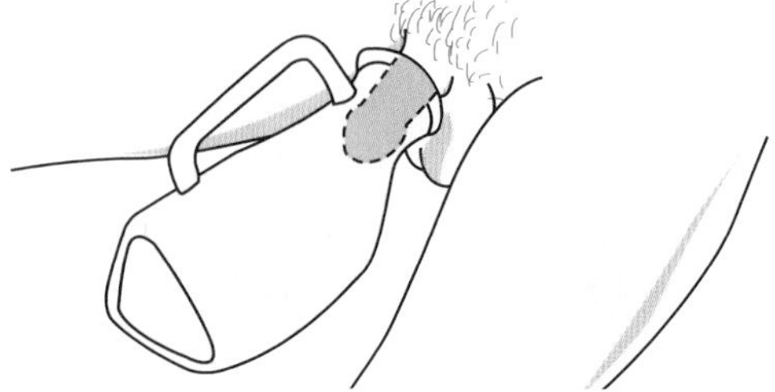

Fig. 16-9. *Position the penis inside the urinal if the resident cannot do it himself.*

9. Remove and discard gloves. Wash your hands.
10. Place disposable wipes within resident's reach. Ask the resident to clean his hands with the hand wipe when finished if he is able. Place the call light within reach while resident is using urinal. Ask resident to signal when done. Leave the room and close the door.
11. When called by the resident, return and put on clean gloves.
12. Discard disposable wipes.
13. Remove urinal or have resident hand it to you. Empty contents into toilet unless specimen is needed or the urine is being measured for intake/output monitoring. Note color, odor, and qualities (for example, cloudiness) of contents.
14. Turn the faucet on with a paper towel. Rinse the urinal with cold water and empty it into the toilet. Flush the toilet. Place urinal in proper area for cleaning or clean it according to facility policy.
15. Remove and discard gloves.
16. Wash your hands.
17. Make resident comfortable.
18. Return bed to lowest position. Remove privacy measures.
19. Place call light within resident's reach.

20. Report any changes in resident to the nurse.
21. Document procedure using facility guidelines.

Some residents are able to get out of bed, but may still need help walking to the bathroom and using the toilet. Others who are able to get out of bed but are unable to walk to the bathroom may use a portable commode, or bedside commode (BSC). A **portable commode** is a chair with a toilet seat and a removable container underneath (Fig. 16-10). Toilets can be fitted with raised seats to make it easier for residents to get up and down. Handrails can also be installed next to the toilet. If these assistive devices are needed but are not present, nursing assistants should report this to the nurse. When residents need assistance to get to the bathroom or use the commode, NAs must offer to help often. This will avoid accidents and embarrassment.

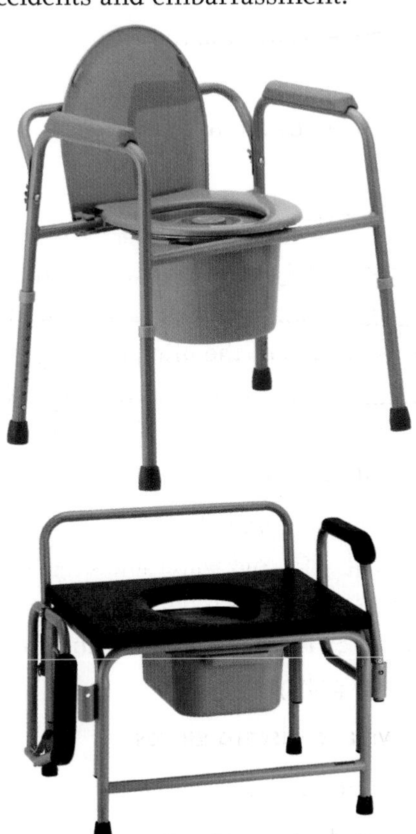

***Fig. 16-10.** The top photo shows a regular portable commode and the bottom photo shows a bariatric portable commode, which can be used for people who are overweight or obese.* (PHOTO COURTESY OF NOVA MEDICAL PRODUCTS, WWW.NOVAMEDICALPRODUCTS.COM)

Assisting a resident to use a portable commode or toilet

Equipment: portable commode with basin, toilet paper, disposable wipes, towel, 3 pairs of gloves

1. Identify yourself by name. Identify the resident by name.
2. Wash your hands.
3. Explain procedure to the resident. Speak clearly, slowly, and directly. Maintain face-to-face contact whenever possible.
4. Provide for resident's privacy with curtain, screen, or door.
5. Lock bed wheels. Make sure resident is wearing non-skid shoes and that the laces are tied. Help resident out of bed and to the portable commode or bathroom.
6. Put on gloves.
7. If needed, help resident remove clothing and sit comfortably on toilet seat. Put toilet paper and disposable wipes within reach. Ask resident to clean his hands with a wipe when finished if he is able.
8. Remove and discard your gloves. Wash your hands.
9. Provide privacy. Place call light within reach while resident is using commode. Ask resident to signal when done. Leave the room and close the door.
10. When called by resident, return and put on clean gloves. Provide perineal care if help is needed. Wipe female residents from front to back. Dry the perineal area with a towel. Help the resident put on clothing.
11. Place the towel in a hamper or bag, and discard disposable supplies.
12. Remove and discard gloves. Wash your hands.
13. Help resident back to bed. Make resident comfortable.

14. Put on clean gloves.
15. When using a portable commode, remove waste container. Empty it into the toilet unless a specimen is needed or the urine is being measured for intake/output monitoring. Empty into toilet. Note color, odor, and consistency of contents.
16. Turn the faucet on with a paper towel. Rinse the container with cold water and empty it into the toilet. Flush the toilet. Place container in proper area for cleaning or clean it according to facility policy.
17. Remove and discard gloves.
18. Wash your hands.
19. Make sure bed is in lowest position. Remove privacy measures.
20. Place call light within resident's reach.
21. Report any changes in resident to the nurse.
22. Document procedure using facility guidelines.

3. Describe common diseases and disorders of the urinary system

Urinary Incontinence

Urinary incontinence is the inability to control the bladder, which leads to an involuntary loss of urine. Incontinence can occur in residents who are confined to bed, ill, elderly, paralyzed, or who have circulatory or nervous system diseases or injuries. There are different types of incontinence, including the following:

- Stress incontinence is the loss of urine due to an increase in intra-abdominal pressure, for example, when sneezing, laughing, or coughing.
- Urge incontinence is involuntary voiding from a sudden urge to void.
- Mixed incontinence is a combination of both urge incontinence and stress incontinence.
- Reflex incontinence is similar to urge incontinence, but usually occurs when a specific bladder volume is reached.
- Functional incontinence is urine loss caused by things outside the urinary tract.
- Overflow incontinence is loss of urine due to overflow or over-distention of the bladder.

Incontinence is *not* a normal part of aging. Nursing assistants should always report incontinence. It may be a sign or symptom of an illness.

Guidelines: Urinary Incontinence

- **G** Offer a bedpan, urinal, commode, or trip to the bathroom often. Follow toileting schedules in the care plan.
- **G** Answer call lights and requests for help immediately.
- **G** Urinary incontinence is a major risk factor for pressure ulcers. Document all episodes of incontinence carefully and accurately.
- **G** Cleanliness and careful skin care are important for residents who are incontinent. Urine is very irritating to the skin. It should be washed off immediately and completely. Keep residents clean, dry, and free from odor. Observe the skin carefully when bathing and giving perineal care.
- **G** Incontinent residents who are bedbound should have a plastic, latex, or disposable sheet placed under them to protect the bed. Place a draw sheet over it to absorb moisture and protect the skin.
- **G** Some residents will wear disposable incontinence pads or briefs for adults. They keep body wastes away from the skin (Fig. 16-11). Assist residents as needed with changing wet briefs immediately. Do not refer to an incontinence brief as a *diaper.* Residents are not children, and doing that is disrespectful.

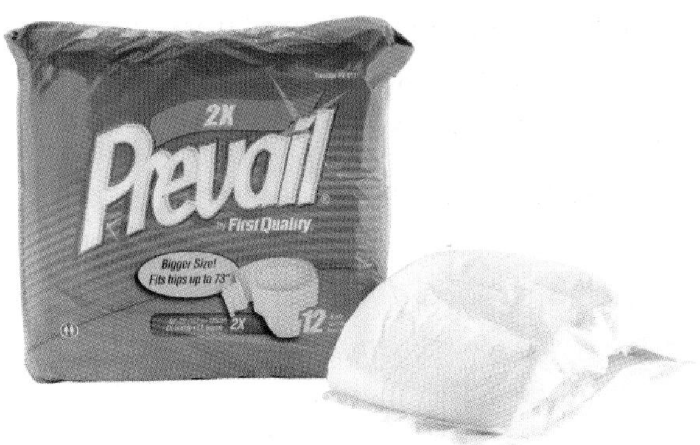

Fig. 16-11. A type of incontinence pad.

- G Encourage residents to drink plenty of fluids.
- G Residents who are incontinent need reassurance and understanding. Be professional and kind when dealing with incontinence. Doing so may help put residents at ease.

Changing Incontinence Briefs

When changing an incontinence brief, the nursing assistant should make sure to assemble all needed items beforehand, including a protective pad, perineal care supplies, disposable wipes, gloves, and a clean brief. He should put on gloves before handling the brief. When removing the soiled brief, the NA should roll it inward, soiled side inside, without spilling its contents. Working from front to back, he should carefully remove all urine and/or feces from the skin. After cleaning the area thoroughly, he should blot it dry and apply the clean brief.

Urinary Tract Infection (UTI)

Urinary tract infection (UTI) causes inflammation of the bladder and the ureters. This results in painful burning during urination and the frequent feeling of needing to urinate. UTI or **cystitis**, also inflammation of the bladder, may be caused by a bacterial infection. Certain situations, such as being bedbound, can cause urine to stay in the bladder too long. This provides an ideal environment for bacteria to grow.

Cystitis is more common in women because the urethra is much shorter in women (three to four inches) than in men (seven to eight inches). Bacteria can reach a woman's bladder more easily. To avoid infection, women should wipe the perineal area from front to back after bladder and bowel elimination.

Guidelines: Preventing UTIs

- G Encourage residents to wipe from front to back after elimination (Fig. 16-12). When giving perineal care, make sure you do this, too.

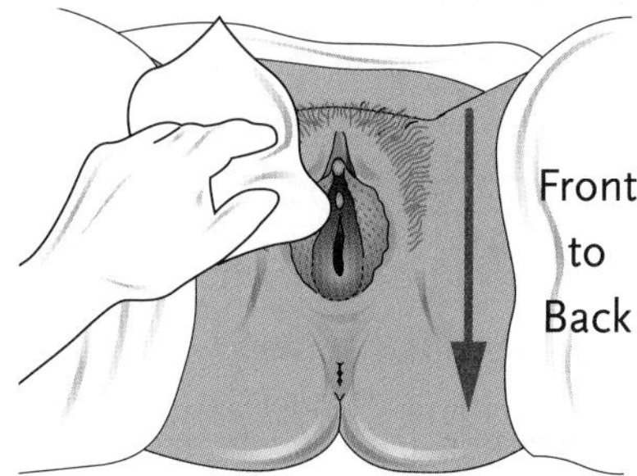

Fig. 16-12. After elimination, wipe from front to back to prevent infection.

- G Give careful perineal care when changing incontinence briefs.
- G Encourage plenty of fluids. Drinking plenty of fluids helps prevent UTIs. Drinking cranberry and blueberry juices acidifies urine, which helps to prevent infection. Vitamin C also has this effect.
- G Offer bedpan or a trip to the toilet at least every two hours. Answer call lights promptly.
- G Taking showers, rather than baths, helps prevent UTIs.
- G Report cloudy, dark, or foul-smelling urine, or if a resident urinates often and in small amounts.

Calculi

Calculi, or kidney stones, form when urine crystallizes in the kidneys. Kidney stones can block the kidneys and ureters, causing severe pain. Kidney stones can result from some of the same conditions that cause cystitis. They can also be the result of a vitamin deficiency, mineral imbalance, structural abnormalities of the urinary tract, or infection.

Symptoms of calculi may not be felt until they begin to move down the ureter, causing pain. Symptoms include the following:

- Abdominal pain
- Flank or back pain
- Groin pain
- Burning during urination, painful urination
- Frequent urination
- Blood in the urine
- Nausea, vomiting
- Chills, fever

Urine straining is the process of pouring all urine through a fine filter to catch any particles. This is done to detect the presence of calculi that can develop in the urinary tract. Kidney stones can be as small as grains of sand or as large as golf balls. If any stones are found, they are saved and then sent to a laboratory for examination.

If straining urine is listed on an assignment sheet, the nursing assistant will first need to collect a routine urine specimen. Then he will go into the bathroom and pour the specimen through a strainer or a 4x4-inch piece of gauze into a specimen container. Any stones that are found are wrapped in the filter and are placed in the specimen container to go to the lab.

Treatment of calculi includes drinking plenty of water to produce greater quantities of urine. Pain relievers may be ordered. Kidney stones usually pass on their own, but if they do not, surgery may be required.

Nephritis

Nephritis is an inflammation of the kidneys. Symptoms include a decrease in urine output, rusty-colored urine, and a burning feeling during urination. A person with nephritis often has a swollen face, eyelids, and hands because she is retaining fluid. Children and young adults usually recover without problems. Older people can develop a chronic form of nephritis.

Renovascular Hypertension

Renovascular hypertension is a condition in which a blockage of arteries in the kidneys causes high blood pressure. Medications may be used to help control blood pressure. Further treatment may include surgery. More information about hypertension and its symptoms, treatment, and related care is found in Chapter 18.

Chronic Renal Failure

Chronic renal failure (CRF) also called **chronic kidney failure**, occurs because the kidneys become unable to eliminate certain waste products from the body. This disease can develop as the result of chronic urinary tract infections, nephritis, or diabetes. Excessive salt in the diet can also cause damage to the kidneys. Over time, the disease becomes worse. Symptoms include the following:

- High blood pressure
- Decreased urine output or no urine output
- Dark urine
- Anemia
- Nausea, vomiting
- Loss of appetite
- Weight changes
- Fatigue and weakness
- Headaches
- Difficulty sleeping
- Back pain
- Edema
- Stool that is bloody or black

Kidney dialysis, an artificial means of removing the body's waste products, is done when the kidneys are no longer able to function properly. Dialysis can improve and extend life for several years. Residents will be on fluid restrictions of different degrees. Chronic renal failure can progress to end-stage renal disease, which is fatal without kidney dialysis or a kidney transplant.

4. Describe guidelines for urinary catheter care

Some residents may have a urinary catheter. A **catheter** is a thin tube inserted into the body that is used to drain fluids or inject fluids. A urinary catheter is used to drain urine from the bladder. A **straight catheter** does not remain inside the person. It is removed immediately after urine is drained. An **indwelling catheter** remains inside the bladder for a period of time (Fig. 16-13). The urine drains into a bag. Nursing assistants do not insert, remove, or irrigate catheters. NAs may be asked to provide daily care for the catheter, cleaning the area around the urethral opening and emptying the drainage bag.

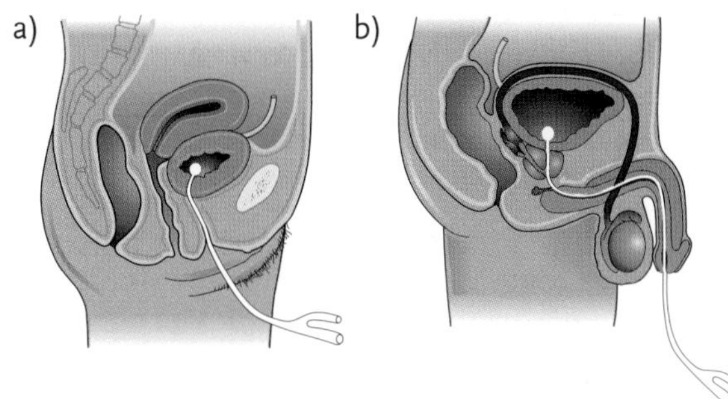

Fig. 16-13. *An illustration of a) an indwelling catheter (female) and b) an indwelling catheter (male).*

An external catheter, or **condom catheter** (also called a *Texas catheter*), has an attachment on the end that fits onto the penis (Fig. 16-14). The attachment is fastened with special tape. Urine drains through the catheter into the tubing, then into the drainage bag. Smaller bags, called *leg bags*, attach to the leg and collect the urine. The condom catheter is changed daily or as needed.

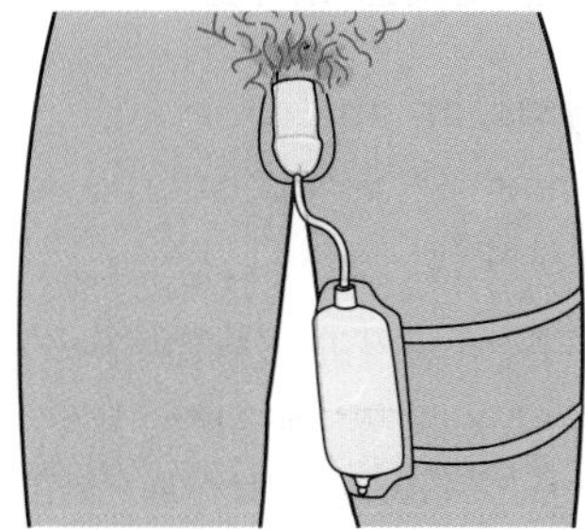

Fig. 16-14. *An illustration of an external, or condom, catheter.*

Guidelines: Urinary Catheters

G Make sure that the drainage bag is always lower than the hips or bladder. Urine must never flow from the bag or tubing back into the bladder. This can cause infection.

G Keep the drainage bag off the floor.

G Keep the tubing as straight as possible. It should not be kinked. Kinks, twists, or pressure on the tubing (such as from the resident sitting or lying on the tubing) can prevent urine from draining.

G Keep the genital area clean to prevent infection. Because the catheter goes all the way into the bladder, bacteria can enter the bladder more easily. Daily care of the genital area is especially important.

Observing and Reporting: Urinary Catheters

Report any of the following to the nurse:

O/R Blood is in the urine or urine looks unusual in any way

O/R Catheter bag does not fill after several hours

O/R Catheter bag fills suddenly

O/R Catheter is not in place

O/R Urine leaks from the catheter

O/R Resident reports pain or pressure

O/R Odor is present

Providing catheter care

Equipment: bath blanket, protective pad, bath basin with warm water, soap, bath thermometer, 2-4 washcloths or disposable wipes, towel, gloves

1. Identify yourself by name. Identify the resident by name.
2. Wash your hands.
3. Explain procedure to the resident. Speak clearly, slowly, and directly. Maintain face-to-face contact whenever possible.

4. Provide for resident's privacy with curtain, screen, or door.
5. Adjust bed to a safe working level, usually waist high. Lock bed wheels.
6. Lower head of bed. Position resident lying flat on her back.
7. Remove or fold back top bedding, keeping resident covered with bath blanket.
8. Test water temperature with thermometer or on the inside of your wrist to ensure it is safe. Water temperature should be no higher than 105°F. Have resident check water temperature. Adjust if necessary.
9. Put on gloves.
10. Ask the resident to flex her knees and raise her buttocks off the bed by pushing against the mattress with her feet. Place clean protective pad under her buttocks.
11. Expose only the area necessary to clean the catheter. Avoid overexposing the resident.
12. Place towel or pad under catheter tubing before washing.
13. Wet washcloth in basin and apply soap to washcloth. Clean area around meatus. Use a clean area of the washcloth for each stroke.
14. Hold catheter near meatus to avoid tugging the catheter.
15. Clean at least four inches of catheter nearest the meatus. Move in only one direction, away from the meatus. Use a clean area of the cloth for each stroke.
16. Dip a clean washcloth in the water. Rinse area around the meatus, using a clean area of washcloth for each stroke.
17. Dip a clean washcloth in the water. Rinse at least four inches of catheter nearest the meatus. Move in only one direction, away from the meatus (Fig. 16-15). Use a clean area of the washcloth for each stroke.

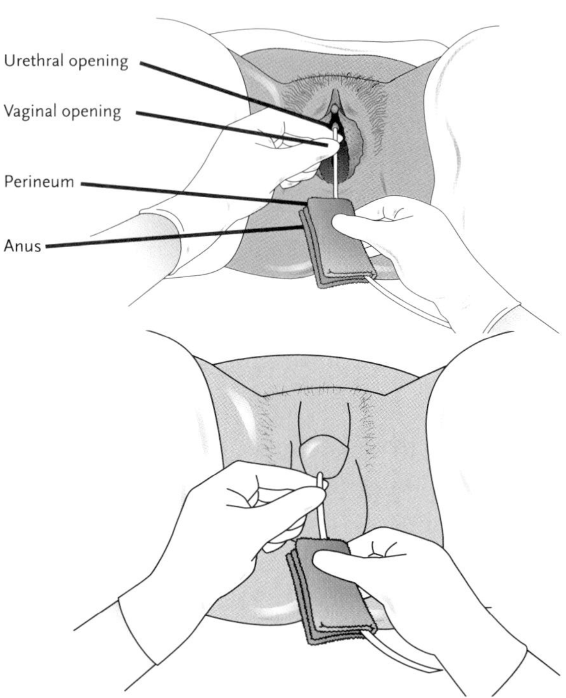

Fig. 16-15. *Hold the catheter near the meatus to avoid tugging the catheter. Moving in only one direction, away from the meatus, helps prevent infection. Use a clean area of the washcloth for each stroke.*

18. Remove towel or pad from under catheter tubing. Replace top covers and remove bath blanket.
19. Dispose of linen in proper containers.
20. Empty basin into the toilet and flush. Place basin in proper area for cleaning or clean and store it according to facility policy.
21. Remove and discard gloves.
22. Wash your hands.
23. Remove bath blanket and replace top covers. Make resident comfortable. Check that the catheter tubing is free from kinks and twists and that it is securely fastened to the leg.
24. Return bed to lowest position. Remove privacy measures.
25. Place call light within resident's reach.
26. Report any changes in resident to the nurse.
27. Document procedure using facility guidelines.

Residents' Rights

Urinary Catheters

The nursing assistant should protect privacy when a resident has a urinary catheter. She should keep the tubing and bag covered and close doors and pull privacy screens when providing catheter care.

Emptying the catheter drainage bag

Equipment: graduate (measuring container), alcohol wipes, paper towels, gloves

1. Identify yourself by name. Identify the resident by name.
2. Wash your hands.
3. Explain procedure to the resident. Speak clearly, slowly, and directly. Maintain face-to-face contact whenever possible.
4. Provide for resident's privacy with curtain, screen, or door.
5. Put on gloves.
6. Place paper towel on the floor under the drainage bag. Place graduate on the paper towel.
7. Open the drain or spout on the bag so that the urine flows out of the bag and into the graduate (Fig. 16-16). Do not let spout or clamp touch the graduate.

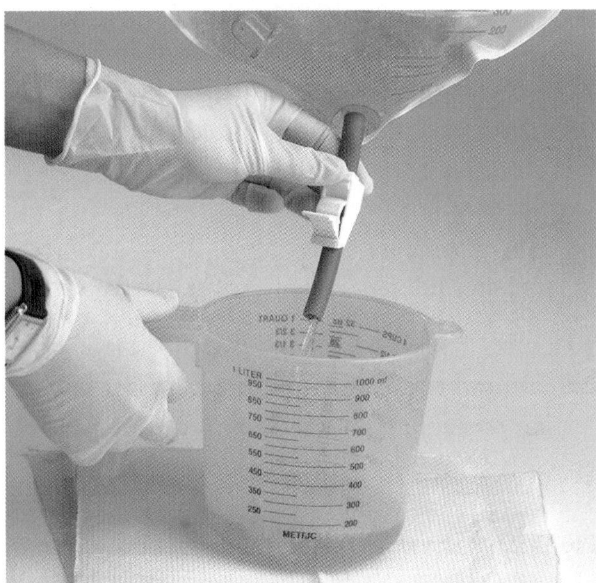

Fig. 16-16. *Keep the spout and clamp from touching the graduate while draining urine.*

8. When urine has drained, close spout. Using alcohol wipes, clean the drain spout. Replace the drain in its holder on the bag.
9. Go into the bathroom. Place graduate on a flat surface and measure at eye level. Note the amount and the appearance of the urine. Empty into toilet and flush toilet.
10. Clean and store graduate. Discard paper towels.
11. Remove and discard gloves.
12. Wash your hands.
13. Document procedure and amount of urine.

Changing a condom catheter

Equipment: condom catheter and collection bag, catheter tape, plastic bag, bath blanket, protective pad, supplies for perineal care, gloves

1. Identify yourself by name. Identify the resident by name.
2. Wash your hands.
3. Explain procedure to the resident. Speak clearly, slowly, and directly. Maintain face-to-face contact whenever possible.
4. Provide for resident's privacy with curtain, screen, or door.
5. Adjust bed to a safe level, usually waist high. Lock bed wheels.
6. Lower head of bed. Position resident lying flat on his back.
7. Remove or fold back top bedding, keeping resident covered with bath blanket.
8. Put on gloves.
9. Place a clean protective pad under his buttocks.
10. Adjust bath blanket to only expose genital area.
11. If condom catheter is present, gently remove it. Place condom and tape in the plastic bag.
12. Assist as necessary with perineal care.

13. Move pubic hair away from the penis so it does not get rolled into the condom.
14. Hold penis firmly. Place condom at tip of penis and roll toward base of penis. Leave space (at least one inch) between the drainage tip and glans of penis to prevent irritation. If resident is not circumcised, be sure that foreskin is in normal position.
15. Gently secure condom to penis with special tape provided. Apply tape in a spiral manner (Fig. 16-17).

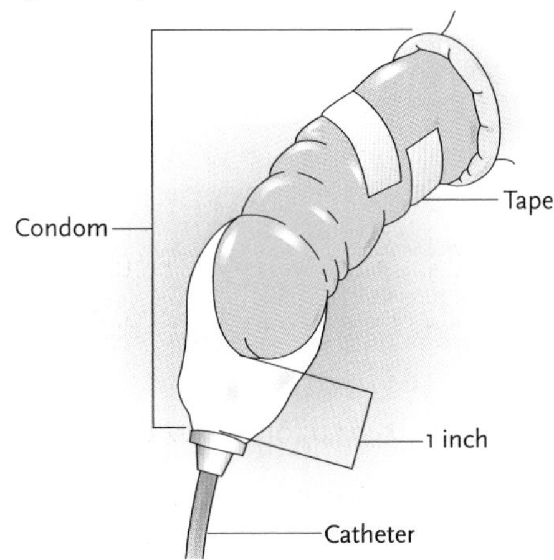

Fig. 16-17. *Gently secure condom to penis with provided tape, applying it in a spiral.*

16. Connect catheter tip to drainage tubing. Make sure tubing is not twisted or kinked.
17. Check to see if collection bag is secured to leg. Make sure drain is closed.
18. Discard used supplies in plastic bag. Place soiled clothing and linens in proper containers. Clean and store supplies.
19. Remove and discard gloves.
20. Wash your hands.
21. Remove bath blanket. Make resident comfortable.
22. Return bed to lowest position. Remove privacy measures.
23. Place call light within resident's reach.
24. Report any changes in resident to the nurse.
25. Document procedure using facility guidelines.

Nursing assistants may be asked to collect a urine specimen from a resident who has a urinary catheter. If this is within an NA's scope of practice, she should follow the nurse's instructions for collecting this type of specimen. If the resident's input and output are being monitored, the NA will need to measure the amount of urine collected. Collecting a specimen this way may take some time.

5. Identify types of urine specimens that are collected

Nursing assistants may need to collect a specimen from a resident. A **specimen** is a sample that is used for analysis in order to try to make a diagnosis. Different types of specimens are used for different tests.

There are several factors to consider when collecting specimens. Body wastes and elimination needs are very private matters for most people. Having another person handle their body wastes may make residents embarrassed and uncomfortable. Nursing assistants should be sensitive to this and should empathize with residents. When collecting specimens, the NA should behave professionally. If she feels that this is an unpleasant task, she should not make it known to the resident. She should not make faces, frown, or use words that let the resident know she feels uncomfortable. Remaining professional when collecting specimens can help put residents at ease.

Urine specimens may be routine, clean-catch (mid-stream), or 24-hour. A **routine urine specimen** is collected any time the resident voids. The resident will void into a bedpan, urinal, commode, or hat. A **hat** is a plastic collection container sometimes put into a toilet to collect and measure urine or stool (Fig. 16-18). Some residents will be able to collect their own urine specimens. Others will need a nursing assistant's help. The NA must be sure to explain exactly how the specimen must be collected (Fig. 16-19).

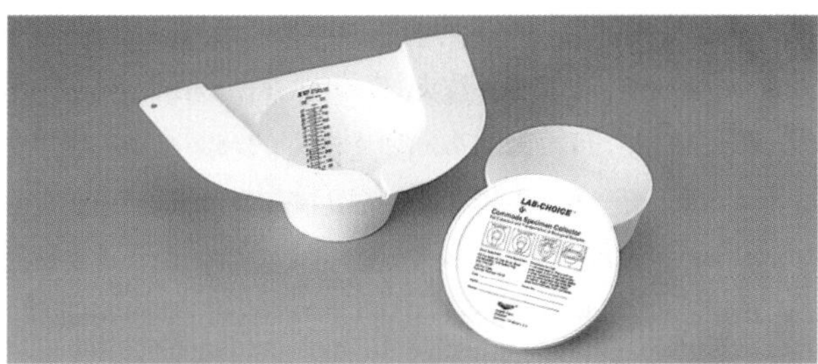

Fig. 16-18. A hat is a container that is sometimes placed under the toilet seat to collect and measure urine or stool. Hats should be labeled and must be cleaned after each use.

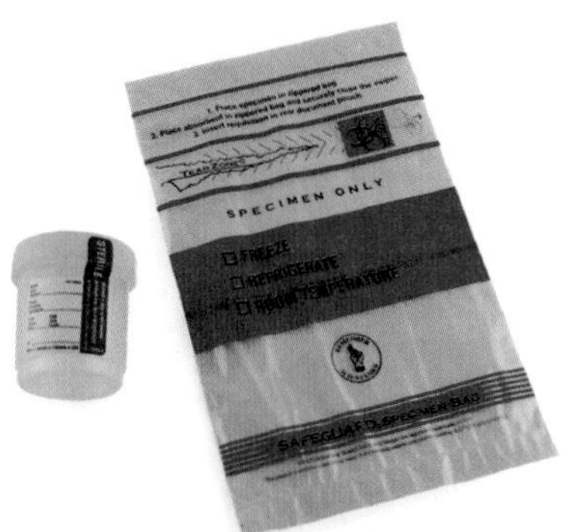

Fig. 16-19. Specimens must always be labeled with the resident's name, date of birth, room number, the date, and time, before being taken to the lab. A specimen may need to be placed in a clean specimen bag before transporting it.

Collecting a routine urine specimen

Equipment: urine specimen container with completed label (labeled with resident's name, date of birth, room number, date, and time) and lid, specimen bag, 2 pairs of gloves, bedpan or urinal (if resident cannot use a portable commode or toilet), hat for toilet (if resident uses portable commode or toilet), plastic bag, toilet paper, disposable wipes, paper towels, supplies for perineal care, laboratory slip

1. Identify yourself by name. Identify the resident by name.
2. Wash your hands.
3. Explain procedure to the resident. Speak clearly, slowly, and directly. Maintain face-to-face contact whenever possible.
4. Provide for resident's privacy with curtain, screen, or door.
5. Put on gloves.
6. Fit hat to toilet or commode, or provide resident with bedpan or urinal.
7. Ask resident to void into hat, urinal, or bedpan. Ask the resident not to put toilet paper in with the sample. Provide a plastic bag to discard toilet paper separately.
8. Place toilet paper and disposable wipes within resident's reach. Ask resident to clean his hands with a wipe when finished if he is able.
9. Remove and discard gloves. Wash your hands.
10. Place the call light within resident's reach. Ask resident to signal when done. Leave the room and close the door.
11. When called by the resident, return and put on clean gloves. Provide perineal care if help is needed.
12. Take bedpan, urinal, or hat to the bathroom.
13. Pour urine into the specimen container. Specimen container should be at least half full.
14. Cover the urine container with its lid. Do not touch the inside of container. Wipe off the outside with a paper towel and apply label.
15. Place the container in a clean specimen bag.
16. Discard extra urine in toilet. Turn the faucet on with a paper towel. Rinse the bedpan, urinal, or hat with cold water and empty it into the toilet. Flush the toilet. Place equipment in proper area for cleaning or clean it according to facility policy.
17. Remove and discard gloves.
18. Wash your hands.
19. Remove privacy measures.
20. Place call light within resident's reach.
21. Report any changes in resident to the nurse.
22. Take specimen and lab slip to proper area. Document procedure using facility guidelines. Note amount and characteristics of urine.

Residents' Rights

Specimens

When collecting specimens, the nursing assistant should first explain how she will be collecting the specimen. The NA should do this in private, keeping her voice low. She should also close the door to the bathroom or bedroom and pull the privacy curtain. In addition, the NA should be discreet when removing the specimen from the room.

The **clean-catch specimen**, or mid-stream specimen (CCMS), is collected by first cleaning the perineal area and then urinating a small amount into the toilet to clear the urethra. Then the person begins urinating again into a clean or sterile container, stopping before urination is complete. The container is removed, and the person finishes urinating into the toilet. This type of specimen is called *mid-stream* because the first and last urine are not included in the sample. Its purpose is to determine the presence of bacteria in the urine.

Collecting a clean-catch (mid-stream) urine specimen

Equipment: specimen kit with container with completed label (labeled with resident's name, date of birth, room number, date, and time) and lid, specimen bag, cleaning solution, gloves, bedpan or urinal (if resident cannot use a portable commode or toilet), plastic bag, toilet paper, disposable wipes, paper towels, supplies for perineal care, lab slip

1. Identify yourself by name. Identify the resident by name.
2. Wash your hands.
3. Explain procedure to the resident. Speak clearly, slowly, and directly. Maintain face-to-face contact whenever possible.
4. Provide for resident's privacy with curtain, screen, or door.
5. Put on gloves.
6. Open the specimen kit. Do not touch the inside of the container or the inside of the lid.
7. If the resident cannot clean his or her perineal area, you will need to do it. Use the wipes and cleaning solution to do this. Be sure to use a clean area of the wipe or a clean wipe for each stroke. See bed bath procedure in Chapter 13 for a reminder on how to give perineal care.
8. Ask the resident to urinate a small amount into the bedpan, urinal, or toilet, and to stop before urination is complete.
9. Place the container under the urine stream and have the resident start urinating again. Fill the container at least half full. Ask the resident to stop urinating and remove the container. Have the resident finish urinating in bedpan, urinal, or toilet.
10. After urination, provide a plastic bag so resident can discard toilet paper. Give perineal care if help is needed. Ask resident to clean his hands with a wipe if he is able.
11. Cover the urine container with its lid. Do not touch the inside of container. Wipe off the outside with a paper towel and apply label.
12. Place the container in a clean specimen bag.
13. Discard extra urine in toilet. Turn the faucet on with a paper towel. Rinse the bedpan or urinal with cold water and empty it into the toilet. Flush the toilet. Place equipment in proper area for cleaning or clean it according to facility policy.
14. Remove and discard gloves.
15. Wash your hands.
16. Make resident comfortable.
17. Return bed to lowest position if adjusted. Remove privacy measures.
18. Place call light within resident's reach.
19. Report any changes in resident to the nurse.
20. Take specimen and lab slip to proper area. Document procedure using facility guidelines. Note amount and characteristics of urine.

A **24-hour urine specimen** collects all the urine voided by a resident in a 24-hour period. It is used to test for certain chemicals and hormones. Usually the collection begins at 7 a.m. and continues until 7 a.m. the next day. When beginning a 24-hour urine specimen collection, the resident must void and discard the first urine so that the collection begins with an empty bladder. All urine must be collected and stored properly. If any is accidentally thrown away or improperly stored, the collection will have to be started over.

Collecting a 24-hour urine specimen

Equipment: 24-hour specimen container with lid, bedpan or urinal (for residents confined to bed), hat for toilet (if resident can use portable commode or toilet), gloves, disposable wipes, supplies for perineal care, sign to alert other team members that a 24-hour urine specimen is being collected, form for recording output, laboratory slip

1. Identify yourself by name. Identify the resident by name.
2. Wash your hands.
3. Explain procedure to the resident. Speak clearly, slowly, and directly. Maintain face-to-face contact whenever possible. Emphasize that all urine must be saved.
4. Provide for resident's privacy with curtain, screen, or door.
5. Place a sign on the resident's bed to let all care team members know that a 24-hour specimen is being collected. Sign may read *Save all urine for 24-hour specimen.*
6. When starting the collection, have the resident completely empty the bladder. Discard the urine. Note the exact time of this voiding. The collection will run until the same time the next day (Fig. 16-20).
7. Label the container with the resident's name, date of birth, room number, and dates and times the collection period begins and ends.

INTAKE-OUTPUT RECORD

Resident/Patient Name			Room No.
	FLUID INTAKE	URINE	EMESIS or DRAINAGE
7:00 A.M. to 3:00 P.M.			
	8-Hour Total		
3:00 P.M. to 11:00 P.M.			
	8-Hour Total		
11:00 P.M. to 7 A.M.			
	8-Hour Total		

Form 3039 © Briggs, Des Moines, IA 50306 PRINTED IN U.S.A. R404
DON'T BREAK THE LAW MAKE THE CALL Save 13%* 1-800-247-2343 www.BriggsCorp.com
*savings on buying vs. copying

Fig. 16-20. *One type of form to record urine output over 24 hours.* (REPRINTED WITH PERMISSION OF BRIGGS CORPORATION, 800-247-2343, WWW.BRIGGSCORP.COM)

8. Wash hands and put on gloves each time the resident voids.

9. Pour urine from bedpan, urinal, or hat into the container. Container may be stored at room temperature, in the refrigerator, or on ice. Follow facility policy.
10. After each voiding, help as necessary with perineal care. Ask the resident to clean his hands with a wipe after each voiding.
11. After each voiding, place equipment in proper area for cleaning or clean it according to facility policy.
12. Remove and discard gloves.
13. Wash your hands.
14. After the last void of the 24-hour period, remove the sign. Take specimen and lab slip to proper area. Document procedure using facility guidelines. Make sure to include the time of the last void before the 24-hour collection period began and the last void of the 24-hour collection period.

6. Explain types of tests performed on urine

Different types of tests can be used to detect different things in urine. Dip strips can be used to test for such things as pH level, glucose, ketones, blood, and specific gravity. These strips, called reagent strips, have different sections that change color when they react with urine (Fig. 16-21).

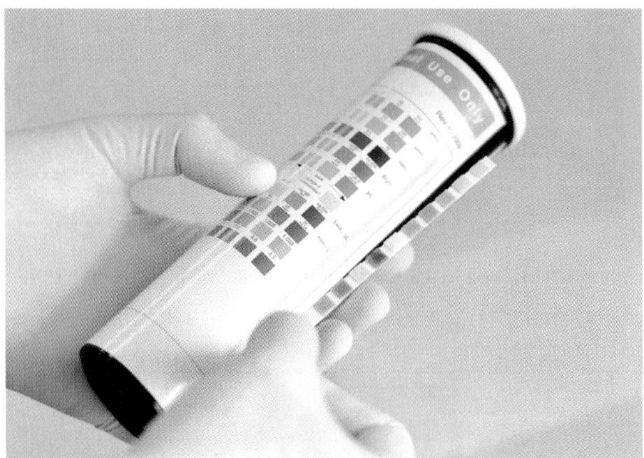

Fig. 16-21. *Reagent strips change color when they react with urine. The color is then compared to a color chart to determine levels of each chemical factor.*

Testing pH levels: The pH scale ranges from 0 to 14. The lower the number, the more acidic the fluid. The higher the number, the more alkaline the fluid. Normal pH range for urine is 4.6–8.0. A pH imbalance may be due to medication, food, or illness.

Testing for glucose and ketones: In diabetes, the pancreas does not produce enough insulin or does not produce any insulin (Chapter 18). Insulin is the substance the body needs to convert glucose, or natural sugar, into energy. Without insulin to process glucose, these sugars collect in the blood. Some sugar appears in the urine.

Diabetics may also have ketones in the urine. Ketones are chemical substances produced when the body burns fat for energy or fuel. Ketones are produced when there is not enough insulin to help the body use sugar for energy. Without enough insulin, glucose builds up in the blood. Since the body cannot use glucose for energy, it breaks down fat instead. When this occurs, ketones form in the blood and spill into the urine.

In addition to strip testing, a double-voided (also called *fresh-fractional*) urine specimen may be used to test for glucose. A double-voided specimen is a urine specimen that is collected after first emptying the bladder and then waiting until another specimen can be collected. This may be ordered because testing urine that has been in the bladder for some time may not accurately reflect the amount of glucose present. With a double-voided specimen, after the person has voided, he is encouraged to drink fluids. Then approximately 30 minutes later, a second (double-voided) specimen is collected and tested.

Testing for blood: In normal urine, blood should not be present. Illness and disease can cause blood to appear in urine. Some blood is hidden, or occult. This blood can be detected by testing the urine.

Specific gravity: A specific gravity (also called *urine density*) test is performed to measure the concentration of particles in the urine. It may be ordered to check kidney function. The test evaluates the body's water balance and urine concentration by showing how the urine compares to water. Normal values range from 1.002 to 1.028. The test usually requires a clean-catch urine specimen.

Testing urine with reagent strips

Equipment: urine specimen as ordered, reagent strip, gloves

1. Wash your hands.
2. Put on gloves.
3. Take a strip from the bottle and recap bottle. Close it tightly.
4. Dip the strip into the specimen.
5. Follow manufacturer's instructions for when to remove strip. Remove strip at correct time.
6. Follow manufacturer's instructions for how long to wait after removing strip. After proper time has passed, compare strip with color chart on bottle. Do not touch bottle with strip.
7. Read results.
8. Discard used items. Discard specimen in the toilet. Flush toilet.
9. Remove and discard gloves.
10. Wash your hands.
11. Document procedure using facility guidelines.

7. Explain guidelines for assisting with bladder retraining

Injury, illness, or inactivity may cause a loss of normal bladder function. Residents may need help in re-establishing a regular routine and normal function. Problems with elimination can be embarrassing or difficult to discuss. Nursing assistants should be sensitive to this and always remain professional when handling incontinence or working to re-establish routines. It is hard enough for residents to handle incontinence without having to worry about caregivers' reactions.

Guidelines: Bladder Retraining

- G Follow Standard Precautions. Wear gloves when handling body wastes.
- G Explain the bladder training schedule to the resident. Follow the schedule carefully.
- G Keep a record of the resident's bladder habits. When you see a pattern of elimination, you can predict when the resident will need a bedpan or a trip to the bathroom.
- G Offer a bedpan or a trip to the bathroom before beginning long procedures (Fig. 16-22).

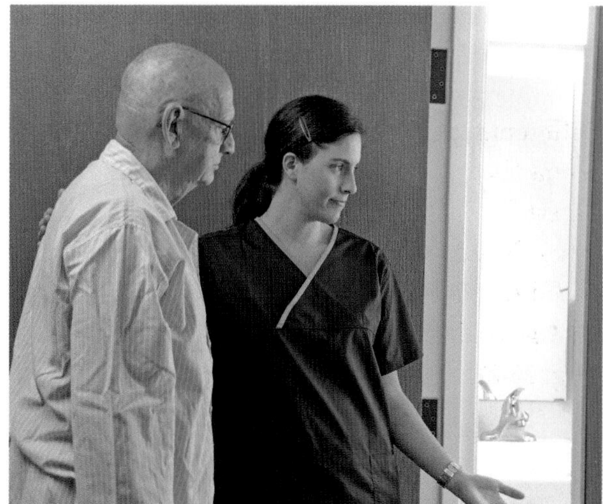

Fig. 16-22. *Offer regular trips to the bathroom.*

- G Encourage the resident to drink plenty of fluids. Do this even if urinary incontinence is a problem. About 30 minutes after fluids are taken, offer a trip to the bathroom or a bedpan or urinal.
- G Answer call lights promptly. Residents cannot wait long when the urge to go to the bathroom occurs. Leave call lights within reach (Fig. 16-23).

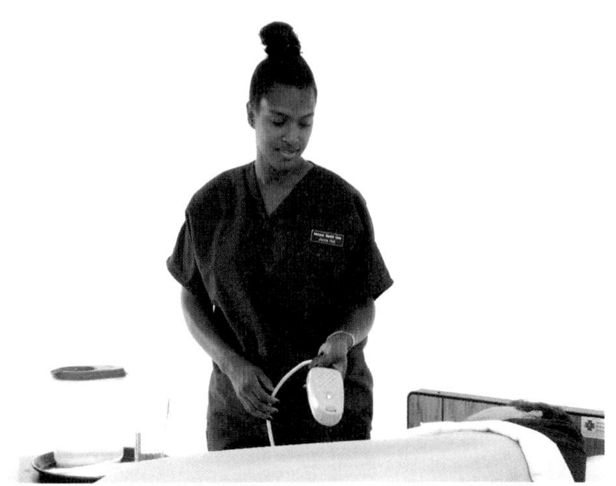

Fig. 16-23. Leave call lights within reach, and answer call lights promptly.

- Provide privacy for elimination—both in the bed and in the bathroom.
- If a resident has trouble urinating, try running water in the sink. Have him lean forward slightly to put pressure on the bladder.
- Do not rush the resident during urination.
- Help residents with careful perineal care. This helps prevents skin breakdown and promotes proper hygiene. Carefully observe for skin changes.
- Discard wastes according to your facility's policies.
- Discard clothing protectors and incontinence briefs properly. Double-bag these items if ordered. This stops odors from collecting.
- Some facilities use washable bed pads or briefs. Follow Standard Precautions when rinsing before placing these items in the laundry.
- Keep an accurate record of urination. This includes any episodes of incontinence (Fig. 16-24).
- Offer positive words for successes or even attempts to control the bladder. However, do not talk to residents as if they were children. Keep your voice low and do not draw attention to any aspect of retraining.

BOWEL & BLADDER RETRAINING PROGRAM

DATE																					
DATE STARTED	INCONTINENT	VOIDED	BM	INCONTINENT	VOIDED	BM	INCONTINENT	VOIDED	BM	INCONTINENT	VOIDED	BM	INCONTINENT	VOIDED	BM	INCONTINENT	VOIDED	BM	INCONTINENT	VOIDED	BM
7 am																					
8 am																					
9 am																					
10 am																					
11 am																					
12 noon																					
1 pm																					
2 pm																					
3 pm																					
4 pm																					
5 pm																					
6 pm																					
7 pm																					
8 pm																					
9 pm																					
10 pm																					
11 pm																					
12 midnight																					
1 am																					
2 am																					
3 am																					
4 am																					
5 am																					
6 am																					
SIGNATURE 7-3																					
3-11																					
11-7																					

S - SUPPOSITORY INSERTED
BM - BOWEL MOVEMENT

LICENSED NURSES INSTRUCTIONS:

NAME - LAST	FIRST	MIDDLE	ROOM NO.	ATTENDING PHYSICIAN	HOSP. NO.

Form 609 BOWEL & BLADDER RETRAINING PROGRAM

Fig. 16-24. A sample bowel/bladder retraining record. (REPRINTED WITH PERMISSION OF BRIGGS CORPORATION, DES MOINES, IOWA, 800-247-2343, BRIGGSCORP.COM)

- Never show frustration or anger toward residents who are incontinent. The problem is out of their control. Your negative reactions will only make things worse. Be professional and positive.
- When the resident is incontinent or cannot urinate when asked, be positive. Never make the resident feel like a failure. Praise and encouragement are essential for a successful program. Some residents will always be incontinent. Be patient. Offer these residents extra care and attention. Skin breakdown may lead to pressure ulcers without proper care. Always report changes in skin.

Chapter Review

1. What is the normal color of urine? Light or pale yellow, clear & not cloudy.
2. List five things to observe and report to the nurse about urine.
   1) Cloudy urine
   2) Dark or rust-colored urine,
   3) Strong, offensive or fruity smelling.
   4) Pain, burning or pressure when urinating
   5) Blood, pus, mucus or discharge in urine

3. What is the best position for women to be in to have normal urination? What is the best position for men?

4. When performing perineal care, in what direction should the nursing assistant wipe the resident?

5. How should a standard bedpan be positioned? How should a fracture pan be positioned?

6. List and define types of incontinence.

7. Is urinary incontinence a normal part of aging?

8. Why should a nursing assistant never refer to an incontinence brief as a diaper?

9. What are four ways that nursing assistants can help prevent urinary tract infections?

10. Why should the catheter drainage bag always be kept lower than the hips or the bladder?

11. Why should catheter tubing be kept as straight as possible?

12. List five signs and symptoms to report to the nurse about catheters.

13. What is a clean-catch urine specimen?

14. How can nursing assistants help reduce discomfort and embarrassment when assisting with specimen collection?

15. List four things reagent strips can test for in urine.

16. Why do residents who are incontinent need careful perineal care?

17. About how long after fluids are taken should the NA offer to take a resident to the bathroom?

18. Out of the list of guidelines for bladder retraining, list two that help promote dignity.

17 Bowel Elimination

1. List qualities of stool and identify signs and symptoms about stool to report

Defecation, or bowel elimination, is the act of passing feces from the large intestine out of the body through the anus. Feces, also called stool or bowel movements, are semi-solid material made up of water, solid waste material, bacteria, and mucus. The number of bowel movements a person has varies with age and with the amount and type of foods consumed.

Stool is normally brown, soft, and formed in a tubular shape from its passage through the colon. However, food, medications, and supplements, as well as illness, can cause a change in the normal color of stool. For example, iron supplements can cause stool to appear black. Red food coloring, beets, and tomato juice can make stool red.

Observing and Reporting: Stool

Report any of these to the nurse:

- O/R Whitish, black, red, or hard stools
- O/R Liquid stools (diarrhea)
- O/R Constipation (the inability to have a bowel movement or the frequent, difficult, and often painful elimination of a hard, dry stool)
- O/R Flatulence/gas
- O/R Pain when having a bowel movement
- O/R Blood, pus, mucus, or discharge in stool
- O/R Fecal incontinence (inability to control the bowels, leading to involuntary passage of stool)

2. List factors affecting bowel elimination

There are many factors that can affect normal bowel elimination, including the following:

Normal changes of aging: As a person ages, peristalsis slows. **Peristalsis** are the involuntary contractions that move food through the gastrointestinal system. Digestion takes longer and is less efficient. Proteins, vitamins, and minerals are not absorbed as well. Decreased saliva production affects the ability to chew and swallow, as does tooth loss. Medication use and a dulled sense of taste may result in poor appetite.

To help promote normal bowel elimination, nursing assistants should encourage fluids and nutritious, appealing meals and should help make mealtimes enjoyable. Dentures should fit properly and be cleaned regularly. Oral care should be given regularly as well. Residents who have trouble chewing and swallowing are at risk of choking. NAs can assist by providing plenty of fluids with meals and cutting food into smaller pieces if ordered. NAs should follow a toileting schedule for residents if there is one.

Residents who have fecal incontinence or diarrhea must be kept clean and dry. When assisting with perineal care, NAs should wipe from front to back to prevent infection. They should help residents wash their hands after having bowel movements.

Psychological factors: Stress, anger, fear, and depression all affect gastrointestinal function. Stress, anger, and fear can increase peristalsis and elimination, while depression may decrease it. A lack of privacy can greatly affect elimination, too.

To promote normal bowel elimination, it is very important for an NA to provide plenty of privacy. She should close the bathroom door if a resident is in the bathroom. If the resident needs to use a bedpan, the NA should pull the privacy curtain and close the door. Residents should not be rushed or interrupted when they are in the bathroom. It is important for an NA to report signs of depression and anxiety (Chapter 20), as well as any changes in frequency of elimination.

Food and fluids: What a person consumes greatly affects bowel elimination. Fiber intake improves bowel elimination. Foods high in fiber include fruits, whole grains, and raw vegetables (Fig. 17-1). Some high-fiber foods cause flatulence, or gas, which can aid elimination, but can also cause discomfort. Foods that may cause gas include the following:

- Beans
- Fruits (e.g., pears, apples, peaches)
- Whole grains
- Vegetables (e.g., broccoli, cabbage, onions, asparagus)
- Dairy products
- Carbonated drinks

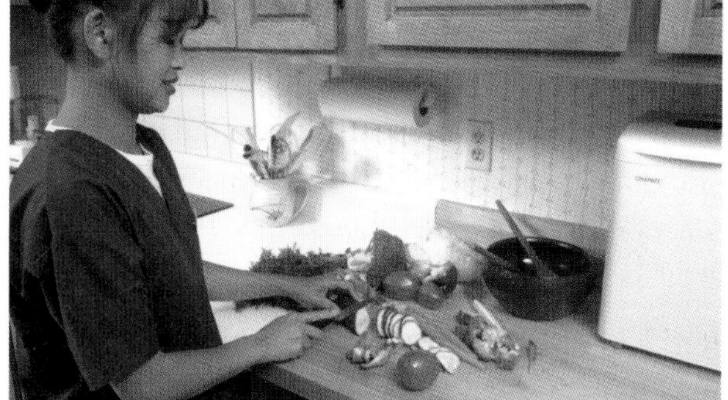

Fig. 17-1. *Raw fruits and vegetables are high in fiber, which helps with bowel elimination.*

Some foods can cause constipation, such as foods high in animal fats (dairy products, meats, and eggs) or foods high in refined sugar but low in fiber. Inadequate fluid intake not only contributes to dehydration, but also can cause constipation.

To promote normal bowel elimination, residents should eat a diet that contains fiber and drink plenty of fluids to help prevent constipation. NAs should offer drinks to residents every time they see them, as long as they are not on fluid restrictions. A healthy person needs at least 64 ounces of fluid each day.

Physical activity: Regular physical activity helps bowel elimination (Fig. 17-2). It strengthens abdominal and pelvic muscles, which helps peristalsis. Immobility and a lack of exercise weakens these muscles and may slow elimination.

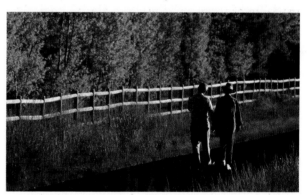

Fig. 17-2. *Regular exercise and activity is important for promoting normal bowel elimination.*

To promote normal bowel elimination, the NA should encourage regular activity and assist as needed. She can try to make it fun for the resident. A walk can be something that the resident enjoys and looks forward to.

Personal habits: The time of day that bowel movements occur varies from person to person. For example, one person may have a bowel movement early in the day, while another has one in the early afternoon. Another person may have a few bowel movements throughout the day. This depends on the person, his habits, and the amount and type of food and drink consumed. Elimination usually occurs after meals.

The position of the body affects elimination. A person who is supine (flat on his back) will have the most trouble with bowel elimination. It is almost impossible to contract muscles in this position.

To promote normal bowel elimination, residents should have an opportunity to have a bowel movement at the time of day that is normal for them. The best position for elimination is squatting and leaning forward. If the person cannot get out of bed, the NA can raise the head of the bed for elimination. That way the resident does not have to work against gravity.

Medications: Medications affect bowel elimination. Laxatives are used to cause bowel movements and may cause excessive elimination. Other medications, such as pain relievers, can slow elimination. Antibiotics may cause diarrhea. To promote normal bowel elimination, the NA can offer a trip to the bathroom or a bedpan often. Any changes in appearance of stool or frequency of bowel elimination should be reported.

Disorders and illnesses affect bowel elimination, and there is more information about them in the next Learning Objective.

3. Describe common diseases and disorders of the gastrointestinal system

Constipation

Constipation is the inability to eliminate stool (have a bowel movement), or the infrequent, difficult, and often painful elimination of a hard, dry stool. Constipation occurs when the feces move too slowly through the intestine. This can result from decreased fluid intake, poor diet, inactivity, medications, aging, certain diseases, or ignoring the urge to eliminate. Signs of constipation include abdominal swelling, gas, irritability, and a record of no recent bowel movement.

Treatment often includes increasing the amount of fiber eaten and fluids consumed, increasing the activity level, and possibly medication. Accurate documentation of bowel movements is important. An enema or suppository may be ordered to help with constipation. An **enema** is a specific amount of water, with or without an additive, that is introduced into the colon to stimulate the elimination of stool. A **suppository** is a medication given rectally to cause a bowel movement.

Fecal Impaction

A **fecal impaction** is a hard stool that is stuck in the rectum and cannot be expelled. It results from unrelieved constipation. Symptoms include no stool for several days, oozing of liquid stool, cramping, abdominal swelling, and rectal pain. When an impaction occurs, a nurse or doctor will insert one or two gloved fingers into the rectum and break the mass into fragments so that it can be passed. Prevention of fecal impactions often includes the same measures as those used for preventing constipation, i.e. high-fiber diet, plenty of fluids, an increase in activity level, and possibly medication.

Hemorrhoids

Hemorrhoids are enlarged veins in the rectum that may also be visible outside the anus. Hemorrhoids can develop from an increase in pressure in the lower rectum due to straining during bowel movements. Chronic constipation, obesity, pregnancy, and sitting for long periods of time on the toilet are other causes. Signs and symptoms include rectal itching, burning, pain, and bleeding. Treatment may include medications, compresses, and sitz baths. Surgery may be necessary. When cleaning the anal area, NAs should be very careful to avoid causing pain and bleeding from hemorrhoids.

Diarrhea

Diarrhea is the frequent elimination of liquid or semi-liquid feces. Abdominal cramps, urgency, nausea, and vomiting can accompany diarrhea, depending on the cause. Bacterial and viral infections, microorganisms in food and water, irritating foods, and medications can cause diarrhea. Treatment of diarrhea usually involves medication, an increase in certain fluids, and a change of diet.

Fecal Incontinence

Fecal incontinence is the inability to control the bowels, leading to an involuntary passage of stool. Common causes are constipation, muscle and nerve damage, loss of storage capacity in the rectum, and diarrhea. Treatment includes a change in diet, medication, bowel training, or surgery.

Flatulence

Flatulence, also called flatus or gas, is air in the intestine that is passed through the rectum, which can result in cramping or abdominal pain. Flatulence may have any of the following causes:

- Swallowing air while eating
- Eating high-fiber foods
- Eating foods that a person cannot tolerate, for example, when a person who has lactose intolerance eats dairy products (**Lactose intolerance** is the inability to digest lactose, a type of sugar found in milk and other dairy products. It is caused by a deficiency of lactase enzyme.)
- Antibiotics
- **Colitis**, or irritable bowel syndrome (IBS), which is a chronic form of stomach upset that gets worse from stress
- **Malabsorption**, which means that the body cannot absorb or digest a particular nutrient properly; it is often accompanied by diarrhea

Excessive flatulence, depending on the cause, is often treated with change of diet, medication, and reducing the amount of air swallowed.

Gastroesophageal Reflux Disease

Gastroesophageal reflux disease, commonly referred to as **GERD**, is a chronic condition in which the liquid contents of the stomach back up into the esophagus. The liquid can inflame and damage the lining of the esophagus. It can cause bleeding or ulcers. In addition, scars from tissue damage can narrow the esophagus and make swallowing difficult.

Heartburn is the most common symptom of GERD. **Heartburn** is the result of a weakening of the sphincter muscle that joins the esophagus and the stomach. When healthy, this muscle prevents the leaking of stomach acid and other contents back into the esophagus. Stomach acid causes a burning sensation, commonly called heartburn, in the esophagus. If heartburn occurs frequently and remains untreated, it can cause scarring or **ulceration**.

Heartburn and GERD must be reported to the nurse. These conditions are usually treated with medications. Serving the evening meal three to four hours before bedtime may help. The resident should not lie down until at least two to three hours after eating. Providing residents with extra pillows so the body is more upright during sleep can help. Serving the largest meal of the day at lunchtime, serving several meals of small portions throughout the day, and reducing fast foods, fatty foods, and spicy foods may also help. Stopping smoking, not drinking alcohol, and wearing loose-fitting clothing are often helpful as well.

Peptic Ulcers

Peptic ulcers are raw sores in the stomach or the small intestine. A dull or gnawing pain occurs one to three hours after eating, accompanied by belching or vomiting. Food, antacids, and medications temporarily relieve the pain. Ulcers are caused by excessive acid production. Residents with peptic ulcers should avoid smoking and drinking too much alcohol and caffeine, which increase the production of gastric acid. A bland diet may be ordered (Chapter 15). Peptic ulcers may cause bleeding. Bowel movements may appear black and tarry because of the bleeding.

Ulcerative Colitis and Colitis

Ulcerative colitis is a chronic inflammatory disease of the large intestine. Symptoms include cramping, diarrhea, pain occurring to one side of the lower abdomen, rectal bleeding, and loss of appetite. Ulcerative colitis is a serious illness that can cause intestinal bleeding and death if left untreated.

Medications can relieve symptoms, but they cannot cure ulcerative colitis. Surgical treatment may include a colostomy, which is the diversion of waste to an artificial opening (**stoma**) through the abdomen. Stool is diverted through the stoma instead of the anus. There is more information on colostomy care later in the chapter.

Colitis, or irritable bowel syndrome (IBS), has symptoms similar to but milder than those of ulcerative colitis. Diet and/or medication can usually control colitis.

Colorectal Cancer

Colorectal cancer, also known as colon cancer, is cancer of the gastrointestinal tract. Signs and symptoms include changes in normal bowel patterns, cramps, abdominal pain, and rectal bleeding. Colorectal cancer must be treated with surgery. Chapter 18 provides more information on cancer.

4. Discuss how enemas are given

Putting fluid into the rectum in order to eliminate stool or feces is called an enema. Enemas may be given prior to surgery or a medical test, or when a person cannot eliminate stool on his own. Nursing assistants may be trained to give enemas, depending upon the state and facility in which they work. If NAs are allowed to give enemas, they must make sure to follow policies and procedures. Any questions an NA may have should be discussed with the nurse before giving an enema.

Doctors will write an enema order. There are four different types of enemas:

- Tap water enema (TWE): 500-1000 mL of water from a faucet
- Soapsuds or soap solution enema (SSE): 500-1000 mL water with 5 mL of mild castile soap added
- Saline enema: 500-1000 mL water with two teaspoons of salt added
- Commercially-prepared enema: 120 mL solution; may have oil or other additives

Tap water, soapsuds, and saline enemas are all considered cleansing enemas. They all require more fluid than commercially-prepared enemas do. Equipment used for giving cleansing enemas includes an IV pole, the enema solution, tubing, and a clamp.

Guidelines: Enemas

G Keep the bedpan nearby or make sure that the bathroom is vacant before assisting with an enema.

G The resident will be placed in Sims' (left side-lying) position (Fig. 17-3). If the person is positioned on the left side, the water does not have to flow against gravity.

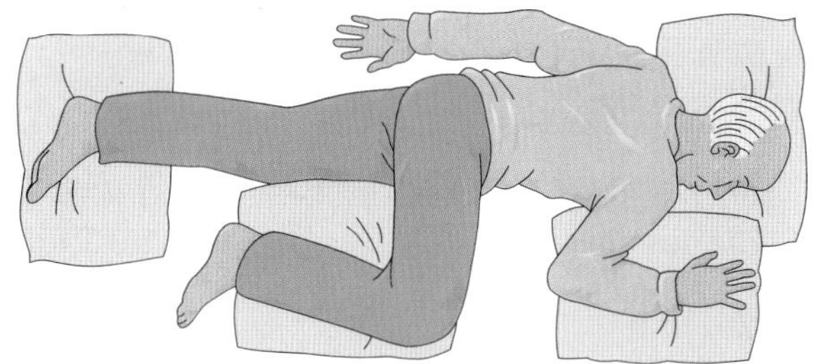

Fig. 17-3. *The Sims' position (left side-lying position) is the proper position for an enema.*

- **G** The enema solution should be warm, not hot or cold.
- **G** The enema bag should not be raised to more than the height listed in the care plan.
- **G** The tip of the tubing should be lubricated with lubricating jelly.
- **G** Unclamp the tube. Allow a small amount of solution to run through the tubing, then re-clamp the tube. This gets rid of the air before it is inserted (the air could cause cramping).
- **G** The solution should flow in slowly; the resident will be less likely to have cramps.
- **G** Hold the enema tubing in place while giving the enema. Stop immediately if the resident has pain or if you feel resistance. Report to the nurse if this happens.
- **G** The resident should take slow deep breaths when taking an enema to help hold the solution longer.
- **G** Report any of the following to the nurse:
  - Resident could not tolerate enema because of cramping.
  - The enema had no results.
  - The amount of stool was very small.
  - Stool was hard, streaked with red, very dark, or black.

Giving a cleansing enema

Equipment: bath blanket, IV pole, enema solution, tubing and clamp, protective pad, bedpan, lubricating jelly, bath thermometer, tape measure, toilet paper, disposable wipes, robe, non-skid footwear, towel, supplies for perineal care, paper towel, 2 pairs of gloves

1. Identify yourself by name. Identify the resident by name.
2. Wash your hands.
3. Explain procedure to the resident. Speak clearly, slowly, and directly. Maintain face-to-face contact whenever possible.
4. Provide for resident's privacy with curtain, screen, or door.
5. Adjust bed to a safe level, usually waist high. Lock bed wheels.
6. Help resident into left side-lying Sims' position. Cover with a bath blanket.
7. Place the IV pole beside the bed.
8. Clamp the enema tube. Prepare the enema solution. Fill bag with 500-1000 mL of warm water (105°F), and mix the solution. Check water temperature with bath thermometer.
9. Unclamp the tube. Let a small amount of solution run through the tubing. Re-clamp the tube.
10. Hang the bag on IV pole. Using the tape measure, make sure the bottom of the enema bag is not more than 12 inches above the resident's anus (Fig. 17-4).

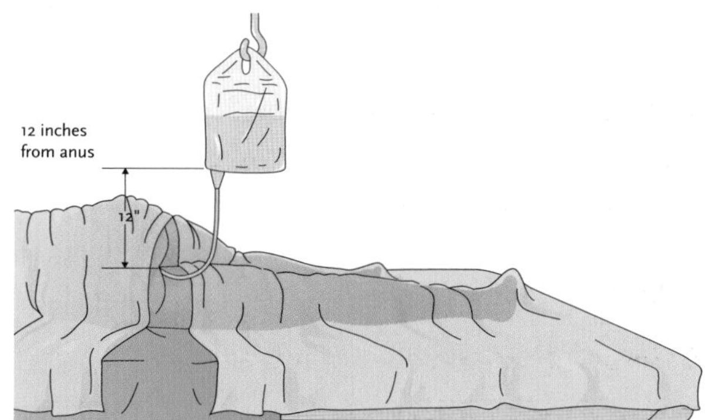

Fig. 17-4. *Bottom of the bag should not be more than 12 inches above the anus.*

11. Put on gloves.
12. Place protective pad under resident. Ask resident to remove undergarments or help him do so. Place bedpan close to resident's body.
13. Lubricate tip of tubing with lubricating jelly.
14. Ask the resident to breathe deeply. This relieves cramps during procedure.
15. Place one hand on the upper buttock. Lift to expose the anus. Ask the resident to take a deep breath and exhale (Fig. 17-5). Using the

other hand, gently insert the tip of the tubing two to four inches into the rectum. Stop immediately if you feel resistance or if the resident complains of pain. If this happens, clamp the tubing. Tell the nurse immediately.

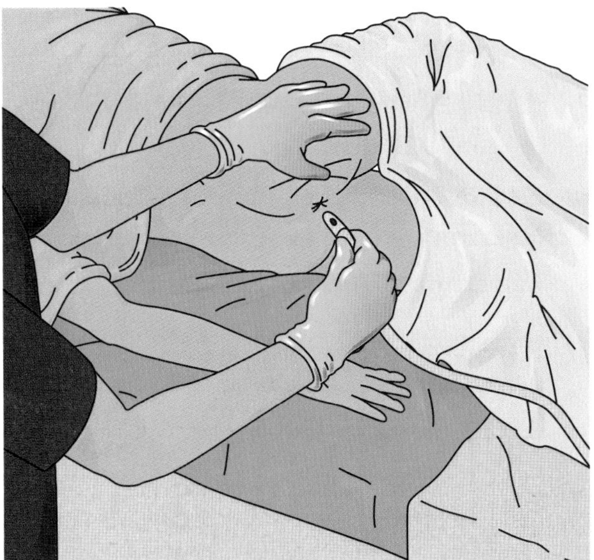

Fig. 17-5. *Lift the upper buttock to expose the anus. Ask the resident to take a deep breath before inserting the tubing.*

16. Unclamp the tubing. Allow the solution to flow slowly into the rectum. Ask resident to take slow, deep breaths. If resident complains of cramping, clamp the tubing and stop for a couple of minutes. Encourage him to take as much of the solution as possible.
17. Clamp the tubing before the bag is empty when the solution is almost gone. Gently remove the tip from the rectum. Place the tip into the enema bag. Do not contaminate yourself, the resident, or the bed linens.
18. Ask the resident to hold the solution inside as long as possible.
19. Help resident to use bedpan, commode, or get to the bathroom. If the resident uses a commode or toilet, put on robe and non-skid footwear. Lower the bed to its lowest position before the resident gets up.
20. Remove and discard gloves. Wash your hands.
21. Place toilet paper and disposable wipes within resident's reach. Ask the resident to clean his hands with the hand wipe when finished if he is able. If the resident is using the toilet, ask him not to flush it when finished.
22. Place the call light within resident's reach. Ask resident to signal when done. Leave the room and close the door.
23. When called by the resident, return and put on clean gloves.
24. Lower the head of the bed. Make sure resident is still covered.
25. Remove bedpan carefully and cover bedpan.
26. Provide perineal care if help is needed. Wipe female residents from front to back. Dry the perineal area with a towel. Help the resident put on undergarment. Cover the resident and remove the bath blanket.
27. Place the towel and bath blanket in a hamper or bag, and discard disposable supplies.
28. Take bedpan to the bathroom. Call the nurse to observe the enema results. Empty the contents of bedpan carefully into the toilet.
29. Turn the faucet on with a paper towel. Rinse the bedpan with cold water and empty it into the toilet. Flush the toilet. Place bedpan in proper area for cleaning or clean it according to facility policy.
30. Remove and discard gloves.
31. Wash your hands.
32. Make resident comfortable.
33. Return bed to lowest position. Remove privacy measures.
34. Place call light within resident's reach.
35. Report any changes in resident to the nurse.
36. Document procedure using facility guidelines.

Residents' Rights

Giving Enemas

Protecting a resident's rights when giving an enema includes providing plenty of privacy during this procedure. The NA should keep the resident covered with a bath blanket or sheet, only exposing the anal area. She should pull the privacy curtain around the bed and close the door. The NA should answer any questions that the resident has about the procedure. However, if any questions are not within the NA's scope of practice to answer, she should refer them to the nurse before beginning.

A commercially-prepared enema usually has 120 mL solution and may have additives (Fig. 17-6). An oil retention enema has a type of oil in it to soften the stool to allow it to pass more easily. It is often used when a person has been constipated for a long time, resulting in a stool that is very hard, or when a person has a fecal impaction. Commercially-prepared enemas do not require an IV pole, tubing, or clamp, because they are prepackaged and pre-mixed.

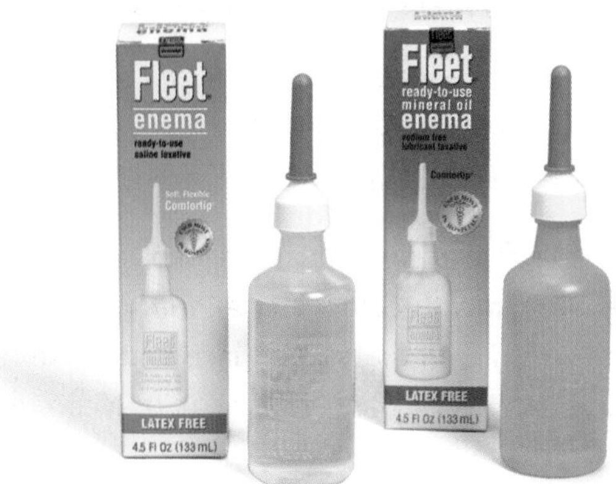

***Fig. 17-6.** Commercially-prepared enemas may come with additives, such as saline and mineral oil.* (REPRINTED WITH PERMISSION OF BRIGGS CORPORATION, 800-247-2343, WWW.BRIGGSCORP.COM)

Giving a commercial enema

Equipment: bath blanket, standard or oil retention commercial enema kit, protective pad, bedpan, lubricating jelly, toilet paper, disposable wipes, robe, non-skid footwear, towel, supplies for perineal care, 2 pairs of gloves

1. Identify yourself by name. Identify the resident by name.
2. Wash your hands.
3. Explain procedure to the resident. Speak clearly, slowly, and directly. Maintain face-to-face contact whenever possible.
4. Provide for resident's privacy with curtain, screen, or door.
5. Adjust bed to a safe level, usually waist high. Lock bed wheels.
6. Help resident into left-sided Sims' position. Cover with a bath blanket.
7. Put on gloves.
8. Place protective pad under resident. Ask resident to remove undergarments or help him do so. Place bedpan close to resident's body.
9. Uncover resident enough to expose anus only.
10. Lubricate tip of bottle with lubricating jelly.
11. Ask resident to breathe deeply to relieve cramps during procedure.
12. Place one hand on the upper buttock. Lift to expose the anus. Ask the resident to take a deep breath and exhale. Using the other hand, gently insert the tip of the tubing about one and a half inches into the rectum. Stop if you feel resistance or if the resident complains of pain. Tell the nurse immediately.
13. Slowly squeeze and roll the enema container so that the solution runs inside the resident. Stop when the container is almost empty.
14. Gently remove the tip from the rectum, and place the bottle inside the box upside down (Fig. 17-7).
15. Ask the resident to hold the solution inside as long as possible.
16. Help resident use bedpan or commode or get to the bathroom. If the resident uses a commode or toilet, put on robe and non-skid footwear. Lower the bed to its lowest position before the resident gets up.

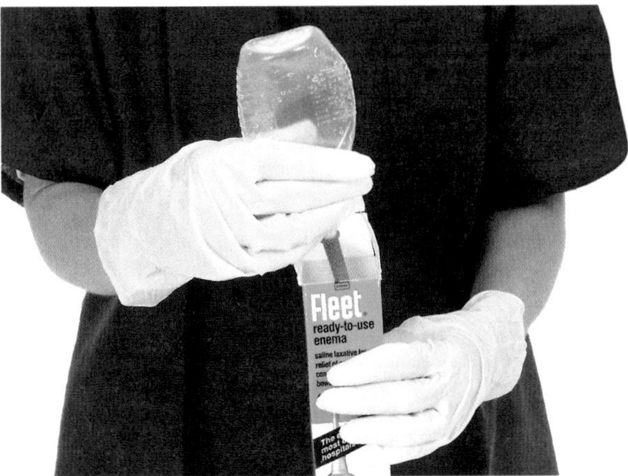

Fig. 17-7. Place enema bottle upside down in the box.

17. Remove and discard gloves. Wash your hands.
18. Place toilet paper and disposable wipes within resident's reach. Ask the resident to clean his hands with the hand wipe when finished if he is able. If the resident is using the toilet, ask him not to flush it when finished.
19. Place the call light within resident's reach. Ask resident to signal when done. Leave the room and close the door.
20. When called by the resident, return and put on clean gloves.
21. Lower the head of the bed. Make sure resident is still covered.
22. Remove bedpan carefully and cover bedpan.
23. Provide perineal care if help is needed. Wipe female residents from front to back. Dry the perineal area with a towel. Help the resident put on undergarment. Cover the resident and remove the bath blanket.
24. Place the towel and bath blanket in a hamper or bag, and discard disposable supplies.
25. Take bedpan to the bathroom. Call the nurse to observe the enema results. Empty the contents of bedpan carefully into the toilet.
26. Turn the faucet on with a paper towel. Rinse the bedpan with cold water and empty it into the toilet. Flush the toilet. Place bedpan in proper area for cleaning or clean it according to facility policy.
27. Remove and discard gloves.
28. Wash your hands.
29. Make resident comfortable.
30. Return bed to lowest position. Remove privacy measures.
31. Place call light within resident's reach.
32. Report any changes in resident to the nurse.
33. Document procedure using facility guidelines.

5. Demonstrate how to collect a stool specimen

Stool (feces) specimens are collected so that the stool can be tested for blood, pathogens, and other things, such as worms or amoebas. Worms and amebas can be detected with an ova and parasites test. If the specimen is to be examined for ova and parasites, it must be taken to the lab immediately. This examination must be made while the stool is still warm.

If the resident uses a bedpan or portable commode for elimination, the nursing assistant will take the stool specimen from there. If the resident uses the toilet, a hat (collection container) should be used for the collection.

The NA should ask the resident to let her know when he can have a bowel movement, and she should be ready to collect the specimen.

Collecting a stool specimen

Equipment: specimen container with completed label (labeled with resident's name, date of birth, room number, date, and time) and lid, specimen bag, 2 pairs of gloves, 2 tongue blades, bedpan (if resident cannot use portable commode or toilet), hat for toilet (if resident uses portable commode or toilet), plastic bag, toilet paper, disposable wipes, paper towels, supplies for perineal care, lab slip

1. Identify yourself by name. Identify the resident by name.

2. Wash your hands.
3. Explain procedure to the resident. Speak clearly, slowly, and directly. Maintain face-to-face contact whenever possible.
4. Provide for resident's privacy with curtain, screen, or door.
5. Put on gloves.
6. Fit hat to toilet or commode, or provide resident with bedpan.
7. When the resident is ready to move bowels, ask him not to urinate at the same time and not to put toilet paper in with the sample. Provide a plastic bag to discard toilet paper separately.
8. Place toilet paper and disposable wipes within resident's reach. Ask resident to clean his hands with a wipe when finished if he is able.
9. Remove and discard gloves. Wash your hands.
10. Place the call light within resident's reach. Ask resident to signal when done. Leave the room and close the door.
11. When called by the resident, return and put on clean gloves. Provide perineal care if help is needed.
12. Using the two tongue blades, take about two tablespoons of stool and put it in the container. Without touching the inside of the container, cover it tightly. Apply label and place container in a clean specimen bag.
13. Wrap the tongue blades in toilet paper and put them in plastic bag with used toilet paper. Discard bag in proper container.
14. Empty the bedpan or container into the toilet. Turn the faucet on with a paper towel. Rinse the bedpan with cold water and empty it into the toilet. Flush the toilet. Place equipment in proper area for cleaning or clean it according to facility policy.
15. Remove and discard gloves.
16. Wash your hands.
17. Remove privacy measures.
18. Place call light within resident's reach.
19. Report any changes in resident to the nurse.
20. Take specimen and lab slip to proper area. Document procedure using facility guidelines. Note amount and characteristics of stool.

6. Explain occult blood testing

Occult blood testing is performed to detect blood in stool. **Occult** means something that is hidden or difficult to see or observe. Hidden, or occult, blood in stool may be an indication of colorectal cancer or of other illnesses.

There are different types of tests to detect occult blood in stool. Stool specimens may be sent to the laboratory for this test; however, in some facilities, nursing assistants may be asked to perform this test if they are trained and allowed to do so.

Testing a stool specimen for occult blood

Equipment: labeled stool specimen, occult blood test kit (Fig. 17-8), 2 tongue blades, plastic bag, gloves

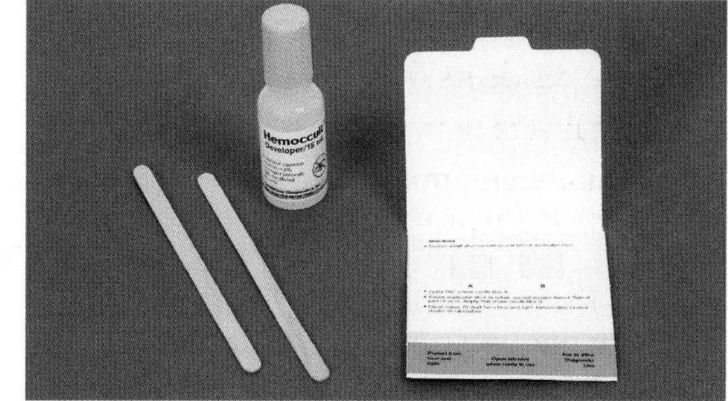

Fig. 17-8. *This is one type of occult blood test kit.*

1. Wash your hands.
2. Put on gloves.
3. Open the test card.
4. Pick up a tongue blade. Get small amount of stool from the specimen container.

5. Using a tongue blade, smear a small amount of stool onto Box A of test card (Fig. 17-9).

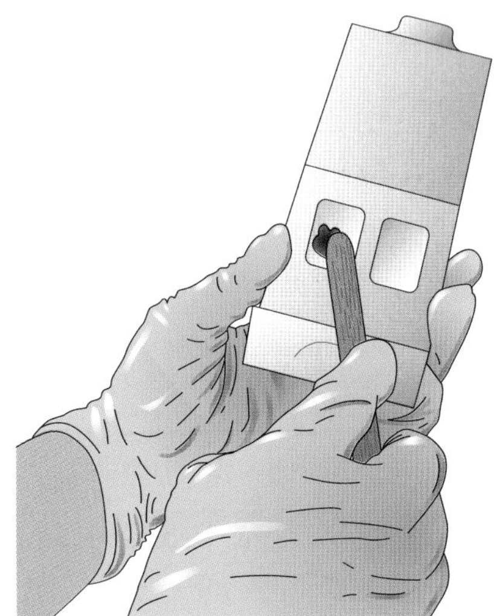

***Fig. 17-9.** Smear a small amount of stool onto Box A.*

6. Flip tongue blade (or use a new tongue blade). Get some stool from another part of specimen. Smear small amount of stool onto Box B of test card.
7. Close the test card. Turn over to other side.
8. Open the flap.
9. Open the developer. Apply developer to each box. Follow manufacturer's instructions.
10. Wait the amount of time listed in instructions, usually between 10 and 60 seconds.
11. Watch the squares for any color changes. Record color changes. Follow instructions.
12. Place tongue blade and test packet in plastic bag, and dispose of plastic bag properly.
13. Remove and discard gloves.
14. Wash your hands.
15. Document procedure using facility guidelines.

7. Define the term *ostomy* and list care guidelines

An **ostomy** is the surgical creation of an opening from an area inside the body to the outside. The terms *colostomy* and *ileostomy* refer to the surgical removal of a portion of the intestines. In a resident with one of these ostomies, the end of the intestine is brought out of the body through an artificial opening in the abdomen. This opening is called a stoma. Stool, or feces, is eliminated through the ostomy rather than through the anus. (When a ureter is opened to the abdomen for urine to be eliminated, it is called a **ureterostomy**.) An ostomy may be necessary due to bowel disease, cancer, or trauma. It may be temporary or permanent.

The terms *colostomy* and *ileostomy* indicate what section of the intestine was removed and the type of stool that will be eliminated. A **colostomy** is a surgically-created opening into the large intestine to allow stool to be expelled. With a colostomy, stool will generally be semi-solid. An **ileostomy** is a surgically-created opening into the end of the small intestine to allow stool to be expelled. Stool will be liquid and may be irritating to the resident's skin.

Residents who have had an ostomy wear a disposable drainage bag, or appliance, that fits over the stoma to collect the feces (Fig. 17-10). The bag is attached to the skin by adhesive. A belt may also be used to secure it.

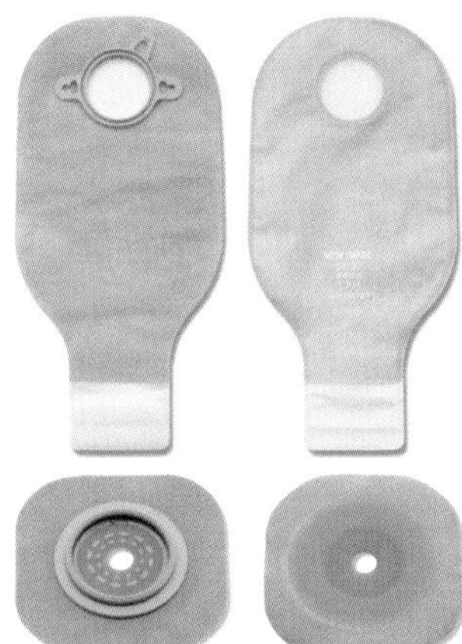

***Fig. 17-10.** This photo shows the front and back of a two-piece system. The top is an ostomy drainage bag, and the bottom is a skin barrier.* (PHOTOS COURTESY OF HOLLISTER INCORPORATED, LIBERTYVILLE, ILLINOIS)

Many people manage the ostomy appliance by themselves. Nursing assistants should receive training before providing ostomy care.

Guidelines: Ostomies

- G Make certain that the resident receives regular, careful skin care. Observe and report any changes in the skin to help prevent skin breakdown.
- G Empty and clean or replace an ostomy bag whenever stool is eliminated.
- G Always wear gloves and wash hands carefully when providing ostomy care. Follow Standard Precautions.
- G Teach proper handwashing techniques to residents with ostomies.
- G Skin barriers protect the skin around the stoma from irritation from the waste products and/or the adhesive material that is used to secure the bag to the body. Barriers may come in the form of a powder, gel, cream, ring, paste, wafer, or square.
- G Residents who have an ileostomy may experience food blockage. A food blockage is a large amount of undigested food, usually high-fiber food, that collects in the small intestine and blocks the passage of stool. Food blockages can occur if the resident eats large amounts of foods that are high-fiber and/or if the resident does not chew the food well. Follow the diet instructions in the care plan and the nurse's instructions for assisting with feeding.
- G Encourage fluids and proper diet. Residents with ileostomies need to drink plenty of fluids because they lose extra liquid in their stools. They may also be on high-potassium diets due to rapid elimination.
- G Many residents with ostomies feel they have lost control of a basic bodily function. They may be embarrassed or angry about the ostomy. Be sensitive and supportive when working with these residents. Always provide privacy for ostomy care.
- G Ostomy pouches are made to be odor resistant. If odors are present, they may be due to a leak or improper cleaning. Report odors to the nurse.
- G Observe how the resident is reacting to the ostomy and his general attitude. Report any emotional or physical problems with adjusting to the ostomy to the nurse.

Observing and Reporting: Ostomies

Report any of the following to the nurse:

- O/R Changes in color, amount, frequency, or odor of stool
- O/R Any skin changes at stoma site, such as sores, excessive redness, or swelling
- O/R Leaking stool
- O/R Absence of stool
- O/R Watery stool with green, stringy material
- O/R Abdominal cramps
- O/R Vomiting

Caring for an ostomy

Equipment: protective pad, bath blanket, clean ostomy drainage bag and belt, disposable wipes, basin of warm water, soap, washcloth, skin cream as ordered, 2 towels, plastic disposable bag, gloves

1. Identify yourself by name. Identify the resident by name.
2. Wash your hands.
3. Explain procedure to the resident. Speak clearly, slowly, and directly. Maintain face-to-face contact whenever possible.
4. Provide for resident's privacy with curtain, screen, or door.
5. Adjust bed to a safe level, usually waist high. Lock bed wheels.
6. Put on gloves.

7. Place protective pad under resident. Cover resident with a bath blanket. Pull down the top sheet and blankets. Expose only the ostomy site. Offer resident a towel to keep clothing dry.
8. Remove ostomy bag carefully. Place it in plastic bag. Note the color, odor, consistency, and amount of stool in the bag.
9. Wipe the area around the stoma with disposable wipes. Discard wipes in plastic bag.
10. Using a washcloth and warm, soapy water, wash the area in one direction, away from the stoma (Fig. 17-11). Rinse. Pat dry with another towel. Apply skin cream as ordered.

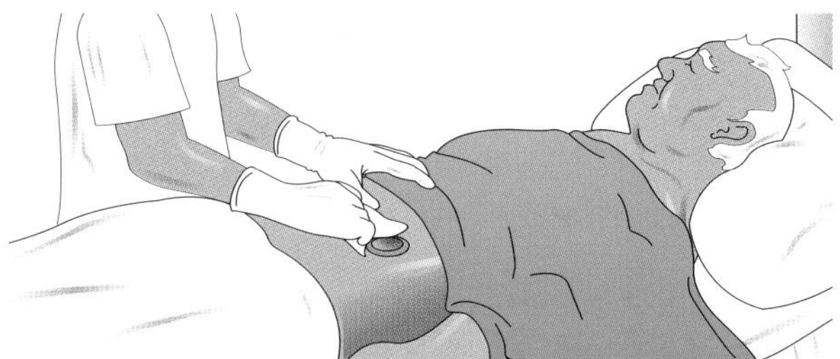

Fig. 17-11. *Wash area gently, moving away from the stoma.*

11. Place the clean ostomy drainage bag on resident. Hold in place and seal securely. Make sure the bottom of the bag is clamped.
12. Remove protective pad and discard. Place soiled linens in proper container. Discard plastic bag properly.
13. Remove and discard gloves.
14. Wash your hands.
15. Make resident comfortable.
16. Return bed to lowest position. Remove privacy measures.
17. Place call light within resident's reach.
18. Report any changes in resident to the nurse. Note any changes to the stoma and surrounding area. A normal stoma is red and moist and looks like the lining of the mouth. Call the nurse if the stoma appears very red or blue or if swelling or bleeding is present.
19. Document procedure using facility guidelines.

8. Explain guidelines for assisting with bowel retraining

Residents who have had a disruption in their bowel routines from illness, injury, or inactivity may need help to re-establish a regular routine and normal function. To assist with bowel retraining, the doctor may order suppositories, laxatives, stool softeners, or enemas. Bowel elimination issues may be difficult for residents to discuss. Nursing assistants should be sensitive to this and should remain professional when assisting residents with bowel retraining.

Residents' Rights

Bowel Retraining

Residents who have problems controlling their bowels need to be treated with dignity. Nursing assistants should think about how they might feel in the same situation. For example, if a resident has a bowel movement in her bed, she probably feels extremely embarrassed about this and the fact that an NA has to clean her and change the sheets. An NA can help the resident maintain her dignity by being kind and supportive. He should promote the resident's right to privacy by keeping his voice low and not discussing her accident in a public area.

Guidelines: Bowel Retraining

- G Follow Standard Precautions. Wear gloves when handling body wastes.
- G Explain the bowel training schedule to the resident. Follow the schedule carefully.
- G Keep a record of the resident's bowel habits. When you see a pattern of elimination, you can predict when the resident will need a bedpan or a trip to the bathroom.
- G Encourage the resident to drink plenty of fluids.

- Encourage the resident to eat foods that are high in fiber. Encourage residents to follow special diets, as ordered. Chapter 15 has more information on diet and nutrition.
- Answer call lights promptly. Leave call lights within reach.
- Provide privacy for elimination—both in the bed and in the bathroom.
- Do not rush the resident during elimination.
- Help residents with careful perineal care. This prevents skin breakdown and promotes proper hygiene. Carefully observe for skin changes.
- Discard wastes according to your facility's policies.
- Discard clothing protectors and incontinence briefs properly. Double-bag these items if ordered.
- Some facilities use washable bed pads or briefs. Follow Standard Precautions when placing these items in the laundry.
- Keep an accurate record of elimination.
- Praise successes or attempts to control bowels. However, do not talk to residents as if they were children. Keep your voice low and do not draw attention to any aspect of bowel retraining.
- Never show frustration or anger toward residents who are incontinent. Remember that the problem is out of their control. Be positive and professional.

Chapter Review

1. How does stool normally appear?
2. List five things to observe and report to the nurse about stool.
3. What is the best position for bowel elimination? What should be done if a person cannot get out of bed for defecation?
4. List three possible treatments for constipation.
5. List three signs of a fecal impaction.
6. List three causes of diarrhea.
7. What is gastroesophageal reflux disease (GERD)?
8. What are two things that people with peptic ulcers should avoid?
9. What are three symptoms of colorectal cancer?
10. In what position must the resident be placed for an enema?
11. What should the nursing assistant do if a resident feels pain or if the nursing assistant feels resistance while giving an enema?
12. What two things should not be included in a stool specimen?
13. If a stool specimen needs to be tested for ova and parasites, what should be done immediately and why?
14. What may occult blood in stool indicate?
15. What are three reasons that a resident may need a colostomy or ileostomy?
16. How often should an ostomy bag be emptied?
17. What kinds of foods may need to be eaten when a resident is going through bowel retraining?

18 Common Chronic and Acute Conditions

Diseases and conditions are either acute or chronic. An **acute illness** means that the illness has severe symptoms; this type of illness is usually short-term and is treated immediately. A **chronic illness** is long-term or long-lasting, even lasting over a lifetime. The symptoms are managed. Chronic conditions may have short periods of severity. The person may be hospitalized to stabilize the disease.

This chapter organizes diseases or conditions under the body system in which they are located. Common diseases of the urinary and gastrointestinal systems are in Chapters 16 and 17.

1. Describe common diseases and disorders of the integumentary system

Pressure ulcers, a common disorder of the integumentary system, are covered in Chapter 13. Burns are covered in Chapter 7.

Scabies

Scabies is a skin infection caused by a tiny mite called *Sarcoptes scabiei*. The mite burrows into the skin, where it lays eggs, which causes intense itching and a skin rash that may look like thin burrow tracks. These tracks typically appear in the folds of the skin.

Scabies is contagious and is spread through direct contact with an infected person. It can spread quickly in crowded places, such as long-term care facilities and child care facilities. Treatment of scabies involves medications, often in the form of prescription creams and lotions (Chapter 13 has information on applying lotions). Oral medications may be used if the person does not respond to the creams and/or lotions.

Shingles

Shingles, also called herpes zoster, is a skin rash caused by the varicella-zoster virus (VZV), which is the same virus that causes chickenpox. (Herpes zoster is not the same virus that causes the sexually-transmitted infection.) Any person who has had chickenpox is at risk for developing shingles. After having chickenpox, the virus remains in the body, where it usually does not cause problems. However, it can reappear later in life and cause shingles.

Initial signs and symptoms of shingles include pain, tingling, or itching in an area, which later develops into a rash of fluid-filled blisters that is similar to chickenpox (Fig. 18-1). The rash usually goes away within two to four weeks.

Shingles cannot be transmitted to other people. However, if a person has never had chickenpox, he may acquire chickenpox from a person who has active shingles (when the rash is in the blister phase). The risk of getting shingles increases as a person ages. People with immune systems weakened by diseases such as cancer and HIV are at greater risk of getting shingles.

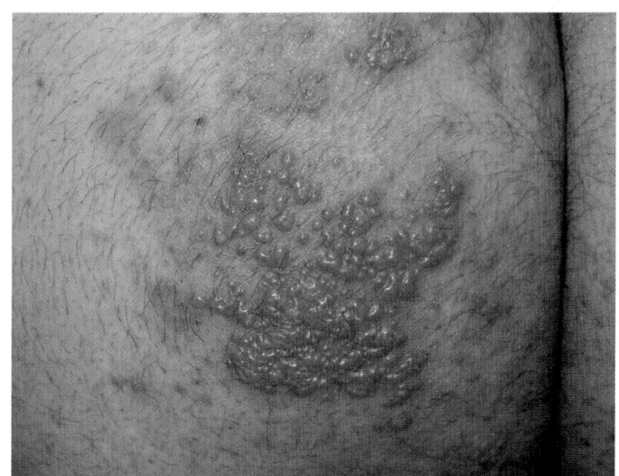

Fig. 18-1. Shingles in blister form. (PHOTO COURTESY OF DR. JERE MAMMINO, DO)

Keeping the rash covered, especially while it is in blister form, is important. Infected people should wash their hands often and should not scratch or touch the rash.

Shingles is treated with medication, which should be started as soon as possible. Starting medication immediately can help reduce the severity of the disease and can shorten the length of the illness. There is a vaccine for shingles that is often recommended for people 60 years or older who have had chickenpox. The vaccine can help reduce the risk of contracting shingles.

Wounds

A **wound** is a type of injury to the skin. Wounds are classified as either open or closed. An open wound has skin that is not intact. Open wounds can be categorized in the following ways: incisions, lacerations, abrasions, and puncture wounds. Incisions are caused by a knife or razor, such as a cut made during surgery with a surgical instrument. Lacerations are irregular wounds caused by ripping or blunt trauma, such as tearing of skin during childbirth. Abrasions are wounds in which the top layer of skin is scraped or worn off, often by coming into moving contact with a rough surface. Puncture wounds are breaks in the skin caused by a nail or a needle.

In a closed wound, the skin's surface has not been broken. Closed wounds can be contusions (bruises) or hematomas. Contusions are caused by blunt force trauma that damages tissue under the skin. Hematomas are caused by damage to a blood vessel that causes blood to collect under the skin.

Wounds are examined and cleaned with various liquids, such as tap water, sterile saline, or antiseptic solution. Bleeding may need to be stopped. Dressings, bandages, sutures, staples, or special strips or glue may need to be applied.

Dermatitis

Dermatitis is a general term that refers to an **inflammation**, or swelling, of the skin. There are different types of dermatitis, including atopic dermatitis, also known as *eczema*, and stasis dermatitis. Dermatitis usually involves swollen, reddened, irritated, and itchy skin.

Eczema commonly occurs along with allergies, including asthma or chronic hay fever. Physical and mental stressors may also cause eczema, and it may be inherited. Eczema usually begins in childhood and may not be as severe later in life. Symptoms include dry, itchy, and inflamed skin, usually on the cheeks, arms, and legs, although it can cover other parts of the body. Symptoms improve and worsen at various times. Atopic dermatitis is not contagious.

Special lotions are used to treat this condition. Further measures to help cracked skin may be prescribed, such as wet dressings. Antihistamines may help intense itching.

Stasis dermatitis is a skin condition that commonly affects the lower legs and ankles. The condition occurs due to a build up of fluid under the skin. This build-up causes problems with circulation, and poor circulation results in skin that is fragile and poorly nourished. Stasis dermatitis can also lead to severe skin problems such as open ulcers and wounds.

Early signs of stasis dermatitis include a rash, a scaly, red area, and itching. Other signs are swelling of the legs, ankles, or other areas; thin, tissue-like skin; darkening skin at ankles or legs; thickening skin at ankles or legs; signs of skin irritation; and leg pain. Nursing assistants should report any of these signs to the nurse.

Ways to treat stasis dermatitis include surgery for varicose veins and medications, such as diuretics, to reduce fluid in the body. The resident should wear stockings and shoes that fit properly and are not too tight. Elevating the feet may be ordered, and the legs should not be crossed. NAs may need to apply special elastic stockings to help promote circulation and should be gentle when handling or cleaning the skin. The resident may be on a low-sodium diet.

Fungal Infections

Mushrooms, mold, and yeasts (*Candida*) are all examples of fungi. Some types of fungi, such as *Candida*, normally live in and on the body, in such places as the skin and in the vagina and intestines. However, sometimes normal balances of fungi can change, resulting in fungal infections, such as *tinea pedis* (athlete's foot), *tinea cruris* (jock itch), or vaginal yeast infections. *Tinea*, often called ringworm, is another example of a fungal infection (Fig. 18-2). These imbalances that result in infections can be caused by a weakened immune system or by taking antibiotics.

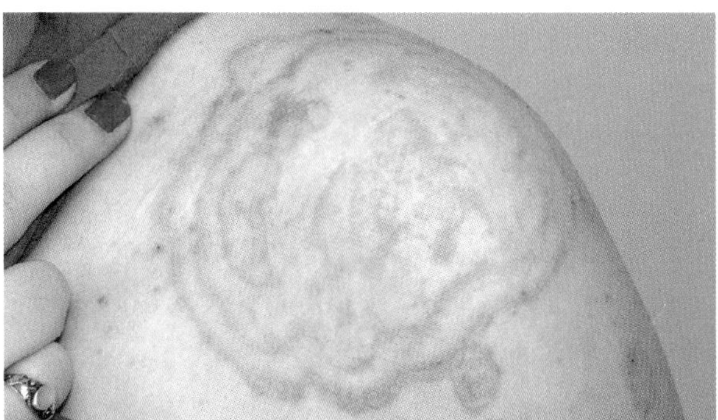

Fig. 18-2. *Tinea is a fungal infection that causes red, ring-like patches to appear on the upper body, hands, and/or feet.* (PHOTO COURTESY OF DR. JERE MAMMINO, DO)

Fungi can be difficult to kill. Treatment generally consists of applying antifungal drugs directly on the infection, such as the skin, inside the mouth, or in the vagina. Medication may also need to be taken orally or injected if the infection is more serious.

Residents' Rights

Diseases and Disorders

Nursing assistants must respect the privacy of residents who are ill. Residents' conditions should not be discussed in public areas. NAs should not make negative comments or show negative facial reactions to unpleasant symptoms, such as vomiting, or to conditions like skin disorders.

2. Describe common diseases and disorders of the musculoskeletal system

Arthritis

Arthritis is a general term that refers to inflammation, or swelling, of the joints. It causes stiffness, pain, and decreased mobility. Arthritis may be the result of aging, injury, or an **autoimmune illness**. An autoimmune illness causes the body's immune system to attack normal tissue in the body. Two common types of arthritis are osteoarthritis and rheumatoid arthritis.

Osteoarthritis, also called degenerative arthritis or degenerative joint disease (DJD), is a common type of arthritis that affects the elderly. It may occur with aging or as the result of joint injury. Hips and knees, which are weight-bearing joints, are usually affected. Joints in the fingers, thumbs, and spine can also be affected. Pain and stiffness seem to increase in cold or damp weather.

Rheumatoid arthritis can affect people of all ages. Joints become red, swollen, and very painful (Fig. 18-3). Deformities can result and may be severe and disabling. Movement is eventually restricted. Fever, fatigue, and weight loss are also symptoms. Rheumatoid arthritis usually affects the smaller joints first, then progresses to larger ones. Other parts of the body that may be affected are the heart, lungs, eyes, kidneys, and skin. Rheumatoid arthritis is considered an autoimmune disease.

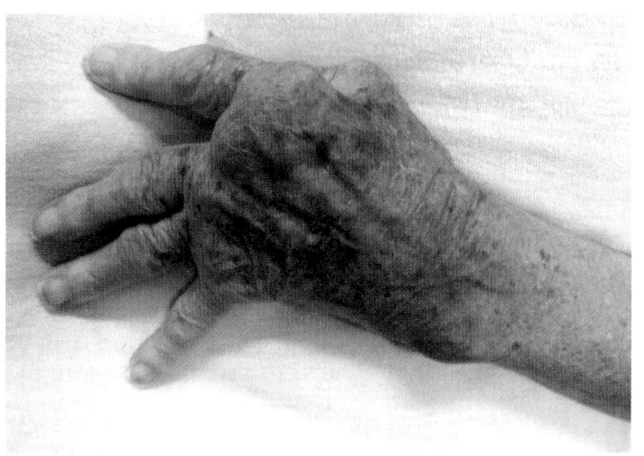

Fig. 18-3. Rheumatoid arthritis. (PHOTO COURTESY OF DR. JAMES HEILMAN, WIKIPEDIA)

Arthritis is generally treated with the following:

- Anti-inflammatory medication such as aspirin or ibuprofen, or other medication
- Local applications of heat to reduce swelling and pain
- Range of motion exercises (Chapter 21)
- Regular exercise and/or activity routine
- Diet to reduce weight or maintain strength

Guidelines: Arthritis

G Watch for stomach irritation or heartburn caused by aspirin or ibuprofen. Some residents cannot take these medications. Report signs of stomach irritation or heartburn immediately.

G Encourage activity. Gentle activity can help reduce the effects of arthritis. Follow care plan instructions carefully. Use canes or other walking aids as needed.

G Adapt activities of daily living (ADLs) to allow independence. Many devices are available to help residents bathe, dress, and feed themselves when they have arthritis (Chapter 21).

G Choose clothing that is easy to put on and fasten. Encourage use of handrails and safety bars in the bathroom. Special utensils make it easier for residents to feed themselves (Fig. 18-4).

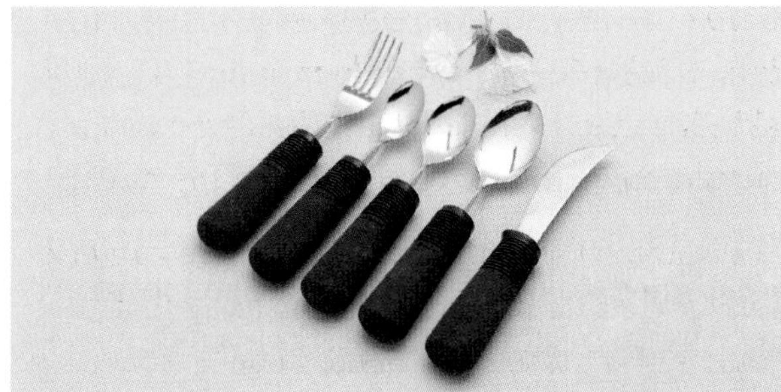

Fig. 18-4. Special equipment can help a person with arthritis remain independent. (PHOTO COURTESY OF NORTH COAST MEDICAL, INC., WWW.NCMEDICAL.COM, 800-821-9319)

G Treat each resident as an individual. Arthritis is very common among elderly residents. Do not assume that each resident has the same symptoms and needs the same care.

G Help maintain resident's self-esteem by encouraging self-care. Maintain a positive attitude. Listen to the resident's feelings. You can help him remain independent as long as possible.

Osteoporosis

Osteoporosis is a disease that causes bones to become porous and brittle. Brittle bones can break easily. Weakness in the bones may be due to age, lack of hormones, lack of calcium in bones, excessive alcohol use, or lack of exercise. It occurs more commonly in women after menopause (the end of menstruation). Extra calcium and regular exercise can help prevent osteoporosis. Signs and symptoms of osteoporosis include low back pain, stooped posture, and becoming shorter over time (Fig. 18-5).

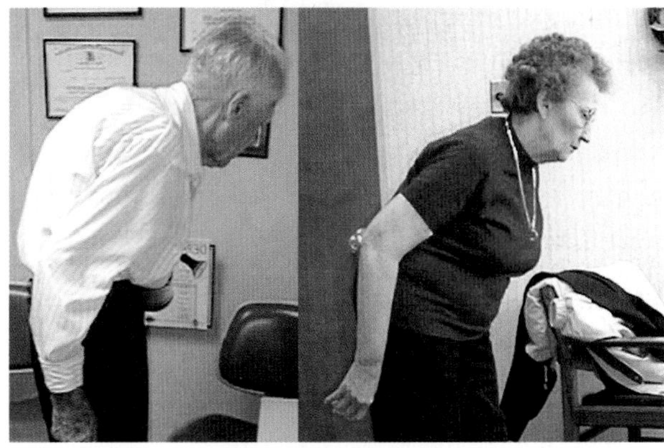

Fig. 18-5. Stooped posture is a common sign of osteoporosis. (PHOTOS COURTESY OF JEFFREY T. BEHR, MD)

To prevent or slow osteoporosis, nursing assistants should encourage residents to walk and do other light exercise as ordered. Exercise can strengthen bones as well as muscles. NAs must move residents with osteoporosis very carefully. Medication, calcium, and fluoride supplements are used to treat osteoporosis.

Fractures

A fracture is a broken bone caused by an accident or by osteoporosis. A **closed fracture** is a broken bone that does not break the skin. An **open fracture**, also known as a compound fracture, is a broken bone that penetrates the skin. An open fracture carries a high risk of infection and usually requires immediate surgery.

Preventing falls, which can lead to fractures, is very important. Fractures of arms, wrists, elbows, legs, and hips are the most common. Signs and symptoms of a fracture are pain, swelling, bruising, changes in skin color at the site, and limited movement.

When bones are fractured, the sections of broken bone must be placed back into alignment so the body can heal. The body can grow new bone tissue and fuse the sections of fractured bone together. The bone must be unable to move to allow this healing to occur. This is often accomplished by the use of a cast.

Two common types of casts are made of plaster and fiberglass. Plaster casts take longer to dry when they are made, up to one to two days. Casts are more often made of fiberglass. Fiberglass casts are lighter than plaster casts, and they dry quickly. A cast must be completely dry before a person can bear weight on it. As a cast dries, it gives off heat. This heat must escape or it will burn the skin. A cast should never be covered with any material until it has completely dried.

Guidelines: Cast Care

- G If caring for a resident who has a wet cast, do not cover the cast until it is dry. Assist the resident to change positions as ordered to allow the cast to dry evenly. Place the cast on pillows. A hard surface alters the shape of the cast. Use the palms of the hands to lift the cast. Fingers will dent it, and dents will cause pressure on the resident's skin.
- G Elevate the extremity that is in a cast. This helps stop swelling (Fig. 18-6). Use pillows to assist with elevation. If the resident is in bed, elevate the arm or leg slightly above the level of the heart.

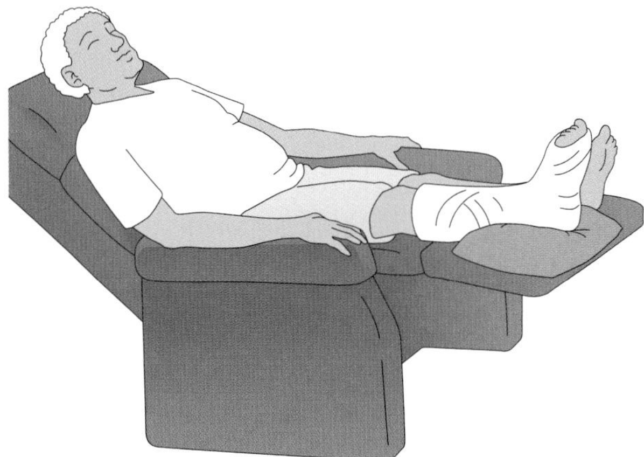

Fig. 18-6. *To help stop swelling, elevate the extremity that is in a cast.*

- G Observe the affected extremity for swelling, skin discoloration, cast tightness or pressure, sores, skin that feels hot or cold, pain, burning, numbness or tingling, drainage, bleeding, or odor. Compare to the extremity that does not have a cast. Report any of these signs or symptoms to the nurse, along with any signs of infection, such as fever or chills.
- G Protect the resident's skin from the rough edges of the cast. The stocking that lines the inside of the cast can be pulled up and over the edges and secured with tape. Tell the nurse if cast edges irritate the resident's skin.
- G Keep the cast dry. Wet casts lose their shape. Keep the cast clean.
- G Do not insert or allow the resident to insert anything inside the cast, even when the skin itches. Pointed or blunt objects may injure

the skin, which is already dry and fragile. Skin can become infected under the cast.

- G Tell the nurse prior to moving or exercising if pain medication is needed. Help with range of motion exercises as ordered. Allow plenty of time for movement. Assist resident with cane, walker, or crutches as needed.
- G Use bed cradles as needed to reduce pressure from bed linens.

Hip Fractures

Weakened bones make hip fractures more common. A sudden fall can result in a fractured hip that takes months to heal. Preventing falls is very important. Hip fractures can also occur because of weakened bones that fracture and then cause a fall. A hip fracture is a serious condition. The elderly heal slowly, and they are at risk for secondary illnesses and disabilities.

Most fractured hips require surgery. Total hip replacement (THR) is the surgical replacement of the head of the long bone of the leg (femur) where it joins the hip. This surgery is often performed for the following reasons:

- Fractured hip from an injury or fall that does not heal properly
- Weakened hip due to aging
- Hip is painful and stiff because the joint is weak and the bones are no longer strong enough to bear the person's weight

After the surgery, the person cannot stand on that leg while the hip heals. A physical therapist will assist after surgery. The goals of care include slowly strengthening the hip muscles and getting the resident to bear weight on that leg.

The resident's care plan will state when the resident may begin putting weight on the hip. It will also give instructions on how much the resident is able to do. It is important for nursing assistants to help with personal care and using assistive devices, such as walkers or canes.

Guidelines: Hip Replacement

- G Keep often-used items, such as medications, telephone, tissues, call lights, and water within easy reach. Avoid placing items in high places.
- G Dress starting with the affected (weaker) side first.
- G Never rush the resident. Use praise and encouragement often. Do this even for small accomplishments.
- G Ask the nurse to give pain medication prior to moving and positioning if needed.
- G Have the resident sit to do tasks in order to save her energy.
- G Follow the care plan exactly, even if the resident wants to do more than is ordered. Follow orders for weight-bearing. After surgery, the doctor's order will be written as *partial weight-bearing (PWB)* or *non-weight-bearing (NWB)*. **Partial weight-bearing** means the resident is able to support some body weight on one or both legs. **Non-weight-bearing** means the resident is unable to touch the floor or support any weight on one or both legs. Once the resident can bear full weight again, the doctor's order will be written for *full weight-bearing (FWB)*. **Full weight-bearing** means that both legs can bear 100 percent of the body weight on a step. Help as needed with cane, walker, or crutches.
- G Never perform range of motion exercises on the operative leg unless directed by the nurse.
- G Caution the resident not to sit with her legs crossed. The hip cannot be bent or flexed more than 90 degrees. It cannot be turned inward or outward (Fig. 18-7).

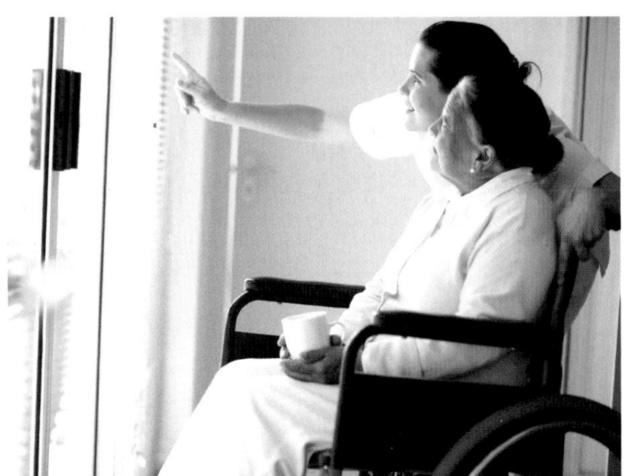

Fig. 18-7. The resident should not sit with her legs crossed.

G An abduction pillow will normally be used for six to 12 weeks after surgery while the resident is sleeping in bed. The abduction pillow immobilizes and positions the hips and lower extremities. The pillow is placed in between the legs, and the legs are secured to the sides of pillow using straps (Fig. 18-8). Follow the nurse's and the care plan's instructions for application and positioning.

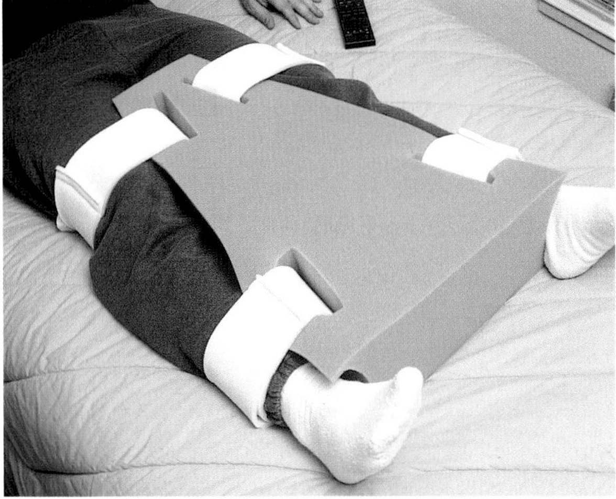

Fig. 18-8. An abduction pillow is placed in between the legs to immobilize and position the hips and lower extremities. (PHOTO COURTESY OF NORTH COAST MEDICAL, INC., WWW.NCMEDICAL.COM, 800-821-9319)

G When transferring from a bed, use a pillow between the thighs to keep the legs separated. Raise the head of the bed to allow the resident to move her legs over the side of the bed with the thighs still separated. Stand on the side of the unaffected hip so that the strong side leads in standing, pivoting, and sitting.

G With chair or toilet transfers, the operative leg/knee should be straightened. The stronger leg should stand first (with a walker or crutches) before bringing the foot of the affected leg back to the walking position.

Observing and Reporting: Hip Replacement

Report any of these to the nurse:

O/R Redness, drainage, bleeding, or warmth in incision area

O/R An increase in pain

O/R Numbness or tingling

O/R Shortening and/or external rotation of affected leg

O/R Abnormal vital signs, especially a change in temperature

O/R Inability of resident to use equipment properly and safely

O/R Unwillingness of resident to follow doctor's orders for activity and exercise

O/R Any problems with appetite

O/R Any improvements, such as increased strength and improved ability to walk

A cast or traction may also be used to immobilize the hip. Traction helps to immobilize a fractured bone, relieve pressure, and lessen muscle spasms due to injury. A resident in traction will require special care that will be included in the care plan. The traction assembly must never be disconnected, and nursing assistants should keep the weights off the floor and not add or remove weights. Proper skin care and repositioning are essential for all residents who are immobilized. Skin will rapidly deteriorate over pressure points. Range of motion exercises should be performed as directed. Nursing assistants should report complaints of pain, numbness or tingling, or burning, as well as presence of swelling, redness, bleeding, or sores.

Knee Replacement

Total knee replacement (TKR) is the surgical replacement of the knee with a prosthetic knee. A **prosthesis** is a device that replaces a body part that is missing or deformed because of an accident, injury, illness, or birth defect. It is used to improve a person's ability to function and/or to improve appearance. Total knee replacement surgery is performed to relieve pain and to restore motion to a knee damaged by injury or arthritis. It can help stabilize a knee that buckles or gives out repeatedly.

Care is similar to that for the hip replacement, but the recovery time is much shorter. These residents have more ability to care for themselves.

Guidelines: Knee Replacement

- G To prevent blood clots, apply special stockings as ordered. One type is a compression stocking. It is a plastic, air-filled, sleeve-like device that is applied to the legs and hooked to a machine. This machine inflates and deflates on its own. It acts in the same way that the muscles usually do during normal circumstances. The sleeves are normally applied after surgery while the resident is in bed. Anti-embolic stockings are another type of special stocking. They aid circulation. See later in the chapter for more information on this type of stocking.
- G Perform ankle pumps as ordered. These are simple exercises that promote circulation to the legs. Ankle pumps are done by raising the toes and feet toward the ceiling and lowering them again.
- G Encourage fluids, especially cranberry and orange juices, which contain vitamin C, to prevent urinary tract infections (UTIs).
- G Assist with deep breathing exercises as ordered.
- G A continuous passive motion (CPM) machine may be used after a knee replacement. This machine constantly moves the knee through its normal range of motion (Fig. 18-9). The person does not have to actively help; the machine does the work. Using a CPM machine can help speed recovery. The goal is to decrease stiffness, increase range of motion, and promote healing. The nurse or physical therapist will set the rate and position the resident. You may be asked to stay with the resident while the machine is on.

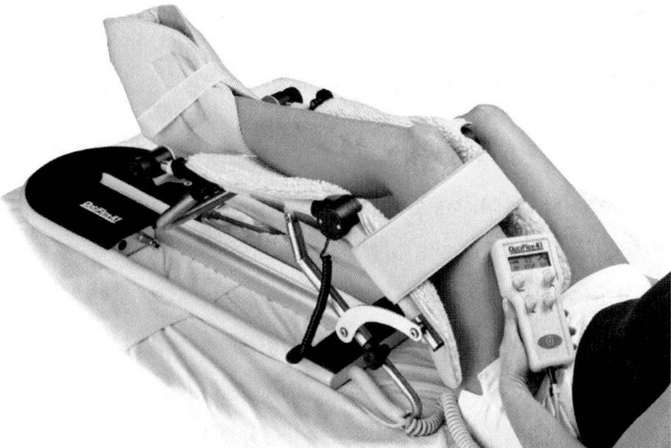

Fig. 18-9. One type of CPM machine. (PHOTO COURTESY OF THE MEDCOM GROUP, LTD., 800-231-4276, WWW.MEDCOMGROUP.COM)

- G Ask the nurse to give pain medication prior to moving and positioning if needed.
- G Report to the nurse if you notice redness, swelling, heat, or deep tenderness in one or both calves.

Muscular Dystrophy (MD)

Muscular dystrophy (MD) refers to a number of progressive diseases that cause a variety of physical disabilities due to muscle weakness. MD is an inherited disease; it causes a gradual wasting away of muscle, weakness, and deformity. The muscles of the hands are impaired, and there may be twitching of the hand and arm muscles. Legs may be weak and stiff. The person may be in a wheelchair.

Most forms of MD are present at birth or become apparent during childhood. Many forms of MD are very slow to progress. Often people with MD can live to middle or even late adulthood.

In the early stages of this disease, nursing assistants should help with activities of daily living

(ADLs) or range of motion (ROM) exercises. In the more advanced stages, assistance with skin care and positioning may be necessary, as well as performing ADLs for the resident.

Amputation

Amputation is the surgical removal of some or all of a body part, usually a hand, arm, foot, or leg. Amputation may be the result of an injury or disease. After amputation, some people feel that the amputated limb is still there, or they feel pain in the part that has been amputated. **Phantom sensation** is the term used when a person feels that the body part is still there. The person may experience warmth, tingling, or itching in the area where the limb existed. **Phantom limb pain** occurs when the person feels pain in a limb (or extremity) that has been amputated. It may persist for a short time or for several years. The pain or sensation, which has various possible causes, including remaining damaged nerve endings, is real. It should not be ignored.

Guidelines: Amputation

G Residents who have had a body part amputated must make many physical, psychological, social, and occupational adjustments due to disability. Be supportive during the continuing process of adjustment. When a body part has been amputated, day-to-day activities may be limited. A resident will need special care to help him adjust to these changes. When the condition is new, a physical and/or occupational therapist may work with the resident.

G Assist residents in performing their ADLs.

G Assist with changes of position as ordered to prevent pressure ulcers.

G Perform range of motion exercises as instructed. These exercises will help prevent contractures and other complications.

G Follow the care plan for care of the prosthesis and the stump. Chapter 21 contains more information on prosthetics and related care.

Complementary or Alternative Health Practices

Many people now use complementary or alternative health practices. **Complementary medicine** refers to treatments that are used in addition to the conventional treatments prescribed by a doctor. **Alternative medicine** refers to practices and treatments used instead of conventional methods. Residents may use any of the following:

- Chiropractic medicine concentrates on the spine and musculoskeletal system. Chiropractors believe that a misaligned spine can interfere with the body's proper function. Chiropractors do not use drugs or surgery; they use hands-on manipulations, also called adjustments, of the spine or other joints. They also teach exercises and provide nutrition and other health counseling.

  Heat, cold, and muscle stimulation are used to improve function. Chiropractors are frequently consulted for back, neck, and joint pain, as well as for headaches.
- Massage therapy manipulates soft body tissues with touch and pressure and is used to reduce stress and to promote relaxation and pain relief.
- Acupuncture is a very old Chinese healing technique. Very fine needles are inserted into specific points on the body in order to restore health, relieve pain, or treat other conditions.
- Homeopathy involves giving small doses of a substance to stimulate the body's ability to heal itself. If given in large doses, the substance would produce symptoms of an illness or the illness itself.
- Herbs and other dietary supplements may be taken for prevention as well as treatment of diseases or conditions. If you know that a resident is taking herbs or supplements, report this to the nurse, as some can cause serious problems if taken with certain medications.

If residents are using complementary or alternative medicine, NAs should not make judgments about treatment or discuss their opinions. They should not make recommendations about these methods. If an NA has concerns, she should talk to the nurse.

3. Describe common diseases and disorders of the nervous system

Chapter 19 provides information on dementia and Alzheimer's disease. Dementia and Alzheimer's disease are common disorders of the nervous system.

CVA or Stroke

The medical term for a stroke is a cerebrovascular accident (CVA). CVA, or stroke, occurs when blood supply to a part of the brain is blocked or a blood vessel leaks or ruptures within the brain. Without blood, part of the brain does not receive oxygen. Brain cells will begin to die, and additional damage can occur due to leaking blood, clots, and swelling of the tissues. Swelling can also cause pressure on other areas of the brain.

Strokes can be mild or severe. Afterward, a resident may experience paralysis, weakness, inability to speak or understand words, trouble swallowing, and loss of bowel or bladder control. Chapter 4 has a more comprehensive list of how a CVA may affect a person.

Each side of the brain controls different functions. Symptoms that a person experiences depend on which side of the brain is affected by the stroke. Weaknesses on the right side of the body show that the left side of the brain was affected. Weaknesses on the left side of the body show that the right side of the brain was affected.

If the stroke was mild, the resident may experience few, if any, complications. Physical therapy may help restore physical abilities. Speech and occupational therapy can also help with communication and performing ADLs.

Guidelines: CVA/Stroke

- G Residents with paralysis, weakness, or loss of movement will usually receive physical or occupational therapy. Range of motion exercises will help strengthen muscles and keep joints mobile. Residents may also need to perform leg exercises to improve circulation. Safety is always important when post-CVA residents are exercising. Assist carefully with exercises as ordered.
- G Never refer to the weaker side as the "bad side" or talk about the "bad" leg or arm. The terms *weaker* or *involved* should be used to refer to the side with paralysis or paresis.
- G Residents with speech loss or communication problems may receive speech therapy. You may be asked to help. This includes helping residents recognize written or spoken words. Speech therapists will also evaluate a resident's swallowing ability. They will decide if swallowing therapy or thickened liquids are needed.
- G Use verbal and nonverbal communication to express your positive attitude. Let the resident know you have confidence in his abilities through smiles, touches, and gestures. Gestures and pointing can also help you convey information or allow the resident to speak to you. More ideas for communicating with residents recovering from stroke are listed in Chapter 4.
- G Experiencing confusion or memory loss is upsetting. People often cry for no apparent reason after suffering a stroke. Be patient and understanding. Your positive attitude will be important. Keeping a routine may help residents feel more secure.
- G Encourage independence and self-esteem. Let the resident do things for himself whenever possible, even if you could do a better or faster job. Make tasks less difficult for the resident to do. Appreciate and acknowledge residents' efforts to do things for themselves even when they are unsuccessful. Praise even the smallest successes to build confidence.
- G Always check on the resident's body alignment. Sometimes an arm or leg can be caught, and the resident is unaware.
- G Pay special attention to skin care and observe for changes in the skin if a resident is unable to move.
- G If residents have a loss of touch or sensation, check for potentially harmful situations (for example, heat and sharp objects). If residents are unable to sense or move a part of the

body, check and change positioning often to prevent pressure ulcers.

- Adapt procedures when caring for residents with one-sided paralysis or weakness. Carefully assist with shaving, grooming, and bathing. Diminished sensation or paralysis causes lack of awareness about such things as water temperature and sharpness of razors. Take care so that injury does not occur.

When assisting with transfers or walking, remember the following:

- Always use a gait belt for safety. Stand on the weaker side. Support the weaker (involved) side. Lead with the stronger (uninvolved) side (Fig. 18-10).

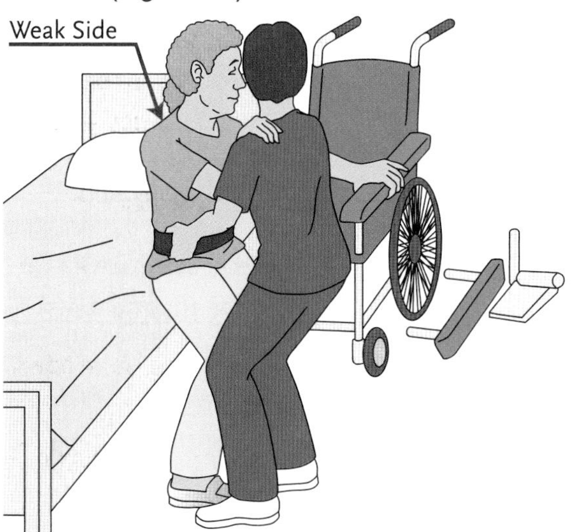

Fig. 18-10. *When helping a resident transfer, support the weaker side while leading with the stronger side.*

When assisting with dressing, remember the following:

- Dress the weaker side first. Place the weaker arm or leg into the clothing first. This prevents unnecessary bending and stretching of the limb. Undress the stronger side first, then remove the weaker arm or leg from clothing to prevent the limb from being stretched and twisted.
- Use assistive equipment to help the resident dress himself (see Chapters 13 and 21). Encourage self-care.

When assisting with eating, remember the following:

- Place food in the resident's field of vision. The nurse will determine a resident's field of vision.
- Use assistive devices such as silverware with built-up handle grips, plate guards, and drinking cups.
- Watch for signs of choking. Report any difficulty with swallowing. Soft foods may be ordered in the care plan if swallowing is difficult.
- Always place food in the unaffected, or non-paralyzed, side of the mouth. Make sure food is swallowed before offering more bites.

Chapters 4 and 7 contain more information about cerebrovascular accidents.

Parkinson's Disease

Parkinson's disease is a progressive, incurable disease that causes a section of the brain to degenerate. Progressive means the disease gets worse with time. Parkinson's disease affects the muscles, causing them to become stiff. In addition, it causes stooped posture and a shuffling gait, or walk. It can also cause pill-rolling. Pill-rolling is a circular movement of the tips of the thumb and the index finger when brought together, which looks like rolling a pill. Tremors or shaking make it very difficult for a person to perform ADLs such as eating and bathing. A person with Parkinson's disease may have a mask-like facial expression. Medications are commonly used to treat this disease. Surgery may be an option for some people.

Guidelines: Parkinson's Disease

- Residents are at a high risk for falls. Protect residents from any unsafe areas and conditions. Assist with ambulation as necessary.
- Help with ADLs as needed.

G Assist with range of motion exercises exactly as ordered to prevent contractures and to strengthen muscles (Fig. 18-11).

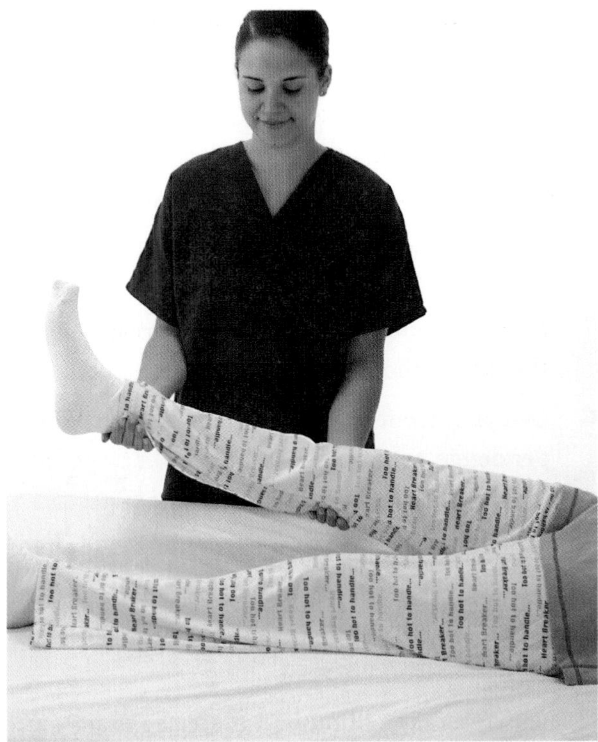

Fig. 18-11. Range of motion exercises help prevent contractures, strengthen muscles, and increase circulation.

G Encourage self-care. Be patient with self-care and communication.

Multiple Sclerosis (MS)

Multiple sclerosis (MS) is a progressive disease that affects the central nervous system. When a person has MS, the protective covering for the nerves, spinal cord, and white matter of the brain breaks down over time. Without this covering, or sheath, nerves cannot send messages to and from the brain in a normal way.

MS progresses slowly and unpredictably. Residents who have this disease will have widely varying abilities. Symptoms will vary as well and may include blurred vision, fatigue, tremors, poor balance, and trouble walking. Weakness, numbness, tingling, incontinence, and behavior changes are also symptoms. MS can eventually cause blindness, contractures, and loss of function in the arms and legs (Fig. 18-12).

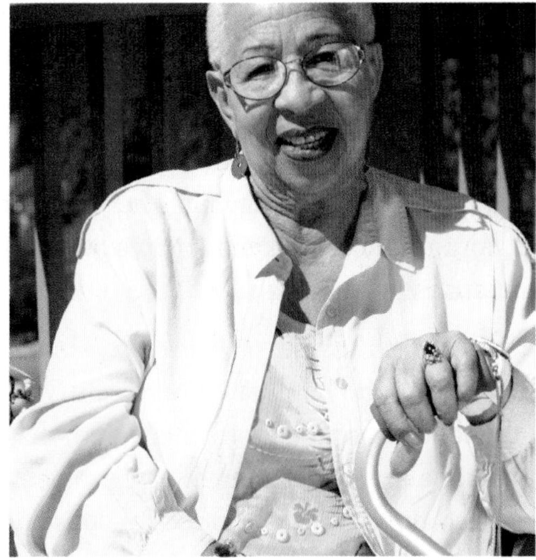

Fig. 18-12. Multiple sclerosis is an unpredictable disease that causes varying symptoms and abilities. MS can cause a range of problems, including fatigue, poor balance, and trouble walking.

Multiple sclerosis is usually diagnosed when a person is in his or her early twenties to thirties. The exact cause is not known, but it may be an autoimmune disease. There is no cure for this disease; it is mostly treated with medication.

Guidelines: Multiple Sclerosis

G Assist with activities of daily living as needed.

G Be patient with self-care and movement. Allow the resident enough time to perform tasks. Offer rest periods as necessary.

G Give the resident plenty of time to communicate. People with MS may have trouble forming their thoughts. Be patient. Do not rush them.

G Prevent falls, which may be due to a lack of coordination, fatigue, or vision problems.

G Stress can worsen the effects of MS. Be calm and listen to residents when they want to talk.

G Encourage a healthy diet with plenty of fluids.

G Give excellent skin care to prevent pressure ulcers.

G Assist with range of motion exercises to prevent contractures and strengthen muscles.

Head and Spinal Cord Injuries

Diving, sports injuries, falls, car and motorcycle accidents, industrial accidents, war, and criminal violence are common causes of head and spinal cord injuries. Problems from these injuries range from mild confusion or memory loss to coma, paralysis, and death.

Head injuries can cause permanent brain damage. Residents who have had a head injury may have the following problems: intellectual disabilities; personality changes; breathing problems; seizures; coma; memory loss; loss of consciousness; paresis; and paralysis. Paresis is paralysis, or loss of muscle function, that affects only part of the body. Often, paresis describes a weakness or loss of ability on one side of the body.

The effects of spinal cord injuries depend on the force of impact and the location of the injury. The higher the injury on the spinal cord, the greater the loss of function. People with head and spinal cord injuries may have **paraplegia**, or loss of function of lower body and legs. These injuries may also cause **quadriplegia**, in which the person is unable to use his legs, trunk, and arms (Fig. 18-13).

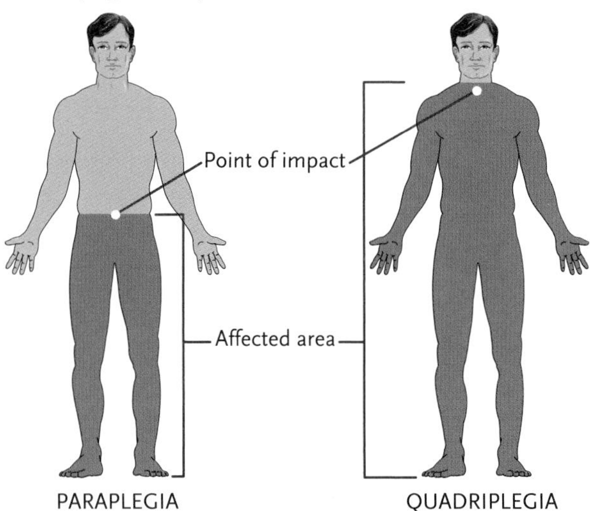

Fig. 18-13. *Loss of function depends on where the spine is injured.*

Rehabilitation is necessary for residents with spinal cord injuries. It will help them maintain the muscle function that remains and to live as independently as possible. Residents will need emotional support as they adjust to their disability. Their specific needs will vary.

Guidelines: Head or Spinal Cord Injury

- G Give emotional support, as well as physical help. Frustration and anger may surface as residents attempt to deal with the reality of their lives. Try not to take it personally.
- G Safety is very important. Be very careful that residents do not fall or burn themselves. Because residents who are paralyzed have no sensation, they are unable to feel a burn.
- G Be patient with self-care. Allow as much independence as possible with ADLs.
- G Give careful skin care. It is essential to prevent pressure ulcers when mobility is limited.
- G Assist residents to change positions at least every two hours to prevent pressure ulcers. Be gentle when repositioning.
- G Perform range of motion exercises exactly as ordered to prevent contractures and strengthen muscles.
- G Immobility leads to constipation. Encourage fluids and a high-fiber diet if ordered in the care plan.
- G Loss of ability to empty the bladder may lead to the need for a urinary catheter. Urinary tract infections are common. Encourage high intake of fluids. Juices high in vitamin C, such as orange juice and cranberry juice, help prevent UTIs. Give extra catheter care as needed.
- G Lack of activity leads to poor circulation and fatigue. Offer rest periods as necessary. Special stockings to help increase circulation may be ordered.
- G Difficulty coughing and shallow breathing can lead to pneumonia. Encourage deep breathing exercises as ordered.
- G Male residents may have involuntary erections. Provide for privacy and be sensitive to this. Be professional.
- G Assist with bowel and bladder training if needed.

Epilepsy

Epilepsy is a brain disorder that results from a disruption in normal electrical impulses in the brain, which causes repeated seizures. However, not all seizures are due to epilepsy. Epileptic seizures can range from mild tremors or brief blackouts to violent convulsions lasting several minutes. Epilepsy may be due to illness or injury that affects the brain, or the cause may be unknown. It is diagnosed by various medical tests, including an electroencephalogram (EEG) to check the electrical activity in the brain. Treatment for epilepsy includes medication or surgery. Chapter 7 contains information on responding to seizures.

Vision Impairment

Vision impairment can affect people of all ages. Some vision impairment causes people to wear corrective lenses, such as eyeglasses or contact lenses (Fig. 18-14). Some people need to wear eyeglasses all the time. Others only need them to read or for activities that require seeing distant objects, such as driving.

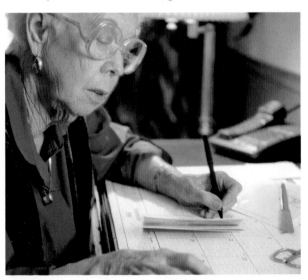

Fig. 18-14. *Nearsightedness (the ability to see objects nearby better than objects in the distance) and farsightedness (the ability to see objects in the distance better than objects nearby) are often corrected through the use of eyeglasses.*

People over the age of 40 are at risk for developing certain serious vision problems. These include cataracts, glaucoma, and blindness. When a **cataract** develops, the lens of the eye, which is normally clear, becomes cloudy. This prevents light from entering the eye (Fig. 18-15). Vision blurs and dims initially, and is eventually lost entirely. This disease process can occur in one or both eyes. It is corrected with surgery, in which a permanent lens implant is usually performed.

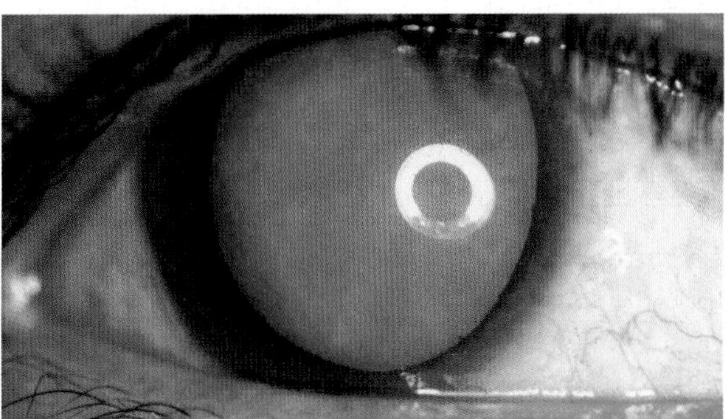

Fig. 18-15. *When a cataract develops, the lens of the eye becomes cloudy. This prevents light from entering the eye.*

Glaucoma is a disease that is the leading cause of blindness in the United States. With glaucoma, the pressure in the eye (intraocular pressure) increases. This eventually damages the retina and the optic nerve. It causes loss of vision and blindness. Glaucoma can occur suddenly, causing severe pain, nausea, and vomiting. It can also occur gradually, with symptoms that include blurred vision, tunnel vision, and blue-green halos around lights. Glaucoma is treated with eye drops and other medication and sometimes with surgery.

Age-related macular degeneration (AMD) is a condition that usually affects older adults (50 and over). It occurs when the macula, which is part of the retina, gradually deteriorates, eventually causing vision loss and such problems as the inability to recognize faces, drive, read, and write. Peripheral (side) vision is not affected.

AMD may evolve slowly, and symptoms may not be apparent in the early stages. A person may experience dark or blurred areas in the center of vision, or objects may appear less bright. AMD occurs in two forms: wet and dry. The dry form is more common.

Risk factors for AMD include age, smoking, race (Caucasians are more likely to develop it), and family history of the disease. There is no cure for AMD, but dry AMD may be treated with zinc and antioxidants. Wet AMD may be treated with injections and laser surgery.

Chapter 4 provides more information on vision and hearing impairments.

4. Describe common diseases and disorders of the circulatory system

Hypertension (HTN) or High Blood Pressure

When blood pressure is consistently 140/90 or higher, a person is diagnosed as having **hypertension (HTN)**, or high blood pressure. Hypertension is often caused by **atherosclerosis**, or a hardening and narrowing of the blood vessels (Fig. 18-16). It can also result from kidney disease, tumors of the adrenal gland, pregnancy, and certain medications.

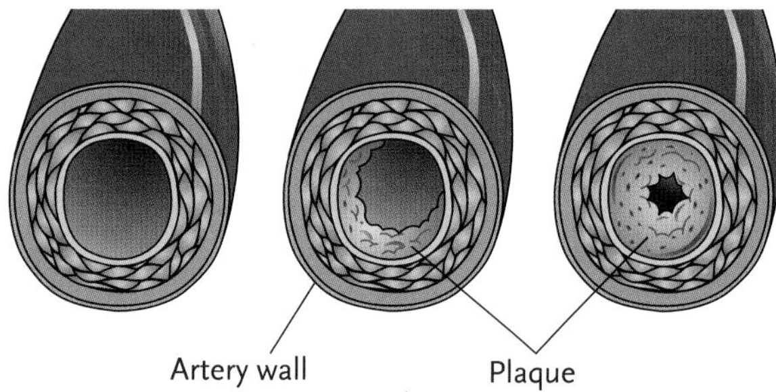

Fig. 18-16. *Arteries may become hardened or narrower because of a build-up of plaque. Hardened arteries are one cause of high blood pressure.*

Hypertension can develop in people of any age. Signs and symptoms of hypertension are not always obvious, especially in the early stages. Often it is only discovered when a blood pressure measurement is taken. Persons with the disease may complain of headaches, blurred vision, and dizziness.

Guidelines: Hypertension

- G Because it can lead to serious conditions such as CVA, heart attack, kidney disease, or blindness, treatment to control hypertension is vital. Residents may take medication that lowers blood pressure or cholesterol. They may take diuretics. Diuretics are a type of medication that reduce fluid in the body. Offer trips to the bathroom regularly. Answer call lights promptly.
- G Residents may also have a prescribed exercise program or a special low-fat, low-sodium diet. You may be required to take frequent blood pressure measurements. Encourage residents to follow their diet and exercise programs.

Coronary Artery Disease (CAD)

Coronary artery disease occurs when the blood vessels in the coronary arteries narrow. This reduces the supply of blood to the heart muscle and deprives it of oxygen and nutrients. Over time, as fatty deposits block the artery, the muscle that was supplied by the blood vessel dies. CAD can lead to heart attack or stroke.

The heart muscle that is not getting enough oxygen causes chest pain, pressure, or discomfort, called **angina pectoris**. The heart needs more oxygen during exercise, stress, excitement, or to digest a heavy meal. In CAD, narrow blood vessels prevent the extra blood with oxygen from getting to the heart (Fig. 18-17).

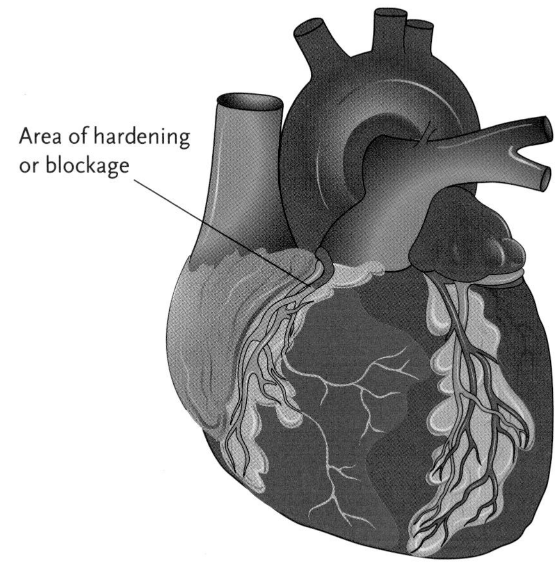

Fig. 18-17. *Angina pectoris results from the heart not getting enough oxygen.*

The pain of angina pectoris is usually described as pressure or tightness in the left side or the center of the chest, behind the sternum or breastbone. Some people complain of pain radiating or extending down the inside of the left arm or to the neck and left side of the jaw. A person suffering from angina pectoris may sweat or appear pale. The person may feel dizzy and have trouble breathing.

Risk factors for coronary artery disease include increasing age, gender (men are more likely to get CAD than women), family history of heart disease, tobacco use, high cholesterol, hypertension, lack of activity, obesity, and diabetes.

Guidelines: Angina Pectoris

- **G** Rest is extremely important. Rest reduces the heart's need for extra oxygen. It helps the blood flow return to normal, often within three to 15 minutes. Encourage residents to rest.
- **G** Medication is also needed to relax the walls of the coronary arteries. This allows them to open and get more blood to the heart. This medication, **nitroglycerin**, is a small tablet that the resident places under the tongue. There it dissolves and is rapidly absorbed. Residents who have angina pectoris may keep nitroglycerin on hand to use as symptoms arise. Nursing assistants are not allowed to give any medication unless they have had special training. Tell the nurse if a resident needs help taking the medication. Nitroglycerin is also available as a patch. Do not remove the patch. Tell the nurse immediately if the patch comes off. Nitroglycerin may also come in the form of a spray that the resident sprays onto or under the tongue.
- **G** Residents may also need to avoid heavy meals, overeating, intense exercise, and exposure to cold or hot and humid weather.

Myocardial Infarction (MI) or Heart Attack

When blood flow to the heart muscle is blocked, oxygen and nutrients fail to reach the cells in that region (Fig. 18-18). Waste products are not removed, and the muscle cells die. This is called a **myocardial infarction (MI)**, or heart attack. The area of dead tissue may be large or small, depending on the artery involved. Someone having a myocardial infarction must receive emergency treatment from medical personnel. This helps minimize damage and may prevent further illness or death. Chapter 7 has a list of warning signs of an MI.

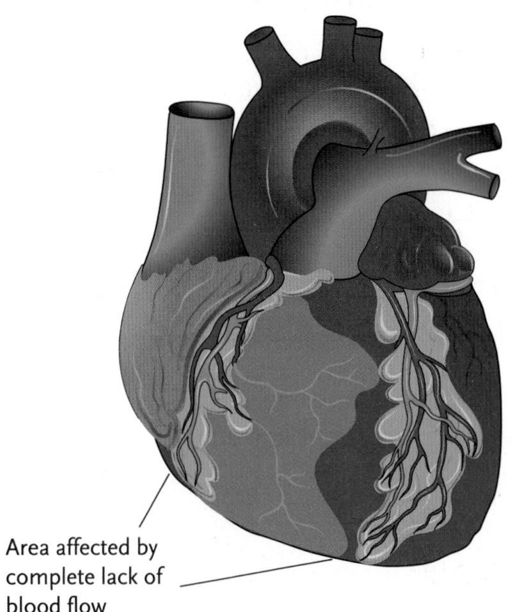

***Fig. 18-18.** A heart attack occurs when all or part of the blood flow to the heart is blocked.*

Guidelines: Myocardial Infarction

- **G** Generally, residents who have had an MI will be placed on a regular exercise program. Encourage residents to follow their exercise programs.
- **G** Residents may be on a diet that is low in fat and cholesterol and/or low in sodium. Encourage residents to follow their special diets.
- **G** Medications may be prescribed to regulate heart rate and blood pressure.

- G Quitting smoking will be encouraged. Be supportive.
- G A stress management program may be started to help reduce stress levels. Help residents avoid stress and listen if they want to talk.
- G Residents recovering from an MI may need to avoid exposure to cold temperatures.

Congestive Heart Failure (CHF)

Coronary artery disease, myocardial infarction, hypertension, or other disorders may all damage the heart. When the heart muscle has been severely damaged, the heart fails to pump effectively. When the left side of the heart is affected, blood backs up into the lungs. When the right side of the heart is affected, blood backs up into the legs, feet, or abdomen. When one or both sides of the heart stop pumping blood effectively, it is called **congestive heart failure** (**CHF**).

Signs and symptoms of congestive heart failure include the following:

- Fatigue
- Trouble breathing, shortness of breath, coughing or gurgling with breathing
- Dizziness, confusion, and fainting
- Pale or cyanotic (blue) skin
- Low blood pressure
- Swelling of the feet and ankles (edema)
- Bulging veins in the neck
- Weight gain

Guidelines: Congestive Heart Failure

- G Although congestive heart failure is a serious illness, it can be treated and controlled. Medications can strengthen the heart muscle and improve its pumping.
- G Medications help remove excess fluids. This means more trips to the bathroom. Answer call lights promptly. Keep a portable commode nearby if the resident is weak and has trouble getting out of bed and walking to the bathroom. Assist resident as needed.
- G A low-sodium diet or fluid restrictions may be ordered. Encourage residents to follow any diet orders or restrictions.
- G A weakened heart may make it hard for residents to walk, carry items, or climb stairs. Limited activity or bedrest may be prescribed. Allow for a period of rest after an activity.
- G Measure intake and output of fluids as ordered (Chapter 15).
- G Resident may need to be weighed daily at the same time to watch for weight gain from fluid retention. Weigh residents as instructed.
- G Apply elastic leg stockings as ordered to reduce swelling in feet and ankles.
- G Range of motion (ROM) exercises improve muscle tone when activity and exercise are limited. Assist with ROM exercises.
- G Extra pillows may help residents who have trouble breathing. Keeping the head of the bed elevated may also help with breathing.
- G Assist with personal care and activities of daily living (ADLs) as needed.
- G A common side effect of medications for congestive heart failure is dizziness. This may result from a lack of potassium. High-potassium foods and drinks such as raisins, prunes, apricots, baked potatoes, spinach, tomatoes, prune juice, and orange juice can help this.

Peripheral Vascular Disease (PVD)

Peripheral vascular disease (**PVD**) is a disease in which the legs, feet, arms, or hands do not have enough blood circulation. This is due to fatty deposits in the blood vessels that harden over time. The legs, feet, arms, and hands feel cool or cold. Nail beds and/or feet become ashen or blue. Swelling occurs in the hands and feet. Ulcers of the legs and feet may develop and can become infected. Pain may be very severe when walking; however, it is usually relieved with rest.

Some changes in health may lead to inactivity. A lack of mobility may contribute to PVD. For some cases of poor circulation to legs and feet, elastic stockings are ordered. These special stockings help prevent swelling and blood clots. They promote blood circulation. Elastic stockings are also known as *anti-embolic* stockings. The stockings need to be put on in the morning, before the resident gets out of bed. Legs are at their smallest size then. Nursing assistants should follow the manufacturer's instructions for how to put on stockings.

Putting elastic stockings on a resident

Equipment: elastic stockings

1. Identify yourself by name. Identify resident by name.
2. Wash your hands.
3. Explain procedure to resident. Speak clearly, slowly, and directly. Maintain face-to-face contact whenever possible.
4. Provide for resident's privacy with curtain, screen, or door.
5. The resident should be in the supine position (on her back) in bed. With resident lying down, remove her socks, shoes, or slippers, and expose one leg. Expose no more than one leg at a time.
6. Turn stocking inside-out at least to heel area (Fig. 18-19).

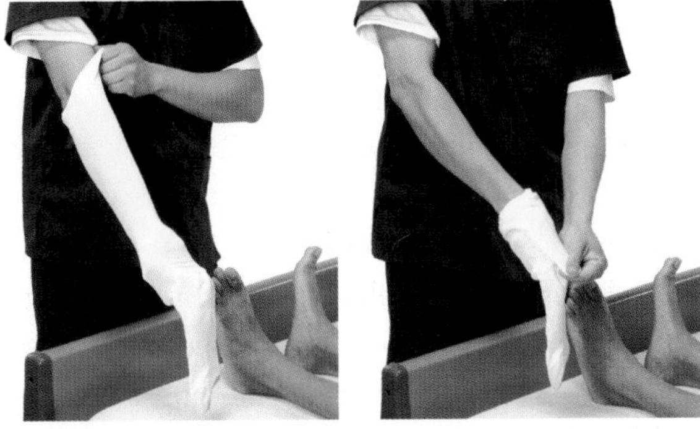

Fig. 18-19. *Turning the stocking inside out allows stocking to roll on gently.*

7. Gently place the foot of the stocking over toes, foot, and heel (Fig. 18-20). Make sure the heel is in the right place (heel of foot should be in heel of stocking).

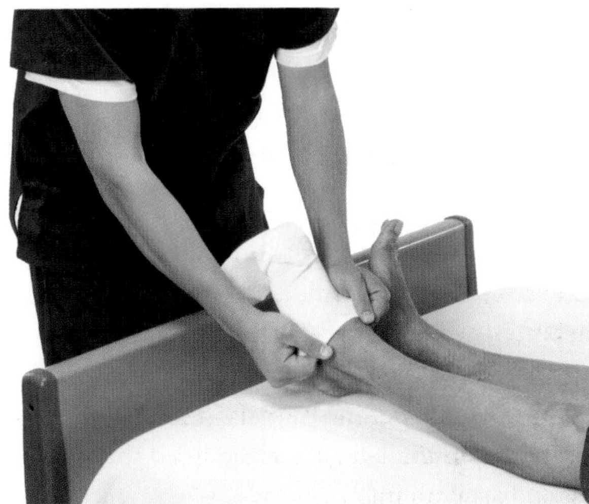

Fig. 18-20. *Gently place the foot of the stocking over the toes, foot, and heel. Promote the resident's comfort and safety. Avoid force and over-extension of joints.*

8. Gently pull the top of stocking over foot, heel, and leg.
9. Make sure there are no twists or wrinkles in stocking after it is applied. It must fit smoothly (Fig. 18-21). Make sure the heel of stocking is over the heel of foot. If the stocking has an opening in the toe area, make sure the opening is either over or under the toe area, depending upon the manufacturer's instructions.

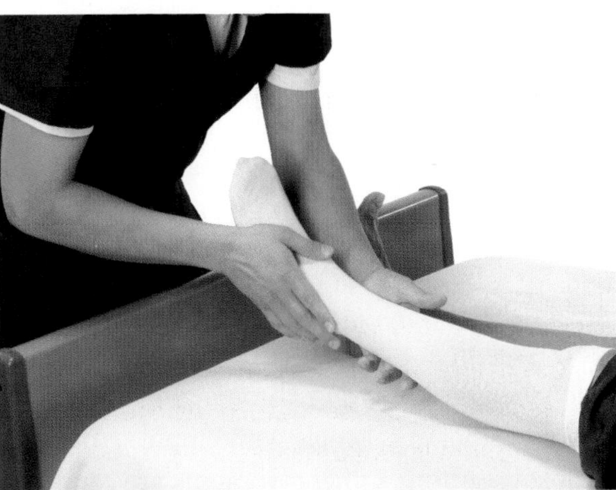

Fig. 18-21. *Make stocking smooth. Twists or wrinkles cause the stocking to be too tight, which reduces circulation.*

10. Repeat for the other leg.
11. Place call light within resident's reach.
12. Wash your hands.
13. Report any changes in resident to nurse.
14. Document procedure using facility guidelines.

Elastic stockings should be removed at least once a day as directed in the care plan. After removing them, the NA should bathe the skin underneath, dry the skin, and reapply them. The skin should be observed for changes in color, temperature, and swelling or sores. The NA should report any changes.

5. Describe common diseases and disorders of the respiratory system

Chronic Obstructive Pulmonary Disease (COPD)

Chronic obstructive pulmonary disease, (**COPD**) is a chronic, progressive disease. This means a person may live for years with it but never be cured. Residents with COPD have trouble breathing, especially with getting air out of the lungs. There are two chronic lung diseases that are grouped under COPD: chronic bronchitis and emphysema.

Bronchitis is an irritation and inflammation of the lining of the bronchi. Chronic bronchitis is a form of bronchitis that is usually caused by cigarette smoking. Symptoms include coughing that brings up sputum (phlegm) and mucus. Breathlessness and wheezing may be present. Treatment includes stopping smoking and possibly medications.

Emphysema is a chronic disease of the lungs that usually results from chronic bronchitis and cigarette smoking. People with emphysema have trouble breathing. Other symptoms are coughing, breathlessness, and a rapid heartbeat. There is no cure for emphysema. Treatment includes managing symptoms and pain. Oxygen therapy, as well as medications, may be ordered. Quitting smoking is very important.

Over time, a resident with either of these lung disorders becomes chronically ill and weakened. There is a high risk for acute lung infections, such as pneumonia. **Pneumonia** is an illness that can be caused by a bacterial, viral, or fungal infection. Acute inflammation occurs in lung tissue. The affected person develops a high fever, chills, cough, greenish or yellow sputum, chest pains, and rapid pulse. Treatment includes antibiotics, along with plenty of fluids. Recovery from pneumonia may take longer for older adults and people with chronic illnesses.

When the lungs and brain do not get enough oxygen, all body systems are affected. Residents may live with a constant fear of not being able to breathe. This can cause them to sit upright in an attempt to improve their ability to expand the lungs. These residents can have poor appetites. They usually do not get enough sleep. All of this can add to feelings of weakness and poor health. They may feel they have lost control of their bodies, particularly their breathing. They may fear suffocation.

Residents with COPD may experience the following symptoms:

- Chronic cough or wheeze
- Difficulty breathing, especially when inhaling and exhaling deeply
- Shortness of breath, especially during physical effort
- Pale, cyanotic, reddish-purple skin
- Confusion
- General state of weakness
- Difficulty completing meals due to shortness of breath
- Fear and anxiety

Guidelines: Chronic Obstructive Pulmonary Disease

G Colds or viruses can make residents very ill quickly. Always observe and report signs of symptoms getting worse.

G Help residents sit upright or lean forward. Offer pillows for support (Fig. 18-22).

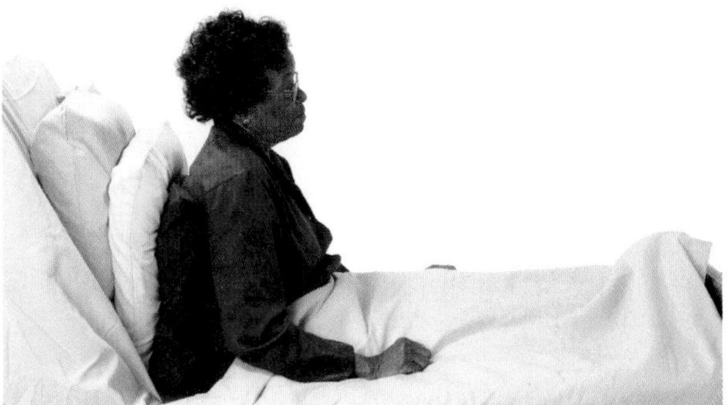

Fig. 18-22. It helps residents with COPD to sit upright and lean forward slightly.

G Offer plenty of fluids and small, frequent meals.

G Encourage a well-balanced diet.

G Keep oxygen supply available as ordered.

G Being unable to breathe or fearing suffocation can be very frightening. Be calm and supportive.

G Use proper infection prevention practices. Wash your hands often and encourage residents to do the same. Dispose of used tissues promptly.

G Encourage as much resident independence with ADLs as possible.

G Remind residents to avoid situations where they may be exposed to infections, especially colds and the flu.

G Encourage pursed-lip breathing. Pursed-lip breathing involves inhaling slowly through the nose and exhaling slowly through pursed lips (as if about to whistle). A nurse should teach residents how to do this.

G Encourage residents to save energy for important tasks. Encourage residents to rest during tasks.

Observing and Reporting: COPD

Report any of the following to the nurse:

O/R Temperature over 101°F

O/R Changes in breathing patterns, including shortness of breath

O/R Changes in color or consistency of lung secretions

O/R Changes in mental state or personality

O/R Refusal to take medications as ordered

O/R Excessive weight loss

O/R Increasing dependence upon caregivers and family

Asthma

Asthma is a chronic inflammatory disease. It occurs when the respiratory system is hyperreactive (that is, reacts quickly and strongly) to irritants, infection, cold air, or allergens such as pollen and dust. Exercise and stress can also cause or worsen asthma. When the bronchi become irritated due to any one of these conditions, they constrict, making it difficult to breathe. As a response to irritation and inflammation, the mucous membrane produces thick mucus. This further inhibits respiration. As a result, air is trapped in the lungs, causing coughing and wheezing.

The exact cause of asthma is unknown. It may be caused by a combination of factors, such as family history and certain environmental exposures. Treatment for asthma includes medications that are given directly into the lungs using sprays or inhalers (Fig. 18-23). Residents with asthma should avoid triggers that bring on asthma attacks, such as allergens, smoke, strong odors, and strenuous exercise.

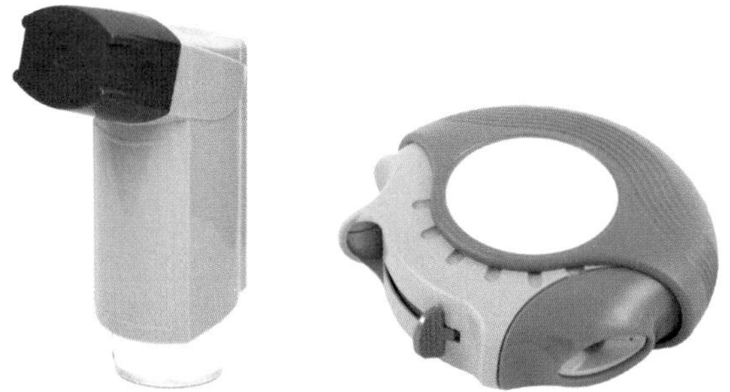

Fig. 18-23. Two different types of asthma inhalers.

Bronchiectasis

Bronchiectasis is a condition in which the bronchial tubes are abnormally enlarged. A person may have it in childhood or may acquire it later in life as a result of chronic infections and inflammation. Cystic fibrosis is a common cause of bronchiectasis. This abnormal state of the bronchial tubes is permanent. Bronchiectasis causes chronic coughing, which produces thick white or green sputum. A person with this disorder may have recurrent pneumonia and weight loss.

Treatment of bronchiectasis includes controlling infections and preventing complications. Antibiotics may be prescribed. Postural drainage may be ordered to eliminate fluid from the lungs. Postural drainage involves using different body positions to drain mucus from the lungs or to loosen it so that it can be coughed up.

Upper Respiratory Infection (URI)

Upper respiratory infection (URI) is commonly called a cold. It is most often caused by a viral infection of the nose, sinuses, and throat. Symptoms usually include nasal discharge, sneezing, sore throat, fever, and fatigue. For most people, it can be dealt with by the body's immune system and by rest and fluids.

Lung Cancer

Lung cancer is the growth of abnormal cells or tumors in the lungs. Symptoms of lung cancer include chronic cough, shortness of breath, and bloody sputum. More information about cancer is located later in the chapter.

Tuberculosis (TB)

Tuberculosis (TB) is a highly contagious lung disease. Symptoms include coughing, low-grade fever, shortness of breath, weight loss, fatigue, and bloody sputum. Chapter 5 includes more information about tuberculosis, care guidelines, and treatment.

Nursing assistants may need to collect a sputum specimen from residents who have TB. Sputum is thick mucus coughed up from the lungs. It is not the same as saliva, which comes from the mouth. People with colds or respiratory illnesses may cough up large amounts of sputum. Sputum specimens may help diagnose respiratory problems or illness or evaluate the effects of medication.

Early morning is the best time to collect sputum. The resident should cough up the sputum and spit it directly into the specimen container. Because sputum may be infectious, the NA should make sure that the resident does not cough on him. Standing behind the resident during the collection process may prevent sputum from coming into contact with the NA. Proper personal protective equipment (PPE) must be worn when collecting sputum. The required PPE are gloves and a mask. It is important that the NA's hands and the specimen container are clean before beginning this procedure.

Collecting a sputum specimen

Equipment: specimen container with completed label (labeled with resident's name, date of birth, room number, date, and time) and lid, specimen bag, tissues, gloves, N95 or other ordered mask, laboratory slip

1. Identify yourself by name. Identify resident by name.
2. Wash your hands.
3. Explain procedure to resident. Speak clearly, slowly, and directly. Maintain face-to-face contact whenever possible.

4. Provide for resident's privacy with curtain, screen, or door.
5. Put on mask and gloves. Coughing is one way that TB bacilli can enter the air. Stand behind the resident if the resident can hold the specimen container by himself.
6. Ask the resident to cough deeply, so that sputum comes up from the lungs. To prevent the spread of infectious material, give the resident tissues to cover his mouth while coughing. Ask the resident to spit the sputum into the specimen container.
7. When you have obtained a good sample (about two tablespoons of sputum), cover the container tightly. Wipe any sputum off the outside of the container with tissues. Discard the tissues. Apply label, and place the container in a clean specimen bag.
8. Remove and discard gloves and mask.
9. Wash your hands.
10. Place call light within resident's reach.
11. Report any changes in resident to the nurse.
12. Take specimen and lab slip to proper area. Document procedure using facility guidelines.

6. Describe common diseases and disorders of the endocrine system

Diabetes

Diabetes mellitus, commonly called **diabetes**, occurs when the pancreas produces too little insulin or does not properly use insulin. **Insulin** is a hormone that converts **glucose**, or natural sugar, into energy for the body. Without insulin to process glucose, these sugars collect in the blood and cannot get to the cells. This causes problems with circulation and can damage vital organs.

Diabetes is common in people with a family history of the illness, in the elderly, and in people who are obese. Diabetes is a chronic disease that has two major types: type 1 and type 2.

Type 1 diabetes is usually diagnosed in children and young adults. It was formerly known as *juvenile diabetes* because it most often appears before age 20. In type 1 diabetes, the pancreas does not produce any insulin. The condition will continue throughout a person's life. Type 1 diabetes is managed with daily injections of insulin or an insulin pump and a special diet. Regular blood glucose testing must be done.

Type 2 diabetes, also called *adult-onset diabetes*, is the most common form of diabetes. In type 2 diabetes, either the body does not produce enough insulin, or the body fails to properly use insulin. This is known as *insulin resistance*. Type 2 diabetes usually develops slowly and is the milder form of diabetes. It typically develops after age 35; the risk of getting this type increases with age. However, the number of children with type 2 diabetes is growing rapidly. Type 2 diabetes often occurs in obese people or those with a family history of the disease (Fig. 18-24). Type 2 diabetes can usually be controlled with diet and/or oral medications. Blood glucose levels should be tested regularly.

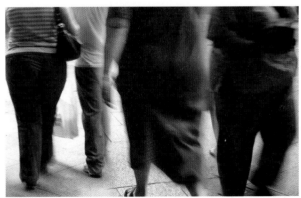

Fig. 18-24. *Being overweight puts a person at risk for type 2 diabetes.*

Pre-diabetes occurs when a person's blood glucose levels are above normal but not high enough for a diagnosis of type 2 diabetes. Research indicates that some damage to the body, especially to the heart and circulatory system, may already be occurring during pre-diabetes.

Pregnant women who have never had diabetes before but who have high blood sugar (glucose) levels during pregnancy are said to have **gestational diabetes**.

People with diabetes may have these signs and symptoms:

- Excessive thirst
- Extreme hunger
- Frequent urination
- Weight loss
- Elevated blood sugar levels
- Glucose (sugar) in the urine
- Sudden vision changes
- Tingling or numbness in hands or feet
- Feeling very tired much of the time
- Very dry skin
- Sores that are slow to heal
- More infections than usual

Diabetes can lead to further complications:

- Changes in the circulatory system can cause heart attack and stroke, reduced circulation to the extremities, poor wound healing, and kidney and nerve damage.
- Damage to the eyes can cause vision loss and blindness.
- Poor circulation and impaired wound healing may cause leg and foot ulcers, infected wounds, and gangrene. Gangrene can lead to amputation.
- Insulin reaction and diabetic ketoacidosis can be serious complications of diabetes. Chapter 7 contains more information.

Diabetes must be carefully controlled to prevent complications and severe illness. When working with people with diabetes, nursing assistants must follow care plan instructions carefully.

Guidelines: Diabetes

G Follow diet instructions exactly. The intake of carbohydrates, including breads, potatoes, grains, pastas, and sugars, must be regulated. Meals must be eaten at the same time each day. The resident must eat all that is served. If a resident will not eat what is served, or if you suspect that he is not following the diet, tell the nurse. More information on diabetic diets is found in Chapter 15.

G Encourage the resident to follow his exercise program. A regular exercise program is important. Exercise affects how quickly bodies use food. Exercise also helps improve circulation. Exercise may include walking or other activities (Fig. 18-25). It may also include passive range of motion exercises. Help with exercises as necessary. Be positive and try to make it fun. A walk can be a chore or it can be the highlight of the day.

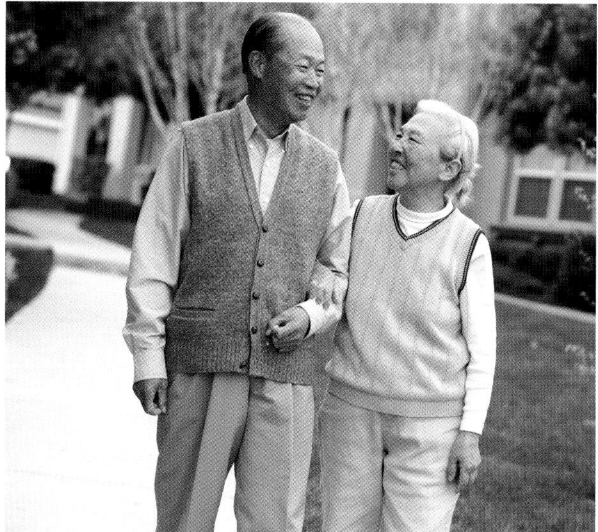

Fig. 18-25. *Exercise is very important for diabetic residents. It helps to increase circulation and maintain a healthy weight.*

G Observe the resident's management of insulin. Doses are calculated exactly. They are given at the same time each day. Nursing assistants are not permitted to inject insulin, but you should know when residents take insulin and when their meals should be served. There must be a balance between the insulin level and food intake.

- G Perform urine and blood tests only as directed. A fingerstick blood glucose test is one type of blood test that may be used to check blood sugar. This is a simple test that is performed by quickly piercing the fingertip, then placing the blood on a chemically active disposable strip. The strip will indicate the result. Another type of test involves using strips, along with a blood glucose meter, a special glucose monitoring machine (Fig. 18-26). Sometimes the care plan will specify a daily blood or urine test for insulin levels. Not all states allow nursing assistants to do this. Know your state's rules. If allowed to assist with this procedure, your facility will provide training for it. Always wear gloves when helping with glucose monitoring. Perform tests only as directed and allowed.

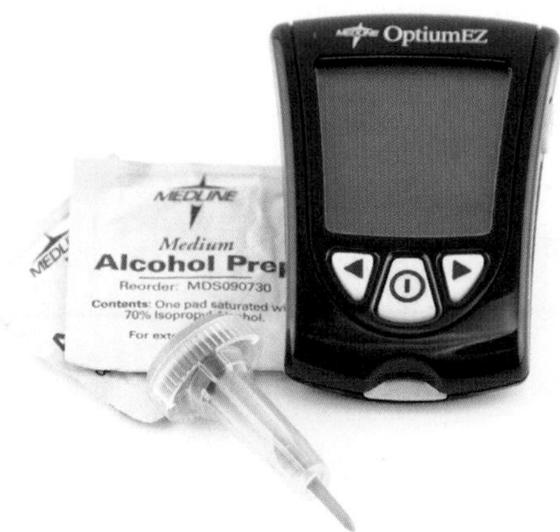

Fig. 18-26. *There are different types of equipment to measure glucose levels in the blood.*

- G Proper foot care is vitally important for people with diabetes. Perform foot care as directed. Because poor circulation occurs in diabetics, even a small sore on the leg or foot can grow into a large wound that may not heal. This can result in amputation. Careful foot care, including regular inspection, is very important (Fig. 18-27). The goals of diabetic foot care are to check for signs of irritation or sores, to promote blood circulation, and to prevent infection.

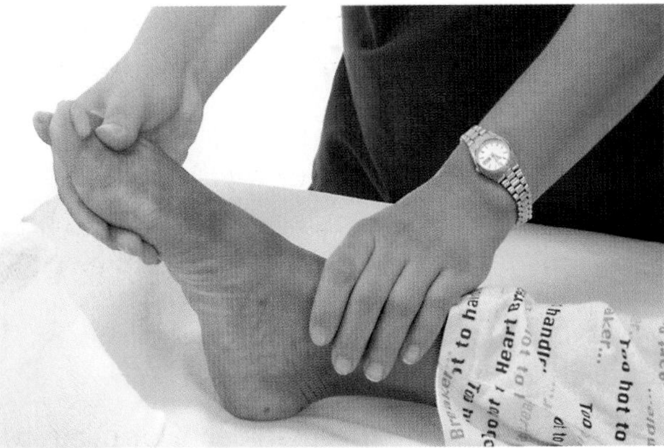

Fig. 18-27. *Observe the legs and feet carefully when giving care. Poor circulation can increase the risk of infection and the loss of toes, feet, or legs to gangrene.*

- G Encourage diabetic residents to wear comfortable, well-fitting leather shoes that do not hurt their feet. Leather shoes breathe and help to prevent build-up of moisture. To avoid injuries to the feet, diabetics should never go barefoot. Cotton socks are best because they absorb sweat. Nursing assistants should never trim or clip any resident's toenails, but especially not a diabetic's toenails. Only a nurse or doctor should do this.

Observing and Reporting: Diabetes

Report any of these to the nurse:

- O/R Any sign of skin breakdown, especially on the feet and toes
- O/R Change in appetite (resident overeating or not eating enough)
- O/R Increased thirst
- O/R Change in urine output
- O/R Nausea or vomiting
- O/R Weight changes
- O/R Change in mental status
- O/R Irritability
- O/R Nervousness or anxiety
- O/R Feeling faint or dizzy
- O/R Visual changes, especially blurred vision
- O/R Change in mobility

- O/R Change in sensation
- O/R Sweet or fruity breath
- O/R Numbness or tingling in arms or legs

Providing foot care for the diabetic resident

Equipment: basin, bath thermometer, mild soap, washcloth, 2 towels, lotion, cotton socks, shoes or slippers, gloves

1. Identify yourself by name. Identify resident by name.
2. Wash your hands.
3. Explain procedure to resident. Speak clearly, slowly, and directly. Maintain face-to-face contact whenever possible.
4. Provide for resident's privacy with curtain, screen, or door.
5. Fill the basin halfway with warm water. Test water temperature with thermometer or against the inside of your wrist. Ensure it is safe. Water temperature should be no higher than 105°F. Have resident check water temperature. Adjust if necessary.
6. Place basin on a bath towel on the floor (if the resident is sitting in a chair) or at the foot of the bed (if the resident is in bed). Make sure basin is in a position that is comfortable for the resident. Support the foot and ankle throughout the procedure.
7. Put on gloves.
8. Remove the resident's socks, and completely submerge the resident's feet in the water. Soak the feet for 10 to 20 minutes.
9. Put soap on a wet washcloth. Remove one foot from the water. Wash the entire foot gently, including between the toes and around nail beds.
10. Rinse the entire foot, including between the toes.
11. Using a towel, pat the foot dry gently, including between the toes.
12. Repeat steps 9 through 11 for other foot.
13. Starting at the toes and working up to the ankles, gently rub lotion into the feet with circular strokes. Your goal is to increase circulation, so take several minutes on each foot. **Do not put lotion between the toes.**
14. Observe the feet, ankles, and legs for dry skin, irritation, blisters, redness, sores, corns, discoloration, or swelling.
15. Help resident put on socks and shoes or slippers.
16. Put soiled linens in appropriate container. Pour water into the toilet and flush it. Place basin in proper area for cleaning or clean and store it according to facility policy. Store supplies.
17. Remove and discard gloves.
18. Wash your hands.
19. Place call light within resident's reach.
20. Report any changes in resident to the nurse.
21. Document procedure using facility guidelines.

Hyperthyroidism

When the thyroid produces too much thyroid hormone, the cells burn too much food. Weight loss, nervousness, and hyperactivity occur. This condition is called **hyperthyroidism**. Hyperthyroidism is usually treated with medication. Occasionally, part of the thyroid is surgically removed.

Hypothyroidism

When the thyroid produces too little thyroid hormone, body processes slow down. Weight gain and physical and mental sluggishness result. This condition is called **hypothyroidism**. Hypothyroidism is sometimes treated with medication.

7. Describe common diseases and disorders of the reproductive system

Sexually-Transmitted Infections (STIs)

Sexually-transmitted infections (STIs), formerly referred to as sexually-transmitted diseases (STDs), are caused by sexual contact with infected people. This contact includes sexual intercourse (vaginal and anal), contact of the mouth with the genitals or anus, and contact of the hands with the genital area.

Sexually-transmitted infections cause a variety of symptoms and health problems, which are detailed below. Using latex condoms during sexual contact can reduce the chances of being infected with or transmitting some STIs (Fig. 18-28). The human immunodeficiency virus (HIV) and some kinds of hepatitis can be sexually transmitted. (HIV and AIDS are discussed in detail in the next learning objective.) STIs are very common. Residents may be unaware of or embarrassed by symptoms of an STI.

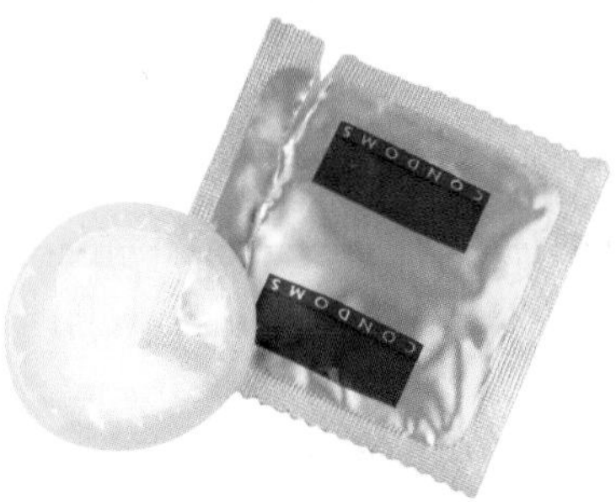

Fig. 18-28. Latex condoms reduce a person's risk of being infected with or transmitting some sexually-transmitted infections.

Chlamydia infection is caused by organisms introduced into the mucous membranes of the reproductive tract. Chlamydia can cause serious infection, including pelvic inflammatory disease (PID) in women. PID can lead to sterility. Signs and symptoms of chlamydia infection include yellow or white discharge from the penis or vagina, burning during urination, swelling of the testes, painful intercourse, and abdominal and low back pain. Chlamydia is treated with antibiotics.

Syphilis is caused by bacteria. It can be treated effectively in the early stages, but if left untreated, it can cause brain damage, mental illness, and even death. Babies born to mothers infected with syphilis may be born blind or with other serious birth defects. Syphilis is easier to detect in men than in women. This is due to open sores called **chancres** that form on the penis soon after infection. In women, these sores may form inside the vagina.

However, the chancres are painless and can go unnoticed. If untreated, the infection progresses to the heart, brain, and other vital organs. Common symptoms at this stage include rash, sore throat, or fever. When detected, syphilis can be treated with penicillin or other antibiotics. The sooner the disease is treated, the better the person's chances of preventing long-term consequences and avoiding infection of sexual partners.

Gonorrhea is caused by bacteria. It, like syphilis, is easier to detect in men than in women because many women with gonorrhea show no early symptoms. This makes it easy for women to spread the disease. Men infected with gonorrhea will typically show a greenish or yellowish discharge from the penis within a week after infection. Painful or swollen testes and burning during urination are other common symptoms in men. If untreated, gonorrhea can cause blindness, joint infection, and sterility in both men and women. Gonorrhea is treated with antibiotics.

Genital herpes, unlike the other STIs discussed here, is caused by a virus—herpes simplex virus type 1 (HSV-1) or type 2 (HSV-2). HSV-2 is generally the cause of genital herpes. Genital herpes cannot be treated with antibiotics, nor can it be cured. Once infected with genital herpes, a person may suffer repeated outbreaks of the disease for the rest of his or her life. A herpes outbreak includes burning, painful, red sores on the genitals that heal in about two weeks. The sores are infectious, but a person with genital herpes can spread the infection even when sores are not present.

Some people infected with genital herpes never experience repeated outbreaks. The later episodes may not be as painful as the initial outbreak. Treatment with antiviral medication can help people stay symptom-free for longer periods of time. The medication can also help lessen the duration and intensity of the episodes. Babies born to women infected with genital herpes can be infected during birth. If a pregnant woman is experiencing an outbreak, the baby is usually delivered by Cesarean section, or C-section.

The human immunodeficiency virus (HIV) can be transmitted sexually as well and is discussed in the next learning objective.

Benign Prostatic Hypertrophy

Benign prostatic hypertrophy (BPH) is a disorder that occurs in men as they age. The prostate becomes enlarged and causes pressure on the urethra. The pressure leads to frequent urination, dribbling of urine, and difficulty in starting the flow of urine. Urinary retention (urine remaining in the bladder) may also occur, causing urinary tract infections. Urine can also back up into the ureters and kidneys, causing damage to these organs. Benign prostatic hypertrophy can be treated with medications or surgery. A test is also available to screen for cancer of the prostate. As men age, they are at increased risk for prostate cancer. Prostate cancer is usually slow-growing and responsive to treatment if detected early.

Vaginitis

Vaginitis is an inflammation of the vagina. It may be caused by a bacteria, protozoa (one-celled animals), or fungus (yeast). Bacterial vaginosis occurs when there is an overgrowth of normal bacteria inside the vagina. Yeast infections are caused by an overproduction of a fungus called *Candida albicans*. Vaginitis may also be the result of hormonal changes after menopause. Women who have vaginitis have a white vaginal discharge, accompanied by itching and burning. Treatment of vaginitis includes oral medications, as well as vaginal creams or suppositories.

8. Describe common diseases and disorders of the immune and lymphatic systems

Acquired Immune Deficiency Syndrome (AIDS)

Acquired immune deficiency syndrome (AIDS) is a disease caused by the human immunodeficiency virus (HIV). HIV attacks the body's immune system and gradually weakens and disables it. AIDS is caused by acquiring the HIV virus through blood or body fluids from an infected person. AIDS is the final stage of HIV infection in which infections, tumors, and central nervous system symptoms appear due to a weakened immune system that is unable to fight infection. It can take years for HIV to develop into AIDS.

HIV is a sexually-transmitted disease. It can also be spread through the blood, from infected needles, or to a fetus from its mother.

In general, HIV affects the body in stages. The first stage involves symptoms similar to the flu, with fever, muscle aches, cough, and fatigue. These symptoms indicate that the immune system is fighting the infection. As the infection worsens, the immune system overreacts and attacks not only the virus, but also normal tissue.

When the virus weakens the immune system in later stages, a group of problems may appear. These include opportunistic infections, tumors, and central nervous system symptoms that would not occur if the immune system were healthy. This stage of the disease is known as AIDS. The diagnosis of AIDS is made when a person's CD4+ lymphocyte (a type of white blood cell) count falls to 200 or below.

In the late stages of AIDS, damage to the central nervous system may cause memory loss, poor coordination, paralysis, and confusion. These symptoms together are known as **AIDS dementia complex**.

The following are signs and symptoms of HIV infection and AIDS:

- Flu-like symptoms, including fever, cough, weakness, and severe or constant fatigue
- Appetite loss
- Weight loss
- Night sweats
- Swollen lymph nodes in the neck, underarms, or groin
- Severe diarrhea
- Dry cough
- Skin rashes
- Painful white spots in the mouth or on the tongue
- Cold sores or fever blisters on the lips and flat, white ulcers on a reddened base in the mouth
- Cauliflower-like warts (caused by the human papilloma virus) on the skin and in the mouth
- Inflamed and bleeding gums
- Bruising that does not go away
- Low resistance to infection, particularly pneumonia, but also tuberculosis, herpes, bacterial infections, and hepatitis
- **Kaposi's sarcoma**, a rare form of skin cancer that appears as purple, red, or brown skin lesions
- Pneumocystis pneumonia, a lung infection
- AIDS dementia complex

Opportunistic infections, such as pneumonia, tuberculosis, or hepatitis, invade the body because the immune system is weak and cannot defend itself. These illnesses complicate AIDS. They further weaken the immune system. It is difficult to treat these infections because generally, over time, a person with AIDS develops resistance to some antibiotics. These infections can cause death in people with AIDS.

There is no cure for this disease, and there is no vaccine to prevent the disease. People who are infected with HIV are treated with drugs that slow the progress of the disease. Without medication, however, the HIV-infected person's weakened resistance to infections may lead to AIDS and eventually to death.

A combination of medications can help people with HIV live longer. The medicines must be taken at precise times. They have many unpleasant side effects. For some people, the medications work less well than for others. Other aspects of HIV treatment include relief of symptoms and prevention and treatment of infection.

Behaviors that put people at high risk for HIV infection/AIDS include the following:

- Sharing drug needles
- Having unprotected or poorly-protected oral, vaginal, or anal sex with an infected person
- Sexual contact with many partners
- Any sexual activity that involves exchange of body fluids with a partner who has not tested negative for HIV or who has had many sexual partners

Ways to protect against the spread of HIV and AIDS include the following:

- Never sharing needles or syringes
- Not having unprotected sex and using condoms during sexual contact
- Staying in a monogamous relationship (being monogamous means having only one sexual partner)
- Practicing abstinence (abstinence means not having sexual contact with anyone)
- Getting tested for HIV and re-tested if necessary (HIV can be detected in most people within two to eight weeks. However, it may take up to three months for HIV to be detectable and up to six months in rare cases. It is especially important that pregnant women get tested.)
- Following Standard Precautions at work

Residents' Rights

The Facts about HIV and AIDS

A handshake or a hug cannot spread the HIV virus. The disease cannot be transmitted by telephones, doorknobs, tables, chairs, toilets, mosquitoes, or by breathing the same air as an infected person. NAs should spend time with residents who have HIV or AIDS and not ignore or avoid them. These residents need the same thoughtful, personal attention that NAs give to all their residents.

Guidelines: HIV/AIDS

- G People with poor immune system function are more sensitive to infections. Wash your hands often and keep everything clean. Follow Standard Precautions.
- G Involuntary weight loss occurs in almost all people who develop AIDS. High-protein, high-calorie, and high-nutrient meals can help maintain a healthy weight.
- G Some people with HIV/AIDS lose their appetites and have difficulty eating. These residents should be encouraged to relax before meals and to eat in a pleasant setting. Familiar and favorite foods should be served. Report appetite loss or difficulty eating to the nurse. If appetite loss continues to be a problem, the doctor may prescribe an appetite stimulant.
- G Residents with infections of the mouth and esophagus may need food that is low in acid and neither cold nor hot. Spicy seasonings should be removed. Soft or pureed foods may be easier to swallow. Drinking liquid meals and fortified drinks, such as milk shakes, may ease the pain of chewing. Warm rinses may help painful sores of the mouth. Careful mouth care is vital.
- G A person who has nausea or vomiting should eat small, frequent meals if possible. The person should eat slowly. The person should avoid high-fat and spicy foods and eat a soft, bland diet. When nausea and vomiting persist, liquids and salty foods should be encouraged. Residents should drink fluids in between meals. Care must be taken to maintain proper intake of fluids to balance lost fluids.
- G Residents who have mild diarrhea may have small, frequent meals that are low in fat, fiber, and milk products. If diarrhea is severe, the doctor may order a BRAT diet (a diet of bananas, rice, applesauce, and toast). This diet is helpful for short-term use.
- G Diarrhea rapidly depletes the body of fluids. Fluid replacement is necessary. Good rehydration fluids include water, juice, caffeine-free soda, and broth. Caffeinated drinks should be avoided.
- G **Neuropathy**, or numbness, tingling, and pain in the feet and legs is usually treated with pain medications. Going barefoot or wearing loose, soft slippers may be helpful. If blankets and sheets cause pain, a bed cradle can keep sheets and blankets from resting on legs and feet (Fig. 18-29).

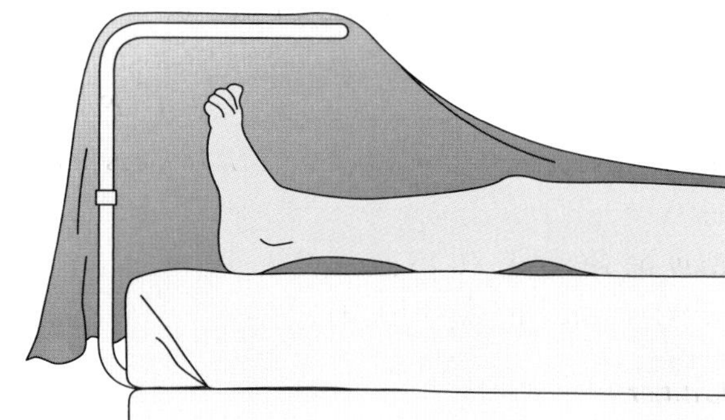

Fig. 18-29. *A bed cradle helps keep covers from resting on the feet.*

- G Give emotional support, as well as physical care. Residents with HIV/AIDS may suffer from anxiety and depression. In addition, they often suffer the judgments of family, friends, and society. Some people avoid a person with AIDS due to homophobia, or a fear of homosexuality. Some people blame the person for his or her illness. People with HIV/AIDS may feel tremendous stress. They may feel uncertainty about their illness, health care, and finances. They may also have lost friends who have died from AIDS. Treat residents with respect and help provide the emotional support they need.

Residents with this disease need support from others. This support may come from family, friends, religious and community groups, and support groups, as well as the care team. Report to the nurse if you feel that residents need more resources and services.

G Withdrawal, apathy, avoidance of tasks, and mental slowness are early symptoms of HIV infection. Medications may also cause side effects of this type. AIDS dementia complex may develop, causing further mental problems. There may also be muscle weakness and loss of muscle control, making falls a risk. Residents in this stage of the disease will need a safe environment and close supervision in their ADLs.

The right to confidentiality is especially important to people with HIV/AIDS. Others may pass judgment on people with this disease. HIV test results are confidential and cannot be shared with a person's family, friends, or employer without his consent. A person with HIV/AIDS cannot be fired from a job because of the disease. However, a healthcare worker with HIV/AIDS may be reassigned to job duties with a lower risk of transmitting the disease.

Cancer

Cancer is a general term used to describe a disease in which abnormal cells grow in an uncontrolled way. Cancer usually occurs in the form of a tumor or tumors growing on or within the body. A **tumor** is a cluster of abnormally-growing cells. **Benign tumors** are considered non-cancerous. They usually grow slowly in local areas. **Malignant tumors** are cancerous. They grow rapidly and invade surrounding tissues.

Cancer invades local tissue and can spread to other parts of the body. When cancer spreads from the site where it first appeared (metastasizes), it can affect other body systems. In general, treatment is more difficult, and cancer is more deadly after this has occurred. Cancer often appears first in the breast, colon, rectum, uterus, prostate, lungs, or skin.

There is no known cure for cancer. However, some treatments are effective. They are discussed later in the chapter.

Risk factors for cancer include the following:

- Age
- Race
- Gender
- Family history
- Tobacco use
- Alcohol use
- Poor diet/obesity
- Lack of physical activity
- Chemicals and food additives
- Radiation
- Exposure to sunlight (Fig. 18-30)

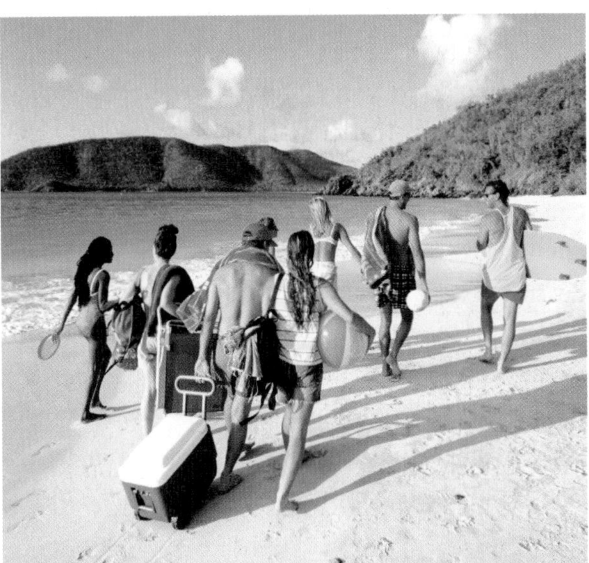

Fig. 18-30. *Prolonged sun exposure puts a person at risk for skin cancer.*

When diagnosed early, cancer can often be treated and controlled. The American Cancer Society has identified some warning signs of cancer:

- Unexplained weight loss

- Fever
- Fatigue
- Pain
- Skin changes
- Change in bowel or bladder function
- Sores that do not heal
- Unusual bleeding or discharge
- Thickening or lump in the breast, scrotum, or other parts of the body
- Indigestion or difficulty swallowing
- New mole or recent change in appearance of a mole or wart
- Nagging cough or hoarseness

People with cancer can live longer and sometimes recover when treated using the following methods. These treatments are most effective when tumors are discovered early. Often these treatments are combined.

Surgery is the front line of defense for most forms of cancer. It is the key treatment for malignant tumors of the skin, breast, bladder, colon, rectum, stomach, and muscle. Surgeons attempt to remove as much of the tumor as possible to prevent cancer from spreading.

Chemotherapy refers to medications given, usually intravenously, to fight cancer. Certain drugs destroy cancer cells and limit the rate of cell growth. However, many of these drugs are toxic to the body. They destroy healthy cells as well as cancer cells. Chemotherapy can have severe side effects, including nausea, vomiting, diarrhea, hair loss, fatigue, and decreased resistance to infection.

Radiation therapy directs radiation to a limited area to kill cancer cells. However, normal or healthy cells in the radiation's path are also destroyed (Fig. 18-31). By controlling cell growth, radiation can reduce pain. Radiation can cause the same side effects as chemotherapy. The skin of the area exposed to radiation may become sore, irritated, and sometimes burned.

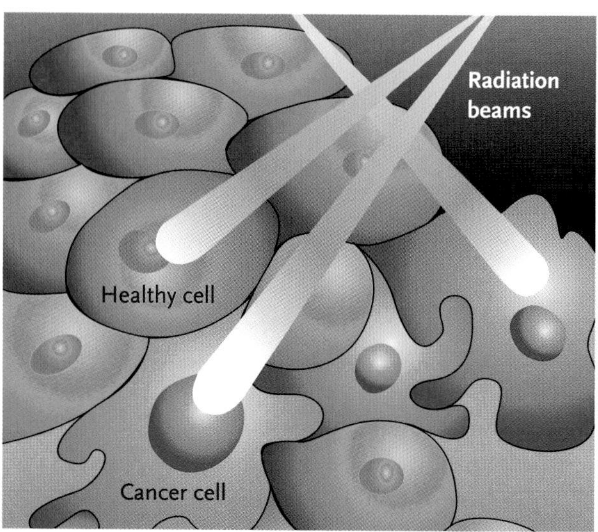

Fig. 18-31. *Radiation is targeted at cancer cells, but it also destroys some healthy cells in its path.*

Guidelines: Cancer

G Each case is different. Cancer is a general term and refers to many separate situations. Residents may expect to live many years or only several months. Treatment affects each person differently. Do not make assumptions about a resident's condition.

G Residents may want to talk or may avoid talking. Respect each resident's needs. Listen if a resident wants to share feelings or experiences with you. However, never push a resident to talk. Be honest. Never tell a resident, "Everything will be okay." Be sensitive. Remember that cancer is a disease, and its cause is unknown. Maintain a positive attitude and focus on concrete details. For example, comment if a resident seems stronger, or mention that the sun is shining outside.

G Proper nutrition is important for residents with cancer. Follow the care plan carefully. Residents frequently have poor appetites. Encourage a variety of food and small portions. Liquid nutrition supplements may be used in addition to, not in place of, meals. If nausea or swallowing is a problem, foods such as soups, gelatins, or starches may appeal to the resident. Use plastic utensils for a resident receiving chemotherapy. It makes food taste better. Metal utensils cause a bitter taste.

- **G** Cancer can cause great pain, especially in the late stages. Watch your resident for signs of pain. Report them to the nurse. Help with comfort measures, such as repositioning and providing distractions, such as conversation, music, or reading materials (Fig. 18-32). Report to the nurse if pain seems to be uncontrolled.

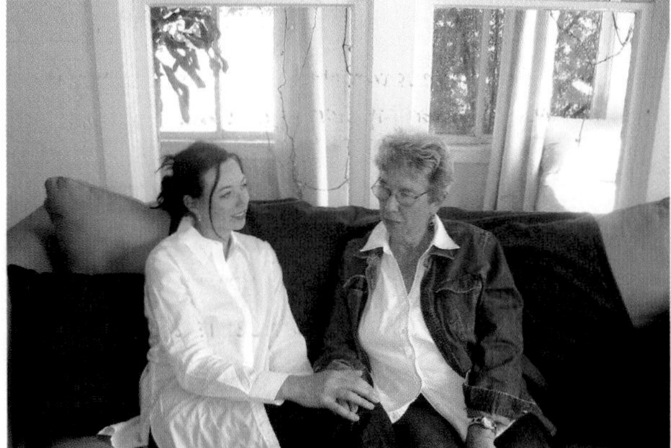

Fig. 18-32. *Give residents with cancer as much emotional support as possible. Distractions such as conversation can help a person deal with pain.*

- **G** Offer back rubs to provide comfort and increase circulation. For residents who spend many hours in bed, moving to a chair for some period of time may improve comfort as well. Residents who are very weak or immobile need to be repositioned at least every two hours.
- **G** Use lotion regularly on dry or delicate skin. Do not apply lotion to areas receiving radiation therapy. Do not remove markings that are used in radiation therapy. Follow any skin care orders (for example: no hot or cold packs, no soap or cosmetics, no tight stockings).
- **G** Help residents brush and floss teeth regularly. Medications, nausea, vomiting, or mouth infections may cause pain and a bad taste in the mouth. You can help ease discomfort by using a soft-bristled toothbrush, rinsing with baking soda and water, or using a prescribed rinse. Do not use a commercial mouthwash if it has alcohol in it. Alcohol in mouthwash can further irritate a resident's mouth. For residents with mouth sores, using oral swabs rather than toothbrushes may be preferable. The swabs can be dipped in a rinse and gently wiped across the gums. Mouth sores can make oral care very painful; be very gentle when giving residents oral care.
- **G** People with cancer may suffer from poor self-image because they are weak and their appearance has changed. For example, hair loss is a common side effect of chemotherapy. Assist with grooming if desired. Your concern and interest can help improve self-image.
- **G** If visitors help cheer your resident, encourage them and do not intrude. If some times of day are better than others, suggest this to visitors. Support groups exist for people with cancer and their families. Check with the nurse for groups in your area. It may help a person with cancer to think of something besides cancer and treatment for a while. Pursue other topics. Get to know what interests your residents have. As always, report any signs of depression immediately.
- **G** Having a family member with cancer can be very difficult. Be alert to needs that are not being met or stresses created by the illness.

Observing and Reporting: Cancer

Report any of these to the nurse:

- O/R Increased weakness or fatigue
- O/R Weight loss
- O/R Nausea, vomiting, or diarrhea
- O/R Changes in appetite
- O/R Fainting
- O/R Signs of depression (Chapter 20)
- O/R Confusion

- O/R Blood in stool or urine
- O/R Change in mental status
- O/R Changes in skin
- O/R New lumps, sores, or rashes
- O/R Increase in pain, or unrelieved pain
- O/R Blood in the mouth

Care after a Mastectomy

A **mastectomy** is the surgical removal of all or part of the breast and sometimes other surrounding tissue. This operation is usually performed because of a tumor.

After a mastectomy, the care plan may include arm exercises for the side of the body on which the surgery was performed. The goal of arm exercises is to strengthen the arm and chest muscles and reduce swelling in the arm and underarm. Exercises may include raising the arm, opening and closing the hand, and bending and straightening the elbow. The resident should wear loose, comfortable clothing while doing any arm exercises.

Nursing assistants should follow the care plan and the nurse's instructions regarding care after a mastectomy. Instructions may include keeping the arm on the affected side raised on pillows to decrease swelling. The resident may use a sling to keep the arm elevated. In addition, deep breathing exercises may be ordered.

9. Identify community resources for residents who are ill

Numerous services and support groups are available for people who are ill and their families or caregivers. These resources can help them through difficult times and help solve problems. Social service agencies, hospitals, hospice programs, churches, and synagogues offer many resources. These include meal services, transportation to doctors' offices or hospitals, counseling, and support groups.

For cancer, a person can visit the American Cancer Society's website at cancer.org or call the local or state chapter. The National Association of Area Agencies on Aging, n4a.org, operates the Eldercare Locator, which is a free national service that links older adults and caregivers to aging information and resources in their own communities.

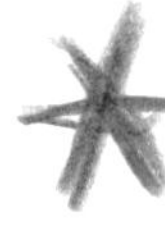

Depending on the community, many resources and services may be available for people with HIV/AIDS. These may include counseling, meal services, access to experimental drugs, and any number of other services. Some online resources for people with HIV or AIDS include the following: aids.gov, cdc.gov/hiv, and aidsinfo.nih.gov.

Chapter Review

1. What is an acute illness? What is a chronic illness?
2. What are signs and symptoms of scabies? How is scabies spread?
3. What causes shingles?
4. What is an open wound? What is a closed wound?
5. What is dermatitis and how does it generally look?
6. What can cause fungal infections?
7. What causes arthritis?
8. What health problems can anti-inflammatory medications cause?
9. What can happen to bones when they are brittle?
10. What can a nursing assistant do to prevent or slow osteoporosis?
11. Why should casts not be covered until they are dry?
12. What type of surface can a cast be placed on?
13. Why should extremities in casts be elevated?
14. Why is a hip fracture a serious condition for an elderly person?
15. When dressing a person who has just had a hip replacement, which side should be dressed first: the affected/weaker side or the unaffected/stronger side?

16. What is the difference between partial weight-bearing (PWB) and non-weight-bearing (NWB)? PWB weight on good foot & gently on affected. NWB – No weight on any foot.

17. List reasons that knee replacements are performed. Knee is bad, injured by accident, birth defect, arthritis. Person can't walk right.

18. List three physical problems that muscular dystrophy can cause. Muscles are weak. There may be twitching of hands or arm. Legs weak & stiff. Wheelchair needed.

19. What is phantom limb pain? What is phantom sensation? Pain is felt in limb that has been removed. The removed body part still feels there.

20. What causes a CVA (stroke)? when blood supply to the brain is blocked or blood leaks into brain tissue, damaging it.

21. What terms should an NA use to refer to the weaker side of a person who has had a stroke? The affected area or involved are. The weaked side. DO NOT USE "BAD" side.

22. When helping a resident who has had a stroke with transfers or walking, on which side should an NA stand—the weaker or stronger side? Use gait belt for safety.

23. When dressing a resident with a one-sided weakness, which side should an NA dress first? The weak side. when undressing go to strong side 1st.

24. In which side of the mouth should food be placed if a resident has a one-sided weakness? Put food in the unaffected side 1st. The non paralyzed side.

25. Why may people with Parkinson's disease have trouble eating and bathing themselves? Muscles are stiff, tremors & shaking. Fingers move involuntary in pill-rolling fashion.

26. List six care guidelines for a person with multiple sclerosis. 1) Be patient. Everything takes longer. 2) Listen carefully as people have trouble expressing their thoughts 3) Do all to prevent falls 4) Diet & encourage fluids 5) Give good skin care 6) Help range of motion exercises.

27. What is paraplegia? What is quadriplegia? Partial paralysis 2 extremities. Quad - All four extremities paralyzed

28. What consistent blood pressure measurement is classified as hypertension? above 140/90 or above

29. List three care guidelines for a resident with angina pectoris. Make sure they rest. Give Nitroglycerin if needed & you are trained to give it. No heavy meals or Extreme exercise. No exposure to extreme heat or cold.

30. List two care guidelines for a resident recovering from a myocardial infarction. Encourage to follow exercise routines. Encourage following diet plans. Help them manage stress. Avoid cold.

31. List seven care guidelines for a resident who has congestive heart failure. ① Answer call lights, keep comode near ② Encourge following diet & drink restrictions ③ Rest after activity ④ Watch fluid intake ⑤ weigh Daily. watch weight. ⑥ Apply stocking if ordered ⑦ Help ROM

32. At what time of day should elastic stockings be put on? Mornings

33. What is a constant fear that a resident with chronic obstructive pulmonary disease (COPD) may have? They fear that they are suffacating and have lost control of their bodies.

34. What is a position that a resident with COPD may prefer to be in? sitting upright and slightly bent forward.

35. What are two causes of emphysema? ① Chronic bronchitis ② smoking

36. How is asthma treated? Medication given directly into lungs. Avoid anything that triggers it.

37. How is bronchiectasis treated? Control infections. Use postural drainage, Meds. Cough up mucus

38. When is the best time of day to collect a sputum specimen? Early Morning.

39. Briefly describe the two major types of diabetes. Type 1 diabetes is inherited. Usually in children & young adults. Type 2 is slowly acquired. Insilin resistance. Obesity. Body not producing enough insulin

40. Why is careful foot care especially important for a resident with diabetes? It's related to poor circulation in the extremities. Small sores can get big & lead to amputation. Gangerene

41. Why is it important for an NA to follow diet instructions exactly for a diabetic resident? The insulin must be regulated & it all depends on carb input.

42. What types of sexual contact can transmit a sexually-transmitted infection (STI)? contact with mucus membranes of infected people & blood too.

43. How is human immunodeficiency virus (HIV) spread? Through sexual intercourse, oral, anal, etc. By a person with a cut in their hand touching the areas of mucus contact. Ex: Dentist

44. Which stage of HIV infection is acquired immune deficiency syndrome (AIDS)? The final stage of the aquired immune deficiency disease

45. Because people who have HIV/AIDS are sensitive to infections, what should the nursing assistant do? Try to prevent the spread of the infection. Keep everything clean. Give high calarie & nutrient meals. Report appetite loss. Encourage Drinking. Give emotional support

46. Is it possible for a person to get AIDS by breathing the same air as an infected person? No. It is passed on by direct contact

47. What are some things that should be done when a person with HIV/AIDS loses his or her appetite and has difficulty eating? Relax before meals. Eat in pleasant setting. Familiar foods.

48. What is a tumor? A tumor is a cluster of abnormally growing cells in an uncontrolled way.

49. List the risk factors for cancer. AGE RACE GENDER FAMILY HISTORY TOBACCO ALCOHOL OBESITY POOR DIET CHEMICALS RADIATION SUNLIGHT

50. What are the side effects of chemotherapy and radiation? They destroy healthy cells along with bad cells. The side effects can be nausea, vomiting, diarrhea, hairloss, fatigue, resistance to infection. Burnin of skin with radiation.

51. List ten signs and symptoms that a nursing assistant should observe and report about cancer. 1) Increased weakness or fatigue 2) weight loss 3) Nausea, vomiting or diarrhea. 4) change in appetite 5) fainting 6) Depression 7) confusion 8) Blood in stool or urine 9) Change in mental status 10) Change in skin 11) new lumps, sores or rashes 12) Increased pain 13) Blood in mouth.

19 Confusion, Dementia, and Alzheimer's Disease

1. Describe normal changes of aging in the brain

As a person ages, some of the ability to think logically and clearly may be lost. This ability is called **cognition**. When some of this ability is lost, a person is said to have **cognitive impairment**. How much ability is lost depends on the individual. Cognitive impairment affects concentration and memory. Elderly residents may lose their memories of recent events, which can be frustrating for them. Nursing assistants can help by encouraging them to make lists of things to remember and writing down names, events, and phone numbers. Other normal changes of aging in the brain include slower reaction time, difficulty finding or using the right words, and sleeping less.

2. Discuss confusion and delirium

Confusion is the inability to think clearly. A confused person has trouble focusing his attention and may feel disoriented. Confusion interferes with the ability to make decisions. The person's personality may change. He may not know his name, the date, other people, or where he is. A confused person may be angry, depressed, or irritable.

Confusion may come on suddenly or gradually. It can be temporary or permanent. Confusion is more common in the elderly. It may occur when a person is in the hospital.

Common causes of confusion include the following:

- Urinary tract infection (UTI)
- Low blood sugar
- Head trauma or head injury
- Dehydration
- Nutritional problems
- Fever
- Sudden drop in body temperature
- Lack of oxygen
- Medications
- Infections
- Brain tumor
- Illness
- Loss of sleep
- Seizures

Guidelines: Confusion

- G Do not leave a confused resident alone.
- G Stay calm. Provide a quiet environment.
- G Speak in a lower tone of voice. Speak clearly and slowly.
- G Introduce yourself each time you see the resident.
- G Remind the resident of his or her location, name, and the date. A calendar can help.
- G Explain what you are going to do, using simple instructions.

- Do not rush the resident.
- Talk to confused residents about plans for the day. Keeping a routine may help.
- Encourage the use of eyeglasses and hearing aids. Make sure they are clean and are not damaged.
- Promote self-care and independence.
- Report observations to the nurse.

Delirium is a state of severe confusion that occurs suddenly; it is usually temporary. Possible causes include infections, disease, fluid imbalances, and poor nutrition. Drugs and alcohol may also cause delirium. Signs and symptoms of delirium include the following:

- Agitation
- Anger
- Depression
- Irritability
- Disorientation
- Trouble focusing
- Problems with speech
- Changes in sensation and perception
- Changes in consciousness
- Decrease in short-term memory

Nursing assistants should report these signs and symptoms to the nurse. The goal of treatment is to control or reverse the cause. Emergency care may be needed, as well as a stay in a hospital.

Confusion and Delirium

When communicating with a person who is confused or disoriented, the nursing assistant should

- Keep her voice low
- Not raise her voice or shout
- Use the person's name, and speak clearly in simple sentences
- Use facial expressions and body language to aid in understanding
- Reduce distractions in the environment by taking action, such as turning down the TV.
- Be gentle and try to decrease fears

3. Describe dementia and define related terms

Dementia is a general term that refers to a serious loss of mental abilities such as thinking, remembering, reasoning, and communicating. As dementia advances, these losses make it difficult to perform ADLs such as eating, bathing, dressing, and toileting. Dementia is not a normal part of aging (Fig. 19-1).

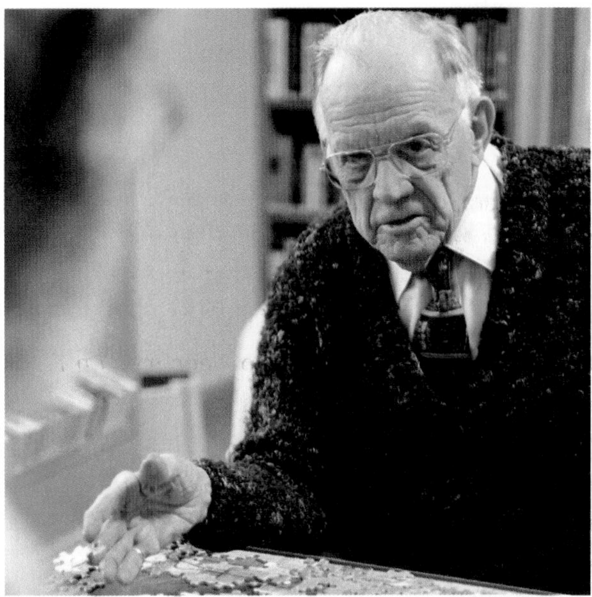

Fig. 19-1. Some loss of cognitive ability is normal; however, dementia is not a normal part of aging.

Here are some terms that are related to dementia:

Progressive: Once they begin, progressive diseases advance. They tend to spread to other parts of the body and affect many body functions.

Degenerative: Degenerative diseases get continually worse. They eventually cause a breakdown of body systems. They cause a greater and greater loss of mental and physical health and abilities. Degenerative diseases can cause death.

Onset: The onset of a disease is the time the signs and symptoms begin.

Irreversible: An irreversible disease or condition cannot be cured. Someone with irreversible dementia (like Alzheimer's disease) will either die from the disease or die with the disease.

The following are a few of the common causes of dementia:

- Alzheimer's disease
- Multi-infarct or vascular dementia (a series of strokes causing damage to the brain)
- Lewy body dementia (abnormal structures, called Lewy bodies, develop in areas of the brain, causing a variety of symptoms)
- Parkinson's disease
- Huntington's disease (an inherited disease that causes certain nerve cells in the brain to waste away)

A diagnosis of dementia involves getting a patient's medical history and having a physical examination, as well as a neurological exam. Blood tests and imaging tests (CT or MRI scan, for example) may be ordered. Electroencephalography (EEG), a test using electrodes on the scalp to trace brain wave activity, may be performed. Diagnosis is a process of ruling out other possible diseases that mimic symptoms of dementia.

4. Describe Alzheimer's disease and identify its stages

Alzheimer's disease (AD) is the most common cause of dementia in the elderly. The Alzheimer's Association (alz.org) estimates that as many as 5.4 million Americans are living with Alzheimer's disease. One in eight older Americans has Alzheimer's disease. Women are more likely than men to have Alzheimer's disease and dementia. The risk of getting AD increases with age, but it is not a normal part of aging.

Alzheimer's disease is a progressive, degenerative, and irreversible disease. AD causes tangled nerve fibers and protein deposits to form in the brain, eventually causing dementia. There is no known cause of AD, and there is no cure. Diagnosis is difficult, involving many physical and mental tests to rule out other causes. However, the only sure way to determine AD at this time is by autopsy. The length of time it takes AD to progress from onset to death varies greatly. It may take anywhere from three to 20 years.

Symptoms of AD appear gradually. It generally begins with memory loss. As the disease progresses, the symptoms get worse. People with AD may get disoriented. They may be confused about time and place. Communication problems are common. They may lose their ability to read, write, speak, or understand. Mood and behavior change. Aggressiveness, wandering, and withdrawal are all part of AD. Alzheimer's disease progresses to complete loss of all ability to care for oneself. The person eventually requires constant care in most cases.

Each person with Alzheimer's disease will show different signs at different times. For example, one resident with Alzheimer's disease may continue to read, but not be able to use the phone. Another may lose the ability to read, but can still do simple math. Skills a person has used often over a lifetime are usually kept longer. Thus some people with Alzheimer's disease can play an instrument with some help long after they have lost much of their memory (Fig. 19-2).

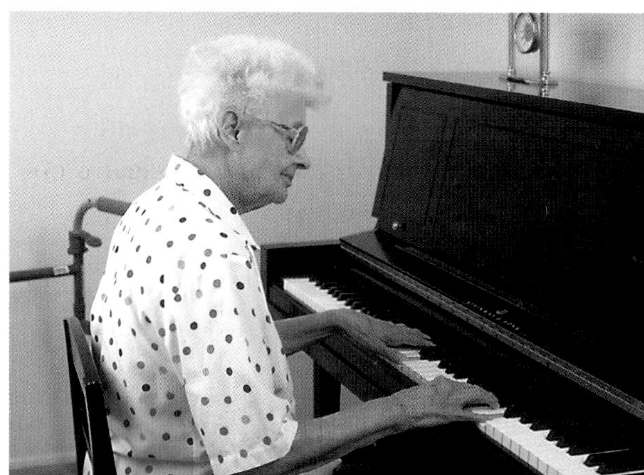

Fig. 19-2. *Even when a person loses much of her memory, she may still keep skills she has used her whole life.*

Alzheimer's disease generally progresses in stages. The Alzheimer's Association identifies seven general stages of Alzheimer's disease, based on a system developed by Barry Reisberg, MD:

Stage 1 - No impairment: At this stage, the person does not show problems with memory loss or other symptoms. No signs of impairment are found during a medical examination.

Stage 2 - Very mild decline: At this stage, the person has mild cognitive loss, which could be due to normal changes of aging or could be the earliest signs of Alzheimer's disease. There may be some memory loss, and the person forgets some words and the location of familiar objects. However, the person's medical examination does not show symptoms, and friends and family members do not notice any symptoms.

Stage 3 - Mild decline: During this stage, people close to the person begin to notice some changes. A medical examination may show problems with memory and concentration. Other problems in this stage include the following:

- Difficulty finding the right word or name
- Trouble remembering peoples' names
- Having a harder time functioning in social and work environments
- Forgetting material that one has just read
- Losing or misplacing objects
- Difficulty with planning or organizing

Stage 4 - Moderate decline: At this stage, the person's medical examination shows clear problems, such as the following:

- Forgetting recent events
- Problems doing more complex arithmetic
- Trouble performing more involved tasks, such as managing finances
- Forgetting some of one's own past experiences and background
- Being moody or withdrawn

Stage 5 - Moderately severe decline: At this stage, cognitive impairment is noticeable. The person starts to need help with some daily activities. Symptoms include the following:

- Inability to recall one's own address, phone number, and other personal details
- Confusion about time and place
- Problems doing less complex arithmetic
- Needing help with some ADLs, such as choosing clothing appropriately

However, the person can often remember many important personal details and usually does not require help with other ADLs, like eating or toileting.

Stage 6 - Severe decline: During this stage, memory loss and other problems worsen. More help is needed with daily activities. Symptoms include the following:

- Forgetting recent events, as well as not being aware of surroundings
- Forgetting one's own past experiences and background (may be able to remember name)
- Having trouble recalling the name of a family member, close friend, or caregiver
- Needing more help with ADLs, such as dressing and toileting
- Trouble controlling bladder or bowels
- Having disruptions in sleep patterns
- Experiencing significant changes in personality and behavior (having delusions, being suspicious, showing compulsive behavior, wandering, or becoming lost)

Stage 7 - Very severe decline: In the final stage of AD, a person may be unable to communicate with others, control movement, or respond to his or her surroundings. The person needs significant help with ADLs, including eating and toileting. Muscles become rigid, and reflexes are abnormal. The person will have difficulty swallowing.

It is important for nursing assistants to encourage independence, regardless of what signs a person with AD is displaying. Residents with

AD should be encouraged to perform their activities of daily living (ADLs). This helps them keep their minds and bodies as active as possible. Working, socializing, reading, problem solving, and exercising should all be encouraged (Fig. 19-3). Having residents with AD do as much as possible for themselves may even help slow the progression of the disease. Tasks should be challenging but not frustrating. Nursing assistants can help residents succeed in doing these tasks.

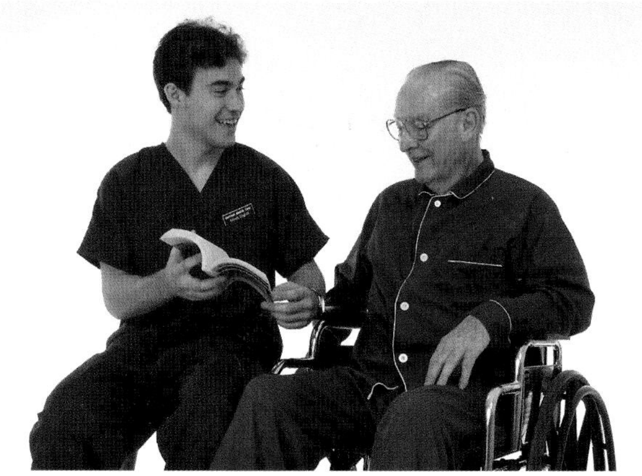

Fig. 19-3. Nursing assistants should encourage reading and thinking activities for residents with AD.

5. Identify personal attitudes helpful in caring for residents with Alzheimer's disease

These attitudes will help nursing assistants give the best possible care to residents with AD:

Do not take things personally. Alzheimer's disease is a devastating mental and physical disorder. It affects everyone who surrounds and cares for the one with AD. People with Alzheimer's disease do not have control over their words and actions. They may often be unaware of what they say or do. A resident with AD may not recognize a caregiver or do what he is supposed to do. He may ignore, accuse, or insult staff members. When this happens, it is important to remember that the behavior is due to the disease.

Be empathetic. It is helpful if the NA thinks about what it would be like to have Alzheimer's disease. She can imagine being unable to do ADLs and being dependent on others for care. It would be very frustrating for anyone to have no memory of recent events or to be unable to find words for what they want to say. NAs should assume that people with AD have insight and are aware of the changes in their abilities. They should treat residents with AD with dignity and respect.

Work with the symptoms and behaviors noted. Each person with Alzheimer's disease is an individual. People with AD will not all show the same symptoms at the same times (Fig. 19-4). Each resident will do some things that others will never do. The best plan is to work with the behaviors that are seen on any particular day. For example, a resident with Alzheimer's disease may want to go for a walk one day, when the day before he did not want to go to the bathroom without help. If it is allowed, the NA should try to go for a walk with him. Nursing assistants should notice and report changes in behavior, mood, and independence.

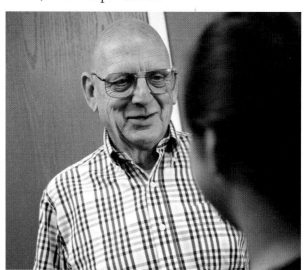

Fig. 19-4. Each resident with AD should be treated as an individual. The NA should work with the symptoms that she sees.

Work as a team. Symptoms and behaviors change daily. When NAs observe and report carefully to all team members, as well as listen to others' reports, it can help the care team develop solutions. For example, a resident with AD may refuse to eat her meals. An NA might discover that if he sits next to the resident and eats something while she has food in front of her, the resident will also eat. The NA may also notice that the resident always eats her bite-sized sandwiches or some other specific food. This is important to report to the team and can help the team provide better nutrition for the resident. Nursing assistants are in a great position to give details about residents. Being with residents often allows them to be experts on each case. NAs should make the most of this opportunity. Residents with AD may not be able to recognize or distinguish between aides, nurses, or administrators. All staff members should be prepared to help when needed.

Be aware of difficulties associated with caregiving. Caring for someone with dementia can be physically and emotionally exhausting, as well as incredibly stressful. NAs should take care of themselves so they can continue to provide the best care (Fig. 19-5). Being aware of the body's signals to slow down, rest, or eat better is important. Each NA's feelings are real; they have a right to them. Mistakes should be viewed as learning experiences. Unmanaged stress can cause physical and emotional problems. NAs can talk to their supervisors if they need help addressing stress or would like to find support groups in their areas. Chapter 24 has more information on handling stress.

Work with family members. Family members can be a wonderful resource. They can help a nursing assistant learn more about a resident. They also give stability and comfort to the resident with Alzheimer's disease. NAs should build relationships with family members and keep the lines of communication open.

In addition, NAs should be reassuring to family members. It is very difficult for families to see a loved one's health and abilities decline. When residents with AD exhibit problem behaviors, it can be stressful for the family. NAs can help by reassuring family members that they understand that this behavior is part of the disease.

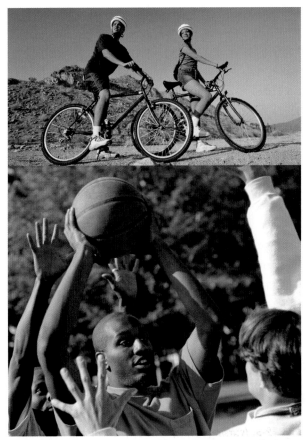

Fig. 19-5. *Regular exercise is an important part of taking care of oneself.*

Remember the goals of the care plan. Along with the practical tasks that nursing assistants will perform, the care plan will also call for maintaining residents' dignity and self-esteem. NAs should help residents to be as independent as possible.

6. List strategies for better communication with residents with Alzheimer's disease

Communication with residents with AD may be simplified if the nursing assistant does the following:

- Always approaches from the front and does not startle the resident.
- Determines how close the resident wants her to be.
- Communicates in a calm area with little background noise and distraction.

- Always identifies herself and uses the resident's name. She should continue to use the resident's name during the conversation.
- Speaks slowly, using a lower tone of voice than normal. This is calming and easier to understand.
- Repeats herself, using the same words and phrases, as often as needed.
- Uses signs, pictures, gestures, or written words to help communicate.
- Breaks complex tasks into smaller, simpler ones. Gives simple, step-by-step instructions as necessary.

In addition, communication with residents with AD can be helped by using these techniques for specific situations:

If the resident is frightened or anxious, the NA should

- Try to keep the resident calm. Speak slowly in a low, calm voice. Get rid of noise and distractions, such as televisions or radios (Fig. 19-6).

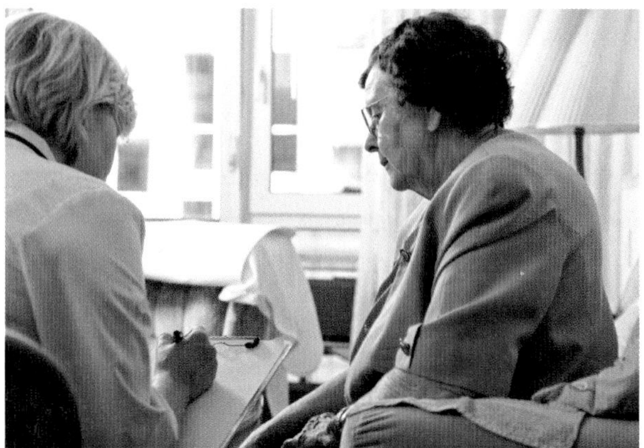

Fig. 19-6. Nursing assistants should try to find a room with little background noise and distraction when communicating with residents with AD.

- Try to see and hear herself as residents might. She should always describe what she is going to do.
- Use simple words and short sentences. If doing a procedure or helping with self-care, it is helpful to list steps one at a time.
- Check her body language to make sure she is not tense or hurried.

If the resident forgets or shows memory loss, the NA should

- Repeat herself, using the same words if she needs to repeat an instruction or question. However, she may be using a word the resident does not understand, such as *tired*. She can try other words like *nap, lie down*, or *rest*.
- Remember that repetition can be soothing for a resident with Alzheimer's disease. Many residents with AD will repeat words, phrases, questions, or actions. This is called **perseveration**. If a resident perseverates, the NA should not try to stop him. She should answer his questions, using the same words each time, until he stops.
- Keep messages simple and break complex tasks into smaller, simpler ones.

If the resident has trouble finding words or names, the NA should

- Suggest a word that sounds correct. If this upsets the resident, the NA can try to learn from it. She should try not to correct a resident who uses an incorrect word. As words (written and spoken) become more difficult, smiling, touching, and hugging can help show care and concern (Fig. 19-7). The NA should remember, however, that some people find touch frightening or unwelcome.

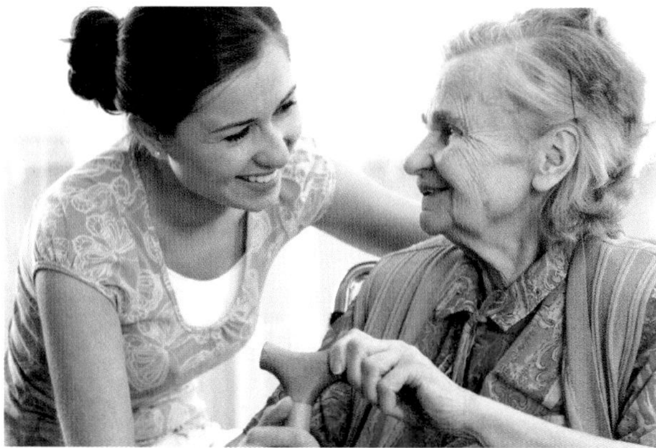

Fig. 19-7. Touch, smiles, and laughter will be understood longer, even after a resident's speaking abilities decline.

If the resident seems not to understand basic instructions or questions, the NA should

- Ask the resident to repeat her words. She should use short words and sentences and allow time to answer.
- Note the communication methods that are effective and use them.
- Watch for nonverbal cues as the ability to talk lessens. She can observe body language—eyes, hands, and face.
- Use signs, pictures, gestures, or written words. For example, a picture of a toilet on the bathroom door can help remind a resident where the bathroom is. The NA can also use gestures, such as holding up a shirt when she wants to help a resident dress. Combining verbal and nonverbal communication is helpful. For example, she can say, "Let's get dressed now," while holding up clothes.

If the resident wants to say something but cannot, the NA should

- Encourage the resident to point, gesture, or act it out.
- If the resident is obviously upset but cannot explain why, she can offer comfort with a smile, or try to distract him. Verbal communication may be frustrating.

If the resident does not remember how to perform basic tasks, the NA should

- Break each activity into simple steps. For instance, she can say, "Let's go for a walk. Stand up. Put on your sweater. First the right arm..." She should always encourage the person to do what he can.

If the resident insists on doing something that is unsafe or not allowed, the NA should

- Try to limit the times she says "don't." Instead, she should redirect activities toward something else.

If the resident hallucinates (sees or hears things that are not really happening) or is paranoid or accusing, the NA should

- Try not to take it personally.
- Try to redirect behavior or ignore it. Attention span is limited. This behavior often passes quickly.

If the resident is depressed or lonely, the NA should

- Take time, one-on-one, to ask how the resident is feeling and really listen to the response.
- Try to involve the resident in activities.
- Always report signs of depression to the nurse. (More information about depression is in Chapter 20.)

If the resident repeatedly asks to "go home," the NA should

- Gently remind him that he is in his home, but not argue if the resident disagrees.
- Redirect or guide the conversation and/or the resident's activities to something he enjoys.
- Expect that the resident may continue to ask to go home and be patient and gentle in her response.

If the resident is verbally abusive or uses bad language, the NA should

- Remember it is the dementia speaking, not the person. She should try to ignore the language and redirect attention to something else.

If the resident has lost most verbal skills, the NA should

- Use nonverbal skills. As speaking abilities decline, people with AD will still understand touch, smiles, and laughter for much longer. However, some people do not like to be touched. The NA should approach touching slowly and be gentle. She can softly touch the hand or place her arm around the resident. A smile can show affection and caring and say she wants to help (Fig. 19-8).

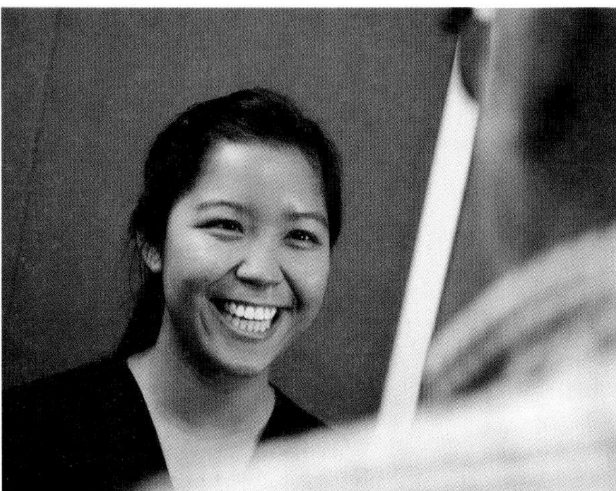

Fig. 19-8. Smiling can communicate positivity and a willingness to help.

- Remember that even after verbal skills are lost, signs, labels, and gestures can reach people with dementia.
- Assume people with AD can understand more than they can express. The NA should never talk about them as though they were not there.

7. Explain general principles that will help assist residents with personal care

Nursing assistants should use the same procedures for personal care and ADLs for residents with Alzheimer's disease as they would with other residents. However, when assisting residents with Alzheimer's disease, NAs should follow these guidelines:

1. **Develop a routine and stick to it.** Being consistent is important for residents who are confused and easily upset.
2. **Promote self-care.** Helping residents care for themselves as much as possible will help them cope with this difficult disease.
3. **Take good care of themselves, both mentally and physically.** This will help NAs give residents the best care.

8. List and describe interventions for problems with common activities of daily living (ADLs)

As Alzheimer's disease worsens, residents will have trouble doing their ADLs. Below are interventions to help residents with these problems. An **intervention** means a way to change an action or development.

If a resident has problems with bathing, the NA should

- Schedule bathing when the resident is least agitated. She should be organized so the bath can be quick. Sponge baths can be given if the resident resists a shower or tub bath.
- Prepare the resident before bathing. Handing the resident the supplies (washcloth, soap, shampoo, towels) serves as a visual aid.
- Take a walk with the resident down the hall, stopping at the tub or shower room, rather than asking directly about the bath.
- Make sure the bathroom is well-lit and is at a comfortable temperature.
- Provide privacy during the bath.
- Be calm and quiet when bathing a resident and keep the process simple.
- Be sensitive when talking to a resident about bathing.
- Give the resident a washcloth to hold. This can distract her while the NA finishes the bath.
- Always follow safety precautions. The NA should ensure safety by using non-slip mats, tub seats, and hand-holds.
- Be flexible about the time to bathe a resident. A resident may not always be in the mood. Also, an NA should be aware that not everyone bathes with the same frequency and

should understand if a resident does not want to bathe.

- Be relaxed and allow the resident to enjoy the bath. The NA should offer encouragement and praise.
- Let the resident do as much as possible during the bath.
- Check the skin regularly for signs of irritation or breakdown during the bath.

If a resident has problems with grooming and dressing, the NA should

- Help with grooming to help residents feel attractive and dignified (Fig. 19-9).

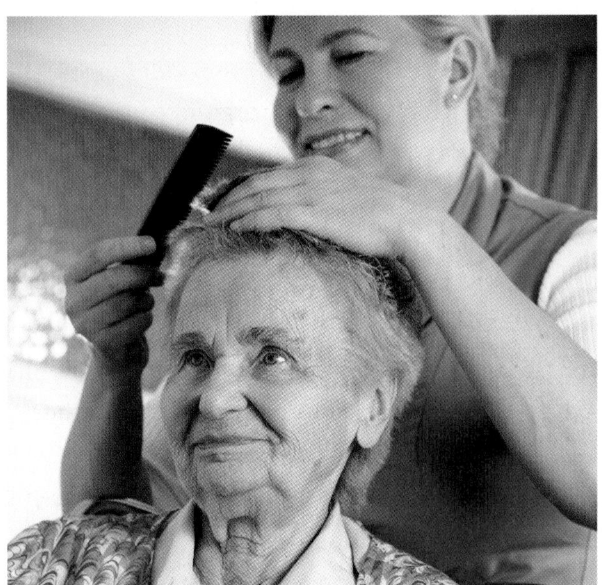

Fig. 19-9. Nursing assistants should assist residents with grooming to promote dignity and self-esteem.

- Avoid delays or interruptions while dressing.
- Show the resident clothing to put on. This brings up the idea of dressing.
- Provide privacy by closing doors and curtains. The resident should be dressed in the resident's room.
- Encourage the resident to pick clothes to wear. A nursing assistant can simplify this by giving just a few choices. She should make sure the clothing is clean and appropriate and lay out clothes in the order in which they are put on (Fig. 19-10). Clothes that are simple to put on are best. Some people with Alzheimer's disease make a habit of layering clothing regardless of the weather.

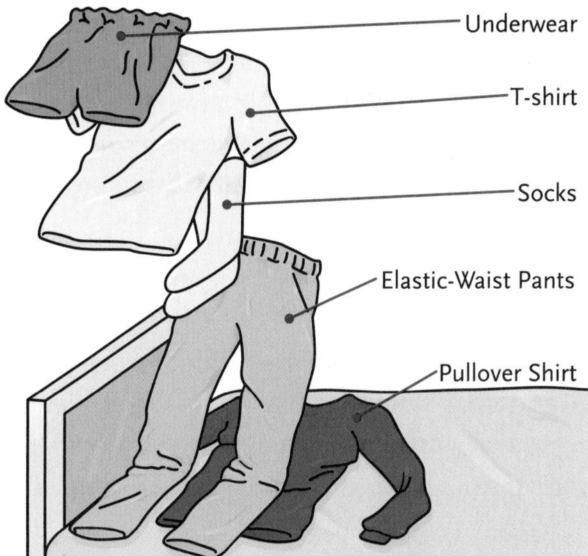

Fig. 19-10. Clothes should be laid out in the order in which they should be put on.

- Break the task down into simple steps. The NA should introduce one step at a time and not rush the resident.
- Use a friendly, calm voice when speaking. The NA should praise and encourage the resident at each step.

Residents' Rights

Rights with Alzheimer's Disease

Nursing assistants should protect the privacy rights of residents with AD by keeping them dressed or covered when in bed. Residents may not be aware that they are exposed. NAs should not discuss their personal information with others. They should allow residents with AD to make the decisions they are able to make, such as what shirt to wear or where to sit to eat.

If a resident has problems with toileting, the NA should

- Encourage fluids. The NA should never withhold or discourage fluids because a resident has problems with urinary incontinence. She should report to the nurse if the resident is not drinking fluids.
- Mark the bathroom with a sign or a picture as a reminder of where it is and to use the toilet.

- Make sure there is enough light in the bathroom and on the way there.
- Note when the resident is incontinent over two to three days and check her every 30 minutes. This can help determine "bathroom times." The NA should take the resident to the bathroom just before her bathroom time.
- Observe toilet patterns for two to three nights for incontinence during the night in order to try to determine nighttime bathroom times.
- Take the resident to the bathroom after drinking fluids and make sure the resident actually urinates before getting off the toilet.
- Take the resident to the bathroom before and after meals and before bedtime.
- Put lids on trash cans, wastebaskets, or other containers if the resident urinates in them.
- Remember that family or friends may be upset by their loved one's incontinence. The NA should be professional when cleaning after episodes of incontinence and not show disgust or irritation.

If a resident has problems with nutrition, the NA should

- Encourage nutritious intake. Food may not interest a resident with Alzheimer's disease at all. It may be of great interest, but a resident may only want to eat a few types of food. A resident with AD is at risk for malnutrition.
- Have meals at regular, consistent times each day. The NA may need to remind the resident that it is mealtime. Familiar foods should be served. Foods should look and smell appetizing.
- Make sure there is adequate lighting.
- Keep noise and distractions to a minimum during meals.
- Keep the task of eating simple. If restlessness prevents getting through an entire meal, the NA can try smaller, more frequent meals. Finger foods (foods that are easy to pick up with the fingers) allow eating while moving around. They allow residents to choose the food they want to eat. Examples of finger foods that may be good to serve are sandwiches cut into fourths, chicken nuggets or small pieces of cooked boneless chicken, fish sticks, cheese cubes, halved hard-boiled eggs, and fresh fruit and soft vegetables cut into bite-sized pieces.
- Avoid serving steaming or very hot foods or drinks.
- Use a simple place setting with a single eating utensil, and remove other items from the table (Fig. 19-11). Plain plates without patterns or colors work best.

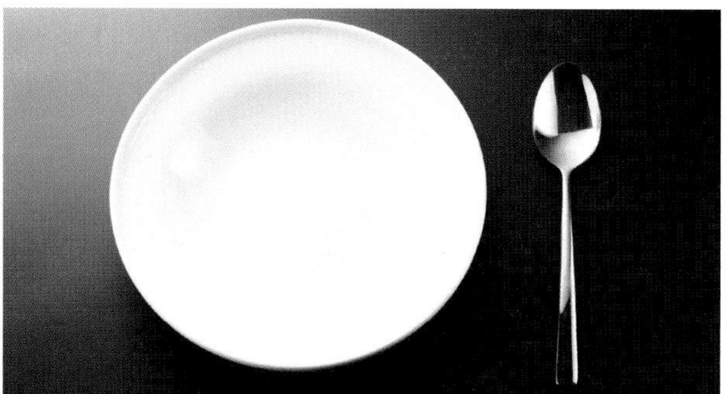

Fig. 19-11. *Plain white plates on a contrasting-colored placemat or surface may help avoid confusion and distraction during eating.*

- Put only one item of food on the plate at a time. Multiple kinds of food on a plate or a tray may be overwhelming.
- Give simple, clear instructions. Residents with AD may not understand how to eat or use utensils. The NA should help the resident taste a sample of the meal first. To get her to eat, she can place a spoon to the lips. This will encourage the resident to open her mouth. She should also ask the resident to open her mouth.
- Guide the resident through the meal, providing simple instructions. The NA should offer regular drinks of water, juice, and other fluids to avoid dehydration.
- Use adaptive equipment, such as special spoons and bowls, as needed.

- Feed the resident slowly, offering small pieces of food.
- Make mealtimes simple and relaxed. The NA should allow plenty of time for eating. She should give the resident time to swallow before the next bite or drink.
- Seat the resident with others at small tables. This encourages socializing.
- Observe for eating or swallowing problems and report them to the nurse as soon as possible. The NA should also observe and report changes or problems in eating habits.

To promote the physical health of residents with AD, the NA should

- Prevent infections and follow Standard Precautions.
- Observe the resident's physical health and report any potential problems. People with dementia may not notice their own health problems.
- Give careful skin care to prevent pressure ulcers.
- Watch for signs of pain. Nonverbal signs that a resident may be in pain include grimacing or clenching fists (Fig. 19-12). Report possible signs of pain to the nurse.
- Maintain a daily exercise routine.

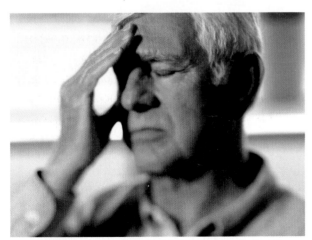

Fig. 19-12. *Be aware of nonverbal signs of pain, such as holding or rubbing a body part. Report these signs to the nurse.*

To promote the mental and emotional health of residents with AD, the NA should

- Maintain self-esteem by encouraging independence in activities of daily living.
- Share in enjoyable activities, such as looking at pictures, talking, and reminiscing.
- Reward positive and independent behavior with smiles and warm touches.

9. List and describe interventions for common difficult behaviors related to Alzheimer's disease

Below are some common difficult behaviors that nursing assistants may face when working with residents with Alzheimer's disease. Each resident is different, and NAs should work with each person as an individual. Details of behavior should be reported to the nurse.

Agitation: A resident who is excited, restless, or troubled is said to be **agitated**. Situations that lead to agitation are **triggers**. Triggers may include a change of routine or caregiver, new or frustrating experiences, or even television. If a resident is agitated, the NA should

- Try to remove triggers, keep routines constant, and avoid frustration.
- Help the resident focus on a soothing, familiar activity, such as sorting things or looking at pictures.
- Stay calm and use a low, soothing voice to speak to and reassure the resident.
- Place an arm around the shoulder, pat, or stroke the resident. This may be soothing for some residents.

Sundowning: When a person gets restless and agitated in the late afternoon, evening, or night, it is called **sundowning**. Sundowning may be caused by hunger or fatigue, a change in routine or caregiver, or any new or frustrating situation. If a resident experiences sundowning, the NA should

- Remove triggers, provide snacks, and encourage rest.
- Avoid stressful situations during this time. Activities, appointments, trips, and visits should be limited.
- Play soft music.
- Set a bedtime routine and keep it.
- Recognize when sundowning occurs and plan a calming activity just before.
- Remove caffeine from the diet.
- Give a soothing back massage.
- Distract the resident with a simple, calm activity like looking at a magazine.
- Maintain a daily exercise routine.

Catastrophic Reactions: When a person with AD overreacts to something, it is called a **catastrophic reaction**. It may be triggered by any of the following:

- Fatigue
- Change of routine, environment, or caregiver
- Overstimulation (too much noise or activity)
- Difficult choices or tasks
- Physical pain
- Hunger
- Need for toileting

Nursing assistants can respond to catastrophic reactions as they would to agitation or sundowning. For example, they can try to remove triggers and help the resident focus on a soothing activity.

Violent Behavior. A resident who attacks, hits, or threatens someone is violent. Violence may be triggered by many situations. These include frustration, overstimulation, or a change in routine, environment, or caregiver. If a resident is violent, the NA should

- Block blows but never hit back.
- Step out of reach.
- Call for help if needed.
- Avoid leaving residents alone.
- Try to remove triggers.
- Use the same techniques to calm residents as for agitation or sundowning.

Pacing and Wandering: A resident who walks back and forth in the same area is **pacing**. A resident who walks aimlessly around the facility or the facility grounds is **wandering** (Fig. 19-13). Pacing and wandering may have some of the following causes:

- Restlessness
- Hunger
- Disorientation
- Need for toileting
- Constipation
- Pain
- Forgetting how or where to sit down
- Too much daytime napping
- Need for exercise

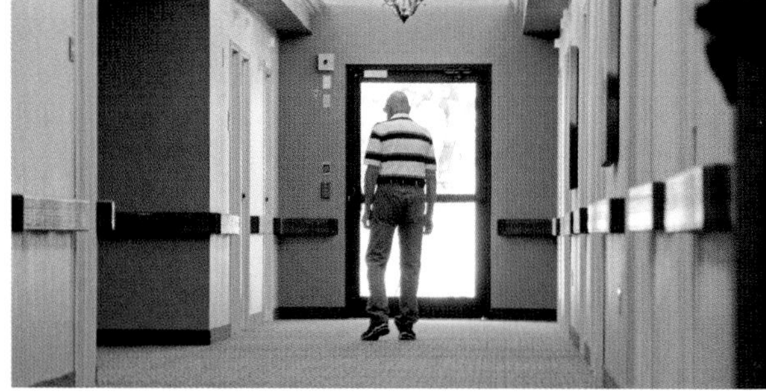

Fig. 19-13. *A resident with AD who is walking aimlessly around the facility is wandering.*

Nursing assistants should remove causes when they can. For example, give nutritious snacks, encourage an exercise routine, and maintain a toileting schedule. If residents pace and wander, they should do so in a safe and secure (locked) area where staff can keep an eye on them (Fig. 19-14). The NA can suggest another activity, such as going for a walk together.

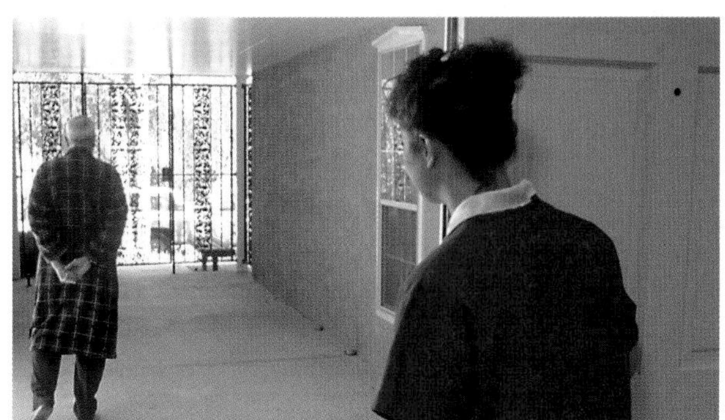

Fig. 19-14. Residents should be in a safe, secured area if they pace or wander.

Marking rooms with signs or pictures may prevent residents from wandering into areas where they should not go. Bed, body, or door alarms can be used in beds or on wheelchairs, chairs, or doors. They help by sounding an alarm when residents who are confused or demented attempt to leave the bed or chair or open a door. They also help prevent falls. If a resident is ordered to have a body alarm (bed or chair), the NA should make sure it is on the resident and is turned on.

Elopement

Residents with Alzheimer's disease or other forms of dementia might try to **elope**, or leave a facility unsupervised and unnoticed. It is very important that residents who elope are located and returned to the facility as quickly as possible. The longer a resident is gone, the greater danger he or she might encounter. If an NA believes a resident might have eloped, she must alert her supervisor immediately. Residents who elope are often found near where they were last seen, and the earlier a search is begun, the more likely the resident is to be found nearby and safe.

Hallucinations or Delusions: A resident who sees, hears, smells, tastes, or feels things that are not there is having **hallucinations**. A resident who believes things that are not true is having **delusions**. If a resident is experiencing hallucinations and/or delusions, the NA should

- Ignore harmless hallucinations and delusions.
- Reassure a resident who seems agitated or worried.
- Not argue with a resident who is imagining things. The feelings are real to him. The NA should not tell the resident that she sees or hears his hallucinations. She should redirect the resident to other activities or thoughts.
- Be calm and reassure resident that she is there to help.

Depression: When residents become withdrawn, have no energy, or do not eat or do things they used to enjoy, they may be depressed. Chapter 20 contains more information on depression and its symptoms. Depression may have many causes, including the following:

- Loss of independence
- Inability to cope
- Feelings of failure or fear
- Reality of facing a progressive, degenerative illness
- Chemical imbalance

If a resident is depressed, the NA should

- Report signs of depression to the nurse immediately. It is an illness that can be treated with medication.
- Encourage independence, self-care, and activity.
- Talk about moods and feelings if the resident is willing, and be a good listener.
- Encourage social interaction.

Perseveration or Repetitive Phrasing: A resident who repeats a word, phrase, question, or activity over and over is perseverating. Repeating a word or phrase is also called **repetitive phrasing**. Such behavior may be caused by several factors, including disorientation or confusion. The NA should be patient with this behavior and not try to silence or stop the resident. She should answer questions each time they are asked, using the same words each time.

Disruptiveness: Disruptive behavior is anything that disturbs others, such as yelling, banging on furniture, slamming doors, etc. Often this behavior is triggered by a wish for attention, by pain or constipation, or by frustration. When a resident is being disruptive, the NA should try to gain his attention. She should be calm and friendly and try to find out why the behavior is occurring. She should ask the resident about it if possible. There may be a physical reason, such as pain or discomfort. If a resident is being disruptive, the NA should

- Gently try to direct the resident to a private area.
- Notice and praise improvements in the resident's behavior. The NA should be tactful and sensitive when doing this to avoid treating the resident like a child.
- Tell the resident about any changes in schedules, routines, or the environment in advance. The NA should involve the resident in developing routine activities and schedules if possible.
- Encourage the resident to join in independent activities that are safe (for example, folding towels). This helps the resident feel in charge and can prevent feelings of powerlessness. Independence is power.
- Help the resident find ways to cope. Focusing on positive activities he or she may still be able to do, such as knitting, crocheting, or crafts, can provide a diversion.

Inappropriate Social Behavior: Inappropriate social behavior may include cursing, name-calling, or other behavior. As with violent or disruptive behavior, there may be many reasons why a resident is behaving in this way. Nursing assistants should try not to take it personally. The resident may only be reacting to frustration or other stress rather than to the NA. The NA should remain calm and be reassuring. She can try to find out what caused the behavior (possible causes include too much noise, too many people, too much stress, pain, or discomfort). If the resident is disturbing others, the NA should gently direct him to a private area if possible. The NA should respond positively to any appropriate behavior. Any physical abuse or serious verbal abuse should be reported to the nurse.

Inappropriate Sexual Behavior: Inappropriate sexual behavior, such as removing clothes, touching one's own genitals, or trying to touch others can be embarrassing to those who see it. It is helpful to be matter-of-fact when dealing with such behavior. Nursing assistants should not overreact, as this may reinforce the behavior. They should be sensitive to the nature of the problem. Is the behavior actually intentional? Is it consistent? If distracting the resident does not work, the NA can gently direct him to a private area and inform the nurse. A resident may be reacting to a need for physical stimulation or affection. Ways to provide physical stimulation include giving backrubs, offering a soft doll or stuffed animal to cuddle, providing comforting blankets, or giving physical touch that is appropriate.

Pillaging and Hoarding: **Pillaging** is taking things that belong to someone else. A person with dementia may honestly think something belongs to him, even when it clearly does not. **Hoarding** is collecting and putting things away in a guarded way. Pillaging and hoarding should not be considered stealing. A person with Alzheimer's disease cannot and does not steal. Stealing is planned and requires a conscious effort. In most cases, the person with AD is only collecting something that catches his attention. It is common for those with AD to wander in and out of rooms collecting things. They may carry these objects around for a while and then leave them in other places. This is not intentional. People with AD will often take their own things and leave them in another room, not knowing what they are doing. The NA can help lessen problems by

- Labeling all personal belongings with the resident's name and room number. This way there is no confusion about what belongs to whom.

- Placing a label, symbol, or object on the resident's door. This helps the resident find his own room.
- Not telling the family that their loved one is stealing from others.
- Preparing the family so they are not upset when they find items that do not belong to their family member.
- Asking the family to tell staff if they notice unfamiliar items in the room.
- Regularly checking areas where residents store items. They may store uneaten food in these places. Providing a rummage drawer—a drawer with items that are safe for the resident to take with him—can help.

Sleep Disturbances: Residents with AD may experience a number of sleep disturbances. If a resident experiences sleep problems, the NA should

- Make sure that the resident gets moderate exercise/activity throughout the day, appropriate to his condition. The NA can encourage him to participate in activities he enjoys.
- Allow the resident to spend some time each day in natural sunlight if possible. Exposure to light and dark at appropriate times can help establish restful sleep patterns.
- Reduce light and noise as much as possible during nighttime hours.
- Discourage sleeping during the day.

10. Describe creative therapies for residents with Alzheimer's disease

Although Alzheimer's disease cannot be cured, there are techniques to improve the quality of life for residents with AD.

Reality orientation involves the use of calendars, clocks, signs, and lists to help residents remember who and where they are. It is useful in the early stages of AD when residents are confused but not totally disoriented. In later stages, reality orientation may only frustrate residents.

Example: Each day when the NA goes into Mrs. Elkin's room, she shows her the calendar and points out what day of the week it is. On the calendar or another piece of paper, the NA lists all the things Mrs. Elkin will do that day. For example, she will take a shower, eat lunch, and go for a walk. When speaking to her, the NA calls her by her name: Mrs. Elkin. When helping with tasks, the NA explains why she does things as she does them. For example, "We use a shower chair in the shower so you don't have to stand up for so long, Mrs. Elkin."

Benefits: Using the calendar, making lists, and using names frequently all help the resident stay in touch with the world around her. This will help her feel more in control of her life. It will also allow her to do as much as possible for herself. Explaining what the NA does and why she does it as she assists her will make the resident feel more like a participant in her care and less like an invalid.

Validation therapy means letting residents believe they live in the past or in imaginary circumstances. **Validating** means giving value to or approving. When using validation therapy, the NA should make no attempt to reorient the resident to actual circumstances. She can explore the resident's beliefs and should not argue with or correct him. Validating can give comfort and reduce agitation. It is useful in cases of moderate to severe disorientation.

Example: Mr. Baldwin tells the NA that he does not want to eat lunch today because he is going out to a restaurant with his wife. The NA knows his wife has been dead for many years and that Mr. Baldwin can no longer eat out. Instead of telling him that he is not going out to eat, the NA asks what restaurant he is going to and what he will have. She suggests that he eat a good lunch now because sometimes the service is slow in restaurants (Fig. 19-15).

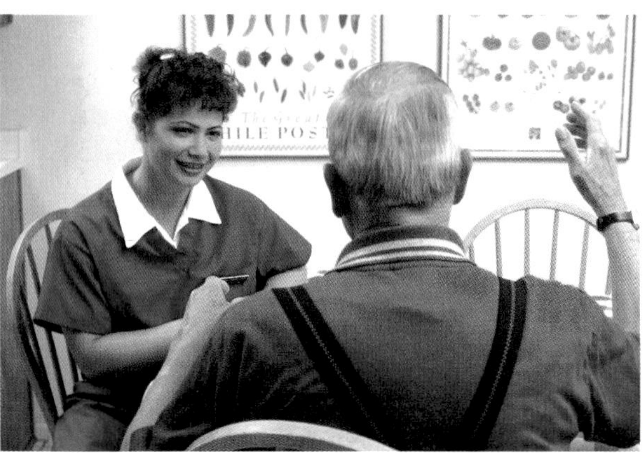

Fig. 19-15. Validation therapy accepts a resident's fantasies without attempting to reorient him to reality.

Benefits: By playing along with Mr. Baldwin's fantasy, the NA lets him know that she takes him seriously. She does not think of him as a crazy person or a child who does not know what is happening in his own life. She also learns more about the resident. He used to enjoy eating out in restaurants. He liked to order certain dishes. Eating out is something he probably associates with being with his wife. These things can help the NA give Mr. Baldwin better care in the future.

Reminiscence therapy involves encouraging residents to remember and talk about the past. Nursing assistants can explore memories by asking about details. They should focus on a time of life that was pleasant. It may help residents work through feelings about a difficult time in the past. It is useful in many stages of AD, but especially with moderate to severe confusion.

Example: Mr. Benton, an 82-year-old man with Alzheimer's disease, fought in World War II. In his room are many mementos of the war—pictures of his war buddies, a medal he was given, and more. The NA asks him to tell him where he was sent in the war. He tells him about being in the Pacific. The NA asks him more detailed questions about his experiences. Eventually the resident shares a lot: the friends he made in the service, why he was given the medal, times when he was scared, and how much he missed his wife and daughter (Fig. 19-16).

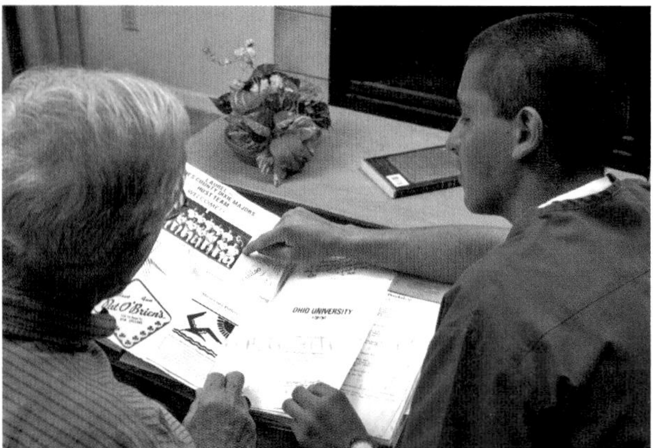

Fig. 19-16. Reminiscence therapy encourages a resident to remember and talk about his past.

Benefits: By asking questions about Mr. Benton's experiences in the war, the NA shows an interest in him as a person, not just as a resident. He lets the resident show him that he is a person who was competent, social, responsible, and brave. This boosts his self-esteem. The NA also learns that Mr. Benton cared very much for his wife and daughter.

Activity therapy uses activities that the resident enjoys to prevent boredom and frustration. These activities also promote self-esteem. The NA can help the resident take walks, do puzzles, listen to music, read, or do other things he or she enjoys (Fig. 19-17). Activities may be done in groups or one-on-one. Activity therapy is useful in most stages of AD.

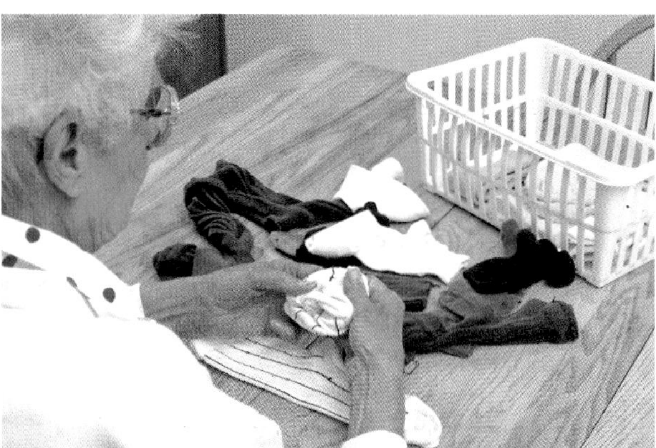

Fig. 19-17. Activities that are not frustrating can be helpful for residents with AD. They promote mental exercise.

Example: Mrs. Hoebel, a 70-year-old woman with AD, was a librarian for almost 45 years. She loves books and reading, but she cannot read much anymore. The NA obtains books from the facility that are filled with pictures. Mrs. Hoebel sits with the books, sorting them, and turning pages and looking at pictures.

Benefits: Mrs. Hoebel can enjoy an activity that always brought her pleasure. She feels competent, because she is sorting books and looking at books, which are tasks she can handle. The NA shows her that she cares about her by taking the time to show an interest in her past. Mrs. Hoebel will associate positive feelings with the NA. That will make caring for her much easier.

Music Therapy

Music therapy involves using music to accomplish specific goals, such as managing stress and improving mood and cognition. This type of therapy has been used successfully with people who have Alzheimer's disease. Music is a form of sensory stimulation. Hearing familiar songs can cause a response in people with dementia who do not respond well or do not respond at all to other treatments. Music & Memory is a nonprofit organization that brings personalized music into the lives of the elderly. Their website, musicandmemory.org, provides more information.

11. Discuss how Alzheimer's disease may affect the family

Alzheimer's disease requires the person's family to make adjustments, which may be difficult. The disease progresses at different rates, and people with AD will need more care as the disease progresses. Eventually most people with AD need constant care. How well the family is able to cope with the effects of the disease depends, in part, on the family's emotional and financial resources.

A person with AD may be living alone, which can cause the family to worry about the person's health and safety. Financial resources may be limited, which adds to stress levels. Finding money needed to pay expenses of home care or adult day services can be difficult. Families do not know what goes on when no one is in the home. They may be afraid that the person is not caring for herself, may not take medications properly, could wander away, or could cause a fire.

A person with AD may be living with the family, which can cause stress and other emotional difficulties for all involved. The household schedule has to change; family members will lose the freedom to come and go as they please. Family members must monitor the loved one's activities and provide constant care. They may lose sleep, as well as lose time to do their own activities and relax.

Alzheimer's disease introduces other stressors, too. It is very difficult to watch a loved one's personality change and her health and abilities deteriorate. It is also hard to switch roles—to go from being a child who was once cared for by the parent to being the one caring for the parent.

Families may make the decision to place a loved one with AD into a long-term care facility for any number of reasons. They may have safety concerns or may not be able to care for the person at home. The family may not be able to handle the issues that AD causes, such as the problem behaviors or the inability to perform personal care. The person with AD may not want her family to do the needed personal care. There may be no available family caregiver.

After making the decision to place a person with AD in a long-term care facility, family members usually feel guilty, even if they know that placement is necessary. The person with AD may be angry and unable to understand the decision. Families worry about mistreatment and are sensitive to being judged by others. They also feel loss and a change in the relationship with their family member.

Family members are making emotional adjustments, just as residents are. They may be experiencing frustration, fear, sadness, anger, loneliness, and depression. It is important for families to be able to express their feelings. Chapter 8 contains information about how to respond to emotional needs of families. Nursing assistants should be sensitive to the big adjustments that residents and their families are making. If help is needed, the NA can refer them to her supervisor.

12. Identify community resources available to people with Alzheimer's disease and their families

There are many resources, such as organizations, books, counseling, and support groups, available for people with Alzheimer's disease and their families. The Alzheimer's Association has a helpline that is available 24 hours a day, seven days at week for information, referral, and support. The number is 800-272-3900, and the Alzheimer's Association website is alz.org. The National Institute on Aging's number is 800-438-4380 and their Alzheimer's Disease Education and Referral (ADEAR) Center website is nia.nih.gov/alzheimers. Healthcare professionals can also be of assistance. Support groups are often helpful because many people in the group are experiencing the same kinds of emotions and problems. People often feel that it is helpful to know that they are not alone in what they are going through. People in support groups often share tips and ideas for care and interventions for problems, which can be beneficial. NAs should inform the nurse if they think residents and/or their families could benefit from a list of community resources.

Chapter Review

1. What does cognitive impairment affect?
2. How can confusion affect a person?
3. Define the term *delirium* and list five causes.
4. What is dementia?
5. Alzheimer's disease is a progressive, degenerative, and irreversible disease. What does this mean?
6. What type of skills does a person with Alzheimer's disease usually retain?
7. What can nursing assistants encourage residents to do that may help slow the progression of AD?
8. Helpful personal attitudes when working with residents who have AD are described in Learning Objective 5. They are:
   - Do not take things personally.
   - Be empathetic.
   - Work with the symptoms and behaviors noted.
   - Work as a team.
   - Be aware of difficulties associated with caregiving.
   - Work with family members.
   - Remember the goals of the care plan.

   List one example of what an NA can do to express each attitude.
9. Possible communication challenges for residents with AD are listed in Learning Objective 6. They include challenges with a resident who may:
   - Be frightened or anxious
   - Forget or show memory loss
   - Have trouble finding words or names
   - Seem not to understand basic questions or instructions
   - Want to say something but cannot
   - Not remember how to perform basic tasks
   - Insist on doing something that is unsafe or not allowed

- Hallucinate or be paranoid or accusing
  Don't take it personally. Redirect attention
- Be depressed or lonely
  Take time one on one. Involve them in other activities Report depression to nurse.
- Ask repeatedly to go home
  Remind them they are home. Think of other activities they might like to do.
- Be verbally abusive or use bad language
  Redirect attention to something else
- Have lost most verbal skills
  Use nonverbal skills. Touch, smile, laugh.

For each communication challenge, list one tip that may help.

10. List three general principles that will assist residents with personal care.
    1) Develope a routine & stick with it.
    2) Help residents in being as independent as possible in caring for themselves.
    3) NA should take good care of themselves.

11. List four interventions for each of the following topics for residents who have AD: bathing, dressing and grooming, toileting, nutrition, physical health, and mental and emotional health.

12. For each of the following common difficult behaviors seen in residents with AD, list one intervention: agitation; sundowning; catastrophic reactions; violent behavior; pacing and wandering; hallucinations and delusions; perseveration; disruptiveness; inappropriate social behavior; inappropriate sexual behavior; pillaging and hoarding; and sleep disturbances.

13. Describe these four creative therapies for AD: reality orientation, validation therapy, reminiscence therapy, and activity therapy.
    REALITY ORIENTATION 1) Use calendars, clocks, signs etc. 2) Lists of things going on.

14. What difficulties might families of people who have AD face?
    Many adjustments will need to be made. Family members lose their freedom. AD person's constant care. Sad to see change in loved one.

15. List two community resources that may help a person who has AD.
    Helping Line: 800-272-3900
    Disease Education (ADEAR) nia.nih.gov/alzheimers

VALIDATION THERAPY
Allow AD people to live in the past in their minds if they want to. Don't correct them. Give value or approve. Do not argue or correct resident. Give comfort. Reduce agitation.

ACTIVITY THERAPY
Let them do simple activity like folding clothes

REMINISCENCE THERAPY - Talk about past.

PILLAGING - Make a drawer of things they can take out & carry around Label things.

HORDING - Prepare family about problem which is diease related

SLEEP DISTURBANCE - More exercise, ↓ Noise

(11)
1) BATHING: Schedule bath time when resident is calm. Prepare everything before the bath. Bathroom should be well lit. Give them a washcloth to hold. Be flexible about bath time. Follow safety precautions
2) DRESSING: Layer clothing in order that it should go on. Help with hair combing, teeth in etc. Provide privacy. Encourage residents to pick out their clothes
3) TOILETING: Report if resident is not drinking fluids. Mark bathroom with a sign or picture of a toilet. Make sure there is adaquate light in bathroom. Take to BR at regular times maybe according to their pattern. Take before and after meals. Be professional about talking about messes, cleaning up messes or messes.
4) NUTRITION: Encourage eating, using familiar foods, Smaller meals, finger foods, good lighting. Keep noise down. No very hot or very cold drinks. Use simple place settings.
5) PHYSICAL HEALTH: Follow standard precautions to slow disease. Report any health concerns or physical appearances. Watch for signs of pain. Exercise routine.
6) MENTAL & EMOTIONAL HEALTH: Maintain self-esteem with independence in ADL's. Share enjoyable activities like looking at pictures, talking, reminiscing etc.

(12) Agitation - Remove triggers. Stay calm.
Sundowning avoid stressful situations. Play music
Catastrophic reactions Watch overstimulation or Difficult tasks
Violent Behaviour - Remove triggers. Call for help.
Pacing & Wandering - check for pain, hunger, boredom, Too much day-time napping, need for exercise.
Hallucinations & Delusions - Ignore harmless ones Be calm, smile, redirect activity
Preseveration - Answer each time with same words.
Disruptiveness - Direct to private room. Remain calm. Report any abuse. Be patient.
SOCIAL MISBEHAVIOR Find out what caused behavior. Stay calm
SEXUAL MISBEHAVIOR - Direct to other area. Calm give a backrub.

20 Mental Health and Mental Illness

1. Identify seven characteristics of mental health

Mental health is the normal functioning of emotional and intellectual abilities. A person who is mentally healthy is able to

- Get along with others (Fig. 20-1)
- Adapt to change
- Care for self and others
- Give and accept love
- Deal with situations that cause anxiety, disappointment, and frustration
- Take responsibility for decisions, feelings, and actions
- Control and fulfill desires and impulses appropriately

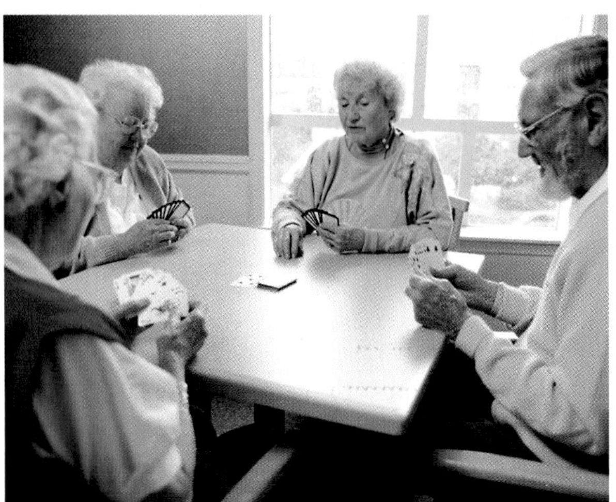

Fig. 20-1. The ability to interact well with other people is a characteristic of mental health.

2. Identify four causes of mental illness

Although it involves the emotions and mental functions, **mental illness** is a disease. It is similar to any physical disease. It produces signs and symptoms and affects the body's ability to function. It responds to proper treatment and care. Mental illness disrupts a person's ability to function at a normal level in the family, home, or community. It often causes inappropriate behavior. Some signs and symptoms of mental illness are confusion, disorientation, agitation, and anxiety.

However, signs and symptoms like those of mental illness can also occur when mental illness is not present. A personal crisis, temporary physical changes in the brain, side effects from medications, or a severe change in the environment may cause a **situation response**. In a situation response, the signs and symptoms are temporary.

Mental illness can be caused or made worse by chronic stress from any of these conditions:

1. **Physical factors**: Illness, disability, or aging can cause stress that may lead to mental illness. Substance abuse or a chemical imbalance can also lead to mental illness. Self-respect and self-worth are the building blocks of mental health. They are challenged when ill or disabled people have difficulty with their activities of daily living (ADLs). Ill or disabled people may become fearful of the future. They may be concerned about their dependence on others.

2. **Environmental factors**: Weak interpersonal or family relationships or traumatic early life experiences (such as suffering abuse as a child) can lead to mental illness.
3. **Heredity**: Mental illness can occur repeatedly in some families. This may be due to inherited traits or family influence.
4. **Stress**: People can tolerate different levels of stress. People have different ways of coping with stress. When the amount of stress becomes too great, a person may not be able to cope with it, and mental illness may arise.

3. Distinguish between fact and fallacy concerning mental illness

A **fallacy** is a false belief. The greatest fallacy about mental illness is that people who are mentally ill can control it. Mentally ill people cannot simply choose to be well. Mental illness is a disease like any other physical illness. Mentally healthy people are usually able to control their emotions and responses. Mentally ill people may not have this control.

Fact and Fallacy

Fact: Mental illness is a disease like any physical illness. People with mental illness cannot control their illness through sheer force of will.

Fallacy: People with mental illness can control their illness or choose to be well.

Intellectual Disability and Mental Illness

Sometimes people confuse the terms *intellectual disability* and *mental illness*. They are not the same. Intellectual disability (formerly called *mental retardation*) is a developmental disability that causes below-average mental functioning. It may affect a person's ability to care for himself, as well as to live independently. It is not a type of mental illness. Here are some ways that it differs from mental illness:

- An intellectual disability is a permanent condition; mental illness can be temporary.
- An intellectual disability is present at birth or emerges in childhood. Mental illness may occur any time during a person's life.
- An intellectual disability affects mental ability. Mental illness may or may not affect mental ability.
- There is no cure for an intellectual disability, although persons who are intellectually disabled can be helped. Many mental illnesses can be cured with treatment, such as medications and therapy.

Although they are different conditions, persons who have either condition need emotional support, as well as care and treatment.

4. Explain the connection between mental and physical wellness

Mental health is important to physical health. Reducing stress can help prevent some physical illnesses (Fig. 20-2). It can help people cope if illness or disability occur. Mental health can help protect and improve physical health. The reverse is also true. Physical illness or disability can cause or worsen mental illness. The stress these conditions create takes a toll on mental health.

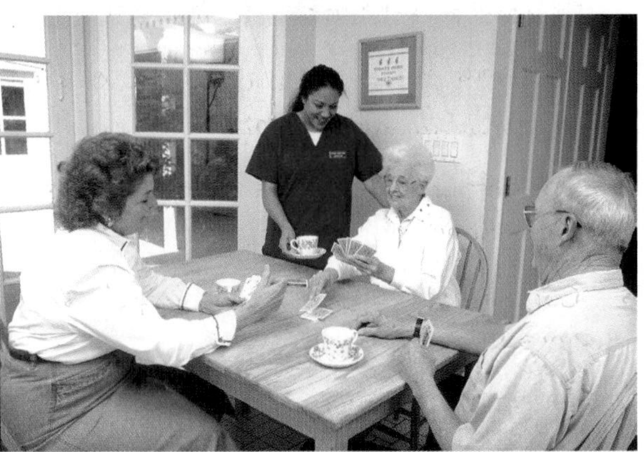

Fig. 20-2. *Social interaction can promote mental and physical health.*

5. List guidelines for communicating with mentally ill residents

Different types of mental illness will affect how well residents communicate. Nursing assistants should treat each resident as an individual and tailor their approach to the situation. The following guidelines can aid communication with residents who are mentally ill:

Guidelines: Communication and Mental Illness

- Do not talk to adults as if they were children.
- Use simple, clear statements and a normal tone of voice.
- Be sure that what you say and how you say it show respect and concern.
- Sit or stand at a normal distance from the resident. Be aware of your body language.
- Be honest and direct, as you would with any resident.
- Avoid arguments.
- Maintain eye contact (Fig. 20-3).
- Listen carefully.

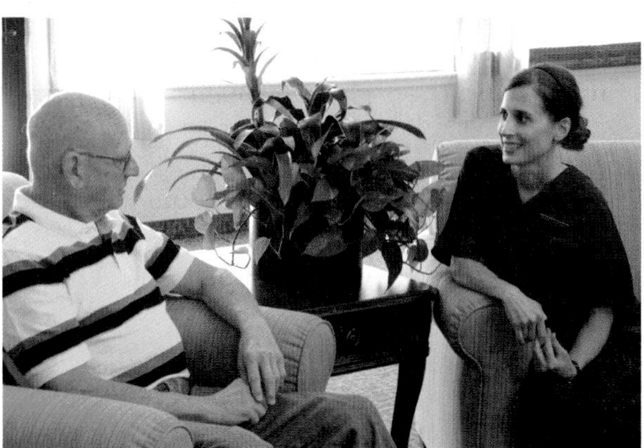

Fig. 20-3. *Nursing assistants should maintain eye contact and sit a normal distance when communicating with residents who are mentally ill.*

6. Identify and define common defense mechanisms

Defense mechanisms are unconscious behaviors used to release tension or cope with stress. They help to block uncomfortable or threatening feelings. All people use defense mechanisms at times. However, people who are mentally ill use them to a greater degree. An overuse of these mechanisms prevents a person from understanding his emotional problems and behaviors. If a person is unable to recognize problems, he will not address them. The problems may get worse. Common defense mechanisms include the following:

Denial: Completely rejecting the thought or feeling—"I'm not upset with you!"

Projection: Seeing feelings in others that are really one's own—"My teacher hates me."

Displacement: Transferring a strong negative feeling to a safer situation—for example, an unhappy employee cannot yell at his boss for fear of losing his job. He later yells at his wife.

Rationalization: Making excuses to justify a situation—for example, after stealing something, saying, "Everybody does it."

Repression: Blocking unacceptable thoughts or painful feelings from the mind—for example, forgetting sexual abuse.

Regression: Going back to an old, usually immature behavior—for example, throwing a temper tantrum as an adult.

7. Describe the symptoms of anxiety, depression, and schizophrenia

There are many degrees of mental illness, from mild to severe. A person with severe mental illness may lose touch with reality and become unable to communicate or make decisions. Some people with mild mental illness, however, seem to function normally. They may sometimes become overwhelmed by stress or overly emotional. Many signs of mental illness are simply extreme behaviors most people occasionally experience. Being able to recognize such behaviors may make it easier to understand residents who are mentally ill.

Anxiety-related Disorders: **Anxiety** is uneasiness or fear, often about a situation or condition. When a mentally healthy person feels anxiety, he can usually identify the cause. The anxiety fades once the cause is removed. A mentally ill person may feel anxiety all the time. He may not know the reason for feeling anxious. Physical signs and symptoms of anxiety-related disorders include shakiness, muscle aches, sweating, cold and clammy hands, dizziness, fatigue, racing heart, cold or hot flashes, a choking or smothering sensation, and a dry mouth (Fig. 20-4).

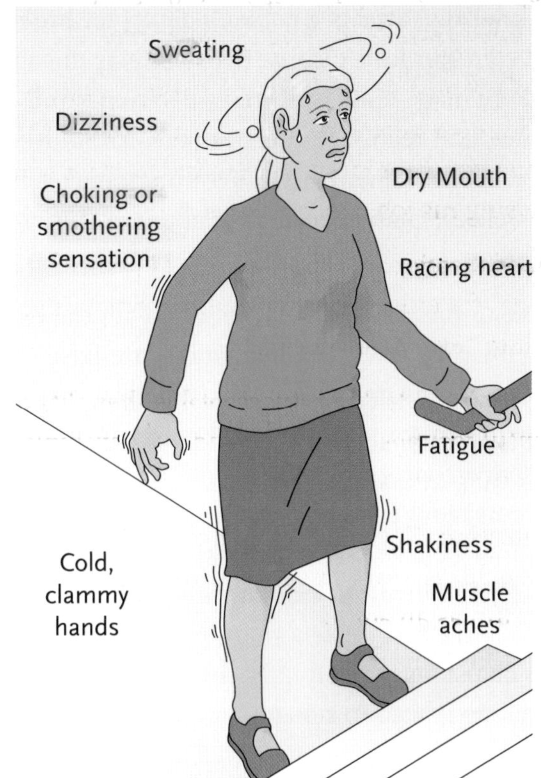

Fig. 20-4. Common symptoms of anxiety.

A **phobia** is an intense form of anxiety or fear. Many people are very afraid of certain things or situations. Examples include a fear of dogs or a fear of flying. For a mentally ill person, a phobia is a disabling terror. It prevents the person from participating in normal activities. For example, the fear of being in a confined space, **claustrophobia**, may make using an elevator a terrifying experience.

Other types of anxiety-related disorders include **panic disorder**, in which a person has repeated episodes of intense fear that something bad will occur. **Obsessive compulsive disorder (OCD)** is an anxiety disorder characterized by obsessive thoughts or behavior. For example, a person may wash his hands over and over again as a way of dealing with anxiety. Anxiety-related disorders may also be caused by a traumatic experience, such as being a victim of a violent crime or being involved in combat while in the military. This type of anxiety is known as **post-traumatic stress disorder (PTSD)**.

Depression: Clinical depression is a serious mental illness. It may cause intense mental, emotional, and physical pain and disability. Depression also makes other illnesses worse. If left untreated, it may result in suicide. The National Institute of Mental Health (NIMH) (the website is nimh.nih.gov) lists depression as one of the most common conditions associated with suicide in older adults.

Clinical depression is not a normal reaction to stress. Sadness is only one sign of this illness. Not all people who have depression complain of sadness or appear sad. Other common symptoms of clinical depression include the following (Fig. 20-5):

- Pain, including headaches, abdominal pain, and other body aches
- Low energy or fatigue
- **Apathy**, or lack of interest in activities
- Irritability
- Anxiety
- Loss of appetite or overeating
- Problems with sexual functioning and desire
- Sleeplessness, difficulty sleeping, or excessive sleeping
- Lack of attention to basic personal care tasks (e.g., bathing, combing hair, changing clothes)
- Intense feelings of despair
- Guilt
- Difficulty concentrating
- Withdrawal and isolation
- Repeated thoughts of suicide and death

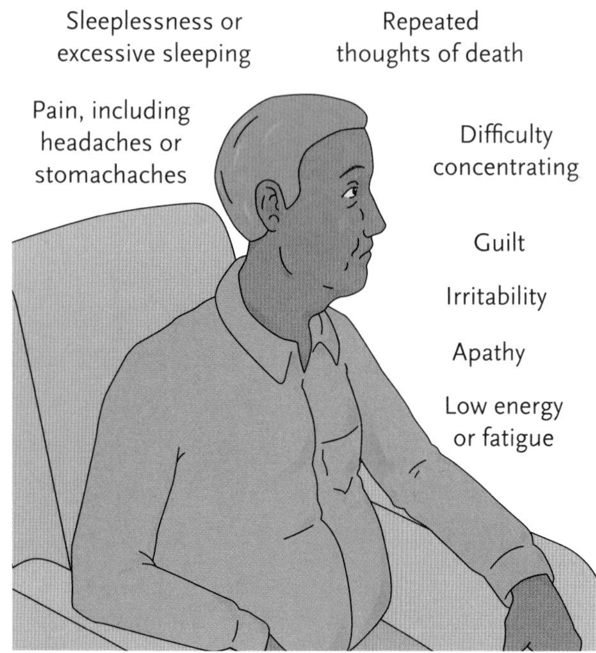

Fig. 20-5. Common symptoms of clinical depression.

Depression is very common in the elderly population. It can occur in conjunction with other illnesses. Cancer, AIDS, Alzheimer's disease, diabetes, and heart attack may be associated with increased rates of depression. It can happen after the death of a loved one. Depression may sometimes be caused by a chemical imbalance.

There are different types and degrees of depression. **Major depressive disorder**, or major depression, may cause a person to lose interest in everything he once cared about. **Bipolar disorder**, also called manic-depressive illness, causes a person to swing from periods of deep depression to periods of extreme activity. Characteristics of these episodes include high energy, little sleep, big speeches, rapidly changing thoughts and moods, inflated self-esteem, overspending, and poor judgment.

People cannot overcome depression through sheer will. Depression is an illness like any other illness. It can be treated successfully. People who suffer from depression need compassion and support. Nursing assistants should know the symptoms so that they can recognize the beginning or worsening of depression. Any suicide threat should be taken seriously and reported immediately. It should not be regarded as an attempt to get attention.

Schizophrenia: Contrary to popular belief, schizophrenia does not mean that a person has a split personality. **Schizophrenia** is a brain disorder that affects a person's ability to think and communicate clearly. It also affects the ability to manage emotions, make decisions, and understand reality. It affects a person's ability to interact with other people. Treatment makes it possible for many people to lead relatively normal lives.

Some of the signs of schizophrenia are easy to observe (Fig. 20-6). Hallucinations are false or distorted sensory perceptions. A person may see someone or something that is not really there or hear a conversation that is not real. Delusions are persistent false beliefs. For example, a person may believe that other people are reading his thoughts. **Paranoid schizophrenia** is a form of the disease that centers mainly on hallucinations and delusions. Not all hallucinations or delusions are related to schizophrenia, though.

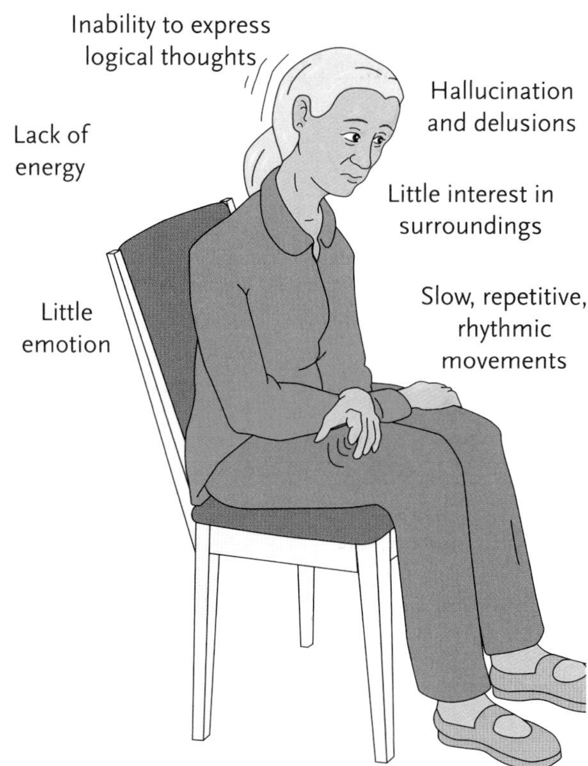

Fig. 20-6. Common symptoms of schizophrenia.

Other symptoms of schizophrenia include disorganized thinking and speech. This makes a person unable to express logical thoughts. Disorganized behavior means a person moves slowly, repeating gestures or movements. People with schizophrenia may also show less emotion. They may seem to have less interest in things around them and lack energy.

8. Explain how mental illness is treated

Mental illness can be treated. Medication and psychotherapy are common treatment methods. Medication is widely used for several diseases and can have a very positive effect. These drugs affect the brain and have been successful in treating the symptoms and behaviors of many people with mental disorders. Medication may allow mentally ill people to function more completely. Medication used to treat mental illness must be taken properly to promote benefits and reduce side effects. NAs may be assigned to observe residents taking their medications.

Psychotherapy is a method of treating mental illness that involves talking about one's problems with mental health professionals. Individuals, groups, couples, or families meet with trained, licensed professionals to work on their problems. Therapists work with their clients to identify problems and causes. They use different techniques to help clients learn more about themselves and to teach them new ways to handle problems and be more in control of their lives.

Residents' Rights

Mental Illness

Residents have the right to participate in the planning of their care. They also have the right to have their medical and personal records handled confidentially. A resident with a history of mental illness has the right to go to his care plan meetings and state his preferences for care and treatment. He also has the right to refuse care and treatment. The fact that the resident has a mental illness is confidential information. Nursing assistants should not share this information with anyone.

9. Explain the nursing assistant's role in caring for residents who are mentally ill

Personal care of residents who are mentally ill is similar to care of any resident. The care plan will state what the nursing assistant should do. The NA will also have some special responsibilities, as described in these guidelines:

Guidelines: Mentally Ill Residents

- Observe residents carefully for changes in condition or abilities. Document and report your observations.
- Support the resident and his or her family and friends. Coping with mental illness can be very frustrating. Your positive, professional attitude encourages the resident and the family. If you need help coping with stress of caring for someone who is mentally ill, speak to the nurse.
- Encourage residents to do as much as possible for themselves. Progress may be very slow. Be patient, supportive, and positive.

10. Identify important observations that should be made and reported

Nursing assistants should carefully observe residents. They should not draw conclusions about the cause of the behavior they see; they should only report the facts of their observations, including what they saw or heard, how long the behavior lasted, and how frequently it occurred.

Observing and Reporting: Mentally Ill Residents

- Changes in ability
- Positive or negative mood changes, especially withdrawal (Fig. 20-7)
- Behavior changes, including changes in personality, extreme behavior, and behavior that is not appropriate to the situation

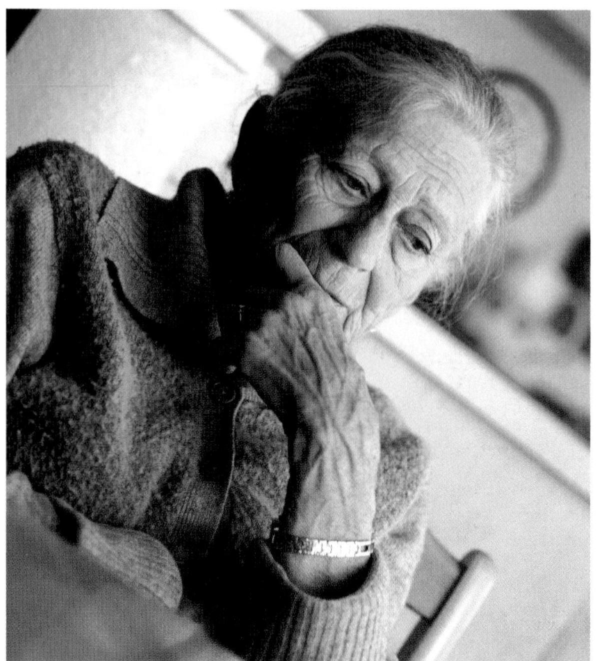

Fig. 20-7. Withdrawal is an important change to report.

- O/R Comments, even jokes, about hurting oneself or others
- O/R Failure to take medicine or improper use of medicine
- O/R Real or imagined physical symptoms
- O/R Events, situations, or people that upset or excite residents

11. List the signs of substance abuse

Substance abuse is the repeated use of legal or illegal drugs, cigarettes, or alcohol in a way that is harmful to oneself or others. The harm caused by substance abuse may come in many forms: damage to the person's health; legal problems; and damage to the person's relationships with family and friends. Chemical dependency is more severe; it may involve needing greater amounts of the drug and having symptoms, even when not using it. Chemical dependency is a disease. It affects a person physically, mentally, and emotionally. Like many other diseases, chemical dependency can develop at any age. It is treatable but frequently requires diagnosis and care by specialists. Treatment is not as simple as just stopping the drug.

It is not necessary for a substance to be illegal for it to be abused (Fig. 20-8). Alcohol and cigarettes are legal for adults, but are often abused. Over-the-counter medications, including diet aids and decongestants, can be addictive and harmful. Even household substances such as paint or glue are abused, causing injury and death.

Nursing assistants may be in a position to observe signs of substance abuse in residents. These signs should be reported to the nurse. NAs can report their observations without accusing anyone. They should simply report what they see, not what they think the cause may be.

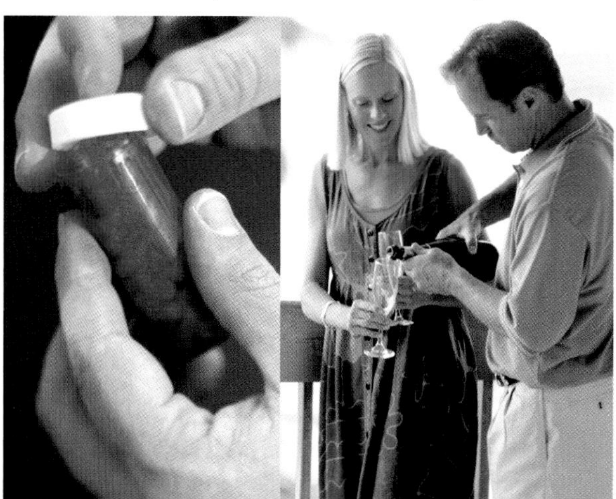

Fig. 20-8. Prescription drugs, cigarettes, and alcohol are examples of legal substances that may be abused.

Observing and Reporting: Substance Abuse

- O/R Changes in physical appearance (red eyes, dilated pupils, weight loss)
- O/R Changes in personality (moodiness, strange behavior, disruption of routines, lying)
- O/R Irritability
- O/R Odor of cigarettes, liquor, or other substances on breath or clothes
- O/R Diminished sense of smell
- O/R Unexplained changes in vital signs
- O/R Loss of appetite
- O/R Inability to function normally

- O/R Need for money
- O/R Confusion or forgetfulness
- O/R Blackouts or memory loss
- O/R Frequent accidents
- O/R Problems with family or friends

Some of the same signs listed above may also indicate other problems. Depression, dementia, medication issues, or medical conditions can also produce many of these same symptoms.

Residents' Rights

Rights with Alcohol

Most residents in long-term care facilities are adults and have the legal right to drink alcohol. However, there are instances when alcohol is not allowed. A doctor may have written an order for a resident not to drink alcohol. A facility may have policies against any alcohol being consumed, which would have been known and agreed to by potential residents before admission.

If a doctor has not written an order stating that a resident may not have alcohol and the facility has no rules against it, a resident may drink alcohol. If a resident is allowed to do so and enjoys having an alcoholic beverage, nursing assistants should not make judgments. They should not gossip about it with other residents or staff members. However, if an NA knows that a resident should not be drinking alcohol, he should report it to the nurse.

Chapter Review

1. For each of the seven characteristics of mental health in Learning Objective 1, give one example of a behavior that demonstrates the characteristic.
2. What are four possible causes of mental illness?
3. What is the most common fallacy about mental illness?
4. Why might a physical illness cause or make a mental illness worse?
5. List six guidelines for communicating with a resident who is mentally ill.
6. What are defense mechanisms?
7. List three signs and symptoms of each of these mental illnesses: anxiety, depression, and schizophrenia.
8. What are the most common treatments for mental illness?
9. List three care guidelines for mentally ill residents.
10. List five important observations to make about a mentally ill resident.
11. List four legal substances that can be abused.
12. List ten signs and symptoms of substance abuse.

21 Rehabilitation and Restorative Care

1. Discuss rehabilitation and restorative care

When a resident loses some ability to function due to an illness or injury, rehabilitation may be ordered. **Rehabilitation** is care that is managed by professionals to help restore a person to his highest possible level of functioning. It involves helping residents move from illness, disability, and dependence toward health, ability, and independence. Rehabilitation involves all parts of the person's disability, including physical needs (e.g., eating, elimination) and psychosocial needs (e.g., independence, self-esteem).

Goals of a rehabilitative program include the following:

- To help a resident regain function or recover from illness
- To develop and promote a resident's independence
- To allow a resident to feel in control of his life
- To help a resident accept or adapt to the limitations of a disability

Rehabilitation will be used for many residents, particularly those who have suffered a stroke, accident, or trauma. Restorative care usually follows rehabilitation. The goal of restorative care is to keep the resident at the level achieved by rehabilitative services.

Both rehabilitation and restorative care take a team approach. The physician and nurses will establish goals of care (Fig. 21-1). These include promoting independence in activities of daily living (ADLs) and restoring health to optimal condition. The physical therapist, occupational therapist, and/or speech-language pathologist will work with the resident to help restore or adapt specific abilities. Social workers or other counselors may see the resident to help promote attitudes of independence and acceptance. The effects of the illness or injury cannot always be reversed. Social workers and counselors help people adjust to trauma and loss.

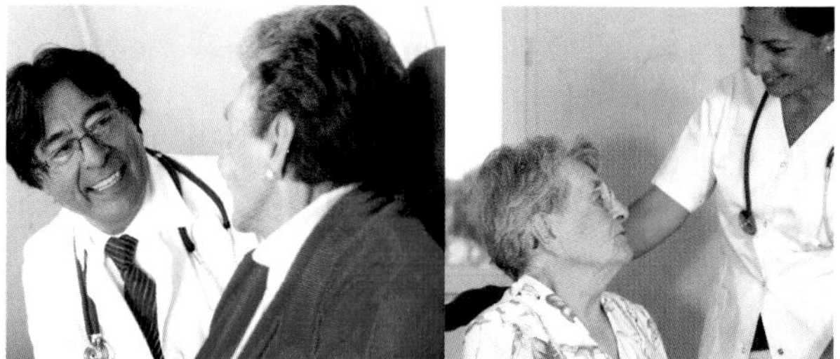

Fig. 21-1. *A team of specialists, including doctors, nurses, physical therapists, and other kinds of therapists, helps residents with rehabilitation.*

Because nursing assistants spend many hours with these residents, they are a very important part of the team. NAs play a critical role in helping residents recover and regain independence. When assisting with restorative care, these guidelines are critical to residents' progress:

Guidelines: Restorative Care

G Be patient. Progress may be slow, and it will seem slower to you and the residents if you are impatient. Residents must do as much as possible for themselves. Encourage independence and self-care, regardless of how long it takes or how poorly they are able to do it. The more patient you are, the easier it will be for them to regain abilities and confidence.

G Be positive and supportive. A positive attitude can set the tone for success. Family members and residents will take cues from you as to how they should behave. If you are encouraging and positive, you help create a supportive atmosphere for rehabilitation.

G Focus on small tasks and small accomplishments. For example, dressing themselves may seem like an overwhelming task to some residents. Break the task down into smaller steps. Today the goal might be putting on a shirt without buttoning it. Next week the goal could be buttoning the shirt if that seems manageable. When the resident can put the shirt on without help, congratulate him on reaching this goal. Take everything one step at a time.

G Recognize that setbacks occur. Progress occurs at different rates. Sometimes a resident can do something one day that he cannot do the next. Reassure residents that setbacks are normal. Focus on the things that the resident can do and not on what he cannot do. However, document any decline in a resident's abilities.

G Be sensitive to the resident's needs. Some residents may need more encouragement than others. Some may feel embarrassed by certain kinds of encouragement. Get to know your residents. Understand what motivates them. Adapt your encouragement to fit each person's personality.

G Encourage independence. A resident's independence may help his ability to be active in the process of rehabilitation. Independence improves self-image and attitude. It also helps speed recovery.

G Involve residents in their care. Residents who feel involved and valued may be more motivated to work hard in rehabilitation. Fears may be eased by including family and friends in the rehabilitation program. A team approach is inspiring.

Residents' Rights

Call Lights

Residents may need help often while going through rehabilitation. No matter how often a resident uses his call light or how demanding he is, it is never acceptable for a nursing assistant to unplug a resident's call light. Staff must respond kindly and promptly to call lights every time they are used. This response can even save lives.

Observing and Reporting: Restorative Care

O/R Any increase or decrease in abilities (For example, note, "Yesterday Mr. Martinez used the bedside commode without help. Today he asked for the bedpan.")

O/R Any change in attitude or motivation, positive or negative

O/R Any change in general health, such as changes in skin condition, appetite, energy level, or general appearance

O/R Signs of depression or mood changes

Working with residents going through rehabilitation and restorative care can be a very rewarding part of caregiving. Nursing assistants should take pride in their contributions to residents' improving health and independence.

Residents' Rights

Rehabilitation

Residents receiving rehabilitation and restorative care services have been ill or injured and are likely to feel tired, afraid, depressed, or be in pain. NAs can help them feel safe and secure by being kind, patient, and helpful. For example, if a resident's therapy schedule interferes with mealtimes, the NA can collect the resident's meal and/or re-heat it cheerfully if needed. A resident who is frightened may benefit from an unrushed conversation. If a resident says she is in pain, the NA should talk to the nurse. She should take action to help the resident. The NA can offer comfort measures, such as a back rub.

2. Describe the importance of promoting independence and list ways that exercise improves health

Maintaining independence is vital during and after rehabilitation and restorative services. When an active and independent person is dependent, physical and mental problems may result. The body becomes less mobile, and the mind is less focused. Studies show that the more active a person is, the better the mind and body work.

Exercise is important for improving and maintaining physical and mental health. Inactivity and immobility can result in loss of self-esteem, depression, pneumonia, urinary tract infection, constipation, blood clots, and dulling of the senses. People who are in bed for long periods of time are more likely to develop muscle atrophy or contractures. When atrophy occurs, the muscle wastes away, decreases in size, and becomes weak. A contracture is the permanent and often very painful shortening of a joint and muscle.

A lack of mobility may cause other problems as well. Immobility reduces the amount of blood that circulates to the skin. Residents who have restricted mobility have an increased risk for pressure ulcers. In addition, a lack of mobility can also cause problems with independence and self-esteem.

The staff's job is to keep residents as active as possible—whether they are bedbound or are able to get out of bed and walk (ambulate). Regular ambulation and exercise help improve the following:

- Quality and health of the skin
- Circulation
- Strength
- Sleep and relaxation
- Mood
- Self-esteem
- Appetite
- Elimination
- Blood flow
- Oxygen level

Promoting social interactions and thinking abilities is important, too. Most facilities have activities geared to residents' ages and abilities. Social involvement should be encouraged. When possible, nursing assistants should join in activities with residents (Fig. 21-2). This promotes independence. It also gives NAs a chance to observe residents' abilities.

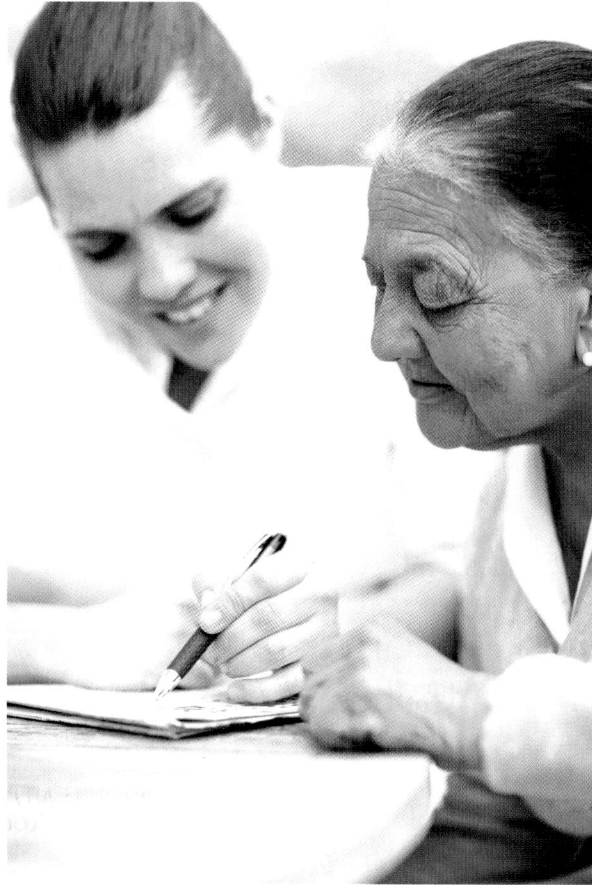

Fig. 21-2. *Promoting mental and physical activity is important. When possible, NAs should join in activities with residents. This NA is helping a resident complete a crossword puzzle.*

Basic Exercise Principles

It is important to get a doctor's approval before starting a new exercise or activity program. It is not safe to exercise with certain heart conditions. Exercising with high blood pressure can be risky. Caution must be used after surgery. It is also necessary to limit exercise if a person has unstable bones, fractures, osteoporosis, or extreme breathing problems.

Warming up should be done before doing any other exercises. This consists of light exercise, such as walking. The warm-up begins to increase heart rate and breathing. It helps prevent injury. Some people like to stretch at the beginning of their workout. Stretching should not be done until the muscles are warm.

Cool-down exercises are done to slowly lower the heart rate. They return other body functions to normal. Suddenly ending an exercise session without cooling down can cause blood to pool in the large leg muscles. This may cause dizziness or even fainting. It is good to stretch after the cool-down, while the muscles are still warm. Stretching keeps muscles flexible and helps them relax.

3. Describe assistive devices and equipment

Many devices are available to help people who are recovering from or adapting to a physical condition. Chapter 2 introduced information about assistive or adaptive equipment. This equipment helps residents perform their activities of daily living (ADLs). Each adaptive device is made to support a particular disability. Raised seating, for example, makes it easier for a resident with weak legs to stand.

Personal care equipment includes long-handled brushes and combs. Plate guards prevent food from being pushed off the plate and make it easier to scoop food onto utensils. Reachers can help put on underwear or pants. A sock aid can pull on socks, and a long-handled shoehorn assists in putting shoes on without bending. Long-handled sponges help with bathing.

Supportive devices, such as canes, walkers, and crutches, are used to assist residents with ambulation (as described in Chapter 10). Safety devices, such as shower chairs and gait or transfer belts, help prevent accidents. Safety bars/grab bars are often installed in and near the tub and toilet to give the resident something to hold on to while changing position. The items shown in Fig. 21-3 can be useful as residents relearn old skills or adapt to new limitations.

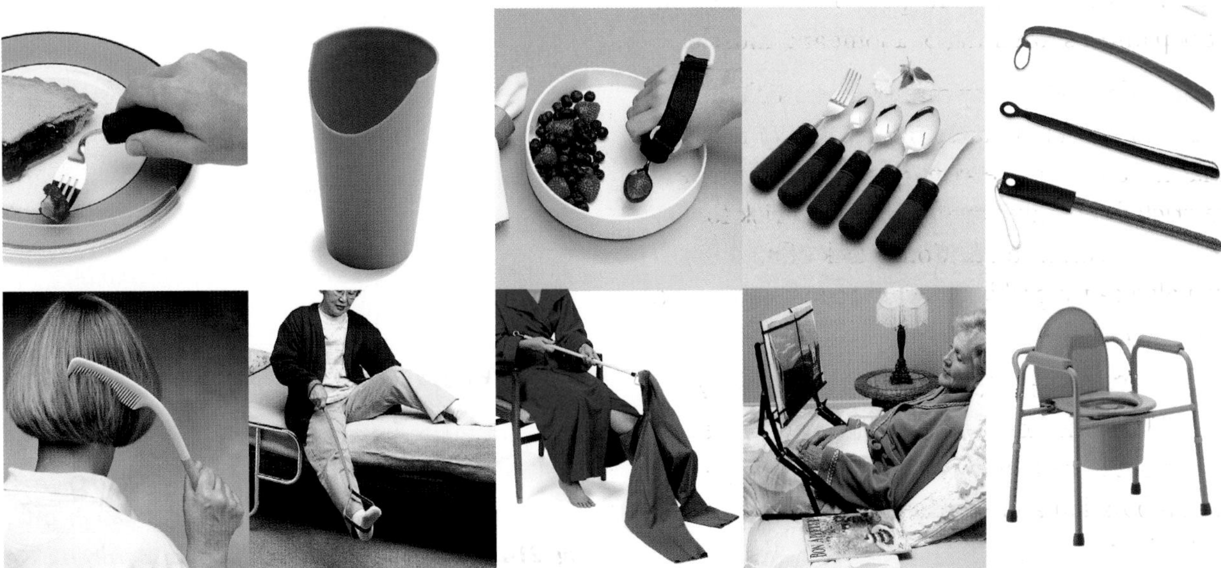

Fig. 21-3. *Many assistive items are available to help residents adapt to physical changes.* (PHOTOS COURTESY OF NORTH COAST MEDICAL, INC., WWW.NCMEDICAL.COM, 800-821-9319)

Residents' Rights

Walking Aids

Residents using new ambulatory aids, such as canes, walkers, boots, crutches, etc., are likely to be off-balance. The nursing assistant should stay close by to be sure they are using these appliances safely. She should observe residents for signs of dizziness. Residents should not be rushed while they are using these devices. The NA should let residents set the pace. To avoid falls, she should clear pathways and wipe up spills immediately.

Trapeze

A trapeze is a triangular piece of equipment that hangs over the head of the bed. It may be mounted to the bed or freestanding. People in bed can grasp the trapeze with their hands, which enables them to lift themselves. The trapeze assists with repositioning and exercise activities.

4. Explain guidelines for maintaining proper body alignment

Residents who are confined to bed need to maintain proper body alignment. This aids recovery and prevents injury to muscles and joints. Chapter 10 includes specific instructions for positioning residents. The following guidelines help residents maintain proper alignment and make progress when they are able to get out of bed.

Guidelines: Alignment and Positioning

- **G** Observe principles of alignment. Remember that proper alignment is based on straight lines. The spine should be in a straight line. Pillows or rolled or folded blankets can support the small of the back and raise the knees or head in the supine position. They can support the head and one leg in the lateral position (Fig. 21-4).
- **G** Keep body parts in natural positions. In a natural hand position, the fingers are slightly curled. Use a rolled washcloth, gauze bandage, or rubber ball inside the palm to support the fingers in this position. Use bed cradles to keep covers from resting on feet if resident is in the supine position.

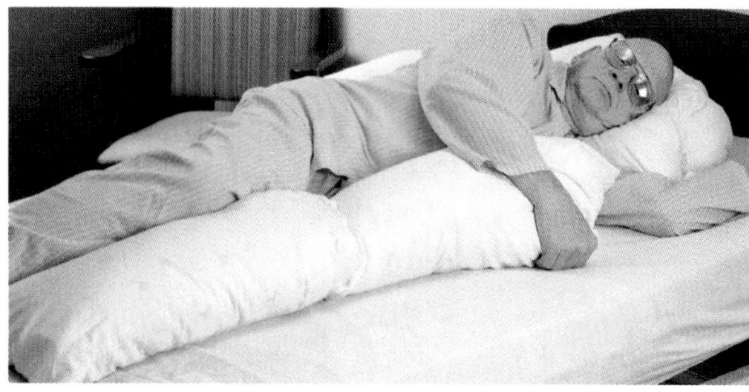

Fig. 21-4. *Pillows or rolled or folded blankets help provide extra support.*

- **G** Prevent external rotation of hips. When legs and hips are allowed to turn outward during long periods of bedrest, hip contractures can result. A rolled blanket or towel tucked alongside the hip and thigh can keep the leg from turning outward.
- **G** Change positions often to prevent muscle stiffness and pressure ulcers. This should be done at least every two hours. Which position the resident uses will depend on the resident's condition and preference. Check the skin every time you reposition the resident.

5. Explain care guidelines for prosthetic devices

A prosthesis is a device that replaces a body part that is missing or deformed because of an accident, injury, illness, or birth defect. It is used to improve a person's ability to function and/or to improve appearance. Examples of prostheses include the following:

- Artificial limbs, such as artificial hands, arms, feet, and legs, are made to resemble the body part that they are replacing (Fig. 21-5). Many advances have been made and continue to be made in the field of prosthetic limbs. Today's artificial limbs are usually made of strong and lightweight plastics and other materials, such as carbon fiber. Most artificial limbs are attached by belts, cuffs, or suction. Direct bone attachment is a newer method of attaching the limb to the body.

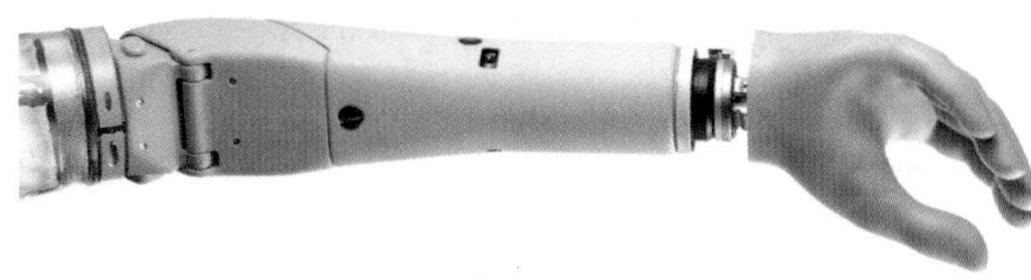

Fig. 21-5. A type of prosthetic arm. (COURTESY: MOTION CONTROL, INC., A SUBSIDIARY OF FILLAUER, SALT LAKE CITY, UT)

- An artificial breast is made of a lightweight, soft, spongy material. It usually fits into a regular bra or in the pocket of a special bra called a mastectomy bra.
- A hearing aid is a small, battery-operated device that amplifies sound for persons with hearing loss. Many elderly residents have hearing aids. Chapter 4 contains more information on hearing aids.
- An artificial eye, or ocular prosthetic, replaces an eye that has been lost to disease or injury. It is usually made of plastic. It is held in place by suction. An ocular prosthetic does not provide vision; it can, however, improve appearance.
- Dentures are artificial teeth. They may be necessary when teeth have been damaged, lost, or must be removed. Many elderly residents have dentures. Chapter 13 has more information on denture care.

Guidelines: Prosthetic Devices

G Because prostheses are specially-fitted, expensive pieces of equipment (some cost tens of thousands of dollars), only care for them as assigned. Handle them carefully. Follow the care plan. Know exactly how to care for the equipment before you begin. If you have any questions, talk to the nurse.

G A therapist or nurse will demonstrate application of a prosthesis. Follow instructions to apply and remove the prosthesis. Follow the manufacturer's care directions.

G Keep the prosthesis and the skin under it dry and clean. The socket of the prosthesis must be cleaned at least daily. Follow the care plan and the nurse's instructions.

G If ordered, apply a stump sock before putting on the prosthesis.

G Observe the skin on the stump. Watch for signs of skin breakdown caused by pressure and abrasion. Report redness or open areas.

G Never try to fix a prosthesis. Report any problems to the nurse.

G Do not show negative feelings about the stump during care.

G If instructed to care for an artificial eye, review the care plan with the nurse. Before handling an artificial eye, wash your hands. Provide privacy for the resident. Put on gloves before beginning care. Artificial eyes are held in by suction. They will come out quickly when pressure is applied below the lower eyelid. Some artificial eyes do not require frequent removal. Others need daily removal and cleaning.

G If the artificial eye is removed, wash the eye with solution and rinse in warm water. Never clean or soak the eye in rubbing alcohol. It will crack the plastic and destroy it.

G When the artificial eye is removed, wash the eye socket with warm water or saline. Use a clean gauze square to clean it. Clean the eyelid with a clean cotton ball. Wipe gently from inner corner (canthus) outward.

G If the artificial eye is to be removed and not reinserted, line an eye cup or basin with a soft cloth or a piece of 4x4 gauze. This prevents scratches and damage. Fill with water or saline solution. Place the artificial eye in the container and close the container. Make sure the container is labeled with the resident's name and room number.

G To reinsert the eye, moisten it and place it far under upper eyelid. Pull down on lower eyelid and the eye should slide into place.

6. Describe how to assist with range of motion exercises

Range of motion (ROM) exercises put a particular joint through its full arc of motion. The goals of range of motion exercises are to decrease or prevent contractures or atrophy, improve strength, and increase circulation. Types of range of motion exercises are as follows:

Active range of motion (AROM) exercises are performed by a resident himself, without help. The nursing assistant's role in AROM exercises is to encourage the resident.

Active assisted range of motion (AAROM) exercises are done by the resident with some assistance and support from the nursing assistant or other caregiver.

Passive range of motion (PROM) exercises are used when residents are not able to move on their own. PROM exercises are performed by the caregiver, without the resident's help.

Range of motion exercises are specific for each body area. They include the following movements (Fig. 21-6):

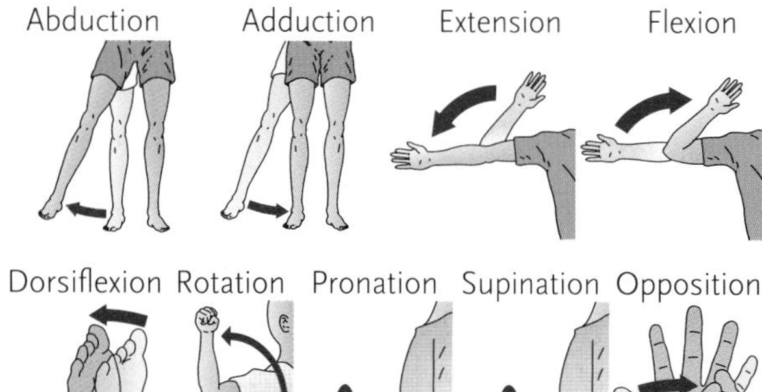

Fig. 21-6. The different range of motion body movements.

- **Abduction**: moving a body part away from the midline of the body
- **Adduction**: moving a body part toward the midline of the body
- **Extension**: straightening a body part
- **Flexion**: bending a body part
- **Dorsiflexion**: bending backward
- **Rotation**: turning a joint
- **Pronation**: turning downward
- **Supination**: turning upward
- **Opposition**: touching the thumb to any other finger

Nursing assistants will not perform ROM exercises without a specific order from a doctor, nurse, or physical therapist. Depending on the care plan, the NA will repeat each exercise three to five times, once or twice a day, working on both sides of the body. When performing ROM exercises, the NA should begin at the resident's head and work down the body. The upper extremities (arms) should be exercised before the lower extremities (legs). The NA should give support above and below the joint. The joints should be moved gently, slowly, and smoothly through the range of motion to the point of resistance. It is important to stop the exercises if the resident complains of pain and to report the pain to the nurse.

Assisting with passive range of motion exercises

1. Identify yourself by name. Identify the resident by name.
2. Wash your hands.
3. Explain procedure to resident. Speak clearly, slowly, and directly. Maintain face-to-face contact whenever possible.
4. Provide for resident's privacy with curtain, screen, or door.
5. Adjust bed to a safe level, usually waist high. Lock bed wheels.
6. Position the resident lying supine—flat on her back—on the bed. Use proper alignment.
7. While supporting the limbs, move all joints

gently, slowly, and smoothly through the range of motion to the point of resistance. Repeat each exercise at least three times unless the resident complains of pain. Stop performing exercises if resident complains of pain and report to the nurse.

8. **Shoulder**. Support the resident's arm at the elbow and wrist while performing ROM for the shoulder. Place one hand under the elbow and the other hand under the wrist. Raise the straightened arm from the side position upward toward head to ear level and return arm down to side of the body (extension/flexion) (Fig. 21-7).

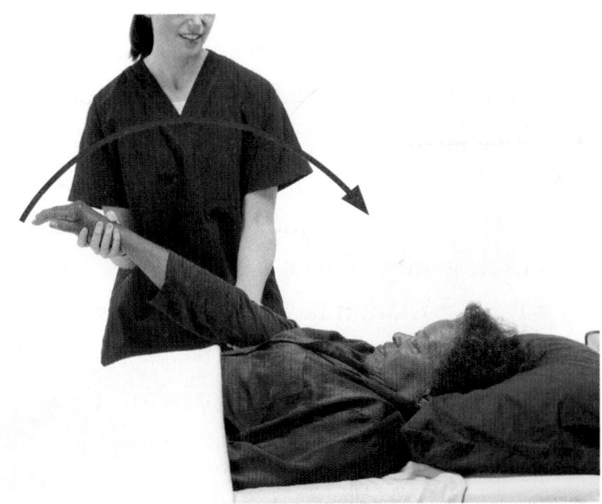

Fig. 21-7. *Raise the straightened arm upward toward head to ear level and return it to the side of the body.*

Move straightened arm away from side of body to shoulder level and return arm to side of body(abduction/adduction)(Fig. 21-8).

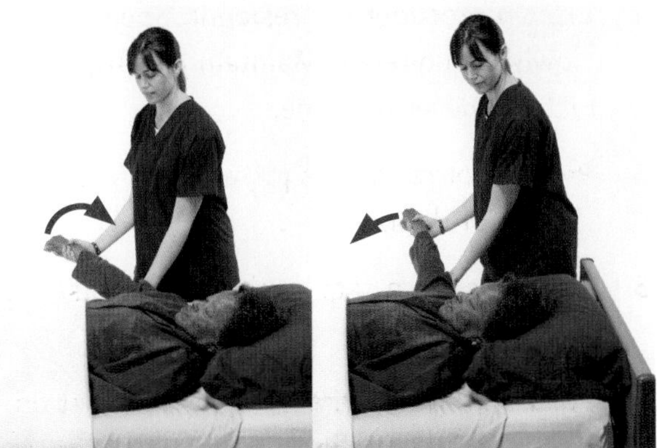

Fig. 21-8. *Move straightened arm away from side of body to shoulder level and return arm to side.*

9. **Elbow**. Hold the resident's wrist with one hand and the elbow with the other hand. Bend the elbow so that the hand touches the shoulder on that same side (flexion). Straighten the arm (extension) (Fig. 21-9).

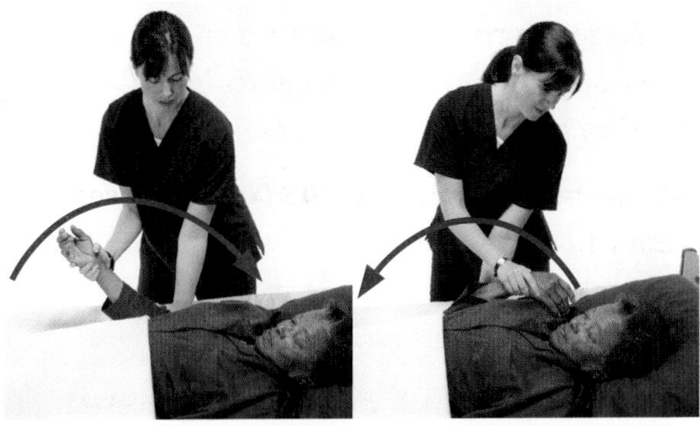

Fig. 21-9. *Bend the elbow so that the hand touches the shoulder on the same side, and then straighten the arm.*

Exercise the forearm by moving it so the palm is facing downward (pronation) and then the palm is facing upward (supination) (Fig. 21-10).

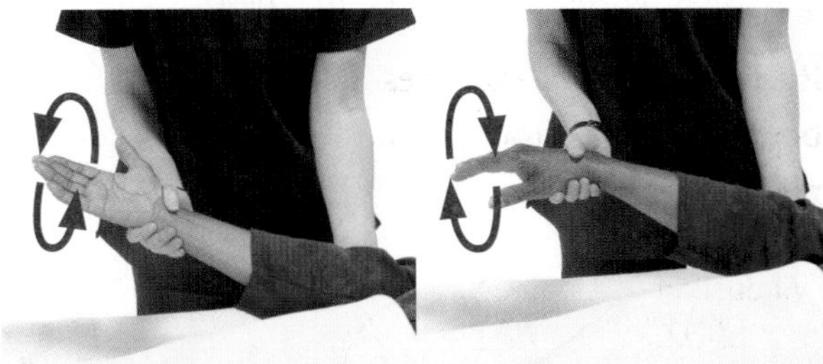

Fig. 21-10. *Exercise the forearm so that the palm is facing downward and then upward.*

10. **Wrist**. Hold the wrist with one hand and use the fingers of the other hand to help move the joint through the motions. Bend the hand down (flexion); bend the hand backward (dorsiflexion) (Fig. 21-11).

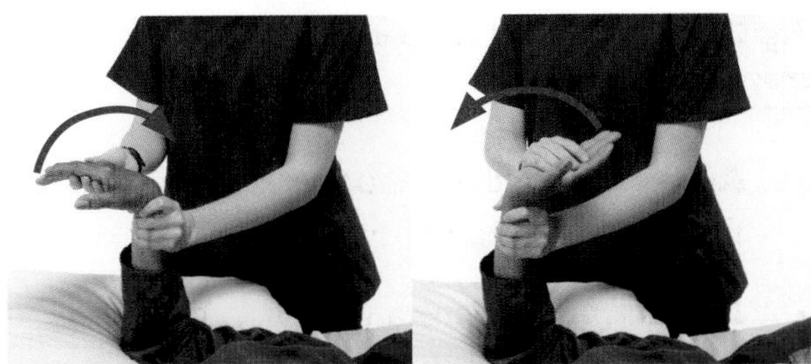

Fig. 21-11. *While supporting the wrist, gently bend the hand down and then backward.*

Turn the hand in the direction of the thumb (radial flexion). Then turn the hand in the direction of the little finger (ulnar flexion) (Fig. 21-12).

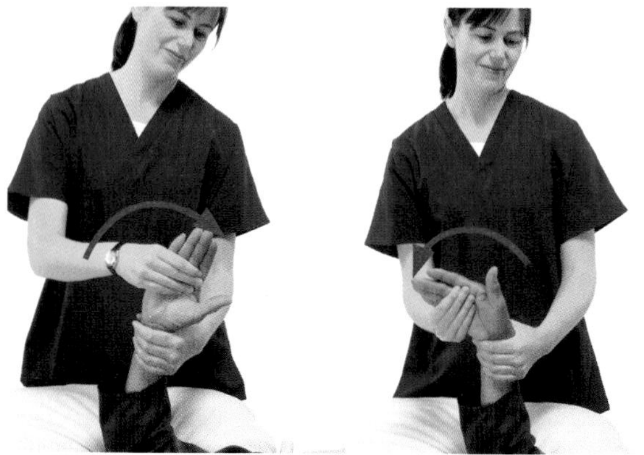

Fig. 21-12. Turn the hand in the direction of the thumb, then turn it in the direction of the little finger.

11. **Thumb**. Move the thumb away from the index finger (abduction). Move the thumb back next to the index finger (adduction) (Fig. 21-13).

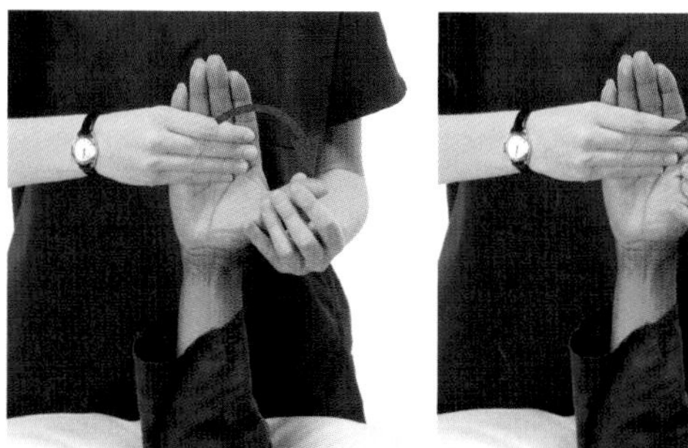

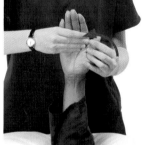

Fig. 21-13. Move the thumb away from the index finger and then back to the index finger.

Touch each fingertip with the thumb (opposition) (Fig. 21-14).

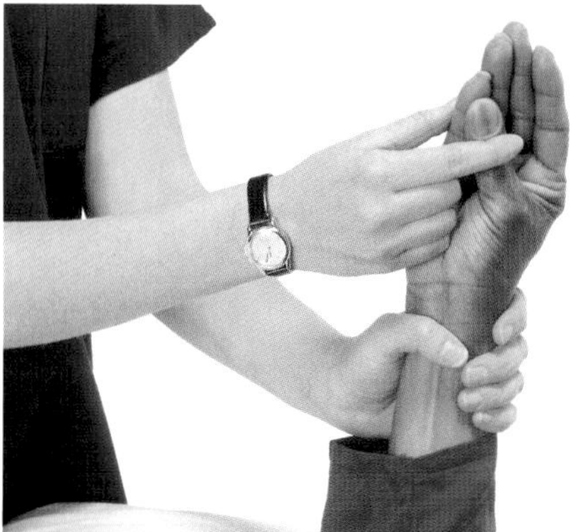

Fig. 21-14. Touch each fingertip with the thumb.

Bend thumb into the palm (flexion) and out to the side (extension) (Fig. 21-15).

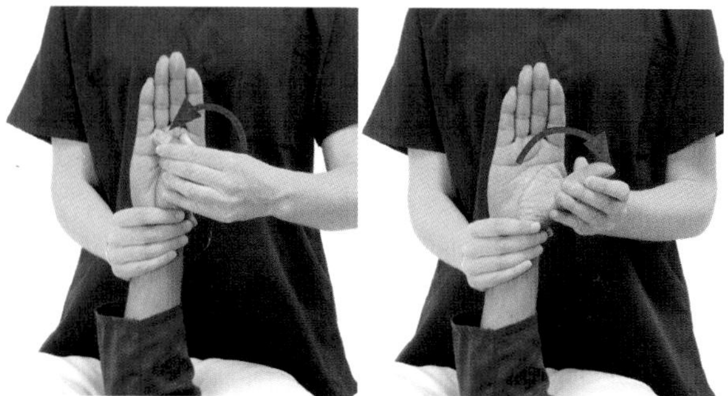

Fig. 21-15. Bend the thumb into the palm and then out to the side.

12. **Fingers**. Make the hand into a fist (flexion). Gently straighten out the fist (extension) (Fig. 21-16).

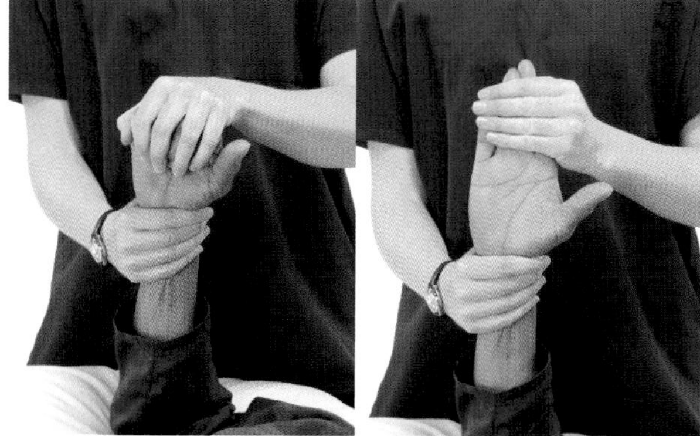

Fig. 21-16. Make the fingers into a fist and then gently straighten out the fist.

Spread the fingers and the thumb far apart from each other (abduction). Bring the fingers back next to each other (adduction) (Fig. 21-17).

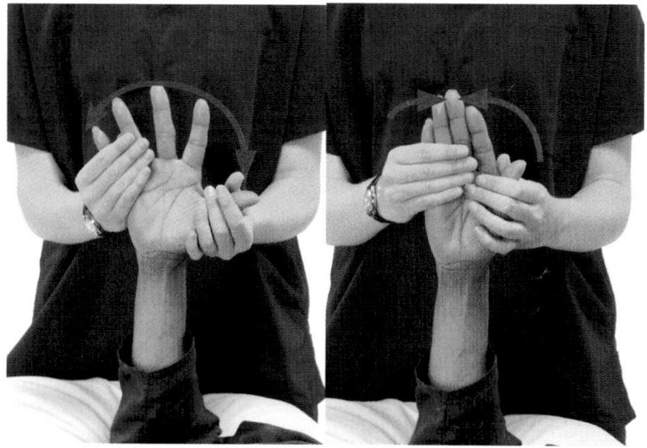

Fig. 21-17. Spread the fingers and thumb far apart from each other and then bring them back next to each other.

13. **Hip**. Support the leg by placing one hand under the knee and one under the ankle. Straighten the leg and raise it gently upward. Move the leg away from the other leg (abduction). Move the leg toward the other leg (adduction) (Fig. 21-18).

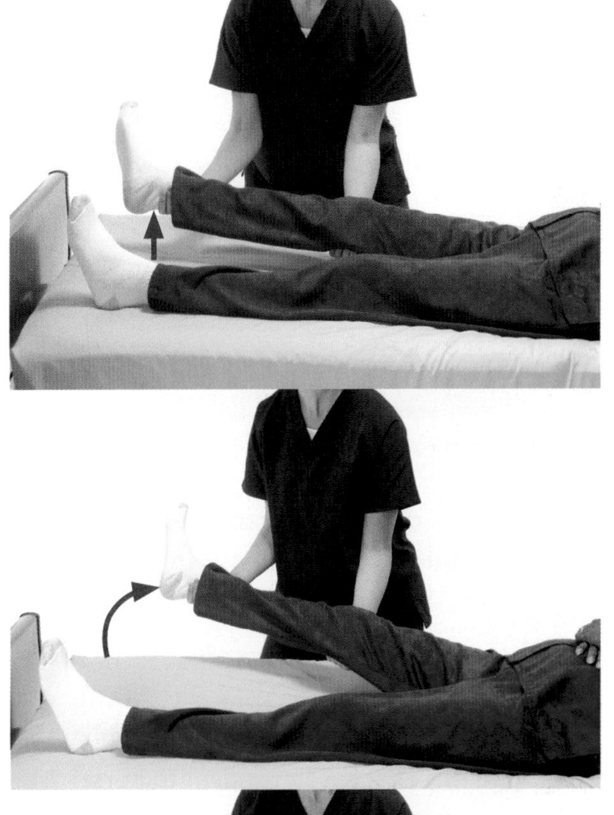

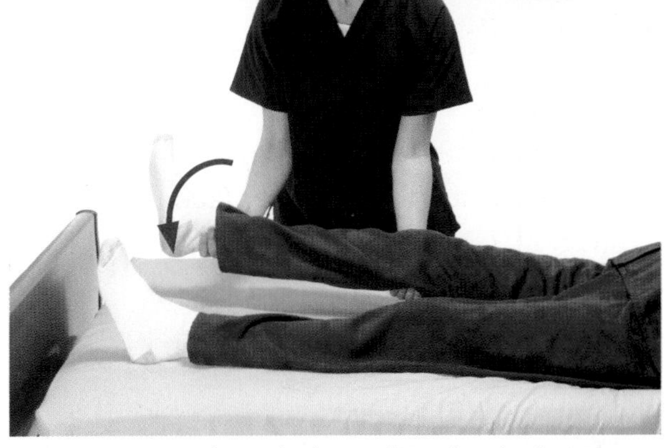

Fig. 21-18. *Straighten the leg and gently raise it. Move the leg away from the other leg and then back toward the other leg.*

Gently turn the leg inward (internal rotation), then turn the leg outward (external rotation) (Fig. 21-19).

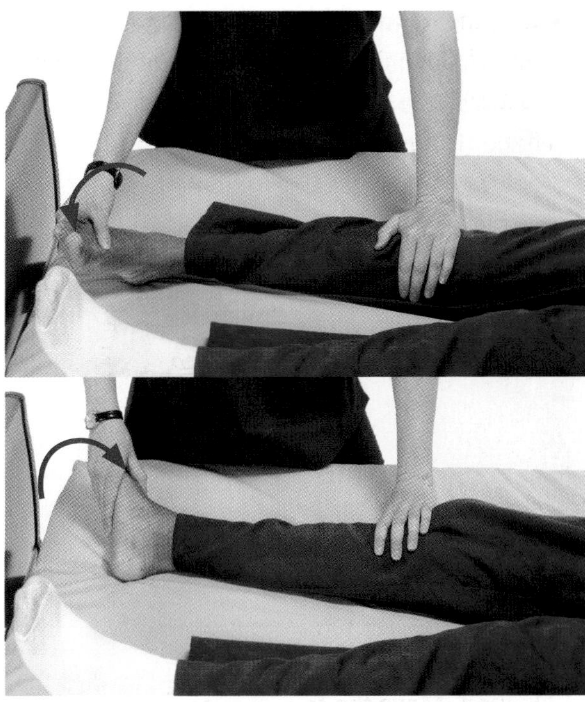

Fig. 21-19. *Gently turn the leg inward and then outward.*

14. **Knee**. Support the leg under the knee and under the ankle while performing ROM for the knee. Bend the knee to the point of resistance (flexion). Return leg to resident's normal position (extension) (Fig. 21-20).

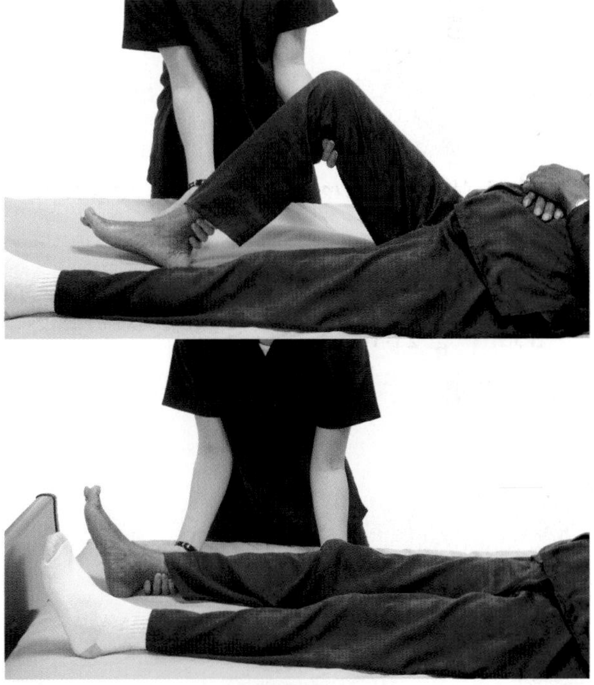

Fig. 21-20. *Gently bend the knee to the point of resistance and return the leg to its normal position.*

15. **Ankle**. Support the foot and ankle close to the bed while performing ROM for the ankle. Push/pull foot up toward the head (dorsiflexion). Push/pull foot down, with the toes pointed down (plantar flexion) (Fig. 21-21).

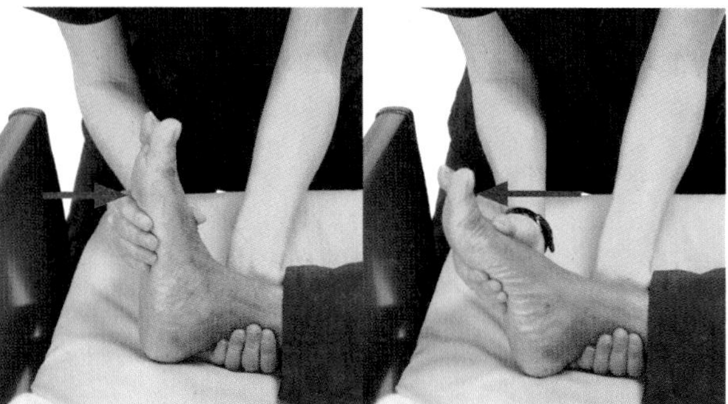

Fig. 21-21. *Push the foot up toward the head and then push it back down.*

Turn the inside of the foot inward toward the body (supination). Bend the sole of the foot so that it faces away from the body (pronation) (Fig. 21-22).

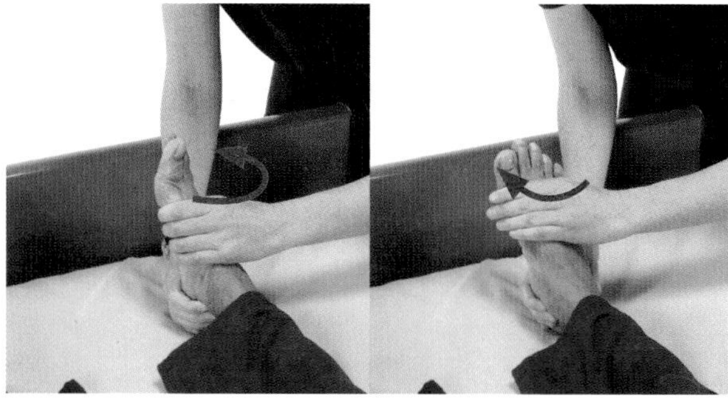

Fig. 21-22. *Turn inside of foot inward, toward the body, and then bend it to face away from the body.*

16. **Toes**. Curl and straighten the toes (flexion and extension) (Fig. 21-23).

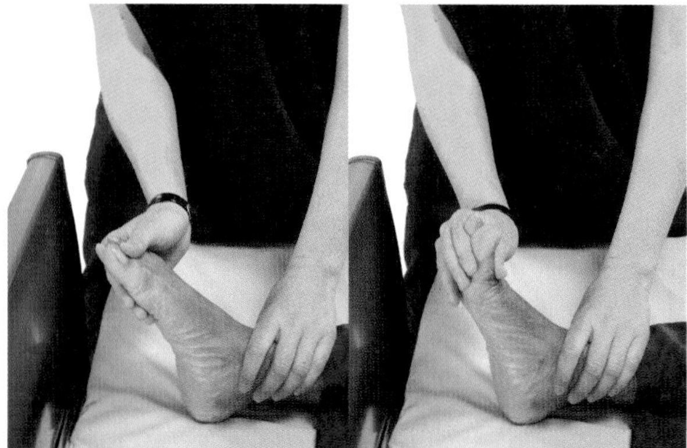

Fig. 21-23. *Curl and straighten the toes.*

Gently spread the toes apart (abduction) (Fig. 21-24).

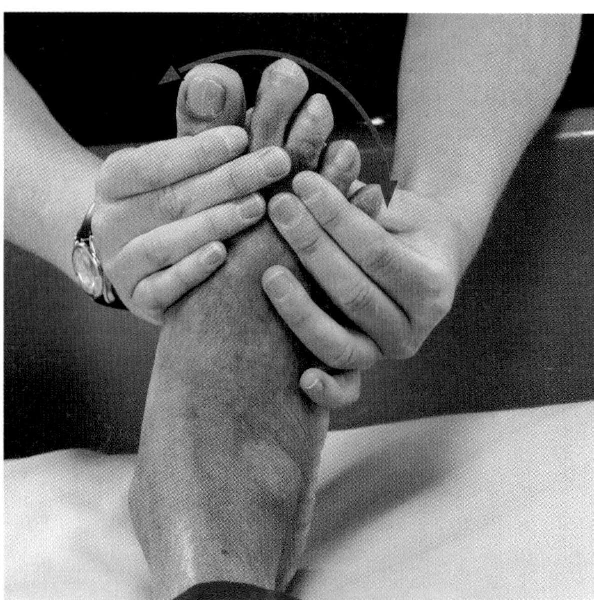

Fig. 21-24. *Gently spread the toes apart.*

17. Return resident to comfortable position. Return bed to lowest position. Remove privacy measures.
18. Place call light within resident's reach.
19. Wash your hands.
20. Report any changes in resident to nurse.
21. Document procedure using facility guidelines. Note any decrease in range of motion or any pain experienced by the resident. Notify the nurse or the physical therapist if you find increased stiffness or physical resistance. Resistance may be a sign that a contracture is developing.

7. Describe the benefits of deep breathing exercises

Deep breathing exercises help expand the lungs, clearing them of mucus and preventing infections (such as pneumonia). Residents who are paralyzed or who have had abdominal surgery are often encouraged to do deep breathing exercises regularly to expand the lungs.

The care plan may include using a deep breathing device called an incentive spirometer (Fig. 21-25). Nursing assistants should not assist with these exercises if they have not been trained; they must ask the nurse for instructions.

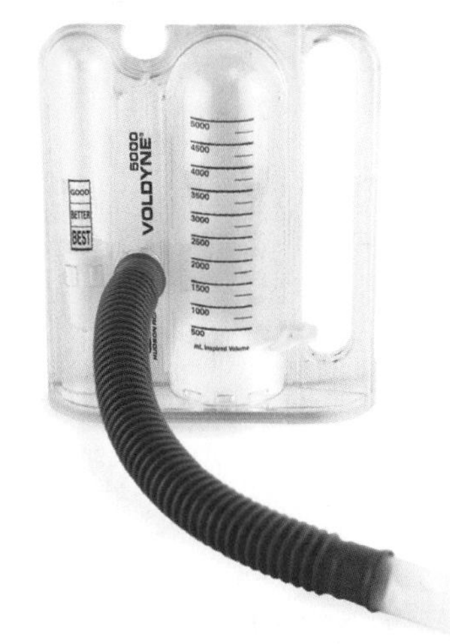

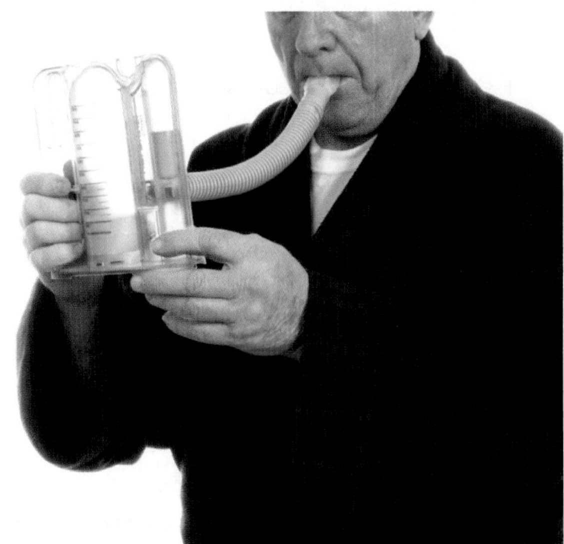

Fig. 21-25. *Incentive spirometers are used for deep breathing exercises.*

Chapter Review

1. What does rehabilitation involve?
   Helping residents moving to health, being more able and independent
2. What attitudes can an NA adopt to assist in residents' restorative care? Give an example of each.
   A) Be patient. ex. Let them try to brush teeth no matter how long it takes
   B) Be cheerful: Comment on how well they did. Smile, laugh
   C) If needed, break down tasks to smaller ones. Don't try to have them totally get dressed themselves
   D) Help them realize setbacks are normal. Don't scold, but have them try again.
   E) Know their personality & what motivates them.
   F) Involve residents in their own care & their family too!
3. List 10 problems that a lack of mobility can cause.
   Lower selfesteem, depression, pneumonia, UTI, constipation, Blood clots, Dullness, Muscle atrophy, contractures, pressure sores
4. What are some benefits of regular exercise?
   Quality of health of the skin, Circulation, Strength, Better sleep & relaxation, Better mood & self esteem, Appetite, Elimination, Blood flow, Oxygen
5. Look at the adaptive devices in Figure 21-3. Choose one and briefly describe how it might help a resident recovering from or adapting to a physical condition.
   A fork that is made with a curve helps get food into mouth
6. List three guidelines to follow to help residents maintain proper alignment.
   The spine should be in a straight line. Body parts should be in natural positions. Prevent external rotation of hips. Change positions often.
7. List and describe four prosthetic devices.
   Artificial limb (leg), Eye, Hearing Aid, Breast, Dentures
8. What should be observed about the skin on the stump of an amputated body part?
   Look for Redness, sores, swelling, abrasion or cuts. ANY SKIN BREAKDOWN
9. Why should alcohol not be used to clean an artificial eye?
   It will cause the plastic to become cloudy or crack & destroy it.
10. What is the purpose of range of motion (ROM) exercises?
    ROM prevents or decreases contractures, or atrophy. They improve strength and help increase circulation & flexibility
11. When performing ROM exercises, where should the NA begin? Which parts of the body should be exercised first?
    Head on down. The arms & hands then legs & feet.
12. Describe the difference between passive, active, and active assisted range of motion exercises.
    passive – No help from patient. active – patient does it all by himself. active assisted – patient does it with help of a NA
13. Why are deep breathing exercises performed?
    To expand the lungs preventing pneumonia. It helps clear mucus. It helps prevent infections.

22 Special Care Skills

1. Understand the types of residents who are in a subacute setting

Subacute care is a kind of specialized care that falls between acute care and long-term care. This type of care can take place in hospitals and in skilled nursing facilities. People in subacute settings require more treatment, monitoring, and services than regular long-term care provides (Fig. 22-1). Subacute care may be necessary due to recent surgery, injuries, or chronic illnesses, such as AIDS.

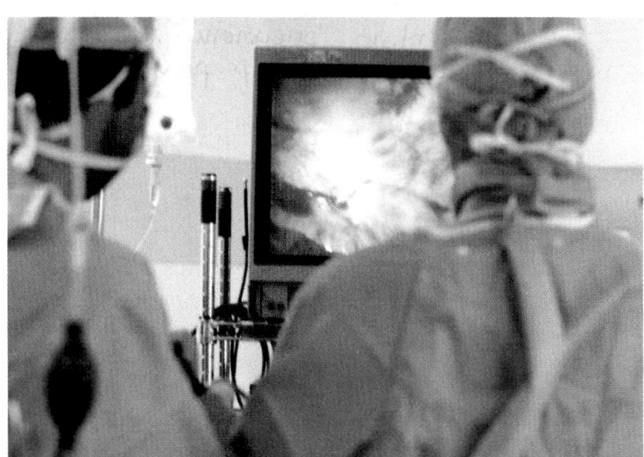

Fig. 22-1. *Subacute care provides a higher level of care; it may be necessary due to surgery, illness, serious wounds, dialysis, or mechanical ventilation.*

Complex wound care, specialized infusion therapy, dialysis, and mechanical ventilation may also require subacute care. Dialysis cleans the body of waste that the kidneys cannot remove due to chronic kidney failure (Fig. 22-2). A mechanical ventilator is a machine that assists with or replaces breathing when a person cannot breathe on his own.

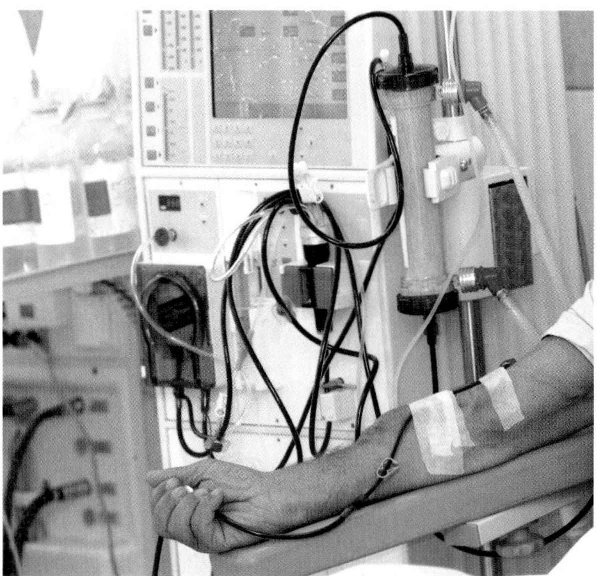

Fig. 22-2. *A patient hooked up to a dialysis machine.*

2. Discuss reasons for and types of surgery

There are many reasons why surgery is performed, including the following:

- To relieve symptoms of a disease
- To repair or remove problem tissues and structures
- To improve appearance or correct function of damaged tissues
- To diagnose disease
- To cure a disease

Surgeries generally fall into three categories: elective, urgent, and emergency. Elective surgery is surgery that is chosen by the patient and is planned in advance. Generally, the surgery is not absolutely necessary. Plastic surgery, such as having a facelift, is an example of an elective surgery.

Urgent surgery is surgery that must be performed for health reasons, but is not an emergency. Urgent surgery may even be planned and scheduled in advance, as with heart surgery such as coronary artery bypass surgery.

Emergency surgery is unexpected and unscheduled surgery that is performed immediately to save a patient's life or a limb. A gunshot wound, car accident, or ruptured appendix are examples of situations that can require emergency surgery.

When a person has surgery, anesthesia will usually be given. **Anesthesia** involves the use of medication to block pain during surgery and other medical procedures. Local anesthesia involves the injection of an anesthetic directly into the surgical site or area to block pain. It is used for minor surgical procedures, and the person may remain awake during the surgery. Regional anesthesia involves injection of an anesthetic into a nerve or group of nerves to block sensation in a particular region of the body. It is limited to an area, but to a larger area than for a local anesthetic. One example of a regional anesthetic is an epidural, which is used during childbirth to block pain in the lower half of the body, from the waist down. General anesthesia is inhaled or injected directly into a vein and affects the brain and the entire body. The person is unaware of his surroundings and does not feel any pain. It blocks any memory of the procedure. This type of anesthesia is stopped when the surgery has been completed.

3. Discuss preoperative care

Depending on where a nursing assistant works, his duties may include giving **preoperative**, or before-surgery, care. Preoperative care includes both physical and psychological preparation. Before a person has surgery, a doctor will explain the procedure, the risks and benefits, and what to expect after surgery. The person will be encouraged to ask questions and give opinions. This is part of informed consent (Chapter 3), a process in which a person, with the help of a doctor, makes informed decisions about her health care. The person must sign a written consent form for surgery or have one signed by a guardian or someone with medical power of attorney.

People who are going to have surgery often experience anxiety, fear, worry, sadness, and other emotions (Fig. 22-3). It is often helpful to express these concerns to members of the healthcare team. Being prepared psychologically may help the resident cope better after surgery. Part of a nursing assistant's role in assisting with this preparation is listening to a resident's concerns. The NA should report any concerns or questions, including requests for a visit from clergy, to the nurse.

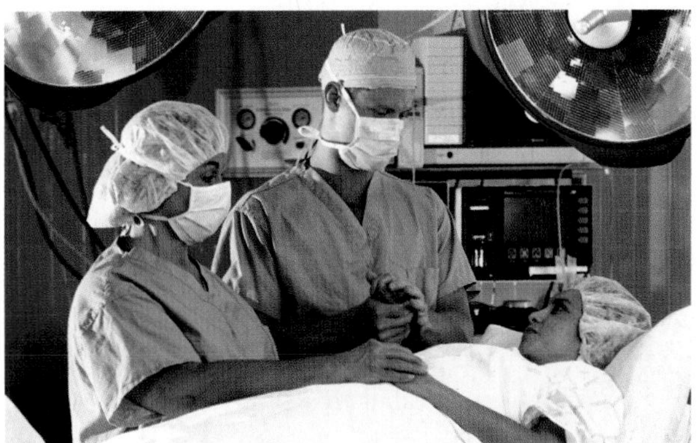

Fig. 22-3. *Patients often have many worries before surgery. A compassionate response by staff may help alleviate concerns.*

A person who is having surgery will require preoperative physical preparation as well. These general guidelines explain physical preparation for surgery:

Guidelines: Preoperative Care

- **G** Before surgery, there will be an order for the resident to receive nothing by mouth (NPO). This time usually ranges anywhere from two to eight hours. Having this medical order means that nothing is allowed by mouth, including water, ice chips, food, etc. Remove the water pitcher, glass, and any other food and fluids from the immediate area. Explain to the resident why you are doing this. Report any concerns to the nurse.

G Assist the resident with urinating before surgery.

G For some residents having surgery of the gastrointestinal tract, the bowels may need to be cleared. An enema or suppository may be ordered. Assist as trained, ordered, and allowed. Be ready to bring the bedpan or portable commode when needed. Provide plenty of privacy.

G Assist with bathing as needed. Dressing the person in loose-fitting clothes may make it easier to change into a gown later.

G Make sure call light is within reach every time before you leave the room.

G Measure and record vital signs as ordered.

G Remove dentures, eyeglasses, contact lenses, hearing aids, jewelry, hairpieces, hairpins, and any other personal items. Store these safely according to policy. For local or regional anesthetic, the doctor may want the person to wear hearing aids and dentures, so that communication will be easier.

G Assist resident to change into gown if required.

G Transfer to a stretcher/gurney if necessary.

G Make sure the resident's identification bracelet is accurate and on the wrist or ankle prior to transport. You may need to verify if the resident has any known allergies by asking this question or verifying what is written on an allergy bracelet.

4. Describe postoperative care

Postoperative, or after-surgery, care begins immediately following surgery. The goal of postoperative care is to prevent infections, promote healing, and return the person to a state of health. Immediate postoperative concerns are problems with breathing, mental status, pain, and wound healing. Complications of surgery can also include urinary retention or infections, constipation, blood pressure variances, and blood clots. Careful postoperative monitoring is critical.

After surgery, the resident is taken to the recovery room and may remain there for some time. This depends on the type of surgery that the resident had, as well as how long the surgery was, what type and how much anesthetic was used, and the resident's level of consciousness.

While the resident is in recovery, the nursing assistant's duties will include changing bed linens and gathering equipment. Equipment needed may include the following:

- Bed protector
- Towels and washcloths
- Vital signs equipment
- Emesis basin
- Pillows and other positioning devices
- Warming blankets
- IV pole
- Oxygen and suction equipment

When the resident returns to the room, the following guidelines are used in providing postoperative care:

Guidelines: Postoperative Care

G Move furniture as needed to allow for the transfer back into bed from the stretcher.

G Assist with transferring the resident back into bed. (Chapter 10 has information on stretcher transfers.)

G Return dentures, eyeglasses, contact lenses, and hearing aids to the resident. Remember that without these items, residents may not be able to talk, eat, see, or hear.

G Measure and record vital signs often after surgery as directed. The schedule may look like this: every 15 minutes for the first hour, every 30 minutes for the next hour to two hours, every hour for the next four hours, and then every four hours. Report any changes immediately.

G Reposition the resident every one to two hours, or as ordered. Elevate the extremities as ordered.

G Assist with deep breathing and coughing exercises (Chapter 21).

G Anti-embolic hose and sequential compression devices (SCDs) may be ordered to increase circulation and reduce the risk of blood clots. A sequential compression device is a plastic, air-filled sleeve that is put on the leg and hooked up to a machine. When turned on, the machine inflates and deflates the sleeve, creating pressure and promoting blood flow. Assist with anti-embolic hose, SCDs, and with leg exercises as instructed.

G Binders are stretchable pieces of fabric that can be fastened. They hold dressings in place and give support to surgical wounds. Binders can also reduce swelling and ease discomfort. Apply binders as ordered.

G Surgical drains may be placed near the incision (Fig. 22-4). These drains help prevent fluid build-up, which can lead to infection. Surgical drains are connected to a collection device such as a bulb, which is emptied regularly. Observe the amount and appearance of the drainage as directed. Sometimes nursing assistants are also responsible for measuring the amount of drainage. If this is part of your responsibilities, the nurse will train you to do it.

G Encourage resident to follow diet orders. A post-operative resident may have an *NPO* order or an order for a clear liquid diet. The resident may be on a high-protein diet to promote wound healing. Following diet orders can help speed the recovery process.

G Assist with elimination. Always provide plenty of privacy for elimination.

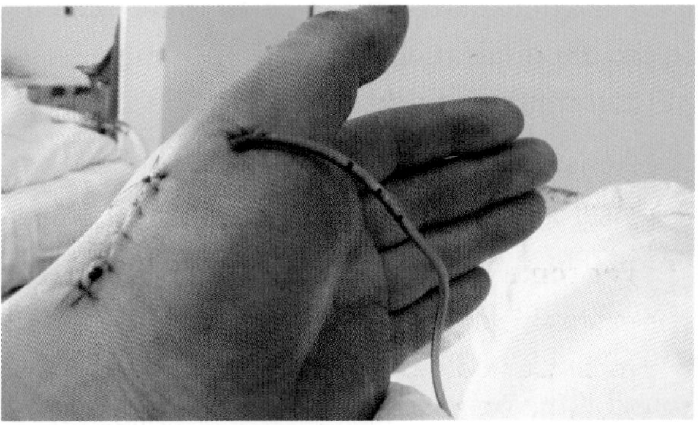

Fig. 22-4. *This photo shows a post-operative hand with a drainage tube in it.* (PHOTO COURTESY OF PAVEL ŠEVELA / WIKIMEDIA COMMONS)

G Help with bathing and grooming as requested and as ordered.

G Assist with ambulation as needed and as ordered. Be encouraging and positive.

Observing and Reporting: Postoperative Care

Report the following signs and symptoms of complications to the nurse immediately:

O/R Changes in vital signs

O/R Difficulty breathing

O/R Mental changes, such as confusion or disorientation

O/R Changes in consciousness

O/R Pale or cyanotic (bluish) skin

O/R Skin that is cold or clammy

O/R Increase in amount of drainage

O/R Swelling at IV site

O/R IV that is not dripping

O/R Nausea or vomiting

O/R Numbness or tingling

O/R Resident complains of pain

5. List care guidelines for pulse oximetry

When residents have had surgery, are on oxygen, are in intensive care, or have cardiac or respiratory problems, a pulse oximeter may be used. A **pulse oximeter** is a noninvasive device that uses a light to determine the amount of oxygen in the blood (also called oxygen saturation). A pulse oximeter also measures a person's pulse rate.

A sensor is clipped on a person's finger, earlobe, or toe (Fig. 22-5). A light passes through the skin, and the percentage of oxygen in the blood and the pulse rate are displayed. An alarm will sound if the oxygen level becomes less than optimal.

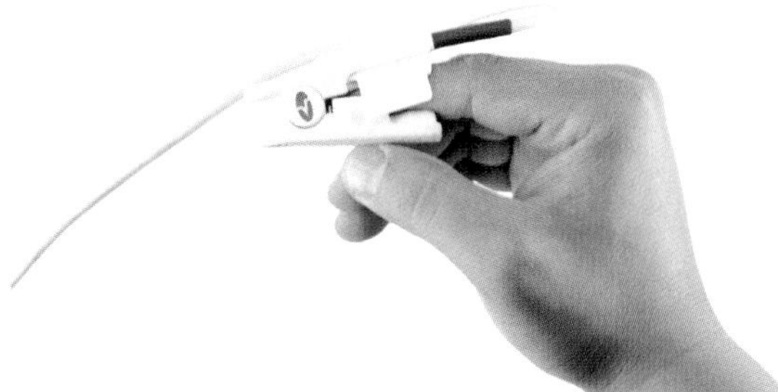

Fig. 22-5. *A pulse oximeter sensor is usually clipped on a person's finger.*

Normal blood oxygen level usually measures between 95% and 100%. However, normal ranges may differ from person to person. Nursing assistants should report any increase or decrease in oxygen levels to the nurse.

Guidelines: Pulse Oximetry

G Report to the nurse immediately if the alarm on the pulse oximeter sounds.

G Tell the nurse if the pulse oximeter falls off or if the resident requests that you remove it.

G Check the skin around the device often. Report any of the following:

- Swelling
- Cyanotic skin
- Shiny, tight skin
- Skin that is cold to the touch
- Sores, redness, or irritation
- Numbness or tingling
- Pain or discomfort

G Check vital signs as ordered. Report changes to the nurse.

6. Describe telemetry and list care guidelines

Telemetry is used to measure the heart rhythm and rate on a continuous basis. Wires are attached to the chest with sticky pads or patches (also called *leads*) (Fig. 22-6). The wires are connected to a battery-powered portable unit, which sends data to computer screens at a monitoring station (Figs. 22-7 and 22-8). This data is monitored and assessed at all times by specially trained staff.

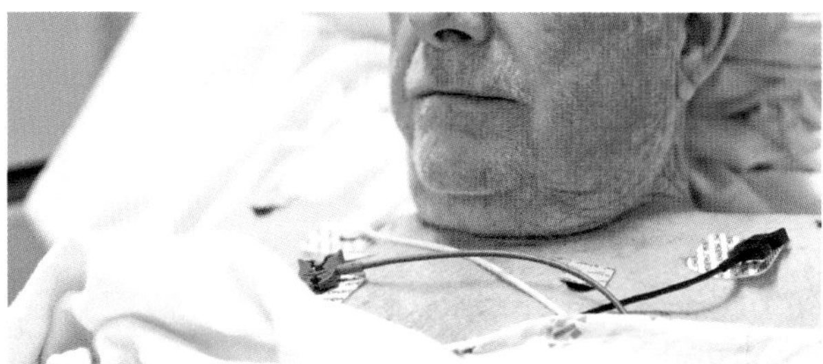

Fig. 22-6. *Pads, or leads, are attached to the person's chest.*

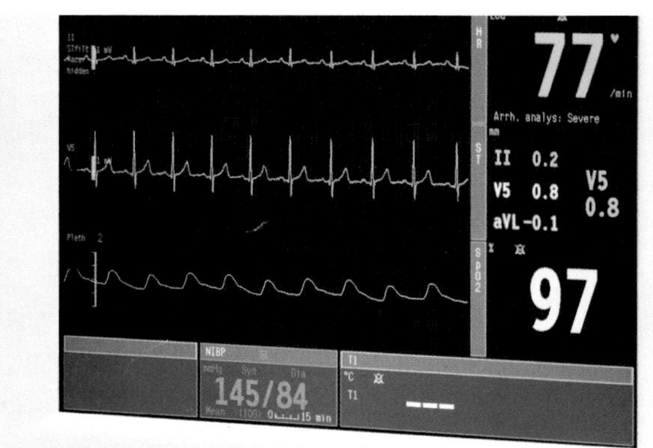

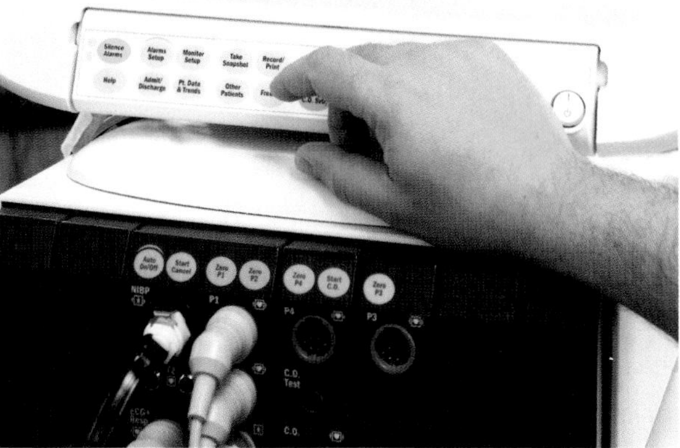

Fig. 22-7. *A telemetry monitoring unit.*

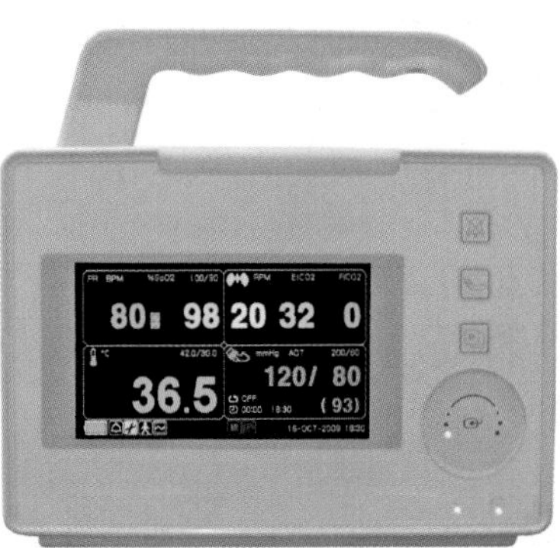

Fig. 22-8. A smaller telemetry monitoring unit that can be carried by the person.

Telemetry may be necessary due to chest pain, heart or lung disease, heart or lung surgery, irregular heartbeats, or certain medications that affect heart rhythm or rate.

Guidelines: Telemetry

- **G** Report to the nurse if the pads become wet or soiled. Report if pads appear loose or fall off.
- **G** Report if the alarm sounds. The alarm may sound if the pads disconnect or if the battery is low.
- **G** Check the skin around the pads often. Report any of the following:
  - Swelling
  - Sores, redness, or irritation
  - Fluid or blood draining from skin
  - Broken skin
- **G** Report resident complaints of chest pain or discomfort, as well as any difficulty breathing.
- **G** Check vital signs as ordered. Report changes to the nurse.

7. Explain artificial airways and list care guidelines

An **artificial airway** is any plastic, metal, or rubber device inserted into the respiratory tract to maintain or promote breathing. Artificial airways keep the airway open. This is necessary when the airway is obstructed due to illness, injury, secretions, or aspiration. Some residents who are unconscious will need an artificial airway.

The artificial airway is inserted using a method called intubation. **Intubation** involves the passage of a plastic tube through the mouth, nose, or an opening in the neck and into the trachea (windpipe). There are different types of artificial airways (Fig. 22-9). One common type is a **tracheostomy**, which is a surgically-created opening through the neck into the trachea. A hollow tube, called a tracheostomy tube or *trach tube,* is inserted through this opening into the trachea. More information on this type of artificial airway may be found in the next Learning Objective.

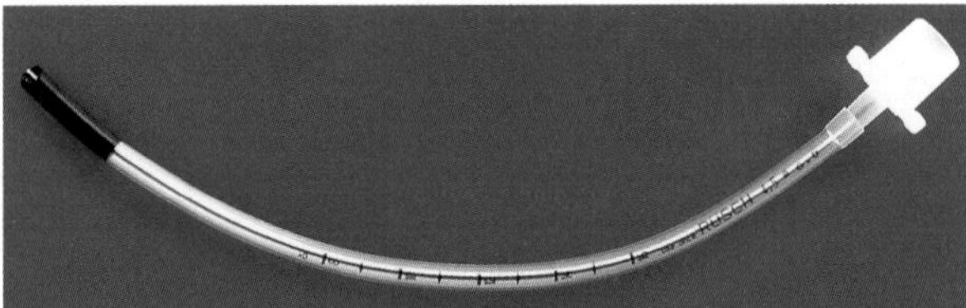

Fig. 22-9. An endotracheal tube is a type of artificial airway that is inserted through the nose or mouth and then into the trachea. (PHOTO COURTESY OF TELEFLEX)

Guidelines: Artificial Airways

- **G** Check the resident regularly. If the tubing falls out, tell the nurse immediately.
- **G** Monitor vital signs as ordered. Report changes to the nurse.
- **G** Perform oral care often, as directed.
- **G** Watch for biting and tugging on tube. If a resident is doing this, tell the nurse.
- **G** Use other methods of communication if the resident cannot speak. Try writing notes, drawing pictures, and using communication boards. Watch for hand and eye signals.
- **G** Be supportive and reassuring. It can be frightening and uncomfortable to have an artificial airway. Some residents may choke or gag. Be empathetic. Imagine how it might feel to have a tube in your nose, mouth, or throat.

8. Discuss care for a resident with a tracheostomy

A tracheostomy is a type of artificial airway commonly seen in long-term care facilities (Fig. 22-10). Tracheostomies may be necessary for many reasons, including the following:

- Tumors/cancer
- Infection
- Severe neck or mouth injuries
- Facial surgery and facial burns
- Long-term unconsciousness or coma
- Obstruction in the airway
- Paralysis of muscles related to breathing
- Aspiration as a result of muscle or sensory problems in the throat
- Severe allergic reaction
- Gunshot wound

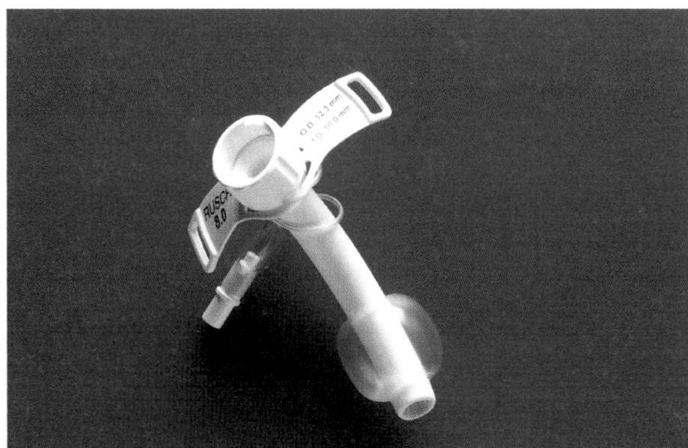

Fig. 22-10. A tracheostomy tube is inserted into the trachea through a surgically-created opening in the neck. (PHOTO COURTESY OF TELEFLEX)

This procedure is usually temporary, but it can be permanent. It is easier to suction and attach respiratory equipment with a tracheostomy than with other artificial airways.

When the tracheostomy is first placed, it may be difficult for the resident to adapt to breathing through the tube. This can cause anxiety and frustration. It may be impossible for the resident to talk or make sounds at first, which also causes fear. During this time, nursing assistants should be especially supportive and encouraging. They can use other methods of communication, such as writing notes, drawing pictures, using communication boards, and using hand and eye signals. Checking on the resident often and answering call lights immediately may help lessen anxiety. People can usually learn to talk through a trach tube.

Care of the tracheostomy may include skin care around the opening, helping with dressing changes, and cleaning the device. Suctioning may be required. Nursing assistants do not perform suctioning or trach care. Their responsibilities will mostly involve observing and reporting.

Observing and Reporting: Tracheostomies

Report any of the following to the nurse:

- O/R Shortness of breath
- O/R Trouble breathing
- O/R Gurgling sounds
- O/R Any signs of skin breakdown around the opening, such as irritation, rash, cracks, breaks, sores, or bleeding on the skin
- O/R The type and amount of discharge that the resident coughs up through the tracheostomy (normal discharge looks like white mucus or saliva)
- O/R Any increase in the amount of discharge
- O/R Discharge that is thick, yellow, green, bloody, or has an odor (this may indicate an infection or other problem in the lungs)
- O/R Mouth sores or discomfort
- O/R Disconnected tubing

It is very important to prevent infection when caring for residents with tracheostomies. They are prone to respiratory infections. Nursing assistants must wash their hands often and wear gloves when indicated. NAs should wear masks if residents are coughing. It is vital that equipment be kept clean. Anything that is dropped on the floor must be sterilized before it can be used in contact with the tubes. Great care must be taken so that nothing gets into the tube which can cause an infection in the lungs.

9. List care guidelines for residents requiring mechanical ventilation

Residents in a subacute unit may be on a mechanical ventilator. **Mechanical ventilation** is using a machine to inflate and deflate the lungs when a person is unable to breathe on his own. A person may require mechanical ventilation due to cardiac or respiratory arrest, lung injuries and diseases, or head and spinal cord injuries.

Residents will not be able to speak while on the mechanical ventilator. This is because air will no longer reach the larynx (vocal cords). Not being able to speak may increase anxiety. The resident may think that no one will know if he is having trouble breathing. Being on a ventilator has been compared to breathing through a straw. Nursing assistants should be empathetic and think about how that might feel. Residents will need a lot of support while connected to the ventilator. NAs should enter the room often so that residents on ventilators can see them. This helps to reassure residents that they are being carefully observed. Clipboards, notepads, and communication boards will help with communication.

Residents on ventilators are often heavily sedated. A **sedative** is an agent or drug that helps calm and soothe a person and may cause sleep. Being sedated helps prevent people on ventilators from feeling discomfort and anxiety. Even if a resident seems unaware of what is happening, the NA must continue to speak to him and explain what she is doing.

Guidelines: Mechanical Ventilator

G Ventilators cause an increased risk for a special type of pneumonia. Wash your hands often when working with residents on mechanical ventilators.

G Report to the nurse if the alarm sounds.

G If you notice tubing that is disconnected or loose, report it immediately.

G Answer the call light promptly.

G Follow the care plan for repositioning instructions. The head of the bed may need to remain elevated.

G Give regular, careful skin care to prevent pressure ulcers. Check the skin around the intubation site often, as well as on the rest of the body. Report any of the following:

- Swelling
- Sores, redness, irritation
- Fluid or blood draining from skin
- Broken skin

G Report if the resident is pulling on or biting the tube. Report if the resident is anxious, fearful, or upset.

G Be patient during communication. Observe body language. Watch for hand or eye signals.

G Check on the resident often, so that the resident can see that you are there. Be supportive, kind, and empathetic.

10. Describe suctioning and list signs of respiratory distress

Subacute care units include residents who require suctioning by nurses or respiratory therapists. Suctioning removes mucus and secretions from the lungs when a person cannot do this on his own. A person who has a tracheostomy may require suctioning. Suctioning can be performed through the nose, mouth, or throat.

Suctioning is normally a sterile procedure. Nursing assistants do not perform suctioning; nurses or respiratory therapists will perform the suctioning. A portable pump, operated on battery power or electrical power, may be used to suction the resident (Fig. 22-11). A canister or bottle on the pump collects the mucus and secretions.

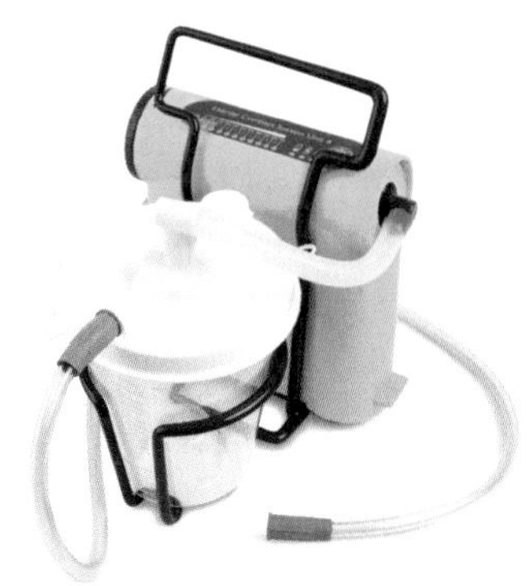

Fig. 22-11. This is one type of suctioning pump. Nursing assistants do not perform suctioning. They help by reporting signs of respiratory distress and monitoring vital signs. (PHOTO COURTESY OF LAERDAL MEDICAL)

A person who needs frequent suctioning may show signs of respiratory distress. Signs of respiratory distress include the following:

- Gurgling sound of secretions
- Difficulty breathing
- Elevated respiratory rate
- Pale, cyanotic, or gray skin around the eyes, mouth, fingernails, or toenails
- Nostrils flaring (nostrils opening wider when breathing in may show that a person is having to work harder to breathe)
- Retracting (chest appears to sink in below the neck with each breath)
- Sweating
- Wheezing

Guidelines: Suctioning

G Report signs of respiratory distress to the nurse immediately.

G Monitor vital signs closely, especially respiratory rate. Report changes.

G Follow Standard Precautions. Don gloves, gown, mask, or goggles as directed.

G Assist the nurse with suctioning as needed. You may be asked to have a towel or washcloth ready to clean the resident after suctioning. Give oral care as ordered.

G Report resident complaints of pain or difficulty breathing.

11. Describe chest tubes and explain related care

Chest tubes are hollow drainage tubes that are inserted into the chest during a sterile procedure (Fig. 22-12). They can be inserted at the bedside or during surgery. Chest tubes drain air, blood or other fluid, or pus that has collected inside the pleural cavity or space. The pleural cavity is the space between the layers of the pleura, the thin membrane that covers and protects the lungs. Chest tubes are also inserted to allow a full expansion of the lungs. Some conditions that require chest tube insertion include the following:

- Air or gas in the pleural space (pneumothorax)
- Blood in the pleural space (hemothorax)
- Pus in the pleural space (empyema)
- Certain types of surgery
- Chest trauma or injuries

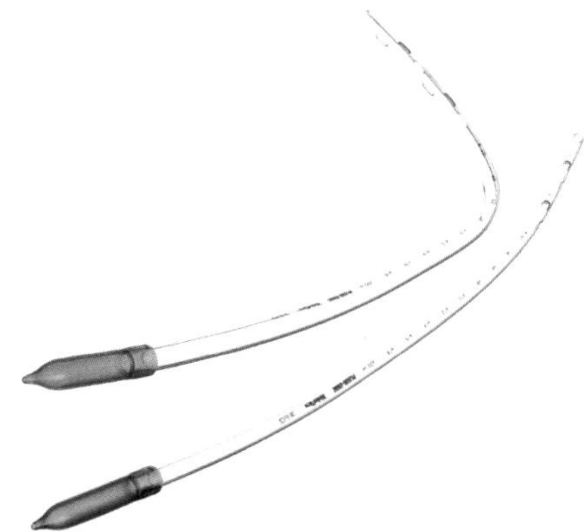

Fig. 22-12. A chest tube is inserted into the chest to drain air, fluid, or pus. (PHOTO COURTESY OF TELEFLEX)

A doctor normally inserts chest tubes. The chest tube is connected to a drainage system. Suction is sometimes attached to the system to encourage drainage. This system must be sealed so that air cannot enter the pleural cavity. The system must be airtight.

When X-rays show that the air, blood, or fluid has been drained, the tube is removed. Medications may be used to prevent or treat infection.

Guidelines: Chest Tubes

- **G** Be aware of the number and location of chest tubes. Tubes may be in the front, back, or on the side of the body.
- **G** Check vital signs as directed. Report any changes immediately to the nurse.
- **G** Report signs of respiratory distress to the nurse immediately. Report complaints of pain.
- **G** Keep the drainage system below the level of the resident's chest.
- **G** Make sure drainage containers remain upright and level at all times.
- **G** Make sure that tubing is not kinked. If tubing becomes kinked, report to the nurse right away.
- **G** Watch for disconnected tubing. If this happens, report it immediately.
- **G** Certain equipment is kept nearby in case tubes are pulled out. Do not remove these items from the area.
- **G** Observe chest drainage for color and amount. Report any changes in color or amount immediately.
- **G** Report if there is an increase or decrease in bubbling in the drainage system. Report if there are clots in the tubing.
- **G** Follow the repositioning schedule. Be very gentle with turning and repositioning. You must move the resident and the tubes at the same time to prevent tubes from coming out. Always get enough help.
- **G** Report odor in the chest tube area.
- **G** Provide rest periods as needed.
- **G** Follow fluid intake orders. Measure intake and output carefully, as ordered.
- **G** If asked to help with coughing and deep breathing exercises, be encouraging and patient.

Other residents who require more direct care and close observation by staff include residents with IVs (Chapter 14) and residents with tube feedings (Chapter 15).

Chapter Review

1. What is different about the type of care provided in a subacute setting as compared to the type of care provided in regular long-term care?
2. Briefly describe three types of surgeries.
3. Which type of anesthesia is inhaled or injected directly into a vein and affects the brain and entire body?
4. List eight guidelines for assisting with pre-operative care.
5. List eight guidelines for assisting with post-operative care.
6. List 10 signs and symptoms to report about a resident after surgery.
7. List two reasons why a resident may need a pulse oximeter.
8. What is important to report about the skin when a resident is using a telemetry unit?
9. What are alternate methods of communication that nursing assistants can use with residents who have artificial airways?
10. What are a nursing assistant's responsibilities with tracheostomy care?
11. In what ways can a nursing assistant show support for a resident who is on a ventilator?
12. Why might a resident be anxious while on a ventilator?
13. List five signs of respiratory distress.
14. What types of fluids are drained by chest tubes?
15. List 12 guidelines for caring for residents with chest tubes.

23 Dying, Death, and Hospice

1. Discuss the stages of grief

Death can occur suddenly without warning, or it can be expected. Older people, or those with terminal illnesses, may have time to prepare for death. A **terminal illness** is a disease or condition that will eventually cause death. Preparing for death is a process that affects the dying person's emotions and behavior.

Dr. Elisabeth Kubler-Ross researched and wrote about the grief process. **Grief** is deep distress or sorrow over a loss. Her book, *On Death and Dying*, describes five stages that dying people and their families or friends may reach before death. These five stages are described below. Not all residents go through all the stages. Some may stay in one stage until death occurs. Residents may move back and forth between stages during the process.

Denial: People in the denial stage may refuse to believe they are dying. They often believe that a mistake has been made. They may demand lab work be repeated. They may talk about the future and avoid discussion about their illnesses. They may simply act like it is not happening. This is the "No, not me" stage.

Anger: Once they start to face the possibility of their death, people may become angry that they are dying. They may be angry because they think they are too young or that they have always taken care of themselves. Anger may be directed at staff, visitors, roommates, family, or friends. Anger is a normal and healthy reaction. Even though it may be upsetting, the caregiver must try not to not take anger personally. This is the "Why me?" stage.

Bargaining: Once people have begun to believe that they really are dying, they may make promises to God or somehow try to bargain for their recovery. This is the "Yes me, but..." stage.

Depression: As dying people become physically weaker and symptoms of the illness get worse, they may become deeply sad or depressed (Fig. 23-1). They may cry or withdraw or be unable to perform even simple activities. They need additional physical and emotional support. Listening to residents and being understanding may be helpful.

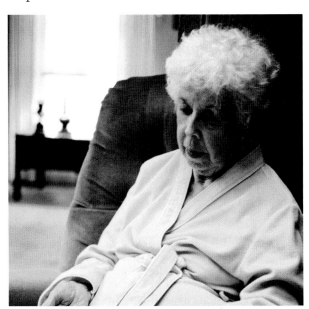

Fig. 23-1. *A person who is dying may become depressed and withdrawn. Giving extra emotional support to these residents may help.*

Acceptance: Most people who are dying are eventually able to accept death and prepare for it. They may ask to see an attorney or accountant. They may arrange with loved ones for the care of important people or things. They may make plans for their last days or for the ceremonies that may follow their death. At this stage, people who are dying may seem emotionally detached.

These stages of dying may not be possible for someone who dies suddenly, unexpectedly, or quickly. Nobody can force anyone to move from stage to stage. Nursing assistants can help by listening and being ready to offer their help.

2. Describe the grief process

Dealing with grief after the death of a loved one is a process as well. Grieving is an individual process. No two people will grieve in exactly the same way. It is also a changing or adaptive process. Clergy, counselors, or social workers can provide help for people who are grieving. Family members or friends may have any of the following reactions to the death of a loved one:

Shock: Even when death is expected, family members and friends may still be shocked after death occurs. Many people do not know what to expect after the death of a loved one and may be surprised by their feelings.

Denial: It is easy to want to believe that everything will quickly return to normal after a death. Denying or refusing to believe they are grieving can help people deal with the initial hours or days after a death. But eventually it is important to face feelings. Grief can be so overwhelming that some people may take years to face their feelings. Professional help can be very valuable.

Anger: Although it is hard to admit it, many people feel angry after a death. They may be angry with themselves, at God, at the doctors, or even at the person who died. There is nothing wrong with feeling anger as a part of grief.

Guilt: It is very common for families, friends, and caregivers to feel guilty after a death. They may wish they had done more for the dying person. They may simply feel that he or she did not deserve to die. They may feel guilty that they are still living.

Regret: Often people regret what they did or did not do for the dying person. They may regret things they said or did not say to the person who has died. Many people have regrets for years.

Sadness: It is very common to feel depressed or emotionally unstable after a death. People may suffer headaches or insomnia when they cannot express their sadness.

Loneliness: Missing someone who has died is very normal. It can bring up other feelings, such as sadness or regret. Many things may remind people of the person who died. The memories may be painful at first. With time, those who survive usually feel less lonely, and memories are less painful.

3. Discuss how feelings and attitudes about death differ

Death is a very sensitive topic; many people find it hard to discuss death. Feelings and attitudes about death can be formed by many factors:

Experience with death: Someone who has been through other deaths may have a different understanding of death than someone who has not.

Personality type: Open, expressive people may have an easier time talking about and coping with death than those who are very reserved or quiet. Sharing feelings is one way of working through fears and concerns.

Religious beliefs: Religious practices and beliefs affect a person's experience with death (Fig. 23-2). These include the process of dying, rituals at the time of death, burial or cremation practices, services held after death, and mourning customs. For example, some Catholics do not believe in cremation. Orthodox Jews may not believe in viewing the body after death. Beliefs about what happens after death can also influence grieving. Those who believe in an afterlife, such as heaven, may be comforted by this belief.

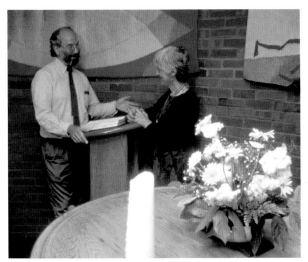

Fig. 23-2. Religious beliefs influence a person's feelings about death.

Cultural background. The practices people grow up with affect how they deal with death. Cultural groups may have different practices to deal with death and grieving. Some groups have meals and other services but say very little about a person's death. In other groups, talking about and remembering the person who has died may be a comfort to family and friends (Fig. 23-3).

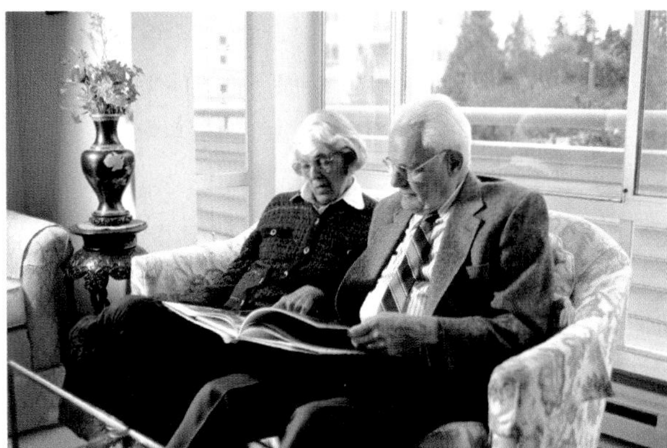

Fig. 23-3. Looking at photos and sharing stories about a person who is dying or who has died is one way that family and friends may grieve.

Learning Objective 10 in this chapter contains more information about different practices relating to death.

4. Discuss how to care for a dying resident

Nursing assistants should follow the care plan when caring for a dying resident. However, they should also keep these guidelines in mind to help make the resident as comfortable as possible:

Guidelines: Caring for the Dying Resident

- G Diminished senses: Reduce glare and keep room lighting low (Fig. 23-4). Hearing is usually the last sense to leave the body, so speak in a normal tone. Tell resident about any procedures that are being done or what is happening in the room. Do not expect an answer. Ask few questions. Encourage family to speak to the resident, but to avoid subjects that are disturbing. Observe body language to anticipate a resident's needs.

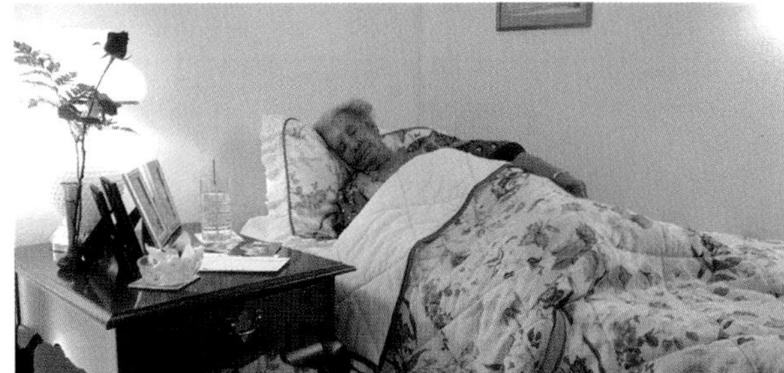

Fig. 23-4. Keep a dying resident's room softly lit without glare.

- G Care of the mouth and nose: Give mouth care often. If the resident is unconscious, give mouth care every two hours. The lips and nostrils may be dry and cracked. Apply lubricant, such as lip balm, to lips and nose.
- G Skin care: Give bed baths and incontinence care as needed. Bathe perspiring residents often. Skin should be kept clean and dry. Change sheets and clothes for comfort. Keep sheets wrinkle-free. Skin care to prevent pressure ulcers is important.
- G Comfort: Pain relief is critical. Residents may not be able to communicate that they are in pain. Observe residents for signs of pain

and report them. Frequent changes of position, back massage, skin care, mouth care, and proper body alignment may help. Body temperature usually rises. Many residents are more comfortable with light covers. However, fever may cause chills. Use extra blankets if residents need more warmth.

To control pain, residents may be connected to a patient-controlled analgesia (PCA) device. A PCA is a method of pain control that allows patients to administer pain medication to themselves. They press a button to give themselves a dose of pain medication. Report any complaints of pain or discomfort to the nurse immediately.

- G Environment: Display favorite objects and photographs where the resident can easily see them. They may provide comfort. Play music if the resident requests it. Make sure the room is comfortable, appropriately lit, and well ventilated. When leaving the room, place the call light within reach, even if the resident is unaware of his surroundings.
- G Emotional and spiritual support: Residents who are dying may be afraid of what is happening and of death. Listening may be one of the most important things you can do for a resident who is dying. Pay attention to these conversations. Report any comments about fear to the nurse.

People who are dying may also need the quiet, reassuring, and loving presence of another person. Touch can be very important. Holding the resident's hand as you sit quietly can be very comforting.

Do not avoid the dying person or his family. Do not deny that death is approaching, and do not tell the resident that anyone knows how or when it will happen. Do give accurate information in a reassuring way. No one can take away a person's fear of death. However, your supportive and reassuring presence can help.

Some residents who are dying may also seek spiritual comfort from clergy. Tell the nurse immediately if resident requests a clergyperson. Provide privacy for visits from clergy and others. Do not discuss your religious or spiritual beliefs with residents or their families or make recommendations.

Take the time to sort out your own feelings about death. If you are not comfortable with the topic, dying residents will feel it. Speak to the nurse if you need resources to help you deal with your feelings.

Advance Directives

Advance directives and DNR orders were introduced in Chapter 3. Advance directives allow people to choose what medical care they want or do not want if they cannot make those decisions themselves. A DNR order tells medical professionals not to perform CPR. DNR orders may be written for a person who has a terminal illness, someone who almost certainly will not be saved by CPR, a person who is not expected to live long, and/or a person who simply wants to let nature take its course.

If a resident has an advance directive in place, the NA may be asked to continue to monitor vital signs, such as temperature, pulse, respirations, and blood pressure, and report the readings to the nurse. Comfort measures, such as pain medication, will continue to be used. However, depending on what the advance directive states, performing CPR or any extraordinary measures may be prohibited, no matter how the vital signs have changed or declined. Extraordinary measures are measures used to prolong life when there is no reasonable expectation of recovery. When a person with a DNR order stops breathing or the heart stops, he or she will die unless the heart or breathing restarts on its own. This is not likely to happen. By law, advance directives and DNR orders must be honored. Nursing assistants should respect each resident's decisions about advance directives.

5. Describe ways to treat dying residents and their families with dignity and how to honor their rights

Nursing assistants can treat residents with dignity when they are approaching death by respecting their rights and their preferences. There are some legal rights to remember when caring for people who are dying:

The right to refuse treatment. Nursing assistants must remember that whether they agree or disagree with a resident's decisions, the choice is not theirs. It belongs to the person involved and/or his or her family. NAs should be supportive of family members and not judge them. The family is most likely following the resident's wishes.

The right to have visitors. When death is close, it is an emotional time for all those involved. Saying goodbye can be a very important part of dealing with a loved one's death. It may also be very reassuring to the dying person to have someone in the room, even if the person does not seem to be aware of his surroundings.

The right to privacy. Privacy is a basic right, but privacy for visiting, or even when the person is alone, may be even more important now.

Other rights of a dying person are listed below in *The Dying Person's Bill of Rights*. This was created at a workshop, *The Terminally Ill Patient and the Helping Person*, sponsored by Southwestern Michigan In-Service Education Council, and appeared in the *American Journal of Nursing*, Vol. 75, January 1975, p. 99.

I have the right to:

- Be treated as a living human being until I die.
- Maintain a sense of hopefulness, however changing its focus may be.
- Be cared for by those who can maintain a sense of hopefulness, however changing this might be.
- Express my feelings and emotions about my approaching death in my own way.
- Participate in decisions concerning my care.
- Expect continuing medical and nursing attentions even though "cure" goals must be changed to "comfort" goals.
- Not die alone.
- Be free from pain.
- Have my questions answered honestly.
- Not be deceived.
- Have help from and for my family in accepting my death.
- Die in peace and dignity.
- Retain my individuality and not be judged for my decisions, which may be contrary to the beliefs of others.
- Discuss and enlarge my religious and/or spiritual experiences, whatever these may mean to others.
- Expect that the sanctity of the human body will be respected after death.
- Be cared for by caring, sensitive, knowledgeable people who will attempt to understand my needs and will be able to gain some satisfaction in helping me face my death.

Guidelines for how nursing assistants should treat their dying residents and their families with dignity include the following:

Guidelines: Treating Dying Residents with Dignity

G Respect their wishes in all possible ways. Communication between staff is extremely important at this time so that everyone understands what the resident's wishes are. Listen carefully for ideas on how to provide simple gestures that may be special and appreciated.

G Do not isolate or avoid a resident who is dying. Enter his room regularly.

G Be careful not to make promises that cannot or should not be kept.

G Continue to involve the dying person in facility activities. Be resident-centered. Do not talk with other staff members about your personal life when caring for a resident.

- Listen if a dying resident wants to talk but do not offer advice. Do not make judgmental comments.
- Do not babble or act especially cheerful or sad. Be professional.
- Keep the resident as comfortable as possible. The nurse needs to know immediately if pain medication is requested. Keep the resident clean and dry.
- Assure privacy when it is desired.
- Respect the privacy of the family and other visitors. They may be upset and not want to be social at this time. They may welcome a friendly smile, however, and should not be isolated, either.
- Help with the family's physical comfort. If requested, get them coffee, water, chairs, blankets, etc.

Residents' Rights

Life Support Measures

Life support measures are used when vital body systems are not working well enough to support life on their own. These measures include feeding tubes, mechanical ventilation, dialysis, etc. The decision to remain on life support or to discontinue life support is often part of a person's advance directives. When the decision is made to discontinue life support and the body is not able to function without these supports, the person will die. This may happen immediately, or the resident may live for a short time. As with any advance directive and personal decision regarding treatment, nursing assistants should not judge a resident's (or a family member's) choice to remain on or discontinue life support. This is a private and personal decision. NAs should respect the resident's wishes and not make comments about his or her choices to anyone, including family members, other residents, or other staff members.

6. Define the goals of a hospice program

Hospice care is the term for the special care that a dying person needs. It is a compassionate way to care for dying people and their families. Hospice care uses a holistic approach. It treats the person's physical, emotional, spiritual, and social needs.

Hospice care can be given seven days a week, 24 hours a day. It is available with a doctor's order. There is always a nurse on call to answer questions, make a visit, or solve a problem. Hospice care may be given in a hospital, at a care facility, or in the home. A hospice can be any location where a person who is dying is treated with dignity by caregivers.

Any caregiver may provide hospice care, but often specially-trained nurses, social workers, and volunteers provide hospice care. The hospice team may include doctors, nurses, social workers, counselors, nursing assistants, therapists, clergy, dietitians, and volunteers.

Hospice care helps meet all needs of the dying resident. The resident, as well as family and friends, are directly involved in care decisions. The resident is encouraged to participate in family life and decision-making as long as possible.

In long-term care, goals focus on the resident's recovery or on the resident's ability to care for herself as much as possible. In hospice care, however, the goals are the comfort and dignity of the resident. This type of care is called **palliative care**. This is an important difference. Nursing assistants will need to change their focus when caring for hospice residents. The focus should be on pain relief and comfort, rather than on teaching residents to care for themselves. Residents who are dying need to feel some independence for as long as possible. Caregivers should allow residents to have as much control over their lives as possible. Eventually, caregivers may have to meet all of the resident's basic needs.

Nursing assistants should remember the following guidelines when working in hospice care:

Guidelines: Hospice Care

- Be a good listener. It is hard to know what to say to someone who is dying or to his loved ones. Most often, people need someone to listen to them (Fig. 23-5). A good listener can be a great comfort. Some people, however, will not want to confide in their caregivers, and you should never push someone to talk.

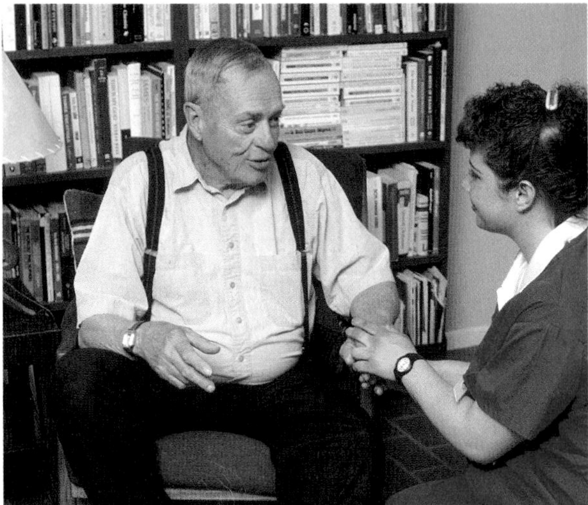

Fig. 23-5. *Being a good listener can be a great help to a dying resident and his family.*

- Respect privacy and independence. Relatives, friends, clergy, and others may visit a dying resident. Make it easy for these difficult visits to take place. Stay out of the way when you can. Do not join in the conversation unless asked to do so. Understand that some people wish to be alone with their dying loved ones. Dying residents can have some independence even when they need total care. Let the resident make choices when possible, such as when to bathe, whether to eat or not, or what to eat or drink.

- Be sensitive to individual needs. Different residents and families will have different needs. The more you know what is needed, the more you can help. Some residents need a quiet and calm atmosphere. Others appreciate a cheery presence and might like you to talk or stay close by. Ask family members or friends how you can help.

- Be aware of your own feelings. Caring for people who are dying can be draining. Know your limits and respect them. Discuss feelings of frustration or grief with another care team member.

- Recognize the stress. Just realizing how stressful it is to work with people who are dying is a first step toward caring for yourself. Talking with a counselor about your experiences at work can help you understand and work through your feelings. Remember, however, that specific information must be kept confidential. A supervisor may be able to make a referral to a counselor or support group.

- Take good care of yourself. Eating right, exercising, and getting enough rest are ways of taking care of yourself (Fig. 23-6). Remember that caring for your emotional health is important too. Talk about and acknowledge your feelings. Take time to do things for yourself, such as reading a book, taking a bubble bath, or another activity that you enjoy. If you are religious or spiritual, these needs may be met by attending religious services, reading, praying, meditating, or just taking a quiet walk. Meeting your needs allows you to best meet other people's needs.

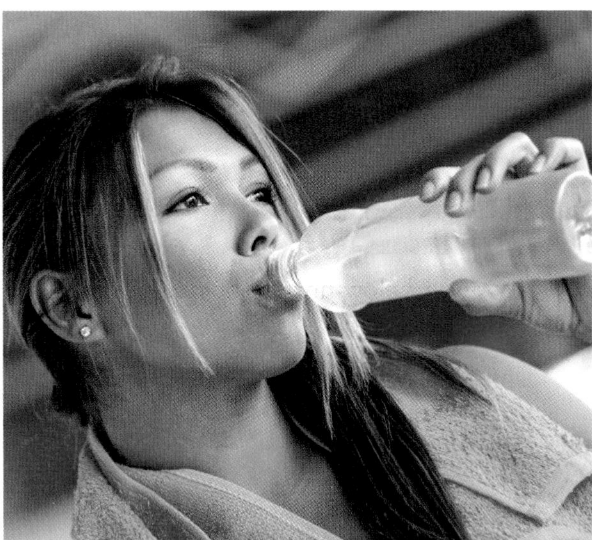

Fig. 23-6. *Nursing assistants should take good care of themselves when caring for people who are dying. This includes eating right, exercising, drinking plenty of water, and finding time to relax.*

- Take a break when you need to. Find ten minutes to sit down and relax or stand up and stretch. This may be enough of a break in some situations.

Hospice Volunteers

According to the National Hospice and Palliative Care Organization, an estimated 458,000 hospice volunteers provided care to over 1.5 million people in the United States in 2010. Hospice volunteers go through a training program to prepare them for hospice work. The volunteers provide a variety of services. This includes caring for the home or family of a dying person, driving or doing errands, and providing emotional support. Their website, nhpco.org, has more information about hospice care.

7. Explain common signs of approaching death

Death can be sudden or gradual. Certain physical changes occur that can be signs and symptoms of approaching death. Vital signs and skin color are often affected. Disorientation, confusion, and reduced responsiveness may occur. Vision, taste, and touch usually diminish. However, it is generally acknowledged that hearing is often present until death occurs.

Common signs of approaching death include the following:

- Blurred and failing vision
- Unfocused eyes
- Impaired speech
- Diminished sense of touch
- Loss of movement, muscle tone, and feeling
- A rising or below-normal body temperature
- Decreasing blood pressure
- Weak pulse that is abnormally slow or rapid
- Alternating periods of slow, irregular respirations and rapid, shallow respirations, called **Cheyne-Stokes** respirations
- A rattling or gurgling sound as the person breathes
- Cold, pale skin
- Mottling (bruised appearance), spotting, or blotching of skin caused by poor circulation
- Perspiration
- Incontinence (both urine and stool)
- Disorientation or confusion

8. List changes that may occur in the human body after death

When death occurs, the body will not have a heartbeat, pulse, respiration, or blood pressure. The muscles in the body become stiff and rigid. This is a temporary condition called ***rigor mortis***, which is Latin for *stiffness of death*. The eyelids may remain open or partially open with the eyes in a fixed stare. The mouth may remain open. The body may be incontinent of both urine and stool.

Though these things are a normal part of death, they can be frightening. Nursing assistants should inform the nurse immediately to help confirm the death.

9. Describe postmortem care

Postmortem care is care of the body after death. It takes place after the resident has been declared dead by a nurse or doctor. It is important for nursing assistants to be sensitive to the needs of the family and friends after death. Family members may wish to sit by the bed to say goodbye. They may wish to stay with the body for a while. They should be allowed to do these things. NAs should be aware of religious and cultural practices that the family wants to observe. Facilities will have different policies on postmortem care. NAs must follow their facility's procedures and only perform assigned tasks.

Guidelines: Postmortem Care

G After death, the muscles in the body become stiff and rigid. This may make the body difficult to move. Talk to the nurse if you need help performing postmortem care.

G Bathe the body. Be very gentle to avoid bruising. Place drainage pads where needed, most often under the head and/or under the perineum (the genital and anal area). Be sure to follow Standard Precautions.

- Do not remove any tubes or other equipment. A nurse or someone at the funeral home will do this.
- If instructed to do so, put dentures back in the mouth and close the mouth. You may need to place a rolled towel under the chin to support the closed mouth position. If this is not possible, place dentures in a denture cup near the resident's head.
- Close the eyes carefully.
- Position the body on the back with legs straight and arms folded across the abdomen. Place a small pillow under the head.
- Follow facility policy on personal items. Check to see if you should remove jewelry. Always have a witness if personal items are removed or given to a family member. Document what was given and to whom.
- Strip the bed after the body has been removed.
- Open windows to air the room as needed and straighten up.
- Document according to your facility's policy.

Organ Donation

Organ donation is the removal of organs and tissues for the purpose of transplanting into someone who needs them. Organ donors can be people who have recently died or living people. If a resident has designated himself an organ donor after death, specific policies and procedures will need be followed. Some organs must be taken from the body very soon after a person dies. NAs should follow the nurse's instructions regarding special preparations or transport.

Residents' Rights

Comforting Others

After a loved one has died, the nursing assistant should show family and friends to a comfortable place to sit and talk privately. She should ask if she can contact anyone for them. She should provide water or another beverage. If family members want to be left alone with the deceased, the NA can provide privacy by leaving the room and closing the door. Family and friends should not feel they are being rushed out of the facility.

It is natural to feel upset and not know what to say when someone has died. Many people talk a lot when feeling stressed. NAs can show their support without talking very much. They should listen patiently and not interrupt (Fig. 23-7). The family may want to repeat what happened and how it occurred. It is helpful for them to repeat this story.

What an NA says is not as important as is being sincere. Simply saying, "I am so sorry," is fine. She should avoid clichés such as, "It is for the better." If the NA can say it honestly, saying something like, "Your mother will be missed here," is supportive and kind.

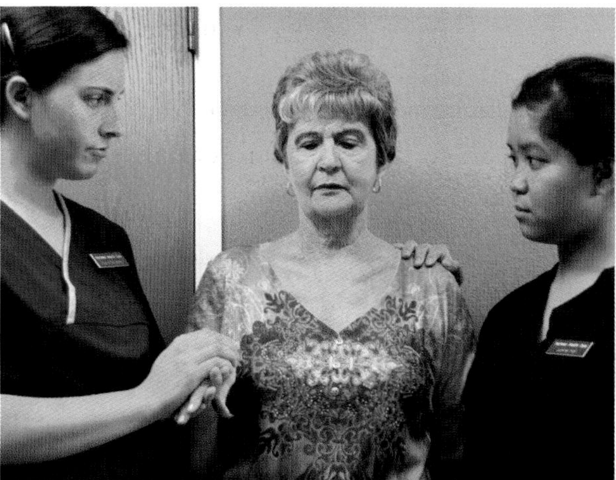

Fig. 23-7. Nursing assistants should be available for family and friends if they want to talk and should allow them to express their feelings.

10. Understand and respect different postmortem practices

When caring for those who are dying, nursing assistants will also interact with families and will witness many different responses to the death of a loved one. Dealing with the loss of a loved one is a monumental task that people face in different ways. It is a process that may begin with the diagnosis of a terminal illness and may not end until years after the loved one's death.

There is no right or wrong way to grieve. A person's initial response to the death of a loved one may be due in part to her cultural or religious background, or it may simply be how that person deals with death. What is important is that when people respond differently than a nursing assistant would, it is the NA's professional duty to respect their responses.

When a death has occurred, some people may respond quietly, with very little obvious emotion, while others may be very vocal. Depending on the preferences of the family, the body may be removed very quickly or the family may wish for the body to remain for some time while people say goodbye, pray, or perform necessary religious rituals. Many cultures forbid leaving the body of the deceased alone. In some cultures and religious traditions, the body must be buried promptly, either on the day of death or within a certain period immediately after. An NA should not be alarmed if this happens or judge the practices of the resident's family.

A nursing assistant may be invited to attend a funeral or other ceremony following the death of a resident. As someone who has cared for the deceased person, the NA may be grieving as well (Fig. 23-8). If she wants to attend the service, she should check with her supervisor first to make sure it is appropriate. It is important to respect professional boundaries.

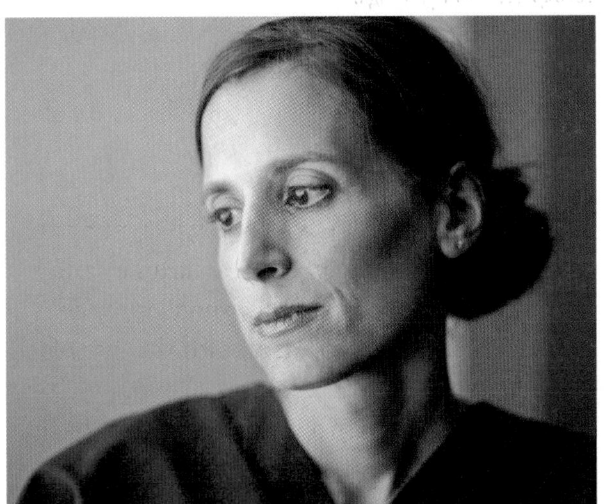

Fig. 23-8. *Nursing assistants should allow themselves to grieve. They will develop close relationships with some residents. It is normal for them to feel sad, angry, or lonely when residents die.*

Just as responses to death vary widely, funeral and burial practices vary from culture to culture and region to region. In some cultures, the family and friends of the deceased person hold a *wake,* or a watch over the body before burial. Traditionally the wake was held in the deceased person's home, and the body was present. Modern wakes may take place at a funeral home. There may be singing, eating, drinking, and storytelling at a wake. The mood is not necessarily sad or somber. A *viewing* is a period of time during which a deceased person's body may be visited by mourners. Viewings may be combined with a celebration of the person's life (as in a wake) or may simply be a time for mourners to pay their quiet respects.

Funerals or memorial services may also involve the display of the dead person's body. This is typically called an open casket funeral. The body will have been preserved for burial by a mortician (a person whose job it is to arrange for the burial or cremation of the dead) and may be dressed formally or in clothing dictated by the person's family, culture, or faith. Some cultures or religious traditions forbid the display of a dead body, and for some it is simply a preference that the body not be displayed. At a closed casket service, the casket, or coffin, is present, but is closed so that the body is not visible.

When a body is not buried in a casket, it may be cremated. Cremation is the burning of a body until it is reduced to ashes. Being cremated may be what the deceased person wanted for personal reasons, or it may be dictated by some religious traditions. An urn, or container for the ashes, may be displayed at a funeral or memorial service rather than a casket.

Most funerals and memorial services are held in a place of worship or at a funeral home. They usually involve readings either of religious scripture and prayers or philosophical excerpts. Many include eulogies, or speeches made in honor of the deceased. Spiritual leaders may offer words of comfort or remembrance. Some funerals are followed by a procession to the place of burial. Often only those closest to the deceased take part in the burial. In some cases, memorial services are entirely separate from the burial, and the deceased person's body is not present at all. A luncheon or reception often follows the service.

Services will incorporate elements of the dead person's religious faith and culture. If an NA is attending a service for a resident who practiced a faith different from her own or who came from a culture different from her own, she should be respectful of the resident's traditions.

The same is true of attending a service for a resident who was an atheist (a person who does not believe in any higher power). Such services will not involve prayers, hymns, or any religious rituals.

No matter what rituals or services take place after a person has died, nursing assistants should not be judgmental or make critical comments. They should be respectful and professional.

Chapter Review

1. Describe one behavior that a nursing assistant might see at each stage of grief.
2. Describe five possible feelings/responses in the grief process.
3. How would you describe your personality type? What helps you work through difficult feelings like those associated with grief?
4. Which sense is usually present until death occurs?
5. What are some of the ways that an NA might provide emotional and spiritual support for a dying resident?
6. What measures may help a dying resident who is in pain?
7. List three legal rights to remember when caring for the terminally ill.
8. What is the focus in palliative care? How does it differ from the usual care NAs provide?
9. List 10 common signs of approaching death.
10. List five changes that may occur in the human body after death.
11. What is postmortem care?
12. Where are drainage pads most often needed during postmortem care?
13. What is a wake?
14. What is cremation?

24 Caring for Your Career and Yourself

The first 23 chapters of this book introduce readers to the long-term care setting. They cover the knowledge, skills, and qualities a person needs to work as a nursing assistant. This final chapter is more personal. It has to do with finding and keeping a job. After a short description of job opportunities in the healthcare field, the chapter addresses the reader directly. It includes a step-by-step job-hunting guide and useful advice about building good relationships with employers and coworkers. It also includes helpful tips for managing stress and staying healthy.

1. Discuss different types of careers in the healthcare field

There are many different types of careers in the healthcare field. Some of these are considered *direct service*. These are the positions that serve the resident or patient directly. Nursing assistants, home health aides, patient care technicians, nurses, physician assistants, and doctors all provide direct service. Professionals in therapeutic services, such as occupational, speech, and physical therapists, also offer direct service.

Some specialized technicians, such as x-ray, lab, and ultrasound technicians, work in diagnostic services (Fig. 24-1). Diagnostic services are procedures performed to determine a condition and/or its cause.

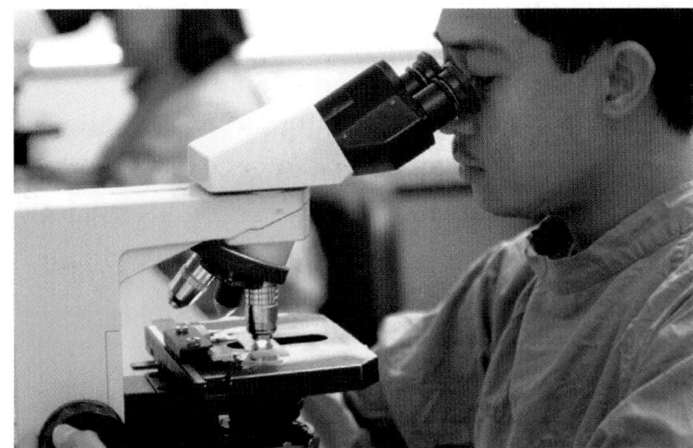

Fig. 24-1. Lab technicians may conduct tests to help diagnose a condition.

Medical social workers and substance abuse counselors are part of psychology, counseling, and social work fields. Activities directors and assistants also work in health care. Administrative and support staff, including directors or other executive staff, medical records personnel, receptionists, office managers, and billing staff are part of the healthcare field.

Career opportunities in health care also include the fields of dentistry, nutrition, and pharmacy. Complementary or alternative healthcare fields include chiropractic medicine, massage therapy, and homeopathic medicine (Fig. 24-2).

There are many opportunities for teachers within health care. Most of the career paths require classes before working in the field, as well as continuing education. Health educators and prevention professionals teach the general population or specific populations, such as people who have diabetes or pregnant women.

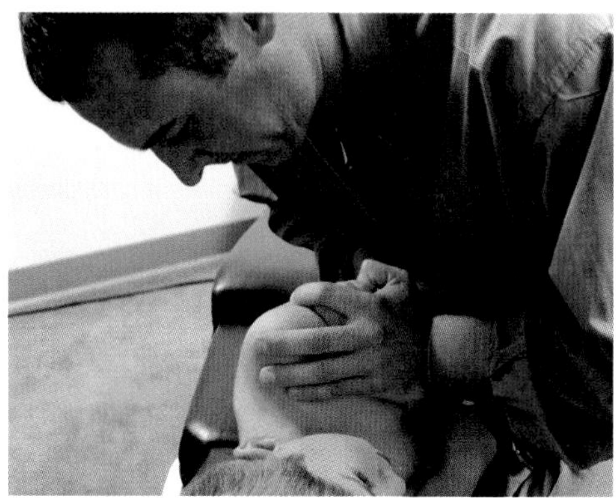

Fig. 24-2. *Chiropractors perform hands-on manipulations, or adjustments, of the spine or joints.*

There are many opportunities available in the healthcare field, depending upon a person's interests, education, and abilities. The careers listed above are only a fraction of the jobs offered in health care. You are reading this textbook most likely because you want to become a nursing assistant. This position may be the best fit for you or, at some point, you may want to try something different. Speak with your supervisor, instructor, or a career counselor if you want more information about other careers in the healthcare field. Review Chapters 1 and 2 for information on the different healthcare settings and educational requirements for care team members.

2. Explain how to find a job and how to write a résumé

You may soon be looking for a job. Nursing assistants may be able to work in long-term care facilities, in assisted living facilities, in hospitals, in the home, and in other settings. To find a job, you must first find potential employers. Then you must contact them to find out about job opportunities. To find potential employers, use the Internet, newspaper, telephone book, or personal contacts. Try these resources:

- Check the Internet (Fig. 24-3). Two websites are jobbankinfo.org and monster.com. You can also visit a search engine: google.com or yahoo.com. Type in nursing assistant or nurse aide and your city. See what employment opportunities are there. Check your local newspaper's website as well.
- Classified or employment sections of the newspaper list jobs currently available. Circle the positions for which you are qualified. Make a list of names, e-mail addresses, and phone numbers to contact.
- Call the state or local Department of Social Services or Department of Aging. Many states hire or place nursing assistants.
- Ask your instructor for potential employers. Some schools maintain a list of employers seeking nursing assistants.

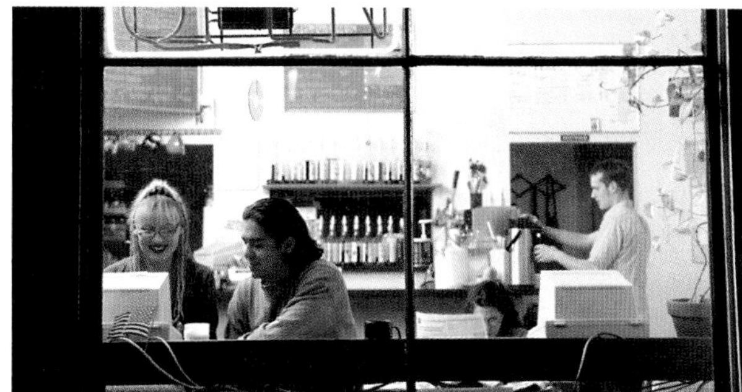

Fig. 24-3. *Searching the Internet is one good way to find a job.*

Once you have a list of potential employers, you need to contact them about job opportunities. Phoning or e-mailing first, unless they mention not to do so, is a good way to find out what opportunities are available. Ask how to apply for a job with each potential employer.

When making an appointment, ask what information to bring with you. Make sure you have this information with you when you go. Some of these documents include the following:

- Identification, including driver's license, social security card, birth certificate, passport, or other official form of identification
- Proof of your legal status in this country and proof that you are legally able to work, even if you are a U.S. citizen. All employers must have files showing that all employees are legally allowed to work in this country. Do not be offended by this request.

- High school diploma or equivalency, school transcripts, and diploma or certificate from your nursing assistant training course. Take your instructor's name, phone number, and e-mail address with you as well.
- References are people who can be called to recommend you as an employee. They include former employers and/or former teachers. Do not use relatives or friends as references. You can ask your references beforehand to write general letters for you, addressed "To whom it may concern," explaining how they know you and describing your skills, qualities, and work habits. Take copies of these with you.

Some potential employers will ask you for a résumé. A **résumé** is a summary or listing of relevant job experience and education. When creating your résumé, include the following information:

- Your contact details: name, address, telephone number, email address
- Your educational experience, starting with the most current first (for example, nursing assistant training course, college degree, high school diploma, or G.E.D. courses)
- Your work experience, starting with the most current first (include name of company or organization, your title, dates worked, and a brief summary of duties)
- Any special skills, such as knowledge of computer software, typing skills, or speaking other languages
- Any memberships in professional organizations
- Volunteer work

State at the end of your résumé that references are available upon request. Try to keep your résumé brief (one page is best) and clear. Use nice white or cream-colored paper for printing your résumé.

The cover letter is a letter included with your résumé. It should be no longer than one page in length. This letter briefly states the position you are seeking and why you would be the best person for the job. Emphasize skills you have that would be a good match. Include the following in a cover letter:

- Date
- Your name, address, phone number, and email address
- Recipient's name, job title, and address
- Salutation (e.g., "Dear Ms. Smith" or "Dear Human Resources Director")
- Introduction (position you are seeking)
- Body (skills/experience that fit job being offered)
- Closing and signature (e.g., "I look forward to hearing from you. Sincerely, Josie Hartman")

3. Demonstrate completing an effective job application

You may need to complete a job application. On one sheet of paper, write down the general information you will need to complete the application. Take this information with you, along with your résumé, if you have one. This will save time and avoid mistakes. Include this information:

- Your address, phone number, and email address
- Your birth date
- Your social security number
- Name and address of the school or program where you were trained and the date you completed your training, as well as your certification number if you have one
- Names, titles, addresses, phone numbers, and email addresses of your previous employers, and the dates you worked there
- Salary information from your former jobs
- Reasons why you left each of your former jobs
- Names, addresses, phone numbers, and e-mail addresses of your references
- Days and hours you are available to work

- A brief statement about why you are changing jobs or why you want to work as a nursing assistant

Fill out the application carefully and neatly (Fig. 24-4). Never lie on a job application. Before you write anything, read it all the way through once.

Employment Application

Personal Information			
Name: Rosie Ferguson		Date: 12/15/2013	
Social Security Number: 555-99-9999			
Home Address: 8529 Indian School Rd. NE			
City, state, Zip: Albuquerque, NM 87112			
Home Phone: 505-291-1274	Business Phone: N/A		
US Citizen? Yes	If Not Give Visa No. & expiration:		

Position Applying For	
Title Certified Nursing Assistant	Salary Desired: $12.00/hr
Referred By: Ms. McClain Instructor, NA Training Center	Date Available: 1/2/2014

Education	
High School (Name, City, State): Laguna High School Albuquerque, NM	
Graduation Date: December 2013	
Technical or Undergraduate School: CNA/HHA Training Center Albuquerque, NM	
Dates Attended: July - December 2012	Degree Major: N/A

References
Mr. Robert Castro, Instructor, NA Training Center, 505-291-1284
Ms. Scott, Health Occupations, Laguna HS, 505-555-6255
Kate Crawford, Instructor, NA Training Center, 505-291-1294

Fig. 31-4. A sample job application.

If you are not sure what is being asked, find out before filling in that space. Fill in all of the blanks. Write *N/A* (not applicable) if the question does not apply to you.

By law, your employer must perform a criminal background check on all new aides hired. You may be asked to sign a form granting permission to do this. Do not take it personally; it is a law intended to protect patients and residents.

4. Demonstrate competence in job interview techniques

To make the best impression at a job interview, be professional and do the following:

- Shower or bathe and use deodorant.
- Brush your teeth.
- Wear only simple makeup and jewelry or none at all.
- Clean and file your nails. Nails should be medium length or shorter.
- Style clean hair simply.
- Shave or trim facial hair before the interview (men).
- Dress neatly and appropriately. Make sure clothing is clean, ironed, and has no holes in it. Do not wear jeans, shorts, or short dresses or skirts (no shorter than knee-length). Make sure your shoes are clean and polished. Do not wear sneakers or flip-flops.
- Do not wear perfume or cologne. Many people dislike or are allergic to scents.
- Do not smoke beforehand because you will smell like smoke during the interview.
- Arrive 10 or 15 minutes early.
- Introduce yourself. Smile and shake hands (Fig. 24-5). Your handshake should be firm and confident.
- Answer questions clearly and completely.
- Make eye contact to show you are sincere (Fig. 24-6).
- Avoid using slang words or expressions.
- Never eat, drink, chew gum, or smoke in an interview.
- Sit up or stand up straight, and look happy to be there.
- Do not bring friends or children to the interview with you.
- Relax and be confident. You have worked hard to get this far.

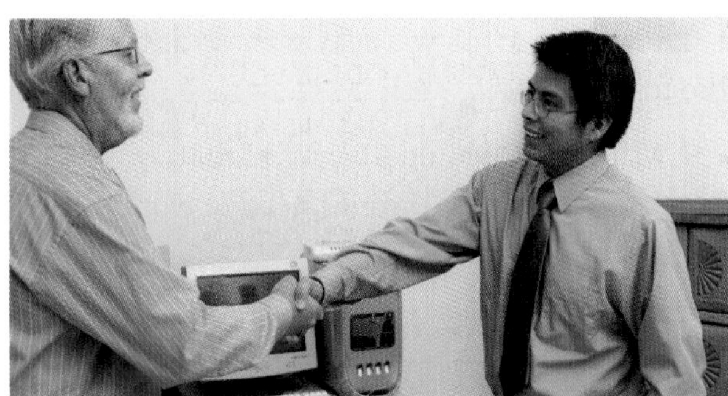

Fig. 24-5. *A person should smile and shake hands confidently when arriving at a job interview.*

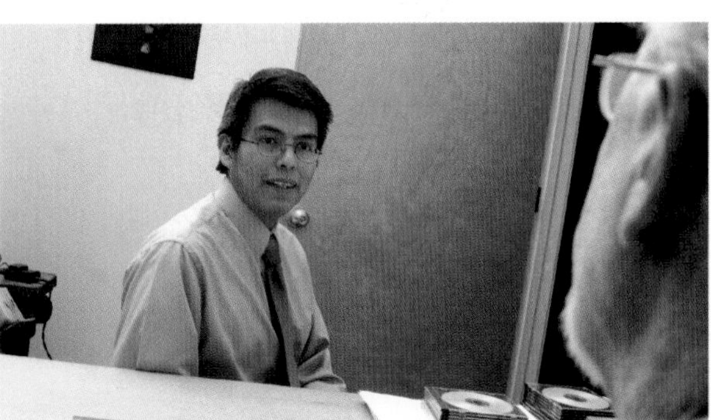

Fig. 24-6. *Being polite and making eye contact during an interview are important.*

Be positive when answering questions. Emphasize what you enjoy or think you will enjoy about the job. Do not complain about any previous jobs you held. Make it clear that you are hardworking and willing to work with all kinds of residents.

The following are some questions you can expect to be asked:

- Why did you become a nursing assistant?
- What do you like about working as an aide?
- What do you not like? (If this is your first job, you may be asked what you expect to like or dislike.)

- What are your best qualities? What are your weaknesses?
- Why did you leave your last job?
- With which kinds of residents do you prefer to work?

Usually interviewers will ask if you have any questions. Have some prepared and written down so you do not forget things you really want to know. Questions you may want to ask include the following:

- What hours would I work? Is there any mandatory overtime I would need to work?
- What benefits does the job include? Is health insurance available? Would I get paid sick days or holidays?
- What is the average caseload for nursing assistants?
- What orientation or training is provided?
- How will I contact my supervisor when I need to do so?
- Are there any policies regarding ongoing education or advancement?
- How soon will you be making a decision about this position?

Later in the interview, you may want to ask about salary or wages if you have not already been given this information. Listen carefully to the answers to your questions. Take notes if needed. At the end of the interview, you will probably be told when you can expect to hear from the employer. Do not expect to be offered a job at the interview. When the interview is over, stand up and shake hands again. Say something like, "Thank you for taking the time to meet with me today. I look forward to hearing from you."

Send a letter after the interview to say thank you and to express your continued interest in the job. If you have not heard anything from the employer within the time frame you discussed with your interviewer, call and ask whether the job has been filled.

5. Describe a standard job description

A job description is an agreement between the employer and the employee. When you start a new job, you will receive a job description. It states your responsibilities and the tasks you will be expected to perform. It also describes the skills required for the job, to whom you must report, and the salary range.

The job description provides protection for you and your employer. It protects you, the employee, from the facility changing duties without notifying you. It protects you from being fired based on something not related to your job description. The employer is protected if ever you were to claim you did not know certain duties were part of the job. The job description reduces misunderstandings and can be used to document what was agreed upon if misunderstandings or legal issues arise.

Tuberculosis Test and Hepatitis B Vaccine

At least once per year, employers are required to test all employees for exposure to tuberculosis. NAs will receive a notice when it is time to have a TB skin test. It is each NA's responsibility to get the test. Once the test has been administered, he or she will be asked to return within 48 to 72 hours for the test results.

Hepatitis B (HBV) is a bloodborne disease that poses a serious threat to healthcare workers. Employers must offer NAs a free vaccine to protect them from hepatitis B. The hepatitis B vaccine is given as a series of three or four shots. An NA will usually get the vaccine when he begins his new job.

6. Discuss how to manage and resolve conflict

Everyone experiences conflict at some point in his or her life. For example, families may argue at home, coworkers may disagree on the job, and so on. If conflict at work is not managed or resolved, it may affect the ability to function well. Productivity and the workplace environment may suffer. When conflict occurs, there is a proper time and place to address it. You may need to talk to your supervisor for help. In general, follow these guidelines for managing conflict:

Guidelines: Resolving Conflict

G Plan to discuss the issue at the right time. Do not start a conversation while you are helping residents. Wait until the supervisor has decided on the right time and place. Privacy is important. Shut the door. Limit distractions, such as television and conversations.

G Agree not to interrupt the person. Do not be rude or sarcastic, or name-call. Use active listening. Take turns speaking.

G Do not get emotional. Some situations may be very upsetting. However, you will be more effective in communicating and problem-solving if you can keep your emotions out of it.

G Check your body language to make sure it is not tense, unwelcoming, or threatening. Maintain eye contact and use a posture that says you are listening and interested. Lean forward slightly and do not slouch.

G Keep the focus on the issue at hand. When discussing conflict, state how you feel when a behavior occurs. Use "I" statements. First describe the actual behavior. Then use "feeling" words to describe how you feel. Let the person know how the problem is affecting you. For example, "When you are late to work, I feel upset because I end up doing your work along with my own."

G People involved in the conflict may need to come up with possible solutions. Think of ways that the conflict can be resolved. A solution may be chosen by a supervisor that does not satisfy everyone. In order to resolve conflict, you may have to compromise. Be prepared to do this.

7. Describe employee evaluations and discuss appropriate responses to criticism

Handling criticism is difficult for most people. Being able to accept criticism and learn from it is important in all relationships, including work relationships. From time to time you will receive evaluations from your employer. These evaluations contain ideas to help you improve your job performance. Here are some ideas for handling criticism and using it to your benefit:

- Listen to the message that is being sent. Do not get so upset that you are unable to understand the message.
- Hostile criticism and constructive criticism are not the same. Hostile criticism is angry and negative. Examples are, "You are useless!" or "You are lazy and slow." Hostile criticism should not come from your employer or supervisor. You may experience hostile criticism from residents, family members, or others. The best response is to say something like, "I'm sorry you are so disappointed," and nothing more. Give the person a chance to calm down before trying to discuss their comments.
- Constructive criticism is intended to help you improve. Constructive criticism may come from your employer, supervisor, or others. Examples are, "You really need to be more accurate in your charting," or "You are late too often. You'll have to make more of an effort to be on time." Listening and acting on constructive criticism can help you be more successful in your job. Pay attention to it (Fig. 24-7).
- If you are not sure how to avoid a mistake you have made, always ask the person criticizing you for suggestions on improving your performance.
- Apologize and move on. If you have made a mistake, apologize as needed (Fig. 24-8).

This may be to a supervisor, a resident, or others. Learn what you can from the incident and put it behind you. Do not dwell on it or hold a grudge. Being able to respond professionally to criticism is important for success in any job.

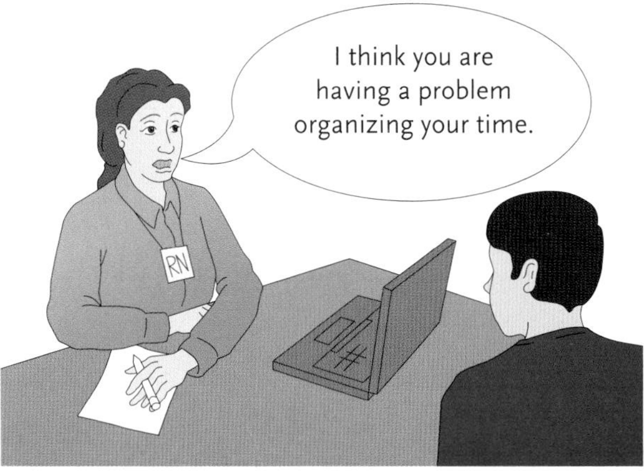
I think you are having a problem organizing your time.
RN

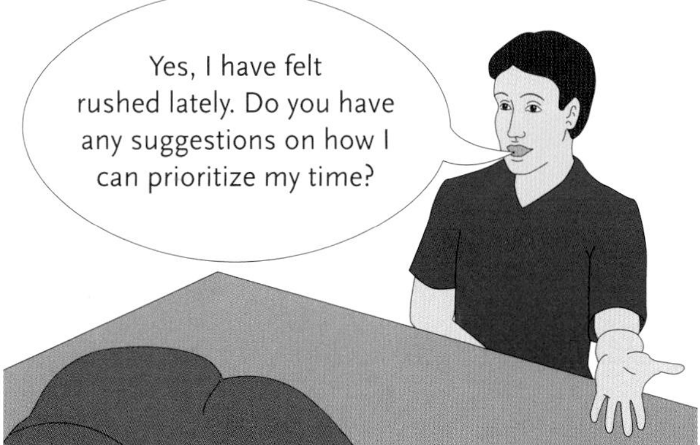
Yes, I have felt rushed lately. Do you have any suggestions on how I can prioritize my time?

Fig. 24-7. *Ask for suggestions when receiving constructive criticism.*

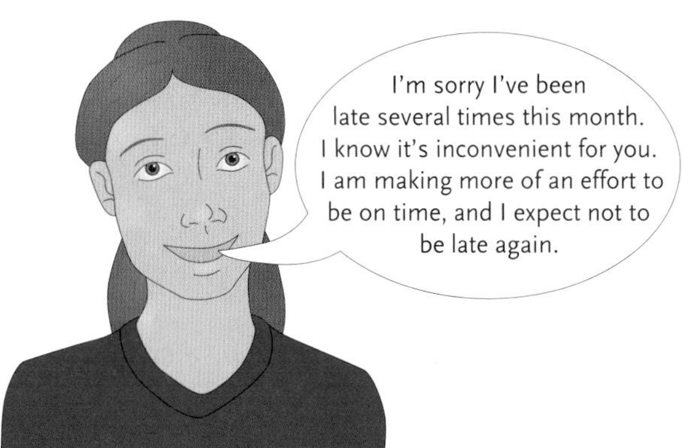
I'm sorry I've been late several times this month. I know it's inconvenient for you. I am making more of an effort to be on time, and I expect not to be late again.

Fig. 24-8. *A person should be willing to apologize if she has made a mistake.*

An evaluation will also cover overall knowledge, conflict resolution, and team effort. Flexibility, friendliness, trustworthiness, and customer service will be considered. Evaluations are often the basis for salary increases. A good evaluation can help you advance within the facility. Being open to criticism and suggestions for improvement will help you be more successful.

8. Explain how to make job changes

If you decide to change jobs, be responsible. Always give your employer at least two weeks' written notice that you will be leaving. Otherwise, your facility may be understaffed. Both the residents and other staff will suffer. In addition, future employers may talk with past supervisors. People who change jobs too often or who do not give notice before leaving are less likely to be hired.

9. Discuss certification and explain the state's registry

To satisfy the requirements set forth in the Omnibus Budget Reconciliation Act (OBRA), states must regulate nursing assistant training, evaluation, and certification. OBRA requires 75 hours as the minimum level of initial training and a 12-hour minimum for annual continuing education (called *in-services*). Many states' requirements exceed the minimum hours. It is a good idea to know your state's rules.

After completing an approved training program, nursing assistants are given a competency evaluation (a certification exam or test) so that they can be certified to work in a state. This exam usually has both a written and skills evaluation. You must pass both parts in order to be certified to work as a nursing assistant.

OBRA also requires that each state keep a registry of nursing assistants. This registry is maintained by a state department, often by the state's Department of Health. The registry contains nursing assistants' training information, results of certification exams, and any findings of abuse, neglect, or theft by nursing assistants.

Employers are able to access this list to verify that you have passed the certification exam, as well as to check if your certification is current. They are also able to see if you have been investigated or found guilty of any abuse or neglect.

Nursing assistant registries are also a good source of information for nursing assistants. By contacting the department that oversees the registry, you can find out how you may be able to move your certification from one state to another state. This is called reciprocity.

Each state has different requirements for maintaining certification. Learn your state's requirements. Follow them exactly, or you will not be able to keep working. Once you are certified, you can lose your certification if you fail to follow your state's rules. Usually this occurs if you do not work in long-term care for a period of time or fail to get the required number of continuing education hours. You can also lose certification due to criminal activities, including abuse and neglect. For your state, make sure you know the following:

- How quickly after completing a training program you must take and pass the certification exam
- How many days per year you must work in long-term care to maintain your certification
- How many hours of continuing education you must take each year

10. Describe continuing education

The federal government requires that nursing assistants have a 12-hour minimum of annual continuing education. Many states may require more. In-service continuing education courses help you keep your knowledge and skills fresh. Classes may also provide you with more information about certain conditions, challenges you face in working with residents, or regulation changes. You need to be up-to-date on the latest that is expected of you.

If you need more instruction in a particular area, speak to your supervisor. Perhaps he or she can arrange for an in-service continuing education class to be offered on that topic. Your employer may be responsible for offering continuing education courses. However, you are responsible for attending and completing them. Specifically, you must do the following:

- Sign up for the course or find out where it is offered.
- Attend all class sessions.
- Pay attention and complete all the class requirements.
- Make the most of your in-service programs. Participate (Fig. 24-9).
- Keep original copies of all certificates and records of your successful attendance so you can prove you took the class.

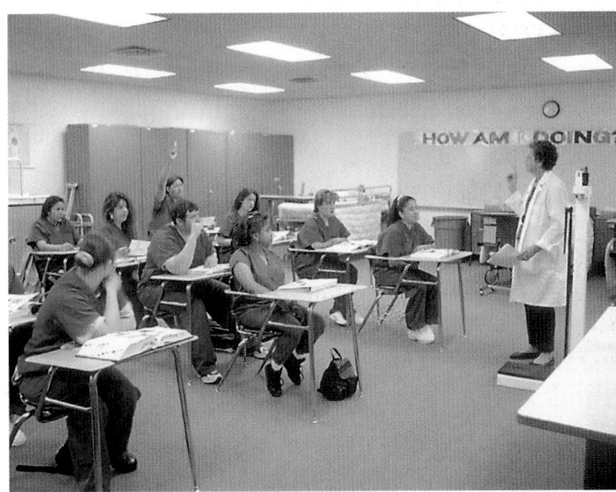

Fig. 24-9. Students should pay attention and participate during continuing education courses.

11. Define *stress* and *stressors*

Stress is the state of being frightened, excited, confused, in danger, or irritated. It is often thought that only bad things cause stress. However, positive situations cause stress, too. For example, getting married or having a new baby are usually positive situations. However, both can cause enormous stress because of the changes they bring to a person's life (Fig. 24-10).

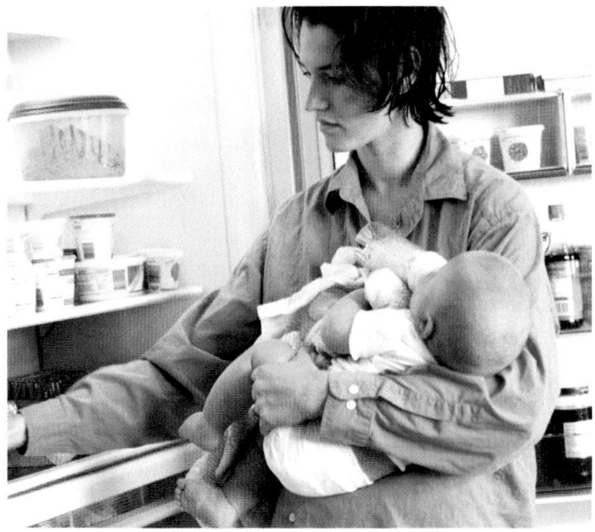

Fig. 24-10. Although having a new baby is usually a happy time, it can also be a stressful one.

You may be thrilled when you get your new job. But starting work may also cause you stress. You may be afraid of making mistakes, excited about earning money or helping people, or confused about your new duties. Learning how to recognize stress and what causes it is helpful. Then you can master a few simple techniques for relaxing and learn to manage stress.

Defense mechanisms are unconscious behaviors used to cope with stress. See Chapter 20 for more information on defense mechanisms.

A **stressor** is something that causes stress. Anything can be a stressor if it causes you stress. Some examples include the following:

- Divorce
- Marriage
- New baby
- Parenthood
- Children growing up
- Children leaving home
- Feeling unprepared for a task
- Starting a new job
- Problems at work
- New responsibilities at work
- Losing a job
- Supervisors
- Coworkers
- Residents
- Illness
- Finances

12. Explain ways to manage stress

Stress is not only an emotional response. It is also a physical response. When a person experiences stress, changes occur in the body. The endocrine system produces more of the hormone adrenaline. This can increase nervous system response, heart rate, respiratory rate, and blood pressure. This is why, in stressful situations, your heart beats quickly, you breathe hard, and you may feel warm or perspire.

Each person has a different tolerance level for stress. In other words, what one person would find overwhelming might not bother another person. A person's tolerance for stress depends on his personality, life experiences, and physical health.

Guidelines: Managing Stress

To manage the stress in your life, develop healthy dietary, exercise, and lifestyle habits:

- G Eat nutritious foods.
- G Exercise regularly. You can exercise alone or with a partner (Fig. 24-11).

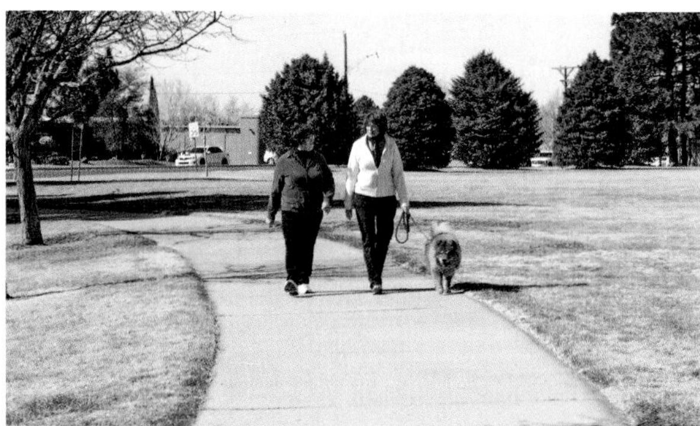

Fig. 24-11. Regular exercise is one healthy way to decrease stress.

- G Get enough sleep.
- G Drink only in moderation.

G Do not smoke.

G Find time at least a few times a week to do something relaxing, such as reading a book, watching a movie, sewing, or any of the following:

- Being in nature
- Doing something artistic (painting, drawing, writing, singing, etc.)
- Doing yoga
- Getting a massage
- Listening to music
- Meditating

Not managing stress can cause many problems. Some of these problems affect how well you do your job. Signs that you are not managing stress include the following:

- Showing anger or being abusive to residents
- Arguing with your supervisor about assignments
- Having poor relationships with coworkers and residents
- Complaining about your job and your responsibilities
- Feeling work-related burnout (burnout is a state of mental or physical exhaustion caused by stress)
- Feeling tired even when you are rested
- Having a difficult time focusing on residents and procedures

Stress can seem overwhelming when you try to handle it yourself. Often just talking about stress can help you manage it better. Sometimes another person can offer helpful suggestions for managing stress. You may be able to think of new ways to handle stress just by talking it through with another person. Get help from one or more of these resources when managing stress:

- Your supervisor or another member of the care team for work-related stress
- Your family
- Your friends
- A support group (Fig. 24-12)
- Your place of worship
- Your doctor
- A local mental health agency
- Any phone hotline that deals with related problems (check the Internet or a phone book)

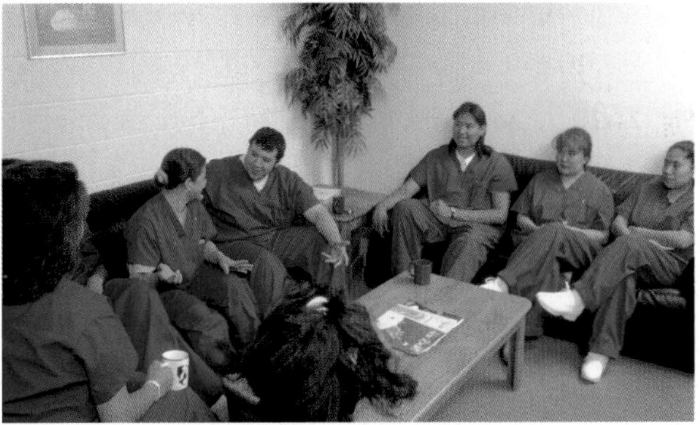

Fig. 24-12. *Support groups can help people deal with different types of stress.*

It is not appropriate to talk to your residents or their family members to help you manage personal or job-related stress.

Developing a plan for managing stress can be very helpful. The plan can include nice things you will do for yourself every day and things to do in stressful situations. When you think about a plan, you first need to answer the following questions:

- What are the sources of stress in my life?
- When do I most often feel stress?
- What effects of stress do I see in my life?
- What can I change to decrease the stress I feel?
- What do I have to learn to cope with because I cannot change it?

When you have answered these questions, you will have a clearer picture of the challenges you face. Then you can try to come up with strategies for managing stress.

13. Describe a relaxation technique

Sometimes a relaxation exercise can help you feel refreshed and relaxed in only a short time. Below is a simple relaxation exercise. Try it out. See if it helps you feel more relaxed.

The body scan. Close your eyes. Focus on your breathing and posture. Be sure you are comfortable. Starting at the balls of your feet, concentrate on your feet. Discover any tension hidden in the feet, and try to relax and release the tension. Continue very slowly. Take a breath between each body part. Move up from the feet, focusing on and relaxing the legs, knees, thighs, hips, stomach, back, shoulders, neck, jaw, eyes, forehead, and scalp. Take a few very deep breaths and open your eyes.

This exercise takes only about two minutes. If it is helpful for you, try it the next time you need a break, at work or at home.

14. List ways to remind yourself of the importance of the work you have chosen to do

Look back over all you have learned in this program. Your work as a caregiver is very important. Every day may be different and challenging. In a hundred ways every week you will offer help that only a caring person like you can give.

Do not forget to value the work you have chosen to do. It is important. Your work can mean the difference between living with independence and dignity and living without them. The difference you make is sometimes life versus death. Look in the face of each of your residents. Know that you are doing important work. Look in a mirror when you get home and be proud of how you make your living (Fig. 24-13).

Being able to reflect on how you spend your time is an important life skill. Learn ways to fully appreciate that what you do has great meaning. Few jobs have the challenges and rewards of working with the elderly, ill, or disabled. Congratulate yourself for choosing a path that includes helping others along the way.

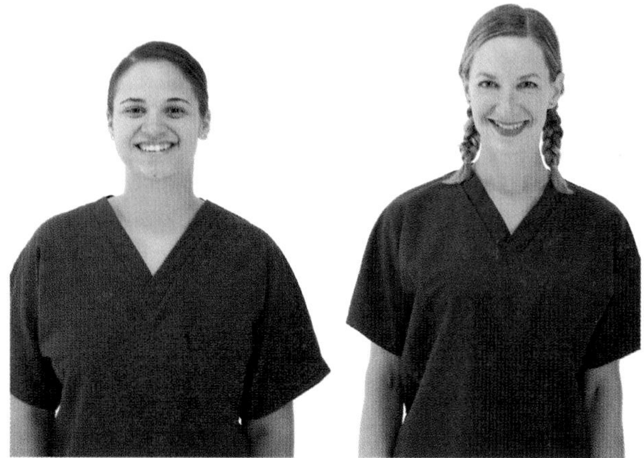

Fig. 24-13. *Being proud of the work a person has chosen to do is important.*

Chapter Review

1. What are direct service positions?
2. What are two good ways to find out about job opportunities with potential employers?
3. List three documents that a person should bring with him when applying for a job.
4. What should be done before writing anything on a job application?
5. List 10 things that show professionalism to potential employers during an interview.
6. How can a nursing assistant follow up on a job interview?
7. What is contained in a job description?
8. List four guidelines to follow while working on resolving conflict.
9. What is the difference between hostile and constructive criticism?
10. Why might an employer not hire a person who has changed jobs often?
11. What information does a registry for certified nursing assistants keep?

12. How many hours of continuing education does the federal government require that NAs have each year?
13. What is stress? Give three examples of stressors you have experienced in the last year. How did you respond to them?
14. List five guidelines for managing stress.
15. What are five resources that are appropriate for an NA to turn to when trying to manage stress?
16. Before developing a stress management plan, what are four questions that a person should ask herself?
17. What do you think you will like best about being a nursing assistant?

Abbreviations

abd	abdomen
ABR	absolute bedrest
ac, a.c.	before meals
ad lib	as desired
ADLs	activities of daily living
adm.	admission
AIDS	acquired immune deficiency syndrome
amb	ambulate, ambulatory
amt	amount
ap	apical
AROM	active range of motion
ASAP	as soon as possible
as tol	as tolerated
ax.	axillary (armpit)
BID, b.i.d.	two times a day
BM	bowel movement
BP, B/P	blood pressure
BPM	beats per minute
BR	bedrest
BRP	bathroom privileges
BSC	bedside commode
c̄	with
C	Centigrade
CA	cancer
cath.	catheter
CBC	complete blood count
CBR	complete bedrest
CCU	cardiac care unit, cardiovascular care unit
CDC	Centers for Disease Control
C. diff	*clostridium difficile*
CHF	congestive heart failure
ck ✓	check
cl liq	clear liquid
CMS	Centers for Medicare and Medicaid Services
CNA	certified nursing assistant
CNS	central nervous system
c/o	complains of, in care of
COPD	chronic obstructive pulmonary disease
CPR	cardiopulmonary resuscitation
CS	Central Supply
CVA	cerebrovascular accident, stroke
CVP	central venous pressure
CVS	cardiovascular system
CXR	chest X-ray
DAT	diet as tolerated
DM	diabetes mellitus
DNR	do not resuscitate
DOA	dead on arrival
DOB	date of birth
DON	director of nursing
Dr., DR	doctor
drsg	dressing
DVT	deep vein thrombosis
Dx, dx	diagnosis
ECG, EKG	electrocardiogram
EMS	emergency medical services
ER	emergency room
exam	examination
F	Fahrenheit
FBS	fasting blood sugar
FF	force fluids
ft	foot
F/U, f/u	follow-up
FWB	full weight-bearing
FYI	for your information
geri chair	geriatric chair
GI	gastrointestinal
H_20	water
h, hr, hr.	hour
H/A, HA	headache
HBV	hepatitis B virus
HHA	home health aide
HIPAA	Health Insurance Portability and Accountability Act
HIV	human immunodeficiency virus
HOB	head of bed
HS, hs	hours of sleep
ht	height
HTN	hypertension
hyper	above normal, too fast, rapid

hypo	low, less than normal
ICU	intensive care unit
inc	incontinent
I&O	intake and output
isol	isolation
IV, I.V.	intravenous (within a vein)
L, lt	left
lab	laboratory
lb.	pound
lg	large
LOC	level of consciousness
LPN	licensed practical nurse
LTC	long-term care
LTCF	long-term care facility
LVN	licensed vocational nurse
MD, M.D.	medical doctor
MDS	minimum data set
meds	medications
MI	myocardial infarction
min	minute
mL	milliliter
mm Hg	millimeters of mercury
mod	moderate
MRSA	methicillin-resistant *staphylococcus aureus*
MSDS	material safety data sheet
NA	nursing assistant
N/A	not applicable
N/C	no complaints, no call
NG, ng	nasogastric
NKA	no known allergies
NPO	nothing by mouth
NVD	nausea, vomiting and diarrhea
NWB	non-weight-bearing
OBRA	Omnibus Budget Reconciliation Act
OOB	out of bed
OR	operating room
OSHA	Occupational Safety and Health Administration
OT	occupational therapist/therapy
oz	ounce
$\bar{p}$	after
pc, p.c.	after meals
PCA	patient-controlled analgesia
PEG	percutaneous endoscopic gastrostomy
peri care	perineal care
per os	by mouth
PHI	protected health information
PNS	peripheral nervous system
PO	by mouth
post-op	after surgery
PPE	personal protective equipment
pre-op	before surgery
p.r.n., prn	when necessary
PROM	passive range of motion
PT	physical therapist/therapy
PVD	peripheral vascular disease
PWB	partial weight-bearing
$\bar{q}$	every
q2h q3h q4h	every two hours every three hours every four hours
qh, qhr	every hour
R	respirations, rectal
R, rt.	right
RBC	red blood cell/count
rehab	rehabilitation
res.	resident
resp.	respiration
RF	restrict fluids
R.I.C.E.	rest, ice, compression, elevation
RN	registered nurse
R/O	rule out
ROM	range of motion
RR	respiratory rate
$\bar{s}$	without
SNF	skilled nursing facility
SOB	shortness of breath
SP	Standard Precautions
spec.	specimen
S&S, S/S	signs and symptoms
SSE	soapsuds enema

staph	*staphylococcus*
stat, STAT	immediately
std. prec.	Standard Precautions
STI	sexually-transmitted infection
strep	*streptococcus*
T., temp	temperature
TB	tuberculosis
TIA	transient ischemic attack
t.i.d., tid	three times a day
TLC	tender loving care
TPN	total parenteral nutrition
TPR	temperature, pulse, and respiration
TWE	tap water enema
U/A, u/a	urinalysis
URI	upper respiratory infection
UTI	urinary tract infection
VRE	vancomycin-resistant *enterococcus*
VS, vs	vital signs
WBC	white blood cell/count
w/c, W/C	wheelchair
WNL	within normal limits
wt.	weight

Symbols

©	copyright
&	and
☣	biohazard
△	change, heat
°	degree
♀	female
♂	male
%	percent
☢	radiation

Appendix

Basic Math Skills

Nursing assistants need math skills when doing certain tasks, such as calculating intake and output. A basic math review is listed below:

Addition

```
    2,905          53,138
+     174     +     3,008
---------     -----------
    3,079          56,146
```

Subtraction

```
   32,542         549,233
–   8,710     –    26,903
---------     -----------
   23,832         522,330
```

Multiplication

```
    4,962              79
x      13     x        41
---------     -----------
   14,886              79
+  49,620     +     3,160
---------     -----------
   64,506           3,239
```

Division

```
       34             39
22 | 748      14 | 546
     - 660         - 420
     -----         -----
        88           126
      - 88         - 126
     -----         -----
         0             0
```

Converting Decimals, Fractions, and Percentages

Decimals, fractions, and percentages are different ways of showing the same value. For example, one-half can be written in the following ways:

As a decimal: 0.5
As a fraction: 1/2
As a percentage: 50%

Here are common values shown in decimal, fraction, and percentage forms:

Decimal	Fraction	Percentage
0.01	1/100	1%
0.1	1/10	10%
0.2	1/5	20%
0.25	1/4	25%
0.333	1/3	33 1/3%
0.5	1/2	50%
0.75	3/4	75%
1	1/1	100%

Follow these rules for converting decimals, fractions, and percentages:

To convert **from decimal to a percentage**, multiply by 100 and add a percent sign (%).

0.25 x 100 = 25%

To convert **from a percentage to decimal**, divide by 100 and delete the percent sign (%).

80% ÷ 100 = 0.8

To convert a **fraction to a decimal**, you will divide the top number by the bottom number.

$$\frac{2}{3} = 2 \div 3 = 0.67$$

To convert a **decimal to a fraction**, write the decimal over the number 1.

Step 1 $\frac{0.5}{1}$

Then multiply top and bottom by 10 for every number after the decimal point (10 for 1 number, 100 for 2 numbers, and so on.)

Step 2 $\frac{0.5}{1} \frac{\times 10}{\times 10} = \frac{5}{10}$

The resulting fraction is 5/10 (or 1/2 if you simplify the fraction).

To convert a **fraction to a percentage**, divide the top number by the bottom number. Then multiply the result by 100, and add a percent sign (%).

Step 1 $\frac{3}{5} = 3 \div 5 = 0.6$

Step 2 $0.6 \times 100 = 60\%$

To convert a **percentage to a fraction**, first convert to a decimal by dividing by 100. Then use the steps for converting a decimal to a fraction.

Step 1 $15\% \div 100 = 0.15$

Step 2 $\frac{0.15}{1}$

Step 3 $\frac{0.15}{1} \frac{\times 100}{\times 100} = \frac{15}{100}$

The resulting fraction is 15/100 (or 3/20 if you simplify the fraction).

Other Useful Information

Multiplication Table

1	2	3	4	5	6	7	8	9	10	11	12
2	4	6	8	10	12	14	16	18	20	22	24
3	6	9	12	15	18	21	24	27	30	33	36
4	8	12	16	20	24	28	32	36	40	44	48
5	10	15	20	25	30	35	40	45	50	55	60
6	12	18	24	30	36	42	48	54	60	66	72
7	14	21	28	35	42	49	56	63	70	77	84
8	16	24	32	40	48	56	64	72	80	88	96
9	18	27	36	45	54	63	72	81	90	99	108
10	20	30	40	50	60	70	80	90	100	110	120
11	22	33	44	55	66	77	88	99	110	121	132
12	24	36	48	60	72	84	96	108	120	132	144

Conversions: Volume

1 milliliter (mL) = 1 cubic centimeter (cc)

1 ounce (oz) = 30 mL (cc)

¼ cup = 2 oz = 60 mL (cc)

½ cup = 4 oz = 120 mL (cc)

1 cup = 8 oz = 240 mL (cc)

1 liter (L) = 1000 mL (cc)

2 pints = 1 quart (qt) = 960 mL (cc)

2 quarts = ½ gallon (gal) = 1920 cc = 2 liters (L)

4 quarts = 1 gallon (gal)

Conversions: Weight

1 kilogram (kg) = 2.2 pounds (lbs)

1 gram (g) = 1000 milligrams (mg)

1 pound (lb) = 16 ounces (oz)

Conversions: Length

1 inch (in) = 2.54 centimeters (cm)
(or round off to 2.5)

12 inches = 1 foot (ft)

3 feet = 1 yard (yd)

10 millimeters (mm) = 1 centimeter (cm)

100 centimeters (cm) = 1 meter

Glossary

24-hour urine specimen: a urine specimen consisting of all urine voided in a 24-hour period.

abdominal thrusts: method of attempting to remove an object from the airway of someone who is choking.

abduction: moving a body part away from the midline of the body.

abrasion: an injury which rubs off the surface of the skin.

abuse: purposeful mistreatment that causes physical, mental, or emotional pain or injury to someone.

acquired immune deficiency syndrome (AIDS): the final stage of HIV infection, in which infections, tumors, and central nervous system symptoms appear due to a weakened immune system that is unable to fight infection.

active assisted range of motion (AAROM): exercises to put a joint through its full arc of motion that are performed by a caregiver with some help from the affected person.

active neglect: the purposeful failure to provide needed care, resulting in harm to a person.

active range of motion (AROM): exercises to put a joint through its full arc of motion that are performed by the affected person alone, without help.

activities of daily living (ADLs): daily personal care tasks, such as bathing; caring for skin, nails, hair, and teeth; dressing; toileting; eating and drinking; walking; and transferring.

acute care: 24-hour skilled care for short-term illnesses or injuries; generally given in hospitals and ambulatory surgical centers.

acute illness: an illness that has severe symptoms, is treated immediately, and is usually short-term.

adaptive devices: special equipment that helps a person who is ill or disabled to perform activities of daily living; also called *assistive devices.*

additive: a substance added to another substance, changing its effect.

adduction: moving a body part toward the midline of the body.

adult day services: care for people who need some assistance or supervision during certain hours, but who do not live in the facility where care is given.

advance directives: legal documents that allow people to choose what medical care they wish to have if they are unable to make those decisions themselves.

affected side: a weakened side from a stroke or injury; also called *weaker* or *involved side.*

ageism: prejudice toward, stereotyping of, and/or discrimination against older persons or the elderly.

age-related macular degeneration (AMD): a condition in which the macula deteriorates, causing vision loss.

agitated: the state of being excited, restless, or troubled.

agnostics: people who believe that they do not know or cannot know if God exists.

AIDS dementia complex: a group of symptoms including memory loss, poor coordination, paralysis, and confusion that occur in the late stages of AIDS due to damage to the central nervous system.

alternative medicine: practices and treatments used instead of conventional healthcare methods.

Alzheimer's disease: a progressive, incurable disease that causes tangled nerve fibers and protein deposits to form in the brain, which eventually cause dementia.

ambulation: walking.

ambulatory: capable of walking.

amputation: the surgical removal of some or all of a body part, usually a hand, arm, leg, or foot.

anesthesia: the use of medication to block pain during surgery and other medical procedures.

angina pectoris: chest pain, pressure, or discomfort.

anorexia: an eating disorder in which a person does not eat or exercises excessively to lose weight.

antimicrobial: an agent that destroys, resists, or prevents the development of pathogens.

anxiety: uneasiness or fear, often about a situation or condition.

apathy: a lack of interest in activities.

apical pulse: the pulse located on the left side of the chest, just below the nipple.

apnea: the absence of breathing.

arthritis: a general term that refers to inflammation of the joints, causing stiffness, pain, and decreased mobility.

artificial airway: any plastic, metal, or rubber device inserted into the respiratory tract to maintain or promote breathing.

aspiration: the inhalation of food, drink, or foreign material into the lungs.

assault: a threat to harm a person, resulting in the person feeling fearful that he or she will be harmed.

assisted living: residences for people who do not need skilled, 24-hour care, but do require some help with daily care.

assistive devices: special equipment that helps a person who is ill or disabled to perform activities of daily living; also called *adaptive devices.*

asthma: a chronic inflammatory disease that causes difficulty with breathing, coughing, and wheezing.

atheists: people who believe that there is no God and actively deny the existence of God.

atherosclerosis: a hardening and narrowing of the blood vessels.

atrophy: the wasting away, decreasing in size, and weakening of muscles from lack of use.

autoimmune illness: an illness in which the body's immune system attacks normal tissue in the body.

axillae: underarms.

baseline: initial values that can be compared to future measurements.

battery: the intentional touching of a person without his or her consent.

benign prostatic hypertrophy (BPH): a disorder that can occur in men as they age, in which the prostate becomes enlarged and causes problems with urination and/or emptying the bladder.

benign tumors: tumors that are considered non-cancerous.

bias: prejudice.

bipolar disorder: a type of depression that causes a person to swing from periods of deep depression to periods of extreme activity; also called *manic-depressive illness.*

bisexual: a person who is sexually attracted to both men and women.

bloodborne pathogens: microorganisms found in human blood, body fluid, draining wounds, and mucous membranes that can cause infection and disease in humans.

Bloodborne Pathogens Standard: federal law that requires that healthcare facilities protect employees from bloodborne health hazards.

body mechanics: the way the parts of the body work together when a person moves.

bones: rigid connective tissues that make up the skeleton, protect organs, and allow the body to move.

bony prominences: areas of the body where bone lies close to the skin.

brachial pulse: the pulse located inside the elbow, about one to one-and-a-half inches above the elbow.

bronchiectasis: condition in which the bronchial tubes are permanently enlarged, causing chronic coughing and thick sputum.

bronchitis: an irritation and inflammation of the lining of the bronchi.

bulimia: an eating disorder in which a person binges, eating huge amounts of foods or very fattening foods, and then purges, eliminating the food by vomiting, using laxatives, or exercising excessively.

calculi: kidney stones that form when urine crystallizes in the kidneys.

cancer: general term to describe a disease in which abnormal cells grow in an uncontrolled way.

cardiopulmonary resuscitation (CPR): medical procedures used when a person's heart or lungs have stopped working.

cataracts: a condition in which milky or cloudy spots develop in the eye, causing vision loss.

catastrophic reaction: reacting to something in an unreasonable, exaggerated way.

catheter: a thin tube inserted into the body to drain fluids or inject fluids.

causative agent: a pathogenic microorganism that causes disease.

C cane: a straight cane with a curved handle at the top.

cells: basic structural units of the body that divide, develop, and die, renewing tissues and organs.

Centers for Disease Control and Prevention (CDC): a government agency under the U.S. Department of Health and Human Services that issues information to protect the health of individuals and communities.

Centers for Medicare & Medicaid Services (CMS): a federal agency within the U.S. Department of Health and Human Services that is responsible for Medicare and Medicaid, among many other responsibilities.

central nervous system (CNS): part of the nervous system that is composed of the brain and spinal cord.

cerebrovascular accident (CVA): a condition that occurs when blood supply to a part of the brain is blocked or a blood vessel leaks or ruptures within the brain; also called *stroke*.

chain of command: the line of authority within a facility or agency.

chain of infection: a way of describing how disease is transmitted from one being to another.

chancres: open sores.

charting: writing down important information and observations about residents.

chest tubes: hollow drainage tubes that are inserted into the chest to drain air, blood or other fluid, or pus that has collected inside the pleural cavity or space.

Cheyne-Stokes: alternating periods of slow, irregular breathing and rapid, shallow breathing.

chickenpox: a highly contagious viral illness that strikes nearly all children.

chlamydia: type of sexually-transmitted infection that is caused by organisms introduced into the mucous membranes of the reproductive tract.

chronic illness: a disease or condition that is long-term or long-lasting and requires management of symptoms.

chronic kidney failure: a condition that occurs when the kidneys cannot eliminate certain waste products from the body; also called *chronic renal failure*.

chronic obstructive pulmonary disease (COPD): a chronic, incurable lung disease that causes difficulty breathing.

chronic renal failure (CRF): a condition that occurs when the kidneys cannot eliminate certain waste products from the body; also called *chronic kidney failure.*

circadian rhythm: the 24-hour day-night cycle.

cite: in a long-term care facility, to find a problem through a survey.

claustrophobia: the fear of being in a confined space.

clean: in health care, a condition in which objects are not contaminated with pathogens.

clean-catch specimen: a urine specimen that does not include the first and last urine voided; also called *mid-stream specimen.*

clichés: phrases that are used over and over again and do not really mean anything.

closed bed: a bed completely made with the bedspread and blankets in place.

closed fracture: a broken bone that does not break the skin.

***Clostridium difficile* (*C. diff, C. difficile*):** bacterial illness that can cause diarrhea and colitis; spread by spores in feces that are difficult to kill.

cognition: the ability to think logically and clearly.

cognitive: related to thinking and learning.

cognitive impairment: loss of ability to think logically; concentration and memory are affected.

colitis: inflammation of the large intestine that causes diarrhea and abdominal pain; also called *irritable bowel syndrome.*

colorectal cancer: cancer of the gastrointestinal tract; also known as colon cancer.

colostomy: surgically-created opening through the abdomen into the large intestine to allow feces to be expelled.

combative: violent or hostile behavior.

combustion: the process of burning.

communication: the process of exchanging information with others by sending and receiving messages.

compassionate: being caring, concerned, considerate, empathetic, and understanding.

complementary medicine: treatments that are used in addition to the conventional treatments prescribed by a doctor.

complex carbohydrates: carbohydrates that are broken down by the body into simple sugars for energy; found in foods such as bread, cereal, potatoes, rice, pasta, and vegetables.

condom catheter: catheter that has an attachment on the end that fits onto the penis; also called *external* or *Texas catheter.*

confidentiality: the legal and ethical principle of keeping information private.

confusion: the inability to think clearly.

congestive heart failure (CHF): a condition in which the heart is no longer able to pump effectively; blood backs up into the heart instead of circulating.

conscientious: guided by a sense of right and wrong; principled.

conscious: the state of being mentally alert and having awareness of surroundings, sensations, and thoughts.

constipation: the inability to eliminate stool, or the infrequent, difficult, and often painful elimination of a hard, dry stool.

constrict: to narrow.

contracture: the permanent and often painful shortening of a muscle, usually due to lack of activity.

cultural diversity: the different groups of people with varied backgrounds and experiences who live together in the world.

culture: a system of learned behaviors, practiced by a group of people, that is considered to be the tradition of that people and is passed on from one generation to the next.

culture change: a term given to the process of transforming services for elders so that they are based on the values and practices of the person receiving care; core values include choice, dignity, respect, self-determination, and purposeful living.

cyanotic: skin that is blue or gray.

cystitis: inflammation of the bladder that may be caused by bacterial infection.

dandruff: an excessive shedding of dead skin cells from the scalp.

dangle: to sit up with the legs hanging over the side of the bed in order to regain balance and stabilize blood pressure.

defecation: the act of passing feces from the large intestine out of the body through the anus.

defense mechanisms: unconscious behaviors used to release tension or cope with stress.

degenerative: something that continually gets worse.

dehydration: a serious condition resulting from inadequate fluid in the body.

delegation: transferring responsibility to a person for a specific task.

delirium: a state of severe confusion that occurs suddenly and is usually temporary.

delusions: false beliefs.

dementia: the serious loss of mental abilities, such as thinking, remembering, reasoning, and communicating.

dental floss: a special kind of string used to clean between teeth.

dentures: artificial teeth.

dermatitis: an inflammation of the skin causing swollen, reddened, irritated, and itchy skin.

developmental disabilities: disabilities that are present at birth or emerge during childhood that restrict physical or mental ability.

diabetes: a condition in which the pancreas produces too little insulin or does not properly use insulin.

diabetic ketoacidosis (DKA): complication of diabetes that is caused by having too little insulin; also called *hyperglycemia*.

diagnoses: physicians' determinations of an illness.

diarrhea: frequent elimination of liquid or semi-liquid feces.

diastole: phase when the heart relaxes or rests.

diastolic: second measurement of blood pressure; phase when the heart relaxes or rests.

dietary restrictions: rules about what and when individuals can eat.

diet cards: cards that list the resident's name and information about special diets, allergies, likes and dislikes, and other dietary instructions.

digestion: the process of preparing food physically and chemically so that it can be absorbed into the cells.

dilate: to widen.

direct contact: a way of transmitting pathogens through touching the infected person or his or her secretions.

dirty: in health care, a condition in which objects have been contaminated with pathogens.

disinfection: process that kills pathogens, but not all pathogens; it reduces the pathogen count to a level that is considered not infectious.

disorientation: confusion about person, place, or time.

disposable: only to be used once and then discarded.

disposable razor: type of razor that is discarded after one use; requires the use of shaving cream or soap.

diuretics: medications that reduce fluid volume in the body.

doff: to remove.

domestic violence: physical, sexual, or emotional abuse by spouses, intimate partners, or family members.

don: to put on.

do-not-resuscitate (DNR): a type of advance directive that instructs medical professionals not to perform CPR if a person's heartbeat or breathing stops.

dorsal recumbent: body position in which a person is flat on her back with her knees flexed and her feet flat on the bed.

dorsiflexion: bending backward.

draw sheet: an extra sheet placed on top of the bottom sheet; used for moving residents.

durable power of attorney for health care: a signed, dated, and witnessed legal document that appoints someone else to make the medical decisions for a person in the event he or she becomes unable to do so.

dysphagia: difficulty swallowing.

dyspnea: difficulty breathing.

edema: swelling caused by excess fluid in body tissues.

edentulous: having no teeth; toothless.

electric razor: type of razor that runs on electricity; does not require the use of soap or shaving cream.

elimination: the process of expelling solid wastes (made up of the waste products of food) that are not absorbed into the cells.

elope: in medicine, when a person with Alzheimer's disease wanders away from a protected area and does not return.

emesis: the act of vomiting, or ejecting stomach contents through the mouth and/or nose.

emotional lability: laughing or crying without any reason or when it is inappropriate.

empathy: identifying with the feelings of others.

emphysema: a chronic disease of the lungs that usually results from chronic bronchitis and cigarette smoking.

enema: a specific amount of water, with or without an additive, that is introduced into the colon to stimulate the elimination of stool.

epilepsy: an illness of the brain that produces seizures.

epistaxis: a nosebleed.

ergonomics: the science of designing equipment, areas, and work tasks to make them safer and to suit the worker's abilities.

ethics: the knowledge of right and wrong.

eupnea: normal breathing.

expiration: exhaling air out of the lungs.

exposure control plan: plan designed to eliminate or reduce employee exposure to infectious material.

expressive aphasia: slurred speech or an inability to speak.

extension: straightening a body part.

facilities: in medicine, places where health care is delivered or administered, including hospitals, long-term care facilities, and treatment centers.

fallacy: a false belief.

false imprisonment: unlawful restraint that affects a person's freedom of movement; includes both the threat of being physically restrained and actually being physically restrained.

farsightedness: the ability to see objects in the distance better than objects nearby; also known as hyperopia.

fasting: not eating food or eating very little food.

fecal impaction: a hard stool that is stuck in the rectum and cannot be expelled.

fecal incontinence: the inability to control the bowels, leading to an involuntary passage of stool.

financial abuse: the improper or illegal use of a person's money, possessions, property, or other assets.

first aid: emergency care given immediately to an injured person.

flammable: easily ignited and capable of burning quickly.

flatulence: air in the intestine that is passed through the rectum, which can result in cramping or abdominal pain; also called *flatus* or *gas*.

flexion: bending a body part.

fluid balance: taking in and eliminating equal amounts of fluid.

fluid overload: a condition that occurs when the body cannot handle the amount of fluid consumed.

foot drop: a weakness of muscles in the feet and ankles that causes difficulty with the ability to flex the ankles and walk normally.

force fluids (FF): a medical order to encourage a person to drink more fluids.

Fowler's: a semi-sitting body position, in which a person's head and shoulders are elevated 45 to 60 degrees.

fracture: a broken bone.

fracture pan: a bedpan that is flatter than the regular bedpan.

full weight-bearing (FWB): a doctor's order stating that a person has the ability to support full body weight (100%) on both legs.

functional grip cane: cane that has a straight grip handle.

gait belt: a belt made of canvas or other heavy material that is used to help people who are weak, unsteady, or uncoordinated to stand, sit, or walk; also called *transfer belt*.

gastroesophageal reflux disease (GERD): a chronic condition in which the liquid contents of the stomach back up into the esophagus.

gastrostomy: a surgically-created opening into the stomach that allows insertion of a tube.

gay: a person whose sexual preference is for people of the same sex, or a man whose sexual preference is for men.

genital herpes: an incurable type of sexually-transmitted infection that is caused by herpes simplex viruses type 1 (HSV-1) or type 2 (HSV-2).

geriatrics: the study of health, wellness, and disease later in life.

gerontology: the study of the aging process in people from mid-life through old age.

gestational diabetes: type of diabetes that appears in pregnant women who have never had diabetes before but who have high glucose levels during pregnancy.

glands: organs that produce and secrete chemicals called hormones.

glaucoma: a condition in which the fluid inside the eyeball is unable to drain; increased pressure inside the eye causes damage that often leads to blindness.

glucose: natural sugar.

gonads: sex glands.

gonorrhea: a type of sexually-transmitted infection caused by bacteria; if left untreated, it can cause blindness, joint infection, and sterility in both men and women.

grief: deep distress or sorrow over a loss.

groin: the area from the pubis (area around the penis and scrotum) to the upper thighs.

grooming: practices to care for oneself, such as caring for fingernails and hair.

halitosis: bad breath.

hallucinations: seeing, hearing, smelling, tasting, or feeling things that are not there.

hand hygiene: washing hands with either plain or antiseptic soap and water and using alcohol-based hand rubs.

hat: in health care, a collection container that can be inserted into a toilet to collect and measure urine or stool.

healthcare-associated infection (HAI): an infection acquired within a healthcare setting during the delivery of medical care.

health maintenance organizations (HMOs): a method of health insurance in which a person has to use a particular doctor or group of doctors except in case of emergency.

heartburn: a condition that results from a weakening of the sphincter muscle that joins the esophagus and the stomach and causes a burning sensation in the esophagus.

hemiparesis: weakness on one side of the body.

hemiplegia: paralysis on one side of the body.

hemorrhoids: enlarged veins in the rectum or outside the anus that can cause rectal itching, burning, pain, and bleeding.

hepatitis: inflammation of the liver caused by certain viruses and other factors, such as alcohol abuse, some medications, and trauma.

heterosexual: a person whose sexual preference is for people of the opposite sex; also known as *straight*.

HIV (human immunodeficiency virus): the virus that attacks the body's immune system and gradually disables it; eventually can cause AIDS.

hoarding: collecting and putting things away in a guarded way.

holistic care: a type of care that involves caring for the whole person—the mind as well as the body.

home health care: care that is provided in a person's home.

homeostasis: the condition in which all of the body's systems are working at their best.

homosexual: a person whose sexual preference is for people of the same sex.

hormones: chemical substances created by the body that control numerous body functions.

hospice care: holistic, compassionate care given to dying people and their families.

hygiene: practices to keep bodies clean and healthy.

hyperglycemia: complication of diabetes that is caused by having too little insulin; also called *diabetic ketoacidosis*.

hypertension (HTN): high blood pressure, measuring 140/90 or higher.

hyperthyroidism: condition in which the thyroid produces too much thyroid hormone, causing the cells to burn too much food.

hypoglycemia: complication of diabetes that can result from either too much insulin or too little food; also known as insulin reaction.

hypotension: low blood pressure, measuring 100/60 or lower.

hypothyroidism: condition in which the thyroid produces too little thyroid hormone, causing the body processes to slow down and resulting in weight gain and physical and mental sluggishness.

ileostomy: a surgically-created opening into the end of the small intestine to allow stool to be expelled.

impairment: a loss of function or ability.

incident: an accident, problem, or unexpected event during the course of care that is not part of the normal routine in a healthcare facility.

incontinence: the inability to control the bladder or bowels.

indirect contact: a way of transmitting pathogens by touching something contaminated by the infected person.

indwelling catheter: a type of catheter that remains inside the bladder for a period of time; urine drains into a bag.

infection: the state resulting from pathogens invading the body and multiplying.

infection prevention: the set of methods practiced in healthcare facilities to prevent and control the spread of disease.

infectious: contagious.

inflammation: swelling.

informed consent: the process by which a person, with the help of a doctor, makes informed decisions about his or her health care.

input: the fluid a person consumes; also called *intake.*

insomnia: inability to fall asleep or remain asleep.

inspiration: breathing in.

insulin: a hormone that converts glucose into energy for the body.

insulin reaction: complication of diabetes that can result from either too much insulin or too little food; also known as hypoglycemia.

intake: the fluid a person consumes; also called *input.*

integument: a natural protective covering.

intervention: a way to change an action or development.

intravenous (IV): into a vein.

intubation: the passage of a plastic tube through the mouth, nose, or opening in the neck and into the trachea.

involuntary seclusion: the separation of a person from others against the person's will.

involved: term used to refer to the weaker, or affected, side of the body after a stroke or injury.

irreversible: unable to be reversed or returned to the original state.

isolate: to keep something separate, or by itself.

jaundice: a condition in which the skin, whites of the eyes, and mucous membranes appear yellow.

joint: the place at which two bones meet.

Joint Commission: an independent, not-for-profit organization that evaluates and accredits healthcare organizations.

Kaposi's sarcoma: a rare form of skin cancer that appears as purple, red, or brown skin lesions.

karma: the belief that all past and present deeds affect one's future and future lives.

kidney dialysis: an artificial means of removing the body's waste products when the kidneys are no longer able to function properly.

knee-chest: body position in which the person is lying on her abdomen with her knees pulled towards the abdomen and her legs separated; arms are pulled up and flexed, and the head is turned to one side.

lactose intolerance: the inability to digest lactose, a type of sugar found in milk and other dairy products.

latent TB infection: type of tuberculosis in which the person carries the disease but does not show symptoms and cannot infect others.

lateral: body position in which a person is lying on either side.

laws: rules set by the government to help people live peacefully together and to ensure order and safety.

length of stay: the number of days a person stays in a healthcare facility.

lesbian: a woman whose sexual preference is for women.

leukemia: form of cancer in which the body's white blood cells are unable to fight disease.

lever: something that moves an object by resting on a base of support.

liability: a legal term that means someone can be held responsible for harming someone else.

lithotomy: body position in which a person lies on her back with her hips at the edge of an exam table; legs are flexed, and feet are in padded stirrups.

living will: a document that outlines the medical care a person wants, or does not want, in case he or she becomes unable to make those decisions.

localized infection: an infection that is limited to a specific location in the body and has local symptoms.

logrolling: moving a person as a unit, without disturbing the alignment of the body.

long-term care (LTC): care given in long-term care facilities (LTCF) for people who need 24-hour skilled care.

lung cancer: the growth of abnormal cells or tumors in the lungs.

lymph: a clear yellowish fluid that carries disease-fighting cells called lymphocytes.

major depressive disorder: a type of depression that causes withdrawal, lack of energy, and loss of interest in activities, as well as other symptoms; also called *major depression.*

malabsorption: inability to absorb or digest a particular nutrient properly.

malignant tumors: tumors that are cancerous.

malnutrition: poor nutrition due to improper diet.

malpractice: injury to a person due to professional misconduct through negligence, carelessness, or lack of skill.

managed care: a system or strategy of managing health care in a way that controls costs.

mandated reporters: people who are legally required to report suspected or observed abuse or neglect because they have regular contact with vulnerable populations, such as the elderly in care facilities.

mastectomy: the surgical removal of all or part of the breast and sometimes other surrounding tissue.

masturbation: to touch or rub sexual organs in order to give oneself or another person sexual pleasure.

mechanical ventilation: the use of a machine to inflate and deflate the lungs when a person is unable to breathe on his own.

Medicaid: a medical assistance program for low-income people.

medical asepsis: refers to practices such as handwashing that reduce, remove, and control the spread of microorganisms.

Medicare: a federal health insurance program for people who are 65 or older, are disabled, or are ill and cannot work.

menopause: the end of menstruation.

mental health: the normal functioning of emotional and intellectual abilities.

mental illness: a disease that affects a person's ability to function at a normal level in the family, home, or community.

metabolism: physical and chemical processes by which substances are produced or broken down into energy or products for use by the body.

microbe: a living thing or organism that is so small that it can be seen only under a microscope; also called *microorganism.*

microorganism (MO): a living thing or organism that is so small that it can be seen only under a microscope; also called *microbe.*

Minimum Data Set (MDS): a detailed form with guidelines for assessing residents in long-term care facilities; also details what to do if resident problems are identified.

mode of transmission: the method of describing how a pathogen travels.

modified diets: diets for people who have certain illnesses; also called *special* or *therapeutic diets.*

MRSA (methicillin-resistant *Staphylococcus aureus*): an infection caused by specific bacteria that have become resistant to many antibiotics.

mucous membranes: the membranes that line body cavities that open to the outside of the body, such as the linings of the mouth, nose, eyes, rectum, or genitals.

multidrug-resistant organisms (MDROs): microorganisms, mostly bacteria, that are resistant to one or more antimicrobial agents that are commonly used for treatment.

multidrug-resistant TB (MDR-TB): type of tuberculosis that can develop when a person with TB disease does not take all the prescribed medication.

multiple sclerosis (MS): a progressive disease in which the myelin sheath breaks down over time; without this protective covering, nerves cannot conduct impulses to and from the brain in a normal way.

muscles: groups of tissues that provide movement of body parts, protection of organs, and creation of body heat.

muscular dystrophy (MD): a progressive, inherited disease that causes a gradual wasting away of muscle, as well as weakness and deformity.

myocardial infarction (MI): a condition that occurs when the heart muscle does not receive enough oxygen because blood vessels are blocked; also called *heart attack.*

nasal cannula: a device used to deliver oxygen; consists of a piece of plastic tubing that fits around the face and is secured by a strap that goes over the ears and around the back of the head.

nasogastric tube: a feeding tube that is inserted into the nose and goes to the stomach.

nearsightedness: the ability to see things near but not far; also known as myopia.

neglect: the failure to provide needed care that results in physical, mental, or emotional harm to a person.

negligence: actions, or the failure to act or provide the proper care, that result in unintended injury to a person.

nephritis: an inflammation of the kidneys.

neuropathy: numbness, tingling, and pain in the feet and legs.

nitroglycerin: medication that helps to relax the walls of the coronary arteries, allowing them to open and get more blood to the heart; comes in tablet, patch, or spray form.

non-intact skin: skin that is broken by abrasions, cuts, rashes, acne, pimples, lesions, surgical incisions, or boils.

nonspecific immunity: a type of immunity that protects the body from disease in general.

nonverbal communication: communicating without using words.

non-weight-bearing (NWB): a doctor's order stating that a person is unable to touch the floor or support any body weight on one or both legs.

NPO (nothing by mouth): medical order to withhold all food and fluids taken orally.

nutrient: something found in food that provides energy, promotes growth and health, and helps regulate metabolism.

nutrition: how the body uses food to maintain health.

objective information: information based on what a person sees, hears, touches, or smells; also called *signs.*

obsessive compulsive disorder (OCD): an anxiety disorder characterized by obsessive behavior or thoughts.

obstructed airway: a condition in which the tube through which air enters the lungs is blocked.

occult: hidden; difficult to see or observe.

Occupational Safety and Health Administration (OSHA): a federal government agency that makes rules to protect workers from hazards on the job.

occupied bed: a bed made while a person is in the bed.

ombudsman: a legal advocate for residents in long-term care facilities; helps resolve disputes and settle conflicts.

Omnibus Budget Reconciliation Act (OBRA): law passed by the federal government that includes minimum standards for nursing assistant training, staffing requirements, resident assessment instructions, and information on rights for residents.

onset: in medicine, the first appearance of the signs or symptoms of an illness.

open bed: a bed made with linen folded down to the foot of the bed.

open fracture: a broken bone that penetrates the skin; also known as a compound fracture.

opportunistic infections: infections that invade the body when the immune system is weak and unable to defend itself.

opposition: touching the thumb to any other finger.

oral care: care of the mouth, teeth, and gums.

organs: structural units in the human body that perform specific functions.

orthopnea: shortness of breath when lying down that is relieved by sitting up.

orthosis: a device that helps support and align a limb and improve its functioning; also called *orthotic device.*

orthotic device: a device that helps support and align a limb and improve its functioning; also called *orthosis.*

osteoarthritis: a common type of arthritis that usually affects the hips, knees, fingers, thumbs, and spine; also called *degenerative joint disease (DJD)* or *degenerative arthritis.*

osteoporosis: a disease that causes bones to become porous and brittle, causing them to break easily.

ostomy: a surgically-created opening from an area inside the body to the outside.

outpatient care: care given for less than 24 hours for people who have had treatments or surgery and need short-term skilled care.

output: all fluid that is eliminated from the body; includes fluid in urine, feces, vomitus, perspiration, moisture that is exhaled in the air, and wound drainage.

oxygen concentrator: a box-like device that changes air in the room into air with more oxygen.

oxygen therapy: the administration of oxygen to increase the supply of oxygen to the lungs.

pacing: walking back and forth in the same area.

palliative care: care that focuses on the comfort and dignity of a person who is very sick and/or dying, rather than on curing him or her.

panic disorder: a disorder in which a person has repeated episodes of intense fear that something bad will occur.

paralysis: the loss of ability to move all or part of the body, and it often includes loss of feeling in the affected area.

paranoid schizophrenia: a form of mental illness characterized by hallucinations and delusions.

paraplegia: loss of function of the lower body and legs.

Parkinson's disease: a progressive disease that causes the brain to degenerate; causes stooped posture, shuffling gait, pill-rolling, and tremors.

partial bath: a bath given on days when a complete bath or shower is not done; includes washing the face, hands, underarms, and perineum.

partial weight-bearing (PWB): a doctor's order stating that a person is able to support some body weight on one or both legs.

passive neglect: the unintentional failure to provide needed care, resulting in physical, mental, or emotional harm to a person.

passive range of motion (PROM): exercises to put a joint through its full arc of motion that are performed by a caregiver alone, without the affected person's help.

pathogens: microorganisms that are capable of causing infection and disease.

payers: people or organizations paying for healthcare services.

pediculosis: an infestation of lice.

peptic ulcers: raw sores in the stomach or the small intestine that cause pain, belching, and vomiting.

percutaneous endoscopic gastrostomy (PEG) tube: a feeding tube placed through the abdominal wall into the stomach.

perineal care: care of the genitals and anal area.

perineum: the genital and anal area.

peripheral nervous system (PNS): part of the nervous system made up of the nerves that extend throughout the body.

peripheral vascular disease (PVD): a disease in which the legs, feet, arms, or hands do not have enough blood circulation due to fatty deposits in the blood vessels that harden over time.

peristalsis: involuntary contractions that move food through the gastrointestinal system.

perseveration: the repetition of words, phrases, questions, or actions.

personal: relating to life outside one's job, such as family, friends, and home life.

personal protective equipment (PPE): equipment that helps protect employees from serious workplace injuries or illnesses resulting from contact with workplace hazards.

person-directed care: a type of care that places the emphasis on the person needing care and his or her individuality and capabilities.

phantom limb pain: pain in a limb (or extremity) that has been amputated.

phantom sensation: warmth, itching, or tingling from a body part that has been amputated.

phlegm: thick mucus from the respiratory passage.

phobia: an intense form of anxiety or fear.

physical abuse: any treatment, intentional or not, that causes harm to a person's body.

pillaging: taking things that belong to someone else.

pneumonia: a bacterial, viral, or fungal infection that causes acute inflammation in lung tissue.

policy: a course of action that should be taken every time a certain situation occurs.

portable commode: a chair with a toilet seat and a removable container underneath; also called *bedside commode.*

portal of entry: any body opening on an uninfected person that allows pathogens to enter.

portal of exit: any body opening on an infected person that allows pathogens to leave.

positioning: the act of helping people into positions that promote comfort and health.

postmortem care: care of the body after death.

postoperative: after surgery.

post-traumatic stress disorder (PTSD): an anxiety disorder caused by a traumatic experience.

posture: the way a person holds and positions his body.

pre-diabetes: a condition that occurs when a person's blood glucose levels are above normal but not high enough for a diagnosis of type 2 diabetes.

preferred provider organizations (PPOs): a network of providers that contract to provide health services to a group of people.

prehypertension: a condition in which a person has a systolic measurement of 120–139 mm Hg and a diastolic measurement of 80–89 mm Hg; indicates that the person does not have high blood pressure now but is likely to have it in the future.

premature: the term for babies who are born before 37 weeks gestation (more than three weeks before the due date).

preoperative: before surgery.

pressure points: areas of the body that bear much of its weight.

pressure ulcer: a serious wound resulting from skin breakdown; also called *pressure sore, bed sore,* or *decubitus ulcer.*

procedure: a method, or way, of doing something.

professional: having to do with work or a job.

professionalism: how a person behaves when he is on the job; it includes how a person dresses, the words he uses, and the things he talks about.

progressive: something that continually gets worse or deteriorates.

pronation: turning downward.

prone: body position in which a person is lying on his stomach, or front side of the body.

prosthesis: a device that replaces a body part that is missing or deformed because of an accident, injury, illness, or birth defect; used to improve a person's ability to function and/or his appearance.

protected health information (PHI): a person's private health information, which includes name, address, telephone number, social security number, e-mail address, and medical record number.

providers: people or organizations that provide health care, including doctors, nurses, clinics, and agencies.

psychological abuse: emotional harm caused by threatening, scaring, humiliating, intimidating, isolating, or insulting a person, or by treating him as a child; also includes verbal abuse.

psychosocial needs: needs that involve social interaction, emotions, intellect, and spirituality.

psychotherapy: a method of treating mental illness that involves talking about one's problems with mental health professionals.

pulse oximeter: a noninvasive device that uses a light to determine the amount of oxygen in the blood.

puree: to chop, blend, or grind food into a thick paste of baby food consistency.

quad cane: cane that has four rubber-tipped feet and a rectangular base.

quadriplegia: loss of function of the legs, trunk, and arms.

rabbi: religious leader of the Jewish faith.

radial pulse: the pulse located on the inside of the wrist, where the radial artery runs just beneath the skin.

range of motion (ROM): exercises that put a particular joint through its full arc of motion.

receptive aphasia: inability to understand spoken or written words.

rehabilitation: care that is given by specialists to help restore or improve function after an illness or injury.

reincarnation: a belief that some part of a living being survives death to be reborn in a new body.

renovascular hypertension: a condition in which a blockage of arteries in the kidneys causes high blood pressure.

repetitive phrasing: repeating words, phrases, or questions.

reproduce: to create new human life.

reservoir: a place where a pathogen lives and grows.

Residents' Rights: numerous rights identified in the OBRA law that relate to how residents must be treated while living in a facility; they provide an ethical code of conduct for healthcare workers.

resistant: a state in which drugs no longer work to kill specific bacteria.

respiration: the process of breathing air into the lungs and exhaling air out of the lungs.

restraint: a physical or chemical way to restrict voluntary movement or behavior.

restraint alternatives: any interventions used in place of a restraint or that reduce the need for a restraint.

restraint-free care: an environment in which restraints are not kept or used for any reason.

restrict fluids (RF): a medical order to limit the amount of fluids a person drinks to the level set by the doctor.

résumé: a summary or listing of relevant job experience and education.

rheumatoid arthritis: a type of arthritis in which joints become inflamed, red, swollen, and very painful, resulting in restricted movement and possible deformities.

***rigor mortis*:** the Latin term for the temporary condition after death in which the muscles in the body become stiff and rigid.

rotation: turning a joint.

routine urine specimen: a urine specimen that can be collected any time a person voids.

safety razor: a type of razor that has a sharp blade with a special safety casing to help prevent cuts; requires the use of shaving cream or soap.

scabies: contagious skin infection caused by a tiny mite burrowing into the skin, where it lays eggs; causes intense itching and a skin rash that may look like thin burrow tracks.

scalds: burns caused by hot liquids.

schizophrenia: a form of mental illness that affects a person's ability to think, communicate, make decisions, and understand reality.

scope of practice: defines the tasks that healthcare providers are legally allowed to do and how to do them correctly.

sedative: an agent or drug that helps calm and soothe a person and may cause sleep.

sentinel event: an accident or incident that results in grave physical or psychological injury or death.

sexual abuse: the forcing of a person to perform or participate in sexual acts against his or her will; includes unwanted touching, exposing oneself, and the sharing of pornographic material.

sexual harassment: any unwelcome sexual advance or behavior that creates an intimidating, hostile, or offensive working environment.

sexually-transmitted infections (STIs): infections caused by sexual contact with infected people; signs and symptoms are not always apparent.

sharps: needles or other sharp objects.

shearing: rubbing or friction that results from the skin moving one way and the bone underneath it remaining fixed or moving in the opposite direction.

shingles: non-contagious skin rash caused by the varicella-zoster virus (VZV), which is the same virus that causes chickenpox; causes pain, tingling, itching, and a rash of fluid-filled blisters.

shock: a condition that occurs when organs and tissues in the body do not receive an adequate blood supply.

shower chair: a sturdy, water- and slip-resistant chair designed to be placed in a bathtub or shower.

simple carbohydrates: carbohydrates that are found in foods such as sugars, sweets, syrups, and jellies and have little nutritional value.

Sims': body position in which a person is lying on his left side with the upper knee flexed and raised toward the chest.

situation response: a temporary condition that has symptoms like those of mental illness; possible causes include a personal crisis, temporary physical changes in the brain, side effects from medications, interactions among medications, and severe changes in the environment.

sitz bath: a warm soak of the perineal area to clean perineal wounds and reduce inflammation and pain.

skilled care: medically-necessary care given by a skilled nurse or therapist.

slide board: a wooden board that helps transfer people who are unable to bear weight on their legs; also called *transfer board.*

special diets: diets for people who have certain illnesses; also called *therapeutic* or *modified diets.*

specific immunity: a type of immunity that protects against a particular disease that is invading the body at a given time.

specimen: a sample that is used for analysis in order to try to make a diagnosis.

sphygmomanometer: a blood pressure cuff.

spiritual: of, or relating to, the spirit or soul.

sputum: thick mucus coughed up from the lungs.

Standard Precautions: a method of infection prevention in which all blood, body fluids, non-intact skin, and mucous membranes are treated as if they were infected with an infectious disease.

sterilization: a method used to decrease the spread of pathogens and disease by destroying all microorganisms, including those that form spores.

stethoscope: an instrument designed to listen to sounds within the body.

stoma: an artificial opening in the body.

straight catheter: a catheter that does not remain inside the person; it is removed immediately after urine is drained or collected.

stress: the state of being frightened, excited, confused, in danger, or irritated.

stressor: something that causes stress.

subacute care: care given in a hospital or in a long-term care facility for people who need less care than for an acute illness, but more care than for a chronic illness.

subjective information: information that a person cannot or did not observe, but is based on something reported to the person that may or may not be true; also called *symptoms.*

substance abuse: the repeated use of legal or illegal drugs, cigarettes, or alcohol in a way that is harmful to oneself or others.

sudden infant death syndrome (SIDS): a condition in which babies stop breathing while asleep and die for no known reason.

suffocation: the stoppage of breathing from a lack of oxygen or an excess of carbon dioxide in the body that may result in unconsciousness or death.

sundowning: becoming restless and agitated in the late afternoon, evening, or night.

supination: turning upward.

supine: body position in which a person lies flat on his back.

suppository: a medication given rectally to cause a bowel movement.

surgical asepsis: the state of being free of all microorganisms; also called *sterile technique.*

surgical bed: a bed made to accept residents who are returning to bed on stretchers.

susceptible host: an uninfected person who could get sick.

sympathy: sharing in the feelings and difficulties of others.

syncope: loss of consciousness; also called *fainting.*

syphilis: a type of sexually-transmitted infection caused by bacteria; if left untreated, it can cause brain damage, mental illness, and death.

systemic infection: an infection that is in the bloodstream and is spread throughout the body, causing general symptoms.

systole: phase where the heart is at work, contracting and pushing blood out of the left ventricle.

systolic: first measurement of blood pressure; phase when the heart is at work, contracting and pushing the blood from the left ventricle of the heart.

tachypnea: rapid breathing.

tactful: showing sensitivity and having a sense of what is appropriate when dealing with others.

TB disease: type of tuberculosis in which the person shows symptoms of the disease and can spread TB to others.

telemetry: the application of a cardiac monitoring device that sends information about the heart's rhythm and rate to a monitoring station.

terminal illness: a disease or condition that will eventually cause death.

therapeutic diets: diets for people who have certain illnesses; also called *special* or *modified diets.*

tissues: groups of cells that perform similar tasks.

total parenteral nutrition (TPN): the intravenous infusion of nutrients administered directly into the bloodstream, bypassing the digestive system.

tracheostomy: a surgically-created opening through the neck into the trachea.

transfer belt: a belt made of canvas or other heavy material that is used to help people who are weak, unsteady, or uncoordinated to stand, sit, or walk; also called *gait belt.*

transgender: a person whose gender identify conflicts with his or her birth sex (sex assigned at birth due to anatomy).

transient ischemic attack (TIA): a warning sign of a CVA/stroke resulting from a temporary lack of oxygen in the brain; symptoms may last up to 24 hours.

transitioning: the process of changing genders.

transmission: passage or transfer.

Transmission-Based Precautions: method of infection prevention used when caring for persons who are infected or suspected of being infected with a disease.

transsexual: 1. one who wishes to be accepted by society as a member of the opposite sex; 2. one who has undergone a sex change operation.

trauma: severe injury.

triggers: situations that lead to agitation.

tuberculosis (TB): a highly contagious lung disease caused by a bacterium that is carried on mucous droplets suspended in the air.

tumor: a cluster of abnormally-growing cells.

type 1 diabetes: type of diabetes in which the pancreas does not produce any insulin; is usually diagnosed in children and young adults and will continue throughout a person's life.

type 2 diabetes: common form of diabetes in which either the body does not produce enough insulin or the body fails to properly use insulin; typically develops after age 35 and is the milder form of diabetes.

ulceration: scarring.

ulcerative colitis: a chronic inflammatory disease of the large intestine that causes cramping, diarrhea, pain, rectal bleeding, and loss of appetite.

unoccupied bed: a bed made while no person is in the bed.

upper respiratory infection (URI): a viral infection of the nose, sinuses, and throat; commonly called a cold.

ureterostomy: a surgically-created opening from a ureter to the abdomen for urine to be eliminated.

urinary incontinence: the inability to control the bladder, which leads to an involuntary loss of urine.

urinary tract infection (UTI): inflammation of the bladder and the ureters that results in a painful burning during urination and the frequent feeling of needing to urinate; also called *cystitis.*

urination: the act of passing urine from the bladder through the urethra to the outside of the body; also known as micturition or voiding.

vaginitis: an infection of the vagina that may be caused by bacteria, protozoa, or a fungus.

validating: giving value to or approving.

vegans: people who do not eat any animals or animal products; vegans may also not use or wear any animal products.

vegetarians: people who do not eat meat, fish, or poultry and may or may not eat eggs and dairy products.

verbal abuse: the use of spoken or written words, pictures, or gestures that threaten, embarrass, or insult a person.

verbal communication: communication involving the use of spoken or written words or sounds.

vital signs: measurements—temperature, pulse, respirations, blood pressure, pain level—that monitor the functioning of the vital organs of the body.

VRE (vancomycin-resistant *enterococus*): bacteria (*enterococci*) that have developed resistance to antibiotics as a result of being exposed to vancomycin.

walker: adaptive equipment used for people who are unsteady or who lack balance; usually has four rubber-tipped feet and/or wheels.

wandering: walking aimlessly around the facility or facility grounds.

workplace violence: verbal, physical, or sexual abuse of staff by other staff members, residents, or visitors.

wound: a type of injury to the skin.

yarmulke: a small skullcap worn by Jewish men as a sign of their faith.

Index

Iowa CNA skills